Obesity and Voice

Obesity and Voice

Abdul-Latif Hamdan, MD, EMBA, MPH, FACS
Robert Thayer Sataloff, MD, DMA, FACS
Mary J. Hawkshaw, RN, BSN, CORLN, FCCP

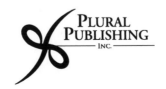

PLURAL
PUBLISHING
INC.

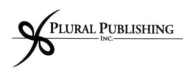

5521 Ruffin Road
San Diego, CA 92123

e-mail: information@pluralpublishing.com
Website: http://www.pluralpublishing.com

Typeset in 10.5/13 Minion Pro by Flanagan's Publishing Services, Inc.
Printed in the United States of America by McNaughton & Gunn, Inc.

For permission to use material from this text, contact us by
Telephone: (866) 758-7251
Fax: (888) 758-7255
e-mail: permissions@pluralpublishing.com

Every attempt has been made to contact the copyright holders for material originally printed in another source. If any have been inadvertently overlooked, the publishers will gladly make the necessary arrangements at the first opportunity.

NOTICE TO THE READER

Care has been taken to confirm the accuracy of the indications, procedures, drug dosages, and diagnosis and remediation protocols presented in this book and to ensure that they conform to the practices of the general medical and health services communities. However, the authors, editors, and publisher are not responsible for errors or omissions or for any consequences from application of the information in this book and make no warranty, expressed or implied, with respect to the currency, completeness, or accuracy of the contents of the publication. The diagnostic and remediation protocols and the medications described do not necessarily have specific approval by the Food and Drug Administration for use in the disorders and/or diseases and dosages for which they are recommended. Application of this information in a particular situation remains the professional responsibility of the practitioner. Because standards of practice and usage change, it is the responsibility of the practitioner to keep abreast of revised recommendations, dosages, and procedures.

Library of Congress Cataloging-in-Publication Data:
Names: Hamdan, A. L. (Abdul Latif), author. | Sataloff, Robert Thayer, author. | Hawkshaw, Mary, author. | Sataloff, Robert Thayer. Professional voice. 4th ed.
Title: Obesity and voice / Abdul-Latif Hamdan, Robert Thayer Sataloff, Mary J. Hawkshaw.
Description: San Diego, CA : Plural Publishing, [2020] | Some chapters are reprinted from Professional voice, 4th ed., by Robert Thayer Sataloff. | Includes bibliographical references and index.
Identifiers: LCCN 2019013066| ISBN 9781635502589 (alk. paper) | ISBN 1635502586 (alk. paper)
Subjects: | MESH: Voice | Obesity--complications | Phonation | Voice Disorders--etiology | Body Weight Changes
Classification: LCC RA645.O23 | NLM WV 500 | DDC 362.1963/98--dc23
LC record available at https://lccn.loc.gov/2019013066

Contents

Preface

Obesity is a worldwide epidemic threat. Its prevalence is rising steadily and currently it affects one-third of the world's population, spanning several countries across the globe.[1] Based on a report published in the *New England Journal of Medicine* 2017, close to 2 billion people are either obese or overweight, and the rate of obesity is higher in children than in adults.[2] The economic implications of obesity-are devastating. In a study by Finkelstein et al,[3] the annual health cost of obese people in the United States was reported to be 60% higher than that of normal-weight subjects, accounting for a significant proportion of the gross national income. In addition to the increase in health care cost, obesity is associated with a reduction in productivity secondary to absenteeism, which in turn might impair the economic competitiveness.[4] In countries like the United States, China, and Mexico, obesity also is considered a threat to the national security as the compromised physical fitness puts military preparedness in jeopardy.[4] Several strategies have been adopted to motivate obese individuals to lose weight. These include publicizing information on healthy dietary behavior and ehealth communication that constitutes mass customization.[5] The "Let's Move" campaign that was launched by former First Lady Michelle Obama was another initiative to prevent obesity in children and foster accessibility to healthy food and diet.[6]

Still, the global spread of obesity continues, and the 2 main related concerns are the self-image/esteem and health-related hazards. The association between poor self-esteem and obesity stems from the emphasis on thinness in our contemporary culture and the labeling of overweight and obese individuals.[7] The stigmatization of overweight and obese individuals in society often leads to psychological disturbances that result in suffering of the affected individual.[8,9] Body image dissatisfaction has become a salient attribute in obese subjects and the negative body image linked to obesity has been associated with appearance anxiety and low self-compassion.[10] The seriousness of this matter has led to the emergence of body image therapy as a psychological approach to alleviate obesity-induced psychological disturbances.[11] In addition, there is a strong association between body image and overall health. The importance of body image in obesity is not confined only to self-esteem and satisfaction. It also can have an impact on physical health-related issues. "Does body satisfaction matter?" is a question that has been addressed by Neumark-Sztainer et al[12] in their investigation on the association between body satisfaction and health behaviors in a sample of 2516 adolescents over the course of 5 years. The results showed that low body satisfaction is associated with unhealthy behaviors such as binge eating, poor weight control, reduced physical activity, and smoking.

Obesity is becoming one the leading causes of disabilities and death. Obese subjects are at a higher risk to develop cardiovascular illnesses, endocrine disorders, and kidney diseases, in addition to psychological disturbances.[13,14] All systems in the body are affected either directly or indirectly to various degrees. The state of meta-inflammation caused by the excess of adipose tissue, a metabolically active organ, is partially responsible for the impairment in function of these systems.[15] As voice is a reflection of our well-being,[16] phonatory effects of obesity are inevitable. All 3 components of voice production, the respiratory system and abdominal back and thoracic muscles as the power source, the vocal folds as the oscillator, and the vocal tract as the resonator, are targets of anatomic and systemic obesity-induced changes. Hence, weight gain affects voice production.

The purpose of this book is to review the current literature on the impact of obesity on phonation and to highlight the various means by which excessive weight may jeopardize voice quality and endurance. Another impetus for writing this book was the unanswered questions regarding the impact of weight loss and weight fluctuation on voice. "Does weight loss affect my voice?" is a frequent question asked by obese patients, particularly professional voice users who are interested in preserving their individual vocal characteristics. This book discusses weight loss and voice, and it suggests future research trends on the link between weight loss, weight gain, obesity, and phonation.

Chapter 1 reviews the increasing prevalence of obesity and its implications for voice dysfunction. Chapter 2 summarizes current understanding of clinical anatomy and physiology of the voice. Chapters 3 and 4 present state-of-the-art information on medical history and physical examination for patients with voice disorders. In Chapter 5, the authors present core information on obesity, and they review literature correlating body size with voice characteristics. Chapter 6 explains the effects of obesity on

sex hormones and the related effects of sex hormone alterations on phonation in obese individuals. Chapter 7 provides insights into basic information about respiration and its importance in phonation. In Chapter 8, the authors explore the relationship between obesity and respiration, explaining the important effects of obesity-related changes in lung function and their consequences for phonation. Chapter 9 includes an exceptionally comprehensive overview of laryngopharyngeal reflux, including more than 600 references. In Chapter 10, the authors highlight what is known about the relationship between reflux and obesity and the effects of obesity-related reflux on the larynx and voice. Chapter 11 is a comprehensive chapter reviewing the most current concepts regarding nutrition and nutrition science, and the relationship between nutrition and voice. In Chapter 12, the authors review the clinically important subject of the effects of weight loss on voice, including "yo-yo" dieting, and bariatric surgery. In the concluding Chapter 13, the authors summarize the information presented in other chapters and highlight the substantial deficits in knowledge about obesity and its impact upon the voice and vocal tract. Clearly, additional research is needed. Considering the epidemic nature of obesity, obesity-related voice research appears to deserve much more attention than it has received, so far.

References

1. Friedrich MJ. Global obesity epidemic worsening. *JAMA*. 2017;318(7):603.
2. Gregg EW, Shaw JE. Global health effects of overweight and obesity. *N Engl J Med*. 2017; 377(1):80–81.
3. Finkelstein EA, DiBonaventura MD, Burgess SM, Hale BC. The costs of obesity in the

workplace. *J Occup Environ Med.* 2010;52:
971–976.

4. Popkin BM. Is the obesity epidemic a
national security issue around the globe?
Curr Opin Endocrinol. 2011;18:328–331.

5. Enwald HPK, Huotari MLA. Preventing
the obesity epidemic by second generation
tailored health communication: an interdisciplinary review. *J Med Internet Res.* 2010;
12(2):e24.

6. Let's Move. America's move to raise a healthier generation of kids. 2010. http://letsmove
.obamawhitehouse.archives.gov/learn-facts/
epidemic-childhood-obesity. Accessed December 10, 2018.

7. Schwartz MB, Brownell KD. Obesity and
body image. *Body Image.* 2004;1(1):43–56.

8. Choi E, Choi I. The associations between
body dissatisfaction, body figure, self-
esteem, and depressed mood in adolescents
in the United States and Korea: a moder-
ated mediation analysis. *J Adolesc.* 2016;53:
249–259.

9. Willows ND, Ridley D, Raine KD, Maxi-
mova K. High adiposity is associated cross-
sectionally with low self-concept and body
size dissatisfaction among indigenous Cree
schoolchildren in Canada. *BMC Pediatr.*
2013;13:118.

10. Seekis V, Bradley GL, Duffy A. The effectiveness of self-compassion and self-esteem

writing tasks in reducing body image concerns. *Body Image.* 2017;23:206–213.

11. Rosen JC. Improving body image in obesity.
In: Thompson, ed. *Body Image Disorders and
Obesity: An Integrative Guide for Assessment
and Treatment.* Washington, DC: American
Psychological Association; 2001:425–440.

12. Neumark-Sztainer D, Paxton SJ, Hannan
PJ, Haines J, Story M. Does body satisfaction matter? Five-year longitudinal associations between body satisfaction and health
behaviors in adolescent females and males.
J Adolesc Health. 2006;39(2):244–251.

13. Field AE, Coakley EH, Must A, et al. Impact
of overweight on the risk of developing
common chronic diseases during a 10-year
period. *Arch Intern Med.* 2001;161(13):
1581–1586.

14. Guh DP, Zhang W, Bansback N, et al. The
incidence of co-morbidities related to obesity and overweight: a systematic review and
meta-analysis. *BMC Public Health.* 2009;
9:88.

15. Fonseca-Alaniz MH, Takada J, Alonso-Vale
MI, Lima FB. Adipose tissue as an endocrine
organ: from theory to practice. *J Pediatr.*
2007;83(5)(suppl):S192–S203.

16. Sataloff RT. Introduction. In *Professional
Voice: The Science and Art of Clinical Care.*
4th ed. San Diego, CA: Plural Publishing;
2017:3–7.

Contributors

Donald O. Castell, MD
Professor of Medicine
Director of Esophageal Disorders Program
Department of Gastroenterology and
   Hepatology
Charleston, South Carolina
Chapter 9

John R. Cohn, MD, FCCP
Professor of Medicine and Pediatrics
Thomas Jefferson University
Philadelphia, Pennsylvania
Chapter 7

**Nyree Dardarian, MS, RD, LDN, CSSD,
FAND**
Assistant Clinical Professor
Director, Center for Nutrition & Performance
Coordinator, Individualized Supervised
   Practice Pathway
Drexel University
Philadelphia, Pennsylvania
Chapter 11

Abigail D. Gilman, MS, RD
Doctoral Candidate and Project Manager
Department of Nutrition Sciences
College of Nursing and Health
Drexel University
Philadelphia, Pennsylvania
Chapter 11

**Abdul-Latif Hamdan, MD, EMBA, MPH,
FACS**
Professor of Otolaryngology, Head and
   Neck Surgery
Head, Division of Laryngology
Director of "Hamdan Voice Unit"

American University of Beirut Medical
   Center
Beirut, Lebanon
Chapters 1, 5, 6, 8, 10, 12, and 13

**Mary J. Hawkshaw, RN, BSN, CORLN,
FCCP**
Research Professor
Department of Otolaryngology-Head and
   Neck Surgery
Drexel University College of Medicine
Philadelphia, Pennsylvania
Chapters 1, 5, 6, 7, 8, 9, 10, 12, and 13

Philip O. Katz, MD
Professor
Department of Medicine
Division of Gastroenterology
Weill Cornell Medical Center
New York, New York
Chapter 9

Jennifer A. Nasser, PhD, RD
Associate Professor
Director
PhD Program in Nutrition Science
Department of Nutrition Science
Drexel University
Philadelphia, Pennsylvania
Chapter 11

Sobhana Ranjan, PhD, RD
Assistant Research Professor
Department of Nutrition Sciences
College of Nursing and Health
Drexel University
Philadelphia, Pennsylvania
Chapter 11

Dahlia M. Sataloff, MD, FACS
Chairman, Department of Surgery
Pennsylvania Hospital
Professor of Clinical Surgery
University of Pennsylvania
Perelman School of Medicine
Philadelphia, Pennsylvania
Chapter 9

Robert Thayer Sataloff, MD, DMA, FACS
Professor and Chairman, Department of
    Otolaryngology-Head and Neck Surgery
Senior Associate Dean for Clinical
    Academic Specialties
Drexel University College of Medicine
Philadelphia, Pennsylvania
Chapters 1, 2, 3, 4, 5, 6, 7, 8, 9, 10, 12, and 13

1

The Epidemic of Obesity: Incidental Dysphonia

Abdul-Latif Hamdan, Mary J. Hawkshaw, and Robert Thayer Sataloff

The Epidemic of Obesity

Several surveys have documented the epidemic nature of obesity as a health crisis worldwide.[1–9] The increase in its prevalence started in the 1960s with adults being affected more than children and women more than men.[4] In the United States, the past 3 decades have witnessed a twofold increase in obesity,[5] with 34.9% of the adult population reported as being obese.[3] Using national survey data, Wang et al[6] projected an increase in the prevalence of overweight or obesity in the United States to 86.3% of the adult population by year 2030 and to 100% by year 2048. This epidemic affects all age groups, including children. Based on multiple National Health and Nutrition Examination Surveys, which included 40,780 children and adolescents between the ages of 2 and 19 years, 17% of the participants were reported to be obese.[7] There are also ethnic disparities, with Hispanic women and non-Hispanic black people being affected the most.[3] According to Li et al,[8] Mexican Americans have the highest mean percent body fat in comparison to non-Hispanic whites. The study was conducted using the National Health and Nutrition Examination Survey, which included 6559 men and 6507 women. The total body fat and fat-free mass were measured using dual-energy x-ray absorptiometry.[8]

Why the rise in obesity prevalence? The pathogenesis of obesity cannot be attributed to one cause. A holistic approach is needed to determine the many factors contributing to this epidemic entity.[10] A thorough understanding of obesity requires understanding not only the dietary volitional behavior but also numerous other issues. Looking at the cause is essential in understanding the interplay between obesity and environmental factors. Numerous etiological models have been developed by many authors.[11–17] Egger and Dixon[11] described a hierarchy of layers of influence in the etiology of obesity. These were stratified as risk factors/markers, immediate determinants, and/or nonimmediate determinants. The hierarchy included an array of factors partly related to lifestyle and behavior and partly to sociocultural influences, relationships, occupation, and environment.[11,12] Based on a report by Swinburn et al,[13] obesogenic environmental factors can be classified as macro and micro factors that include small

1

air, soil, and water-polluted particles. These latter have been shown to play a major role in oxidative stress and in disrupting various body systems.[14–16] The same authors had also previously described an ecological model consisting of 3 main pillars that maintain the energy balance in a human subject. These include biological influence, behavioral influence, and environmental influence.[17] Thus, widespread obesity is the result of many factors that can interact with each other.

But how does it all start? Obesity is the result of a mismatch between the environment we are programed for and the one we live in.[11] This mismatch creates stress that is fueled by manmade inducers referred to as anthropogens.[18] The interface with or adoption of these anthropogens leads to a state of chronic inflammation that worsens with time.[17–20] Several have been identified in the literature, the most important of which are nutrition and inactivity. The intake of processed food, in addition to excessive sugar, has been shown to induce meta-inflammation.[19] Similarly, sedentary activity or physical inactivity has been linked to several inflammatory biomarkers, whereas exercise, irrespective of its type and duration, has been shown to be of health benefit.[21] Other important anthropogens that were linked to obesity include sleep deprivation, stress, anxiety, and depression.[22–24]

Obesity, a Prelude to Systemic Diseases

The anthropogens that induce obesity incite a metabolic response that becomes systemic over time and leads to low-grade chronic inflammation.[11,18,25] When compounded with genetic predisposition, these events predispose to chronic diseases such as cardiac, respiratory, renal, and endocrine disorders.[26,27] A large study by Field et al[28] investigating the association between overweight and health risks revealed an increase in the incidence of diabetes (DM), hypertension, and heart illnesses with an increase in body weight. The study was conducted on men and women between the ages of 30 and 55 years followed over a period of 10 years.

Several studies concur that obesity and overweight are among the most important risk factors associated with the development of DM and its complications.[29–31] Guh et al[29] reported that obese men and women have 7- and 12-fold increased risk for DM type 2, respectively. A systemic review on the prevalence of obesity and DM by Colosia et al[30] showed that 30% to 50% of patients with DM are obese. Weight loss following bariatric surgery has been shown to reverse DM type 2 and is considered a management strategy preferable to medical therapy.[31] Similar to the association between obesity and DM, obesity is associated also with higher risk of cardiovascular diseases.[32–40] A body mass index (BMI) of less than 25 kg/m^2 is considered ideal for cardiovascular health,[41] whereas excessive weight is an independent risk factor that increases the odds for coronary artery diseases (1.46 for men and 1.64 for women).[34] The effect is mediated through several mechanisms: (1) obesity-induced structural changes, where the increase in weight leads to an increase in peripheral resistance, which in turn leads to hypertrophy of cardiac muscles and worsening of their function[33]; (2) the effect of obesity on systemic diseases such as hypertension, diabetes, and dyslipidemia, which impact cardiac function adversely and are considered as cardiac risk factors[34,35]; and (3) adipose tissue-induced inflammatory response and its known systemic impact.[42] Numerous studies also have documented that obesity is associated with abnormal kidney function and high prevalence of kidney diseases.[43–53] The effect of obesity on kidney function is direct and indirect. The direct effect is mediated by the release of inflammatory mediators such as adiponectin and leptin, which lead to abnormal metabolic response and oxidative stress, whereas the indirect effect is induced by exacerbation of comorbid conditions such as hypertension and diabetes.[35,54–58] Commonly reported kidney diseases in obese subjects include nephrolithiasis, glomerulomegaly, glomerulosclerosis, and kidney stones. Scales et al[59] described a higher prevalence of kidney stones in obese subjects than in normal-weight subjects (11.2% vs 6.1%), and Curhan et al[60] reported an odds ratio of developing kidney stones of 1.76 when BMI exceeds 32 kg/m^2.

Obesity also is linked to various types of cancer. According to the International Agency for Research on Cancer (IARC), adding weight increases the risk of developing cancer, whereas losing weight by dieting and physical activity can mitigate that risk.[61] Obesity is considered as an independent prognostic factor that impacts not only prevalence of cancer but also disease-free survival, stage of disease, response to chemotherapy, and overall mortality.[62–66] The association between obesity and cancer is not surprising given the chronic state of inflammation induced by adipose tissue, which acts as a favorable milieu for tumor cell growth and proliferation. Several mechanisms that link cancer to obesity have been proposed. These include (1) high blood level of insulin and IGF-1, which have been associated with a higher risk of cancer by facilitating tumor proliferation;[67–69] (2) the release of inflammatory biomarkers such as adiponectin, adipokines, and leptin;[70,71] and (3) obesity-induced angiogenesis.[72] Presumably as a consequence of the above, obesity has been associated with an increased risk of death. Epidemiologic studies have found that obesity diminishes life expectancy and increases the risk of death[73–76] up to 40%

in overweight subjects and 3-fold in obese patients.[76] A prospective study by Adams et al,[76] conducted on a cohort of 527 625 men and women between the ages of 50 and 71 years, identified a strong association between risk of death, as well as obesity and overweight in all ethnic and racial groups.

Incidental Dysphonia in Obesity

The impact of obesity on voice has scarcely been discussed in the literature. There are studies on the phonatory characteristics of obese patients in comparison to normal-weight subjects, and on vocal parameters' predictive value of body size and contour,[77–84] with only a few studies on the impact of weight loss on voice.[85–87] The impact of weight gain on voice has not been investigated thoroughly. This scarcity of reports is surprising given that voice is a reflection of our well-being. The complexity of voice production and the multiplicity of factors that contribute to phonation are indisputable. In addition to our genetic background and phonatory habits, body traits and health are important influences on acoustic cues that determine one's vocal identity. Numerous reviews highlight the vulnerability of voice vis-à-vis systemic diseases[88,89] and the importance of adipose tissue as an endocrine organ.[90] Review of 3 facets of the interplay between obesity and voice helps clarify clinical issues, as summarized in the next section.

The Systemic Effect

It is well established that obesity leads to numerous metabolic disorders through its immune-modulatory effect. The release of adipokines results in systemic inflammation that predisposes to numerous diseases.[90] In addition to playing a major role in energy homeostasis and its metabolic effect, obesity impacts systems in the body that are integral to voice production. Excessive weight can adversely affect breathing by mechanical impairment, reduction in chest compliance, and alteration in lung perfusion.[91-96] Obesity also can alter the sex hormone environment in both men and women.[97-103] There is reduction in total and free testosterone levels in men and peripheral conversion of androgen to estrogen via several enzymes.[99,100] In menopausal women, the excess fat can act as a reservoir for estrogen replenishment to mitigate the postmenopausal androgenic state.[102,104,105] Obesity also can affect the gastrointestinal system. It has been proven to exacerbate the symptoms and signs of reflux disease by delaying gastric emptying time, altering the function of the lower esophageal sphincter, displacing the gastroesophageal junction zone, and increasing the risk of hiatal hernia.[106-113]

As phonation is a complex process intimately linked to these systems, it is reasonable to infer that obesity-induced alterations in the function of these systems may jeopardize phonation and lead to voice disorders. Further discussion on this topic is presented in Chapters 5, 6, 7, and 8 of this book.

The Positive Energy Imbalance

As previously mentioned in this chapter, obesity is the result of excessive energy intake and/or decrease in energy use (activity level). Both factors are linked to voice production. Diet and voice are discussed in Chapter 58, "Nutrition and the Professional Voice," of the fourth edition of *Professional Voice*,[114] republished for the readers' convenience as Chapter 11 of this book. In summary, dietary behavior in terms of amount and type of nutrients as well as fluid

intake is important for vocal performance. A nutrition strategy based on a balanced diet is often needed in order to meet the dietary requirements of professional voice users just as it is to meet the requirements of other professional athletes. For instance, a meal rich in carbohydrate and low in fat often is recommended a few hours prior to a long performance. Similarly, consumption of fruits and vegetables with lean proteins is always advised.[115] The eating pattern and dietary behavior of obese subjects may have an adverse effect on their vocal performance.[116,117] The imbalance in energy intake and energy expenditure in obese subjects may put the singer at risk of vocal fatigue, hunger, or gastrointestinal discomfort. By the same reasoning, the sedentary activity experienced by obese patients may also affect vocal performance adversely. Jarosz et al[118] examined the correlation between BMI, physical inactivity, and fatigue in 69 African American women (BMI greater than 30 kg/m^2). The results indicated a significant correlation between obesity and body fatigue, which substantiates the deterrent effect of obesity on body activity and lifestyle. Vgontzas et al[119] correlated the excessive daytime sleepiness and fatigue in obese subjects with metabolic disorders even in the absence of obstructive sleep apnea. Given that professional voice users are vocal athletes,[120] body fatigue associated with obesity may have a detrimental effect on voice performance and lead to vocal disorders.[118-120] Further research on this topic is needed to elucidate the relationship between obesity, body fatigue, and voice.

The Vocal Tract and the Bottleneck

Although the vocal signal is energized by breathing and is emitted at the level of the vocal folds, what shapes our vocal identity is the morphology and contour of the supraglottic vocal tract, the bottleneck for sound production. With obesity, there is alteration in the shape and cross-sectional area of the pharyngeal lumen, as well as the configuration of other regions of the vocal tract, which may affect voice quality.[121–124] The upper airway is a target for morphologic changes in obese subjects. Weight-induced fat deposition at various sites of the vocal tract has been described by numerous authors. For example, a study by Busetto et al[125] conducted on female obese subjects showed a strong correlation between weight, fat distribution, and size of the upper airway. Accumulation of fat was noted at the base of tongue, lateral pharyngeal walls, and at the palatopharyngeal folds. Several other studies also have documented an association between obesity and upper airway fat distribution.[123,126] Similarly, Pahkala et al[127] reported hypertrophy of the pharyngeal fat pad in obese subjects scheduled for bariatric surgery. This alteration in the size and configuration of the vocal tract in relation to BMI certainly carries acoustic implications given that formants' dispersion and position depend heavily on the shape of the vocal tract.[128–132] A more thorough discussion on the correlation between vocal tract morphology in obese subjects and phonatory output is reviewed in Chapter 5 of this book, namely, on obesity, body size, and vocal tract.

References

1. An R. Prevalence and trends of adult obesity in the US, 1999–2012. *ISRN Obes.* 2014;2014:185132.
2. Ogden CL, Carroll MD, Kit BK, Flegal KM. Prevalence of obesity and trends in body mass index among US children and adolescents, 1999–2010. *JAMA.* 2012;307(5): 483–490.
3. Ogden CL, Carroll MD, Kit BK, Flegal KM. Prevalence of childhood and adult obesity in the United States, 2011–2012. *JAMA.* 2014;311(8):806–814.
4. Bhupathiraju SN, Hu FB. Epidemiology of obesity and diabetes and their cardiovascular complications. *Circ Res.* 2016;118(11): 1723–1735.
5. World Health Organization. Obesity and overweight. http://www.who.int/mediacentre/factsheets/fs311/en/. Retrieved December 14, 2018.
6. Wang Y, Beydoun MA, Liang L, Caballero B, Kumanyika SK. Will all Americans become overweight or obese? Estimating the progression and cost of the US obesity epidemic. *Obesity (Silver Spring).* 2008;16(10):2323–2330.
7. Ogden CL, Carroll MD, Lawman HG, et al. Trends in obesity prevalence among children and adolescents in the United States, 1988–1994 through 2013–2014. *JAMA.* 2016;315(21):2292–2299.
8. Li C, Ford ES, Zhao G, Balluz LS, Giles WH. Estimates of body composition with dual-energy X-ray absorptiometry in adults. *Am J Clin Nutr.* 2009;90(6):1457–1465.
9. Skinner AC, Skelton JA. Prevalence and trends in obesity and severe obesity among children in the United States, 1999–2012. *JAMA Pediatr.* 2014;168(6):561–566.
10. Have MT, Van der Heide, Machenbach JP, De Beaufort ID. An ethical framework for the prevention of overweight and obesity: a tool for thinking through a programme's ethical aspects. *Eur J Public Health.* 2013; 23(2):299–305.
11. Egger G, Dixon J. Beyond obesity and lifestyle: a review of 21st century chronic disease determinants. *BioMed Res Int.* 2014; 2014(5):731685.
12. Brownell KD, Wadden TA. Etiology and treatment of obesity: understanding a serious, prevalent and refractory disorder. *J Consult Clin Psychol.* 1992;60(4):505–517.
13. Swinburn B, Egger G, and Raza F. Dissecting obesogenic environments: the development and application of a framework for identifying and prioritizing environmental interventions for obesity. *Prev Med.* 1999; 29(6, pt 1):563–570.

14. Laumbach RJ, Kipen HM. Acute effects of motor vehicle traffic-related air pollution exposures on measures of oxidative stress in human airways. *Ann N Y Acad Sci.* 2010;1203:107–112.

15. Sears ME, Genuis SJ. Environmental determinants of chronic disease and medical approaches: recognition, avoidance, supportive therapy, and detoxification. *J Environ Public Health.* 2012;2012:356798.

16. Dietert RR. Misregulated inflammation as an outcome of early-life exposure to endocrine-disrupting chemicals. *Rev Environ Health.* 2012;27(2–3):117–131.

17. Egger G, Swinburn B. An "ecological" approach to the obesity pandemic. *BMJ.* 1997;315(7106):477–480.

18. Egger G. In search of a "germ theory" equivalent for chronic disease. *Prev Chronic Dis.* 2012;9:E95.

19. Egger G, Dixon J. Inflammatory effects of nutritional stimuli: further support for the need for a big picture approach to tackling obesity and chronic disease. *Obes Rev.* 2010;11(2):137–149.

20. Egger G, Dixon J. Non-nutrient causes of low-grade, systemic inflammation: support for a "canary in the mineshaft" view of obesity in chronic disease. *Obes Rev.* 2011; 12(5):339–345.

21. Booth FW, Chakravarthy MV, Gordon SE, Spangenburg EE. Waging war on physical inactivity: using modern molecular ammunition against an ancient enemy. *J Appl Physiol.* 2002;93(1):3–30.

22. Ferrie JE, Kivimaki M, Akbaraly TN, et al. Associations between change in sleep duration and inflammation: findings on C-reactive protein and interleukin 6 in the Whitehall II study. *Am J Epidemiol.* 2013; 178(6):956–961.

23. Colten HR, Altevogt BM, eds. *Sleep Disorders and Sleep Deprivation: An Unmet Public Health Problem.* Institute of Medicine (US) Committee on Sleep Medicine and Research. Washington, DC: National Academies Press; 2006.

24. Almadi T, Cathers I, Chow CM. Associations among work-related stress, cortisol, inflammation, and metabolic syndrome. *Psychophysiology.* 2013;50(9):821–830.

25. Gregor MF, Hotamisligil GS. Inflammatory mechanisms in obesity. *Annu Rev Immunol.* 2011;29:415–445.

26. Manna P, Jain SK. Obesity, oxidative stress, adipose tissue dysfunction, and the associated health risks: causes and therapeutic strategies. *Metab Syndr Relat Disord.* 2015; 13(10):423–444.

27. Pi-Sunyer FX. Health implications of obesity. *Am J Clin Nutr.* 1991;53(6)(suppl): 1595S–1603S.

28. Field AE, Coakley EH, Must A, et al. Impact of overweight on the risk of developing common chronic diseases during a 10-year period. *Arch Intern Med.* 2001;161(13): 1581–1586.

29. Guh DP, Zhang W, Bansback N, Amarsi Z, Birmingham CL, Anis AH. The incidence of co-morbidities related to obesity and overweight: a systematic review and meta-analysis. *BMC Public Health.* 2009;9:88.

30. Colosia AD, Palencia R, Khan S. Prevalence of hypertension and obesity in patients with type 2 diabetes mellitus in observational studies: a systematic literature review. *Diabetes Metab Syndr Obes.* 2013;6:327–338.

31. Ang GY. Reversibility of diabetes mellitus: narrative review of the evidence. *World J Diabetes.* 2018;9(7):127–131.

32. Poirier P, Eckel RH. Obesity and cardiovascular disease. *Curr Atheroscler Rep.* 2002; 4(6):448–453.

33. Bastien M, Poirier P, Lemieux I, Despres JP. Overview of epidemiology and contribution of obesity to cardiovascular disease. *Prog Cardiovasc Dis.* 2014;56(4):369–381.

34. Wilson PW, D'Agostino RB, Sullivan L, Parise H, Kannel WB. Overweight and obesity as determinants of cardiovascular risk: the Framingham experience. *Arch Intern Med.* 2002;162(16):1867–1872.

35. Bastard JP, Maachi M, Lagathu C, et al. Recent advances in the relationship between obesity, inflammation, and insulin resistance. *Eur Cytokine Netw.* 2006;17(1): 4–12.

36. Gregg EW, Cheng YJ, Cadwell BL, et al. Secular trends in cardiovascular disease risk factors according to body mass index in US adults. *JAMA*. 2005;293(15):1868–1874.

37. Saydah S, Bullard KM, Cheng Y, et al. Trends in cardiovascular disease risk factors by obesity level in adults in the United States, NHANES 1999–2010. *Obesity (Silver Spring)*. 2014;22(8):1888–1895.

38. Hubert HB, Feinleib M, McNamara PM, Castelli WP. Obesity as an independent risk factor for cardiovascular disease: a 26-year follow-up of participants in the Framingham heart study. *Circulation*. 1983;67(5):968–977.

39. Manson JE, Colditz GA, Stampfer MJ, et al. A prospective study of obesity and risk of coronary heart disease in women. *N Engl J Med*. 1990;322(13):882–889.

40. Rabkin SW, Mathewson FA, Hsu PH. Relation of body weight to development of ischemic heart disease in a cohort of young North American men after a 26 year observation period: the Manitoba study. *Am J Cardiol*. 1977;39(3):452–458.

41. Lloyd-Jones DM, Hong Y, Labarthe D, et al. Defining and setting national goals for cardiovascular health promotion and disease reduction: the American Heart Association's strategic impact goal through 2020 and beyond. *Circulation*. 2010;121(4): 586–613.

42. Fernández-Sánchez A, Madrigal-Santillán E, Bautista M, et al. Inflammation, oxidative stress, and obesity. *Int J Mol Sci*. 2011; 12(5):3117–3132.

43. Pinto-Sietsma SJ, Navis G, Janssen WM, de Zeeuw D, Gans RO, de Jong PE. A central body fat distribution is related to renal function impairment, even in lean subjects. *Am J Kidney Dis*. 2003;41(4):733–741.

44. Foster MC, Hwang SJ, Larson MG, et al. Overweight, obesity, and the development of stage 3 CKD: the Framingham Heart Study. *Am J Kidney Dis*. 2008;52(1):39–48.

45. Kramer H, Luke A, Bidani A, Cao G, Cooper R, McGee D. Obesity and prevalent and incident CKD: the Hypertension Detection and Follow-Up Program. *Am J Kidney Dis*. 2005;46(4):587–594.

46. Chang A, Van Horn L, Jacobs DR Jr, et al. Lifestyle-related factors, obesity, and incident microalbuminuria: the CARDIA (Coronary Artery Risk Development in Young Adults) study. *Am J Kidney Dis*. 2013;62(2):267–275.

47. Ejerblad E, Fored CM, Lindblad P, Fryzek J, McLaughlin JK, Nyren O. Obesity and risk for chronic renal failure. *J Am Soc Nephrol*. 2006;17(6):1695–1702.

48. Gelber RP, Kurth T, Kausz AT, et al. Association between body mass index and CKD in apparently healthy men. *Am J Kidney Dis*. 2005;46(5): 871–880.

49. Lu JL, Molnar MZ, Naseer A, Mikkelsen MK, Kalantar-Zadeh K, Kovesdy CP. Association of age and BMI with kidney function and mortality: a cohort study. *Lancet Diabetes Endocrinol*. 2015;3(9):704–714.

50. Munkhaugen J, Lydersen S, Wideroe TE, Hallan S. Prehypertension, obesity, and risk of kidney disease: 20-year follow-up of the HUNT I study in Norway. *Am J Kidney Dis*. 2009;54(4):638–646.

51. Iseki K, Ikemiya Y, Kinjo K, Inoue T, Iseki C, Takishita S. Body mass index and the risk of development of end-stage renal disease in a screened cohort. *Kidney Int*. 2004; 65(5):1870–1876.

52. Vivante A, Golan E, Tzur D, et al. Body mass index in 1.2 million adolescents and risk for end-stage renal disease. *Arch Intern Med*. 2012;172(21):1644–1650.

53. Hsu C, McCulloch C, Iribarren C, Darbinian J, Go AS. Body mass index and risk for end-stage renal disease. *Ann Intern Med*. 2006;144(1):21–28.

54. Sharma K. The link between obesity and albuminuria: adiponectin and podocyte dysfunction. *Kidney Int*. 2009;76(2):145–148.

55. Wolf G, Ziyadeh FN. Leptin and renal fibrosis. *Contrib Nephrol*. 2006;151:175–183.

56. Ellington AA, Malik AR, Klee GG, et al. Association of plasma resistin with glomerular filtration rate and albuminuria in hypertensive adults. *Hypertension*. 2007; 50(4):708–714.

57. Furukawa S, Fujita T, Shimabukuro M, et al. Increased oxidative stress in obesity and

its impact on metabolic syndrome. *J Clin Invest.* 2004;114(12):1752–1761.

58. Kambham N, Markowitz GS, Valeri AM, Lin J, D'Agati VD. Obesity-related glomerulopathy: an emerging epidemic. *Kidney Int.* 2001;59(4):1498–1509.

59. Scales CD Jr, Smith AC, Hanley JM, Saigal CS; Urologic Diseases in America Project. Prevalence of kidney stones in the United States. *Eur Urol.* 2012;62(1):160–165.

60. Curhan GC, Willett WC, Rimm EB, Speizer FE, Stampfer MJ. Body size and risk of kidney stones. *J Am Soc Nephrol.* 1998;9(9):1645–1652.

61. Vainio H, Kaaks R, Bianchini F. Weight control and physical activity in cancer prevention: international evaluation of the evidence. *Eur J Cancer Prev.* 2002;11(2): S94–S100.

62. Franks PW, Atabaki-Pasdar N. Causal inference in obesity research. *J Intern Med.* 2017;281(3):222–232.

63. Preziosi G, Oben JA, Fusai G. Obesity and pancreatic cancer. *Surg Oncol.* 2014; 23(2):61–71.

64. Maccio A, Madeddu C, Gramignano G, et al. Correlation of body mass index and leptin with tumor size and stage of disease in hormone-dependent postmenopausal breast cancer: preliminary results and therapeutic implications. *J Mol Med (Berl).* 2010;88(7):677–686.

65. Hursting SD. Minireview: the year in obesity and cancer. *Mol Endocrinol.* 2012; 26(12):1961–1966.

66. Ramos-Nino ME. The role of chronic inflammation in obesity-associated cancers. *ISRN Oncol.* 2013;2013:697521.

67. Pollak M. The insulin and insulin-like growth factor receptor family in neoplasia: an update. *Nat Rev Cancer.* 2012;12(3):159–169.

68. Osborne CK, Bolan G, Monaco ME, Lippman ME. Hormone responsive human breast cancer in long-term tissue culture: effect of insulin. *Proc Natl Acad Sci USA.* 1976;73(12):4536–4540.

69. Gerozissis K. Brain insulin, energy and glucose homeostasis; genes, environment and metabolic pathologies. *Eur J Pharmacol.* 2008;585(1):38–49.

70. Tamakoshi K, Toyoshima H, Wakai K, et al. Leptin is associated with an increased female colorectal cancer risk: a nested case-control study in Japan. *Oncology.* 2005; 68(4–6):454–461.

71. Barb D, Williams CJ, Neuwirth AK, Mantzoros CS. Adiponectin in relation to malignancies: a review of existing basic research and clinical evidence. *Am J Clin Nutr.* 2007; 86(3):s858–s866.

72. Costa C, Incio J, Soares R. Angiogenesis and chronic inflammation: cause or consequence? *Angiogenesis.* 2007;10(3):149–166.

73. Adams KF, Leitzmann MF, Ballard-Barbash R, et al. Body mass and weight change in adults in relation to mortality risk. *Am J Epidemiol.* 2014;179(2):135–144.

74. Corrada MM, Kawas CH, Mozaffar F, Paganini-Hill A. Association of body mass index and weight change with all-cause mortality in the elderly. *Am J Epidemiol.* 2006;163(10):938–949.

75. Calle EE, Thun MJ, Petrelli JM, Rodriguez C, Heath CW Jr. Body-mass index and mortality in a prospective cohort of US adults. *N Engl J Med.* 1999;341(15):1097–1105.

76. Adams KF, Schatzkin A, Harris TB, et al. Overweight, obesity, and mortality in a large prospective cohort of persons 50 to 71 years old. *N Engl J Med.* 2006;355(8): 763–778.

77. Da Cunha MG, Passerotti GH, Weber R, Zilberstein B, Cecconello I. Voice feature characteristic in morbid obese population. *Obesity Surg.* 2011;21(3):340–344.

78. Barsties B, Verfaillie R, Roy N, Maryn Y. Do body mass index and fat volume influence vocal quality, phonatory range, and aerodynamics in females? *Codas.* 2013; 25(4):310–318.

79. Künzel HJ. How well does average fundamental frequency correlate with speaker height and weight? *Phonetica.* 1989;46(1–3):117–125.

80. Evans S, Neave N, Wakelin D. Relationships between vocal characteristics and

body size and shape in human males: an evolutionary explanation for a deep male voice. *Biol Psychol.* 2006;72(2):160–163.

81. Hamdan AL, Al-Barazi R, Tabri D, et al. Relationship between acoustic parameters and body mass analysis in young males. *J Voice.* 2012;26(2):144–147.

82. van Dommelen WA. Speaker height and weight identification: a re-evaluation of some old data. *J Phonetics.* 1993;21(3):337–341.

83. van Dommelen WA, Moxness BH. Acoustic parameters in speaker height and weight identification: sex-specific behavior. *Lang Speech.* 1995;38(pt 3):267–287.

84. Gunter CD, Manning WH. Listener estimations of speaker height and weight in unfiltered and filtered conditions. *J Phonetics.* 1982;10(3):251–257.

85. Solomon NP, Helou LB, Dietrich-Burns K, Stojadinovic A. Do obesity and weight loss affect vocal function? *Semin Speech Lang.* 2011;32(1):31–42.

86. Hamdan AL, Safadi B, Chamseddine G, Kasty M, Turfe ZA, Ziade G. Effect of weight loss on voice after bariatric surgery. *J Voice.* 2014;28(5):618–623.

87. De Souza LB, dos Santos MM, Pernambuco LA, de Almeida Godoy CM, da Silva Lima DM. Effects of weight loss on acoustic parameters after bariatric surgery. *Obes Surg.* 2018;28(5):1372–1376.

88. Sataloff RT. *Professional Voice: The Science and Art of Clinical Care.* 4th ed. San Diego, CA: Plural Publishing; 2017.

89. Sapienza C, Ruddy BH. *Voice Disorders: A Textbook.* San Diego, CA: Plural Publishing; 2009.

90. Fonseca-Alaniz MH, Takada J, Alonso-Vale MI, Lima FB. Adipose tissue as an endocrine organ: from theory to practice. *J Pediatr (Rio J).* 2007;83(5)(suppl):S192–S203.

91. Unterborn J. Pulmonary function testing in obesity, pregnancy, and extremes of body habitus. *Clin Chest Med.* 2001;22(4):759–767.

92. Sampson MG, Grassino AE. Load compensation in obese patients during quiet tidal breathing. *J Appl Physiol Respir Environ Exerc Physiol.* 1983;55(4):1269–1276.

93. Lotti P, Gigliotti F, Tesi F, et al. Respiratory muscles and dyspnea in obese nonsmoking subjects. *Lung.* 2005;183(5):311–323.

94. Naimark A, Cherniack RM. Compliance of the respiratory system and its components in health and obesity. *J Appl Physiol.* 1960;15:377–382.

95. Mafort TT, Rufino R, Costa CH, Lopes AJ. Obesity: systemic and pulmonary complications, biochemical abnormalities, and impairment of lung function. *Multidiscip Respir Med.* 2016;11:28.

96. Farebrother MJ, McHardy GJ, Munro JF. Relation between pulmonary gas exchange and closing volume before and after substantial weight loss in obese subjects. *BMJ.* 1974;3(5927):391–393.

97. Seidell JC, Bjorntorp P, Sjostrom L, Kvist H, Sannerstedt R. Visceral fat accumulation in men is positively associated with insulin, glucose, and C-peptide levels, but negatively with testosterone levels. *Metabolism.* 1990;39(9):897–901.

98. Deslypere JP, Verdonck L, Vermeulen A. Fat tissue: a steroid reservoir and site of steroid metabolism. *J Clin Endocrinol Metab.* 1985;61(3):564–570.

99. López M, Tena-Sempere M. Estradiol and brown fat. *Best Prac Res Clin Endocrinol Metab.* 2016;30(4):527–536.

100. Blouin K, Boivin A, Tchernof A. Androgens and body fat distribution. *J Steroid Biochem Mol Biol.* 2008;108(3–5):272–280.

101. Sattler FR, Castaneda-Sceppa C, Binder EF, et al. Testosterone and growth hormone improve body composition and muscle performance in older men. *J Clin Endocrinol Metab.* 2009;94(6):1991–2001.

102. Kim JH, Cho HT, Kim YJ. The role of estrogen in adipose tissue metabolism: insights into glucose homeostasis regulation. *Endocr J.* 2014;61(11):1055–1067.

103. Woodhouse LJ, Gupta N, Bhasin M, et al. Dose-dependent effects of testosterone on regional adipose tissue distribution

in healthy young men. *J Clin Endocrinol Metab.* 2004;89(2):718–726.

104. Abitbol J, Abitbol P, Abitbol B. Sex hormones and the female voice. *J Voice.* 1999; 13(3):424–446.

105. Gambacciani M, Ciaponi M, Cappagli B, et al. Body weight, body fat distribution, and hormonal replacement therapy in early postmenopausal women. *J Clin Endocrinol Metab.* 1997;82(2):414–417.

106. Barak N, Ehrenpreis ED, Harrison JR, Sitrin MD. Gastro-oesophageal reflux disease in obesity: pathophysiological and therapeutic considerations. *Obes Rev.* 2002; 3(1):9–15.

107. Pandolfino JE, El-Serag HB, Zhang Q, Shah N, Ghosh SK, Kahrilas PJ. Obesity: a challenge to esophagogastric junction integrity. *Gastroenterology.* 2006;130(3):639–649.

108. Merrouche M, Sabaté JM, Jouet P, et al. Gastro-esophageal reflux and esophageal motility disorders in morbidly obese patients before and after bariatric surgery. *Obes Surg.* 2007;17(7):894–900.

109. Ayazi S, Hagen JA, Chan LS, et al. Obesity and gastroesophageal reflux: quantifying the association between body mass index, esophageal acid exposure, and lower esophageal sphincter status in a large series of patients with reflux symptoms. *J Gastrointest Surg.* 2009;13(8):1440–1447.

110. Mittal RK, Balaban DH. The esophagogastric junction. *N Engl J Med.* 1997;336(13): 924–932.

111. Kahrilas PJ, Shi G. Pathophysiology of gastroesophageal reflux disease: the antireflux barrier and luminal clearance mechanisms. In: Orlando RC, ed. *Gastroesophageal Reflux Disease.* New York, NY: Marcel Dekker; 2000:137–164.

112. Wilson LJ, Ma W, Hirschowitz BI. Association of obesity with hiatal hernia and esophagitis. *Am J Gastroenterol.* 1999; 94(10):2840–2844.

113. Maddox A, Horowitz M, Wishart J, Collins P. Gastric and oesophageal emptying in obesity. *Scand J Gastroenterol.* 1989;24(5): 593–598.

114. Nasser J, Dardarian N. Nutrition and the professional voice. In: Sataloff RT, ed. *Professional Voice: The Science and Art of Clinical Care.* 4th ed. San Diego, CA: Plural Publishing; 2017:885–907.

115. Dick RW, Berning JR, Dawson W, Ginsburg RD, Miller C, Shybut GT. Athletes and the arts—the role of sports medicine in the performing arts. *Curr Sports Med Rep.* 2013;12(6):397–403.

116. Fox M, Barr C, Nolan S, Lomer M, Anggiansah A, Wong T. The effects of dietary fat and calorie density on esophageal acid exposure and reflux symptoms. *Clin Gastroenterol Hepatol.* 2007;5(4):439–444.

117. El-Serag HB, Satia JA, Rabeneck L. Dietary intake and the risk of gastro-oesophageal reflux disease: a cross sectional study in volunteers. *Gut.* 2005;54(1):11–17.

118. Jarosz PA, Davis JE, Yarandi HN, et al. Obesity in urban women: associations with sleep and sleepiness, fatigue and activity. *Womens Health Issues.* 2014;24(4): e447–e454.

119. Vgontzas AN, Bixler EO, Chrousos GP. Obesity-related sleepiness and fatigue: the role of the stress system and cytokines. *Ann N Y Acad Sci.* 2006;1083(1):329–344.

120. Stavrides K, Sataloff RT, Emerich K. Chronic fatigue syndrome in singers. In: Sataloff RT, ed. *Professional Voice: The Science and Art of Clinical Care.* 4th ed. San Diego, CA: Plural Publishing; 2017: 877–884.

121. Shakakibara H, Tong M, Matsushita K, Hirata M, Konishi Y, Suetsugu S. Cephalometric abnormalities in non-obese and obese patients with obstructive sleep apnoea. *Eur Respir J.* 1999;13:403–410.

122. Mortimore IL, Marshall I, Wraith PK, Sellar RJ, Douglas NJ. Neck and total body fat deposition in non obese and obese patients with sleep apnea compared with that in control subjects. *Am J Respir Crit Care Med.* 1998;157(1):280–283.

123. Horner RL, Mohiaddin RH, Lowell DG, et al. Sites and sizes of fat deposits around the pharynx in obese patients with obstructive

sleep apnoea and weight matched controls. *Eur Respir J.* 1989;2(7):613–622.

124. Shelton KE, Woodson H, Gay S, Suratt PM. Pharyngeal fat in obstructive sleep apnea. *Am Rev Respir Dis.* 1993;148(2):462–466.

125. Busetto L, Calo E, Mazza M, et al. Upper airway size is related to obesity and body fat distribution in women. *Eur Arch Otorhinolaryngol.* 2009;266(4):559–563.

126. Turnbull CD, Wang SH, Manuel AR, et al. Relationships between MRI fat distributions and sleep apnea and obesity hypoventilation syndrome in very obese patients. *Sleep Breath.* 2018;22(3):673–681.

127. Pahkala R, Seppä J, Ikonen A, Smirnov G, Tuomilehto H. The impact of pharyngeal fat tissue on the pathogenesis of obstructive sleep apnea. *Sleep Breath.* 2014;18(2):275–282.

128. Fitch WT, Giedd J. Morphology and development of the human vocal tract: a study using magnetic resonance imaging. *J Acoust Soc Am.* 1999;106(3, pt 1):1511–1522.

129. Titze IR. *Principles of Vocal Production.* Englewood Cliffs, NJ: Prentice Hall; 1994.

130. Roers F, Mürbe D, Sundberg J. Voice classification and vocal tract of singers: a study of x-ray images and morphology. *J Acoust Soc Am.* 2009;125(1):503–512.

131. Cleveland TF. Acoustic properties of voice timbre types and their influence on voice classification. *J Acoust Soc Am.* 1977;61(6):1622–1629.

132. Dmitriev L, Kiselev A. Relationship between the formant structure of different types of singing voices and the dimensions of supraglottic cavities. *Folia Phoniatr (Basel).* 1979;31(4):238–241.

2

Clinical Anatomy and Physiology of the Voice

Robert Thayer Sataloff

Anatomy

The anatomy of the voice is not limited to the region between the suprasternal notch and the hyoid bone. Practically all body systems affect the voice. The larynx receives the greatest attention because it is the most sensitive and expressive component of the vocal mechanism, but anatomic interactions throughout the patient's body must be considered in treating voice disorders. It is helpful to think of the larynx as composed of 4 anatomic units—skeleton, mucosa, intrinsic muscles, and extrinsic muscles—as well as vascular, neurological, and other related structures. The glottis is the space between the vocal folds. The term *vocal cords* was abandoned in favor of the term *vocal folds* more than 3 decades ago. Vocal folds is a more accurate description of the structure, as described below (although not quite so accurate as the German term "vocal lips"). Moreover, the word "cord" often makes people think of a string-like structure, and vocal fold motion is not similar to a vibrating string.

Laryngeal Skeleton: Cartilages, Ligaments, and Membranes

The most important parts of the laryngeal skeleton are the thyroid cartilage, the cricoid cartilage, and the 2 arytenoid cartilages (Figure 2–1). The laryngeal cartilages are connected by soft attachments that allow changes in their relative angles and distances, thereby permitting alterations in the shape and tension of the tissues extended between them. The intrinsic muscles of the larynx are connected to these cartilages. For example, one of the intrinsic muscles, the thyroarytenoid (TA), extends on each side from the arytenoid cartilage to the inside of the thyroid cartilage just below and behind the thyroid prominence. The medial belly of the TA is also known as the vocalis muscle, and it forms the body of the vocal fold.

The pyramidal, paired arytenoid cartilages sit atop the superior edge of the cricoid cartilage. They each include a muscular process, a vocal process and an apex, a body, and a complex, concave articular surface. They are hyaline cartilages, except for the vocal process, and the apices in some cases, which

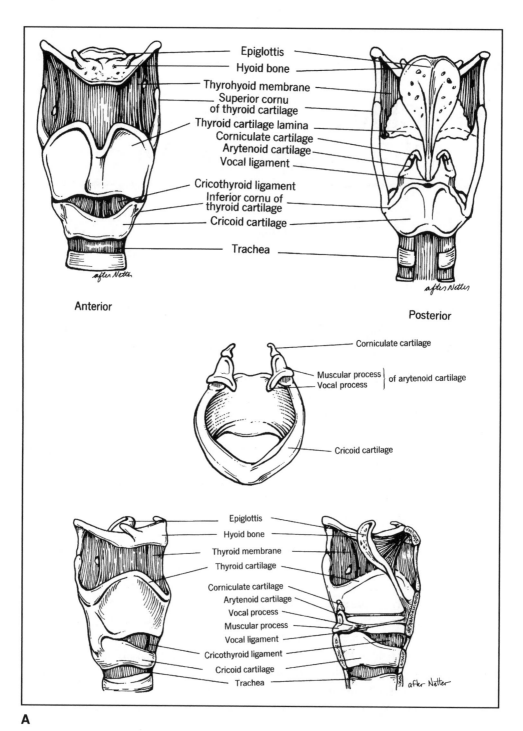

Epiglottis
Hyoid bone
Thyrohyoid membrane
Superior cornu
of thyroid cartilage
Thyroid cartilage lamina
Corniculate cartilage
Arytenoid cartilage
Vocal ligament
Cricothyroid ligament
Inferior cornu of
thyroid cartilage
Cricoid cartilage

Trachea

Anterior

Posterior

Corniculate cartilage

Muscular process
Vocal process } of arytenoid cartilage

Cricoid cartilage

Epiglottis
Hyoid bone
Thyroid membrane
Thyroid cartilage
Corniculate cartilage
Arytenoid cartilage
Vocal process
Muscular process
Vocal ligament
Cricothyroid ligament
Cricoid cartilage
Trachea

A

Figure 2–1. A. Cartilages of the larynx. *(continues)*

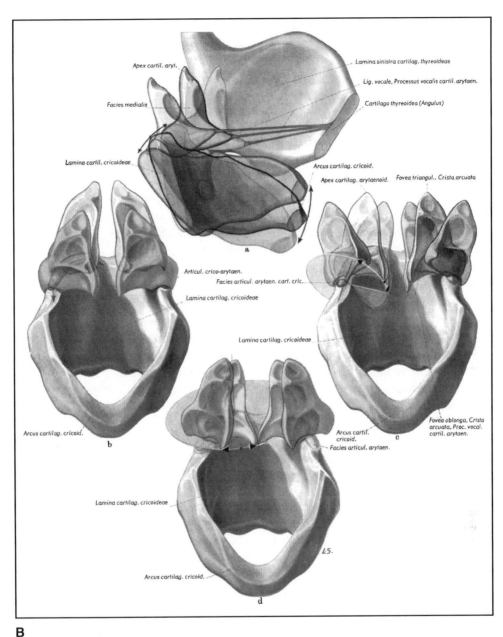

B

Figure 2–1. *(continued)* **B.** Schematic representation of position changes of laryngeal cartilages illustrating the most extreme positions achieved by each. (Reproduced with permission from Pernkopf.[1])

are composed of fibroelastic cartilage. The hyaline portions generally begin to ossify at around 30 years of age.[2] Clinically, arytenoid asymmetry is common. Hamdan et al

studied 110 singers (male-to-female ratio of 2:1) and found no correlation between arytenoid asymmetry and vocal symptoms.[3] In a later study, they also found no correlation between arytenoid asymmetry and posture, neck tension, or glottal attack.[4] Bonilha et al also found that arytenoid asymmetry was common, but there were no statistically significant differences in prevalence of arytenoid asymmetries comparing subjects with normal voices and those with dysphonia.[5]

Ossification of the thyroid cartilage begins earlier, usually at around 20 years of age, and usually begins posteriorly and inferiorly.[2] The 2 thyroid laminae join in the midline, forming an angle of approximately 120° in women and approximately 90° in men. The thyroid prominence is also more noticeable in men and is commonly known as the "Adam's apple." Just above the thyroid prominence, the thyroid laminae form a "V," the thyroid notch. Posteriorly, the laminae extend to form superior and inferior cornua (horns). The superior cornu connects to the hyoid bone via the thyrohyoid ligament. The inferior cornu is connected to the cricoid cartilage by a synovial cricothyroid joint. The joint is encased in a capsular ligament, which is strengthened posteriorly by a fibrous band. Movement of the paired cricothyroid joints is diarthrodial. The primary movement is rotary, with the cricoid rotating around a transverse axis passing through both joints. Gliding in various directions also occurs to a limited extent. This joint tends to move anteromedially during vocal fold adduction and posterolaterally during vocal fold abduction and permits the anterior aspects of the cricoid and thyroid cartilages to be brought more closely together to increase vocal fold length (and frequency of phonation, or pitch) in response to cricothyroid (CT) muscle contraction.

The perichondrium of the thyroid cartilage is thinner internally than externally. Externally, in the midline, there is a tiny landmark that can be helpful in identifying the position of the anterior commissure.[6]

This small, diamond-shaped surface depression is associated with a slightly lighter color compared to the adjacent thyroid cartilage. It is found in the anterior midline, approximately halfway between the thyroid notch and the inferior border of the thyroid cartilage, and a small, unnamed artery travels through this tiny depression, as described by Adams et al.[6] The landmark is referred to sometimes as Montgomery's aperture. At a corresponding location on the inner surface, there is a small protrusion that is devoid of perichondrium. This is the point of attachment of Broyles ligament and the anterior commissure tendon. The rest of the thyroid cartilage is covered with fairly thick perichondrium, and the smooth, concave inner surface is covered by a mucosal membrane. Broyles ligament is formed by the vocal ligament (which is also the upper border of the conus elasticus), the internal perichondrium of the thyroid cartilage, and the thyroepiglottic ligament.

The oblique line is another important external landmark of the thyroid cartilage. It runs anteroinferiorly from a superior thyroid tubercle located just inferior to the superior cornu, and it extends to the inferior thyroid tubercle located at the lower border of the thyroid lamina. The oblique line is actually a ridge to which the thyrohyoid, sternothyroid, and inferior pharyngeal constrictor muscles attach. Fibers from the palatopharyngeus and stylopharyngeus muscles attach to the posterior border of the thyroid cartilage.

The signet ring–shaped cricoid cartilage is the only circumferential cartilaginous structure in the airway. Its posterior lamina may rise to a height of approximately 30 millimeters (mm), and its anterior arch may be only a few millimeters in height. Not only is the anterior aspect of the arch thin, but it also ossifies later than the posterior aspect of the cricoid cartilage, which begins to ossify in the early to mid-20s. Because the anterior portion of the arch is both thin and tends to ossify later, it is particularly prone to fracture during surgical manipulation. This should be remembered in procedures such as cricothyroid approximation; traction should always be centered laterally on the cricoid arch, rather than near the midline. The cricoid and thyroid cartilages are joined through the cricothyroid joints. These synovial joints vary among individuals. They have been divided into 3 groups.[7] In group 1, the rotation axis of the cricothyroid joint is located in the lower third of the joint (13 of 24 specimens studied); in group 2, it is located in the middle third of the joint (5/23); and in group 3 the effective axis of rotation is located in the lower third of the cricoid cartilage. Elongations of the vocal fold were 12% in group 1, 8% in group 2, and 3% in group 3. These differences may be important for patients undergoing cricothyroid approximation surgery, but more research is needed to confirm these findings and investigate their clinical implications. The cricoid is connected to the thyroid cartilage not only through the cricothyroid joints, but also through the cricothyroid membrane and its midline thickening known as the cricothyroid ligament.

Internal dimensions of the cricoid cartilage and trachea vary substantially. Such information is important with regard to tracheal intubation, dilatation, stenting, endoscopy, anastomosis, and transplantation. The luminal cross sections vary between and among men and women. The smallest dimension occurs in the frontal plane.[8] In women, this measures approximately 11.6 mm, with a range of 8.9 to 17 mm. In men, it is about 15 mm, with a range of 11 to 21.5 mm. The distance between the cricoarytenoid joint facets varies from person to person, as well as does the angle between longitudinal axes of the cricoarytenoid

joint facets (42°–74° in women, 37°–75° in men).[8] Morphometric characteristics of the larynx have also been studied by Jotz et al.[9] They examined larynges of 50 male and 50 female fresh cadavers of humans older than 40 years. All laryngeal measurements were greater in men than in women except for the thyroid angle that was greater in women. There was no significant difference in morphological comparison between men and women among various age groups.

The cross section of the trachea is also highly variable, with a frontal diameter reported as narrow as 9.9 mm in women and 12 mm in men.[8] The marked variation in size and shape highlights the difficulty in creating a standardized rigid stent. It should also be noted that the diameter of the cricoid ring in some women is too narrow to permit the atraumatic passage of an endotracheal tube with a 7-mm internal diameter. Anatomic variation also must be taken into consideration during laryngotracheal replacement or transplantation.

In addition to the cricoid, thyroid, and paired arytenoid cartilages, there are numerous other components of the laryngeal skeleton and the related structures. The superior aspect of the laryngeal skeleton is the hyoid bone, which is usually ossified by age 2. The hyoid bone attaches to the mylohyoid, geniohyoid, and hyoglossus muscles superiorly and inferiorly connects to the thyroid cartilage via the thyrohyoid membrane. This U-shaped bone has an inferiorly located lesser cornu and a superiorly located greater cornu on each side.

The epiglottis is a fibroelastic cartilage that is shaped like a leaf and narrows inferiorly where it becomes the petiole. The petiole attaches to the inner surface of the thyroid cartilage immediately below the thyroid notch by the thyroepiglottic ligament. The superior aspect of the epiglottis faces the base of the tongue anteriorly and the laryngeal inlet posteriorly. The hyo-epiglottic ligament connects the posterior surface of the hyoid bone to the lingual surface of the epiglottis. On its laryngeal surface, the epiglottis contains a protuberance that sometimes obscures view of the anterior commissure. This is the epiglottic tubercle. Perichondrium is less densely adherent to the epiglottic cartilage on the lingual surface than on the laryngeal surface, explaining why epiglottic edema tends to be more prominent in the vallecula than in the laryngeal inlet. However, edema on the lingual surface can push the epiglottis posteriorly, resulting in airway obstruction. The preepiglottic space is formed by the mucosa of the vallecula superiorly, the thyroid cartilage and thyrohyoid membrane anteriorly, and the epiglottis posteriorly and inferiorly. Blood vessels and lymphatic channels course through this space.

There are several cartilages of less functional importance located above the thyroid cartilage. The cartilages of Santorini, or corniculate cartilages, are fibroelastic and are found above the arytenoid cartilages. They help improve the rigidity of the aryepiglottic folds. Like the epiglottis and many other elastic cartilages, they do not ossify. The cuneiform cartilages (cartilages of Wrisberg) also do not ossify, even though they consist of hyaline cartilage. They are located in the aryepiglottic folds and also improve rigidity, helping to direct swallowing toward the piriform sinuses. The triticeal cartilages are located laterally within the thyrohyoid ligaments. These structures are hyaline cartilages and often do ossify (as may the lateral thyrohyoid ligaments themselves). They may easily be mistaken on x-rays for foreign bodies. The lateral thyrohyoid ligaments are actually thickenings of the thyrohyoid membrane. There is also more central thickening called the medial thyrohyoid ligament. The laryngeal vessels and the internal branches of the superior laryngeal nerves enter the thyrohyoid membrane posterior to the lateral thyrohyoid ligaments. The thyrohyoid ligaments and membranes are among the structures that suspend the larynx directly or indirectly from the skull base. The other structures that do so include the stylohyoid ligaments, the thyrohyoid ligaments and membrane, the thyroepiglottic ligaments, the cricothyroid ligaments and membrane, the cricoarytenoid ligaments, and the cricotracheal ligament and membrane.

The arytenoid cartilages are capable of complex motion. Previously, it was believed that the arytenoids rock, glide, and rotate. More accurately, the cartilages are brought together in the midline and revolve over the cricoid. It appears as if individuals use different strategies for approximating the arytenoids, and these strategies may influence a person's susceptibility to laryngeal trauma that can cause vocal process ulcers and laryngeal granulomas.

The larynx contains 2 important, large, paired "membranes," the triangular membranes and the quadrangular membranes (Figure 2–2). The paired triangular membranes form the conus elasticus. Each triangular membrane is attached to the cricoid and thyroid cartilages anteriorly (the base of the triangular membrane), to the cricoid cartilage inferiorly, and to the vocal process of the arytenoid cartilage posteriorly (the apex of the triangular membrane). The superior edge of each fibroelastic triangular membrane is the vocal ligament, forming the intermediate and deep layers of lamina propria of the vocal folds, as discussed below. These structures extend anteriorly to form a portion of Broyles ligament. More anteriorly, a portion of the conus elasticus constitutes the cricothyroid ligament.

Like the upper border of the triangular membrane, the upper and lower borders of the quadrangular membrane are free edges.

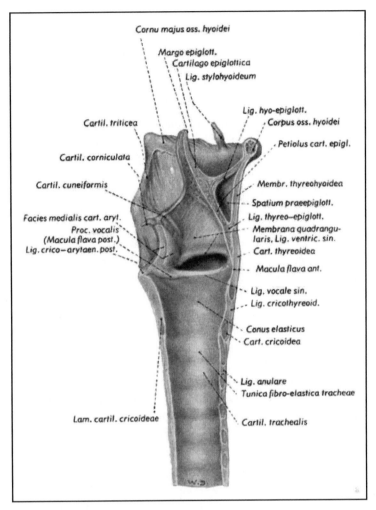

Cornu majus oss. hyoidei

Margo epiglott.
Cartilago epiglottica
Lig. stylohyoideum

Cartil. triticea

Cartil. corniculata

Cartil. cuneiformis

Facies medialis cart. aryt.
Proc. vocalis
(Macula flava post.)
Lig. crico–arytaen. post.

Lig. hyo-epiglott.
Corpus oss. hyoidei

Petiolus cart. epigl.

Membr. thyreohyoidea

Spatium praeepiglott.
Lig. thyreo–epiglott.
Membrana quadrangu-
laris, Lig. ventric. sin.
Cart. thyreoidea

Macula flava ant.

Lig. vocale sin.
Lig. cricothyreoid.

Conus elasticus
Cart. cricoidea

Lig. anulare
Tunica fibro-elastica tracheae

Lam. cartil. cricoideae

Cartil. trachealis

Figure 2–2. Internal view of the larynx illustrating the position of the quadrangular and triangular membranes. (Reproduced with permission from Pernkopf.[1])

The upper border of each quadrangular membrane is the aryepiglottic fold, bilaterally. The lower border extends from the inferior aspect of the epiglottis to the vocal process of the arytenoid cartilages and forms part of the vestibular (or ventricular) fold, or false vocal fold. Superior and inferior thickenings in the quadrangular membrane form the aryepiglottic ligament and the vestibular ligament, respectively. The quadrangular membrane is shorter in vertical height posteriorly than anteriorly. Lateral to these structures is a region called the paraglottic space. It is bounded laterally by the thyroid lamina and medially by the supraglottic mucosa covering the vestibular fold from the ventricle to the aryepiglottic fold. There is a thin, elastic membrane that is contiguous above with the quadrangular membrane and below with the conus elasticus, forming an intermediate segment of elastic tissue that encloses the laryngeal ventricle.

The paraglottic space is contiguous with the space between the cricoid and thyroid cartilages. The laryngeal inlet lies between the aryepiglottic folds.

The region formed by the paired ventricular and aryepiglottic folds is designated as "supraglottis." A pouch of mucosa between the under surface of the false vocal folds and the upper surface of the true vocal folds is called the ventricle of Morgagni, or the laryngeal ventricle. The superior aspect of the laryngeal ventricle is known as the saccule of Hilton. The supraglottis extends from the tip of the epiglottis to the junction between the floor and lateral wall of the laryngeal ventricle. Hence, most clinicians define the floor of the ventricle as part of the glottic larynx. A detailed understanding of the supraglottic larynx is becoming more important clinically because of advances in transoral robotic surgery (TORS), as illustrated by Goyal et al who described anatomic variations in the superior laryngeal neurovascular bundle and differences in anatomic perspective using a robot.[10] The glottic larynx also includes the true vocal folds, anterior commissure, and interarytenoid region at the level of the vocal folds posteriorly (commonly, and incorrectly, referred to as the posterior commissure). The subglottis begins at the junction of squamous and respiratory epithelium under the vibratory margin of the vocal folds, about 5 mm below the beginning of the vibratory margin. The subglottis ends at the inferior border of the cricoid cartilage.

Larynx: Mucosa

With the exception of the vocal folds, the epithelial lining of most of the vocal tract is pseudostratified, ciliated columnar epithelium, typical respiratory epithelium involved in handling mucous secretions. The vibratory margin of the vocal fold is covered with nonkeratinizing, stratified squamous epithelium, better suited than respiratory epithelium to withstand the trauma of vocal fold contact. Vocal fold lubrication is created by cells in several areas. The saccule, the posterior surface of the epiglottis, and the aryepiglottic folds contain seromucinous, tubuloalveolar glands that secrete serous and/or mucinous lubricant. There are also goblet cells within the respiratory epithelium that secrete mucus. These are especially common in the area of the false vocal folds. The goblet cells and glands also secrete glycoproteins, lysozymes, and other materials essential to healthy vocal fold function. The laryngeal mucosa also contains immunologically active Langerhans cells.[11] In most people, secretory glands are not located near the vibratory margin.

The vibratory margin of the vocal folds is much more complicated than simply mucosa overlying muscle. It consists of 5 layers (Figure 2–3).[15] The thin, lubricated epithelium covering the vocal folds forms the area of contact between the vibrating vocal folds and acts somewhat like a capsule, helping to maintain vocal fold shape. The superficial layer of the lamina propria, also known as Reinke space, is composed of loose fibrous components and matrix and lies immediately below the epithelial layer. It contains very few fibroblasts and consists of a network of mucopolysaccharides, hyaluronic acid, and decorin that provide for the flexibility required of the vocal fold cover layer.[16–19] In normal vocal folds the superficial lamina propria also contains fibronectin. Fibronectin is also thought to be deposited as a response to tissue injury.[20] The superficial lamina propria also contains elastin precursors (elaunin and oxytalin), but relatively few mature elastin or collagen fibers. Ordinarily, it has few or no lymphatics, secretory glands, or capillaries. Myo-

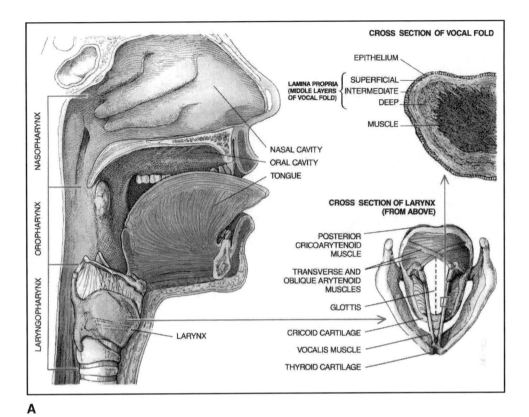

CROSS SECTION OF VOCAL FOLD

EPITHELIUM

LAMINA PROPRIA (MIDDLE LAYERS OF VOCAL FOLD) { SUPERFICIAL / INTERMEDIATE / DEEP

MUSCLE

NASAL CAVITY
ORAL CAVITY
TONGUE

NASOPHARYNX

OROPHARYNX

LARYNGOPHARYNX

CROSS SECTION OF LARYNX (FROM ABOVE)

POSTERIOR CRICOARYTENOID MUSCLE

TRANSVERSE AND OBLIQUE ARYTENOID MUSCLES

GLOTTIS

LARYNX

CRICOID CARTILAGE
VOCALIS MUSCLE
THYROID CARTILAGE

A

Figure 2–3. A. An overview of the larynx and vocal tract, showing the vocal folds, and the region from which the vocal fold was sampled to obtain the cross section showing the layered structure. (Reprinted with permission from Sataloff.[12]) *(continues)*

fibroblasts and macrophages were found in the superficial lamina propria in about one-third of laryngeal specimens studied by Catten et al[19] and were more common in women than in men. The third layer of the vocal folds is the intermediate layer of the lamina propria. Mature elastin fibers make up most of the intermediate layer. They are arranged longitudinally. This layer also contains large quantities of hyaluronic acid, a relatively inflexible space filler that is hydrophilic and is believed to act as a shock absorber.[17] Fibromodulin also is present in the intermediate layer.[18] The deep layer of the lamina propria, the fourth layer, is composed primarily of longitudinally arranged collagenous fibers and is rich in fibroblasts.

De Melo et al analyzed the distribution of collagen in the lamina propria.[21] They described a layer of thick collagen type 1 immediately below the epithelium, and a second, more dense layer superficial to the thyroarytenoid muscle and penetrating between muscle fibers. A layer of collagen type 3 was located between the 2 collagen type 1 layers. The collagen fibers formed an intertwined "wicker basket" network within the lamina propria which helps explain how the vocal fold is able to stretch, despite containing nonstretchable fibers. Interestingly, the authors also noted segmental areas of disarray in the intertwining collagen layers in older patients, suggesting that the variation in histoarchitecture might be related

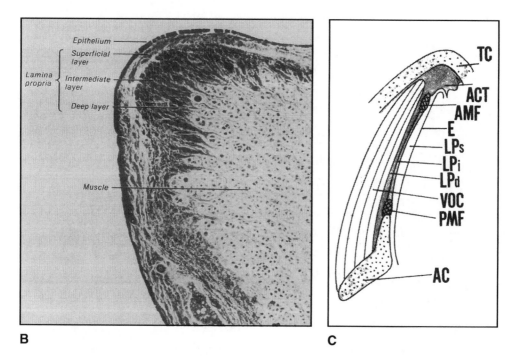

B   **C**

Figure 2–3. *(continued)* **B.** The structure of the vocal fold. (Reprinted with permission from Hirano.[13(p5)]) **C.** Schematic representation of a horizontal section of the vocal fold. TC, thyroid cartilage; ACT, anterior commissure tendon; AMF, anterior macula flava; PMF, posterior macula flava; AC, arytenoid cartilage; E, epithelium; LP, lamina propria; s, superficial layer; i, intermediate layer; d, deep layer; VOC, vocalis muscle. (Reproduced with permission from Gray et al.[14])

to voice changes common among elderly patients. Prades et al reported similar findings and noted that the mean thickness of the superficial layer of lamina propria is about 13% of the total lamina propria.[22] The intermediate layer constitutes about 51%, and the deep layer makes up about 36% of the lamina propria. The TA or vocalis muscle constitutes the body of the vocal fold and is the fifth layer, as well as one of the intrinsic laryngeal muscles. The region that consists of the intermediate and deep layers of the lamina propria is called the vocal ligament and lies immediately below Reinke space. It is important to note that this layered structure of the vocal folds is not present at birth, but rather begins developing at around the age of 7 or 8 years and is not completed until the end of adolescence.[23,24] There are

other differences between the pediatric and adult larynx that are not reviewed in this chapter, but many are discussed elsewhere in this book in connection with relevant clinical entities. A great deal more information is available about the ultrastructure of human vocal folds and may be found in other literature.[25]

Although variations along the length of the membranous vocal fold are important in only a few situations, the surgeon, in particular, should be aware that they exist. The mucosa (epithelium and lamina propria, together) of the normal adult male has been described as being approximately 1.1-mm thick. The superficial layer is about 0.3 mm, the vocal ligament is about 0.8 mm,[26] and the epithelium is about 5 to 25 cells (about 50 microns) in thickness.[27] However, particularly interesting research by Friedrich et al shows additional interesting complexity and variation in the anatomy of the vocal fold.[28] Friedrich et al divided the vocal fold into 5 histological and functional portions. Three of the portions included the musculomembranous vocal fold, and the other 2 regions were divisions of the posterior glottic region and included the region of the vocal process of the arytenoids, which constitutes the cartilaginous portion of the vocal folds and the lateral wall of the posterior glottis. They also found significant differences between men and women in terms of not only absolute measurements, but also relative dimensions of various portions of the vocal fold. In particular, the middle portion of the musculomembranous vocal fold was twice as long in men (8.5 mm) as in women (4.6 mm), accounting for 37% of total glottic length in men and only 29% in women. The authors speculate that this difference in the length of the vibrating portions of the vocal folds may explain why the fundamental frequency ratio between men and women is approximately 1:2, while the overall laryngeal dimensions are only 1:1.5. In addition to variations in length, Friedrich et al also found that the thickness of the lamina propria varied depending on location along the length of the vocal fold and on gender (Figure 2–4). Friedrich's elegant research should be interpreted in the historical context of earlier observations, some of which appear to provide data that are contradictory to his. Actually, the methods of observation and intent of the studies differed; most of the findings in the various studies are reconcilable.

The vocal folds join anteriorly. The area of union is known as the anterior commissure. A "commissure" is a point of coming together. Hence, the term *posterior commissure* has been discouraged, because the vocal folds do not come together in posterior lar-

ynx. However, this terminology has been challenged by Tucker and Tucker,[29] who argue that histologic data showing the posterior union the cricoid cartilage justify the use of the term *posterior commissure*. Their view has not been accepted widely, and most laryngologists still agree with Hirano et al[30] and refer to "the posterior glottis" or "the posterior larynx," rather than the posterior commissure. In 1986, Hirano et al[30] studied the posterior glottis in 20 specimens obtained from autopsy, photographing the larynges from above and below in neutral, adducted, and abducted conditions. They also studied the histology of the posterior glottis in the same 3 conditions. Hirano et al defined the posterior glottis as consisting of 3 portions: the posterior wall of the glottis, the lateral wall of the posterior glottis, and the cartilaginous portion of the vocal fold. They noted that the posterior larynx closes at the supraglottis during vocal fold adduction, rather than at the glottis, thus producing a conical space that can be seen only from below. Using this methodology, they calculated that the posterior glottis accounted for 35% to 45% of the entire glottic length, and 50% to 65% of the entire glottic area. The mucosa covering the posterior glottis consisted of ciliated epithelium, and the lamina propria consisted of only 2 layers. The superficial layer was looser in structure, and the deep layer was composed of dense elastic and collagenous fibers with numerous mucosecretory glands. Many of the fibers in the deep layer ran vertically in the region of the posterior wall of the glottis, but the fibers on the lateral wall were found to run obliquely. This study provided useful, interesting anatomic information. However, in interpreting its physiological significance, it should be remembered that abduction and adduction were accomplished by threads attached to the muscular processes of the arytenoid cartilages; the

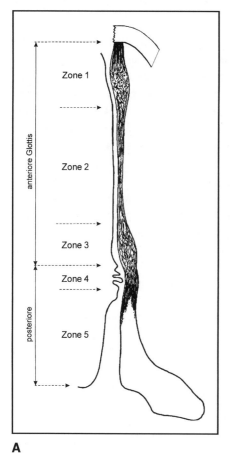

A

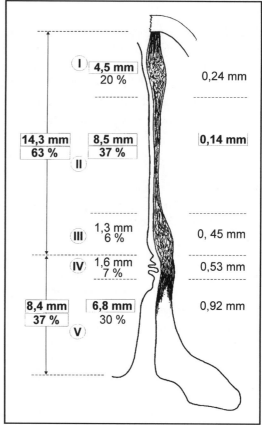

B

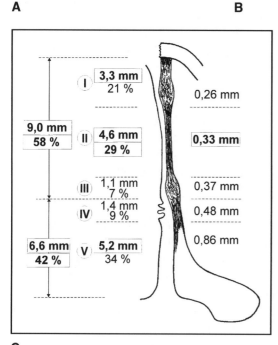

C

Figure 2–4. A. Vocal fold divided into zones. **B.** Proportions of the vocal fold constituted by each zone in men. **C.** Thickness of the lamina propria in millimeters in women. Note that the European numbering system is used in which 0.45 mm is written as 0,45 mm. (Courtesy of Gerhardt Friederich, MD.)

results may or may not be identical to the complex motions that occur during phonation in a living human.[30]

It has long been recognized that particularly striking variations occur at the anterior and posterior portions of the musculomembranous vocal fold, the region between the vocal process and attachment of the vocal fold to the thyroid cartilage.[31] Anteriorly, the intermediate layer of the lamina propria becomes thick, forming an oval mass called the anterior macula flava. This structure is composed of stroma, fibroblasts, and elastic fibers. Anteriorly, the anterior macula flava inserts into the anterior commissure tendon (Broyles ligament). The anterior commissure tendon is a mass of collagenous fibers, which is connected to the midpoint of the thyroid cartilage anteriorly, the anterior macula flava posteriorly, and the deep layer of the lamina propria laterally. As Hirano has pointed out, this arrangement allows the stiffness to change gradually from the pliable musculomembranous vocal fold to the stiffer thyroid cartilage.[31] Sato et al have described stellate cells in the macula flava that are related to fibroblasts, but which appear to constantly synthesize extracellular matrices that are required for normal human vocal fold mucosal function.[32-34] Changes in extracellular matrices alter vocal fold function, particularly viscoelasticity, and these changes are associated with some aspects of vocal aging. Aging changes in the vocal fold stellate cells in the macula flava may be responsible for some of the age-related extracellular matrices alterations.[35-38] Sato also demonstrated that stellate cells of the macula flava were more sensitive to radiation-induced change than many of the other components of vocal folds.[39] These findings suggest that radiation may damage the ability of stellate cells to generate precursors of collagenous and elastic fibers,

indicating that radiation causes changes not only in fiberblasts and other components of the lamina propria, but also in the ability of the stellate cells in the macula flava to maintain normal vocal fold homeostasis. Fuja et al cultured vocal fold stellate cells and demonstrated induced deactivation.[40] Their data suggest that the stellate cells are a potential target for research on the physical elastic properties of vocal fold mucosa during normal phonation, aging, scar, fibrosis, and other conditions.

A similar gradual change in stiffness occurs posteriorly where the intermediate layer of the lamina propria also thickens to form the posterior macula flava, another oval mass that is structurally similar to the anterior macula flava. The posterior macula flava attaches to the vocal process of the arytenoid cartilage through a transitional structure that consists of chondrocytes, fibroblasts, and intermediate cells.[41] Thus, the stiffness progresses from the flexible musculomembranous vocal fold to the slightly stiffer macula flava, to the stiffer transitional structure, to the elastic cartilage of the vocal process, and to the hyalin cartilage of the arytenoid body. It is believed that this gradual change in stiffness serves as a cushion that may protect the vocal folds from mechanical damage caused by contact or vibrations.[41] It may also act as a controlled damper that smooths mechanical changes during vocal fold movements. This arrangement seems particularly well suited to vibration, as are other aspects of the vocal fold architecture. For example, blood vessels in the vocal folds begin posteriorly and anteriorly and run parallel to the vibratory margin, with very few vessels entering the mucosa perpendicular to the free edge of the vibratory margin or from the underlying muscle. Even the elastic and collagenous fibers of the lamina propria run approximately parallel to the vibratory margin, allowing them to compress against each other or pull apart from each other flexibly and parallel with the forces of the mucosal wave. The more one studies the vocal fold, the more one appreciates the beauty of its engineering.

Functionally, the 5 layers have different mechanical properties and are analogous to ball bearings of different sizes that allow the smooth shearing action necessary for proper vocal fold vibration. The posterior two-fifths (approximately) of the vocal folds are cartilaginous, and the anterior three-fifths are musculomembranous (from the vocal process forward) in adults. Under normal circumstances, most of the vibratory function critical to voice quality occurs in the musculomembranous portion.

Mechanically, the vocal fold structures act more like 3 layers consisting of the cover (epithelium and superficial layer of the lamina propria), transition (intermediate and deep layers of the lamina propria), and the body (the vocalis muscles). Understanding this anatomy is important because different pathologic entities occur in different layers and require different approaches to treatment. For example, fibroblasts are responsible for scar formation. Therefore, lesions that occur superficially in the vocal folds (eg, nodules, cysts, and most polyps) should permit treatment without disturbance of the intermediate and deep layers, where fibroblast proliferation, or scar formation, occurs.

In addition to the 5 layers of the vocal fold, there is a complex basement membrane connecting the epithelium to the superficial layer of the lamina propria.[42] The basement membrane is a multilayered, chemically complex structure. It gives rise to type VII collagen loops that encircle type III collagen fibers in the superficial layer of the lamina propria (Figure 2–5). Current research has changed substantially our understanding of vocal fold composition and function. For example, in his description of the basement membrane zone, Gray described a chain link–fence arrangement of anchoring fibers, which he believes permits tissue compression and bending.[16] The density of the anchoring fibers is greatest in the area of greatest vibration and shearing stresses, in the middle of the musculomembranous portion of the vocal folds. Knowledge of the basement membrane has already been important in changing surgical techniques, as discussed later in this book. It also appears important in other matters, such as the ability to heal following trauma, the development of certain kinds of vocal fold pathology, and in histopathologic differential diagnosis.

The vocal folds may be thought of as the oscillators of the vocal mechanism.[43] Above the true vocal folds are tissues known as the "false vocal folds." Unlike the true vocal folds, they do not make contact during normal speaking or singing. However, they may produce voice during certain abnormal circumstances. This phenomenon is called dysphonia plica ventricularis. Until recently, the importance of the false vocal folds during normal phonation was not appreciated. In general, they are considered to be used primarily for forceful laryngeal closure; they come into play during pathological conditions. However, contrary to popular practice, surgeons should recognize that they cannot be removed without affecting phonation. The physics of airflow through the larynx is very complex, involving vortex formation and sophisticated turbulence patterns that are essential to normal phonation. The false vocal folds provide a downstream resistance, which is important in this process, and they probably play a role in vocal tract resonance, as well.

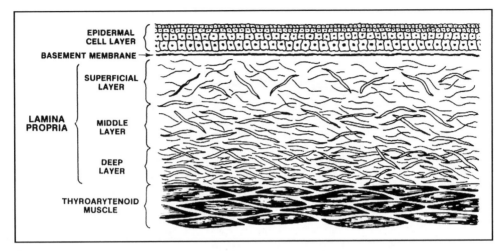

A

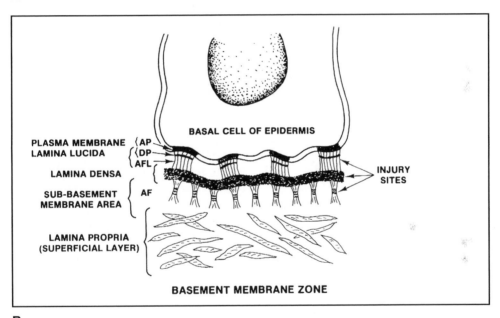

B

Figure 2–5. A. Structure of the vocal fold (not drawn to scale). The basement membrane lies between the epithelium and the superficial layer of the lamina propria. (Reproduced with permission from Gray,[42]) **B.** Basement membrane zone. Basal cells are connected to the lamina densa by attachment plax (AP) in the plasma membrane of the epidermis. Anchoring filaments (AFL) extend from the attachment plax through the subbasal densa plate (DP) and attach to the lamina densa (dark single-layer, electron-dense band just beneath the basal cell layer.) The subbasement membrane zone consists of anchoring fibers (AFs) that attach to the lamina densa and extend into the superficial layer of the lamina propria. Type VII collagen fibers attach to the network of the lamina propria by looping around type III collagen fibers. (Reproduced with permission from Gray.[42]) *(continues)*

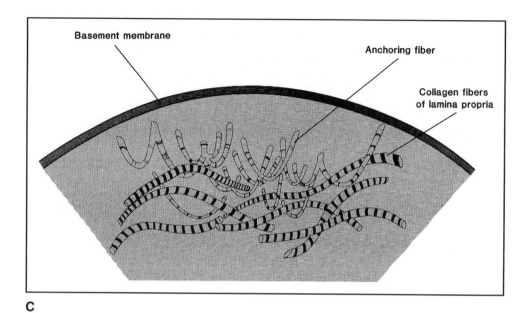

C

Figure 2–5. *(continued)* **C.** Type VII collagen anchoring fibers pass from the basement membrane, reinserting into it. Through the anchoring fiber loops pass type III collagen fibers of the superficial layer of lamina propria. (Courtesy of Steven Gray, MD.)

Laryngeal: Blood Supply and Lymphatic Drainage

The larynx receives its blood supply primarily from the inferior and superior laryngeal arteries and the cricothyroid artery. The superior laryngeal arteries arise from the superior thyroid arteries, which are branches of the external carotid arteries. The superior laryngeal arteries course with the superior laryngeal nerves, piercing the thyrohyoid membrane with the internal branch of the superior laryngeal nerve. The superior laryngeal arteries supply the structures related to the quadrangular membranes and piriform sinuses, primarily above the cricoid cartilage. These include the epiglottis, aryepiglottic fold, thyroarytenoid (TA) muscle, lateral cricoarytenoid (LCA) muscle, interarytenoid (IA) muscle, and vocal fold mucosa. There are anasto-moses with the superior laryngeal artery on the contralateral side and with the inferior laryngeal artery. The cricothyroid (CT) artery also arises from the superior thyroid artery and supplies the CT muscle and membrane, some of the extrinsic laryngeal musculature, and portions of the subglottic pharynx (after penetrating the cricothyroid membrane). The inferior laryngeal arteries arise from the inferior thyroid arteries, branches of the thyrocervical trunk. On the left, the inferior thyroid artery may arise directly from the subclavian artery. The inferior laryngeal arteries travel with the recurrent laryngeal nerves to supply the posterior cricoarytenoid (PCA) muscle, and probably portions of the true vocal fold ventricles and false vocal folds, in some cases. The superior laryngeal veins join the internal jugular veins, and the inferior laryngeal veins empty into the thyrocervical trunks and from there communicate with the subclavian venous system.

The blood supply to the vocal fold mucosa deserves special attention. It is unusual in several ways. The vocal folds contain only small vessels including arterioles, venules, and capillaries. They run parallel to the vibratory margin of the vocal fold, entering from anterior or posterior, and they have frequent arteriovenous anastomoses.[44] This arrangement appears to optimize vessel patency and blood flow even in the presence of the substantial shearing forces encountered during high-pressure phonation. Although Franz and Aharinejad have suggested that there are venous connections between the mucosa and muscle,[44] other authors disagree.[45,46] There appear to be no direct communications between the microvasculature of the superficial lamina propria and the medial belly of the thyroarytenoid (vocalis) muscle. However, Franz and Aharinejad appear to have been correct in suggesting that the serpentine course of subepithelial vessels is engineered to accommodate safely the extreme changes in length and tension that may occur during phonation.[45] The appearance of blood vessels on the superior surfaces of vocal folds may vary in the presence of laryngeal pathology. For example, De Biase and Pontes[47] reviewed 280 videolaryngoscopic images divided into groups of 70 patients each with vocal nodules (VNs), polyps, minimal structural alterations (MSAs) or no abnormalities (control group). Visible superior surface vessels were found in 91.4% of the MSA group, 77.1% of patients with polyps, 44.7% of VN subjects, and 31.4% of controls. Longitudinal and transverse vessels were present in 74.3% and 37.1% (respectively) of the MSA group, 65.7% and 22.9% of subjects with polyps, 34.3% and 12.9% of VN patients, and only 25.7% and 5.7% of controls. Tangled vessels were present

in only the MSA subjects (8.6%). Abrupt changes in vessel caliber and sinuous vessels were found in the subjects with polyps (21.4% and 5.7%, respectively) and MSA subjects (61.4% and 27.1%).

The vessels along the vibratory margin have a different structure than those on the superior surface of the vocal fold or in the TA muscle.[24] For example, capillaries along the vibratory margin are lined by endothelial cells and encircled by pericytes with tight intercellular junctions. The endothelial cells have intermediate-thickness filaments near the cell nucleus and bundles of thick filaments adjacent to the luminal cell membrane.[46] These filaments, together with the lamellate structure of the basement membrane and its interspersed myocytes and pericytes, form a lattice that stabilizes the structure of the microvessels, helping them to tolerate the high shearing forces that can be generated during phonation.[46] This structure enhances mechanical support and helps explain the relative infrequency with which vocal fold hemorrhage occurs, even during forceful phonation. The other vessels of the vocal fold and laryngeal muscles are composed mainly of simple, endothelial-lined capillaries of the continuous (non-fenestrated) variety (the most common type of capillary).[48]

Lymphatic drainage from the larynx occurs through superficial and deep systems, although the deep system is most important. The superficial lymphatic system communicates bilaterally and provides only intramucosal drainage. Each deep system is submucosal and drains its lateral structures. Lymphatic drainage from the larynx courses superiorly and inferiorly. Supraglottic lymphatic vessels travel with the superior laryngeal and superior thyroid vessels to deep cervical lymph nodes (levels II and III) associated with the internal jugular veins. This drainage may be bilateral. There are also lymphatic vessels from the laryngeal ventricles that course through the cricothyroid membrane and thyroid gland en route to the prelaryngeal, prethyroid, supraclavicular, pretracheal, and paratracheal lymph nodes. Inferiorly, lymphatic vessels from the glottic and subglottic larynx form 2 posterolateral pedicles and a middle pedicle. The posterolateral pedicles travel unilaterally with the inferior thyroid artery to the deep lateral cervical (levels III and IV), subclavian, paratracheal, and tracheoesophageal lymph nodes. The middle pedicle courses through the cricothyroid membrane, communicating with pretracheal and delphian nodes, which drain into the deep cervical lymph nodes. There is scant lymphatic drainage from the true vocal folds.

Larynx: Intrinsic Muscles

The intrinsic muscles are responsible for abduction, adduction, and tension of the vocal folds (Figures 2–6 and 2–7). All but one of the muscles on each side of the larynx are innervated by the 2 recurrent (or inferior) laryngeal nerves, which are discussed in detail below. Because these nerves usually run long courses from the neck down into the chest and back up to the larynx (hence, the name "recurrent"), they are easily injured

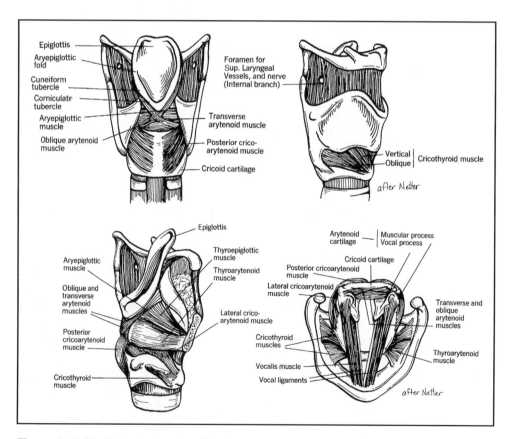

Figure 2–6. The intrinsic muscles of the larynx.

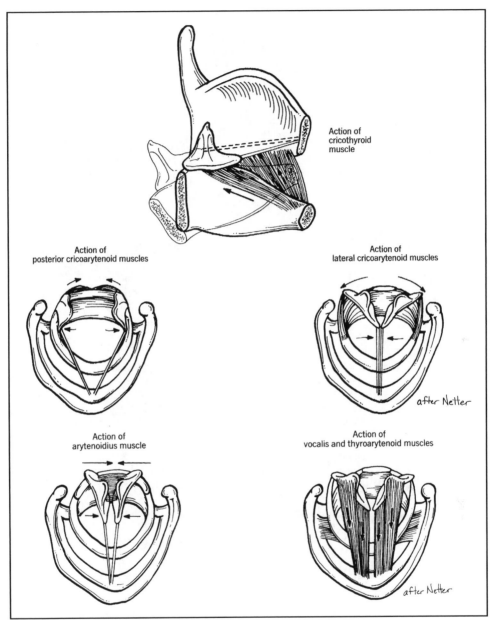

Action of
cricothyroid
muscle

Action of
posterior cricoarytenoid muscles

Action of
lateral cricoarytenoid muscles

after Netter

Action of
arytenoidius muscle

Action of
vocalis and thyroarytenoid muscles

after Netter

A

Figure 2–7. A. Action of the intrinsic muscles. In the bottom 4 figures, the directional arrows suggest muscle actions but may give a misleading impression of arytenoid motion. These drawings should not be misinterpreted as indicating that the arytenoid cartilage rotates around a vertical axis. The angle of the long axis of the cricoid facets does not permit some of the motion implied in this figure. However, the drawing still provides a useful conceptualization of the effect of individual intrinsic muscles, so long as the limitations are recognized. *(continues)*

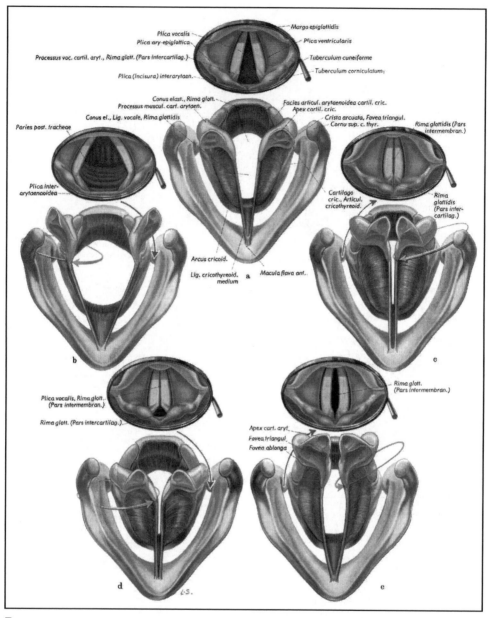

B

Figure 2–7. *(continued)* **B.** The shapes of the glottis as seen on mirror examination and on anatomic preparations during rest (a), inspiration (b), phonation (c), whispering (d), and falsetto singing (e). (Reproduced with permission from Pernkopf.[1])

by trauma, neck surgery, and thoracic surgery. The left recurrent laryngeal nerve is more susceptible to injury during chest surgery because of its course around the aortic arch. The right recurrent laryngeal nerve, however, is more likely to have an oblique course laterally in the neck and thus may be at greater risk for injury in neck surgery.

Such injuries may result in abductor and adductor paralysis of the vocal fold. The remaining muscle, the CT muscle, is innervated by the superior laryngeal nerve on each side, which is especially susceptible to viral and traumatic injury.

For some purposes, including electromyography and surgery, it is important to understand the function of individual laryngeal muscles in detail. The muscles of primary functional importance are those innervated by the recurrent laryngeal nerves including the thyroarytenoid (TA), posterior cricoarytenoid (PCA), lateral cricoarytenoid (LCA), and interarytenoid or arytenoideus (IA), and the superior laryngeal nerves including the cricothyroid (CT) (Figures 2–6, 2–7, and 2–8).

The TA muscle adducts, lowers, shortens, and thickens the vocal folds, thus rounding the vocal fold's edge. Thus, the cover (epithelium and superficial layer of lamina propria) and transition (intermediate and deep layers of lamina propria) are effectively made slacker, while the body is stiffened. Adduction from vocalis muscle (the medial belly of the TA) contraction is active, particularly in the musculomembranous segment of the vocal folds. Contraction of the vocalis muscle tends to lower vocal pitch. The thyroarytenoid originates anteriorly from the posterior (interior) surface of the thyroid cartilage and inserts into the lateral base of the arytenoid cartilage, from the vocal process to the muscular process. More specifically, the superior bundles of the muscle insert into the lateral and inferior aspects of the vocal process and run primarily in a horizontal direction. The anteroinferior bundles insert into the anterolateral aspect of the arytenoid cartilage from its tip to an area lateral to the vocal process. (These fibers are associated primarily with the lateral belly.) The most medial fibers run parallel to the vocal liga-

ment and insert onto the medial aspect of the vocal process. There are also cranial fibers that extend into the aryepiglottic fold. Anteriorly, the vertical organization of the muscle results in a twisted configuration of muscle fibers when the vocal fold is adducted. The neuromuscular organization of the medial belly of the TA muscle is more complex than previously believed. Research by Sanders helped clarify these complexities. He has shown, for example, that muscle groups along the superior and inferior margin of the medial (contact) surface of the vocal folds function differently from one another.[49] The thyroarytenoid is the third largest intrinsic muscle of the larynx. The TA muscle is divided into 2 compartments. The medial compartment is also known as the vocalis muscle. It contains a high percentage of slow-twitch muscle fibers. The lateral compartment has predominantly fast-twitch muscle fibers. One may suspect that the medial compartment (vocalis) is specialized for phonation, whereas the lateral compartment (muscularis) is specialized for vocal fold adduction, but these suppositions are unproven. De Campos et al studied TA muscle in comparison with tongue, because the tongue muscle is considered the most complex structure in the body with regard to movements and muscle fiber orientation.[50] The authors speculated that TA complexities might be correlated with similar muscle structure. They found that both tongue and TA muscle showed the same percentage of transverse (about 72%), undefined (about 15%), and longitudinal (about 10%) fibers. In contrast to these similarities, they found no morphometric correlation comparing the structures of the recurrent laryngeal nerve and the hypoglossal nerve. Studies of TA muscle using myosin antibodies have shown that TA muscle contains unique extrafusal fibers containing tonic myosin, but no muscle spindles.[51]

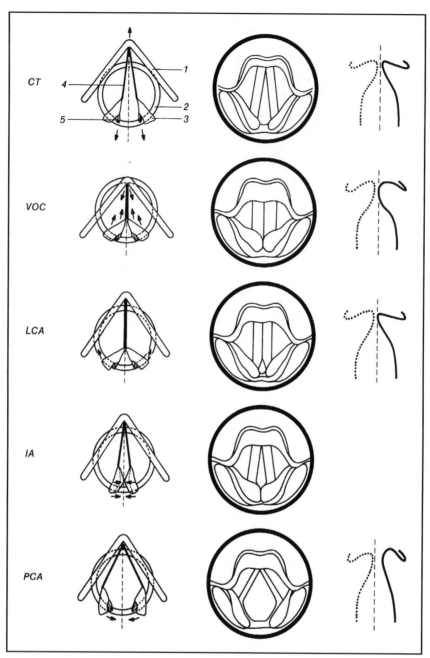

A

Figure 2–8. A. Schematic presentation of the function of the laryngeal muscles. The left column shows the location of the cartilages and the edge of the vocal folds when the laryngeal muscles are activated individually. The arrows indicate the direction of the force exerted. 1, thyroid cartilage; 2, cricoid cartilage; 3, arytenoid cartilage; 4, vocal ligament; 5, posterior cricoarytenoid ligament. The middle column shows the views from above. The right column illustrates contours of frontal sections at the middle of the musculomembranous portion of the vocal fold. The dotted line illustrates the vocal fold position when no muscle is activated. CT, cricothyroid; VOC, vocalis; LCA, lateral cricoarytenoid; IA, interarytenoid; PCA, posterior cricoarytenoid. (Reproduced with permission from Hirano M.[13(p8)]) *(continues)*

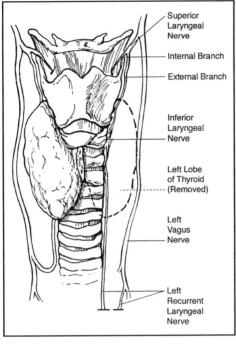

Superior
Laryngeal
Nerve

Internal Branch

External Branch

Inferior
Laryngeal
Nerve

Left Lobe
of Thyroid
(Removed)

Left
Vagus
Nerve

Left
Recurrent
Laryngeal
Nerve

B

Figure 2–8. *(continued)* **B.** The superior and recurrent laryngeal nerve branch from the vagus nerve and enter the larynx.

These findings suggest similarities between thyroarytenoid muscle function and extraocular muscles, both of which perform unloaded (non-weight-bearing) contractions without afferent information from native muscle spindles.

The LCA muscle is a small muscle that adducts, lowers, elongates, and thins the vocal fold. All layers are stiffened, and the vocal fold edge takes on a more angular or sharp contour in response to LCA muscle contraction. It originates on the superior lateral border of the cricoid cartilage and inserts into the anterior lateral surface of the muscular process of the arytenoid. It is an extremely important adductor and is especially important in the initial movement from abduction to adduction. The bilaterally innervated IA muscle (arytenoi-

deus, or interarytenoid muscle, a medium-sized intrinsic muscle) primarily adducts the cartilaginous portion of the vocal folds. It is particularly important in providing medial compression to close the posterior glottis. It has relatively little effect on the stiffness of the musculomembranous portion. The interarytenoid muscle is the only unpaired laryngeal muscle. It is innervated by the recurrent laryngeal nerve and receives fibers from the internal branch of the superior laryngeal nerve (although there is no evidence that the internal branch of the superior laryngeal nerve provides motor innervation to this muscle. The IA muscle consists of transverse and oblique fibers. The transverse fibers originate from the lateral margin of one arytenoid and insert into the lateral margin of the opposite arytenoid. The oblique fibers originate posteriorly and inferiorly from the base of the cricoid cartilage, but they extend around the apex of the arytenoid cartilage to continue as the aryepiglottic musculature.

The PCA muscle abducts, elevates, elongates, and thins the vocal fold by rocking the arytenoid cartilage posterolaterally. All layers are stiffened, and the edge of the vocal fold is rounded during PCA muscle contraction. It is the second largest intrinsic muscle. It originates over a broad area of the posterolateral portion of the cricoid lamina and inserts on the posterior surface of the muscular process of the arytenoid cartilage, forming a short tendon that covers the cranial aspect of the muscular process. Asanau et al studied the PCA.[52] They found 2 separate muscle bellies in all cases. They contained 1, 1-11A, and 11A fibers, but comparing the vertical and horizontal bellies of the PCA revealed differences in the fiber-type composition. They also noted regional differences in both bellies of the PCA. They suggested that the PCA should be considered as a combination of

2 functional subunits differing significantly in muscle fiber-type composition, rather than as a single muscle.

When the superior laryngeal nerves are stimulated, the CT muscles move the vocal folds into the paramedian position. They also lower, stretch, elongate, and thin the vocal folds, stiffening all layers and sharpening the vocal folds' contours. It is the largest intrinsic laryngeal muscle and is largely responsible for longitudinal tension, a very important factor in control of pitch. Contraction of the CT muscles tends to increase vocal pitch through their lengthening effect on the vocal folds. The CT muscle originates from the anterior and lateral portions of the arch of the cricoid cartilage and has 2 bellies. The oblique belly inserts into the posterior half of the thyroid lamina and the anterior portion of the inferior cornu of the thyroid cartilage. The vertical (erect) belly inserts into the inferior border of the anterior aspect of the thyroid lamina.

Intrinsic laryngeal muscles are skeletal muscles. Skeletal muscles are composed primarily of 3 types of fibers. Type I fibers are highly resistant to fatigue, contract slowly, and utilize aerobic (oxidative) metabolism. They have low glycogen levels, high levels of oxidative enzymes, and are relatively smaller in diameter. Fast-contracting type IIB fibers are subdivided into types IIA, IIB, and IIX. The myosin heavy-chain isoform in each fiber type is primarily responsible for determining contraction speed. Only type I, IIA, and IIX fibers are present in humans. Type IIA fibers use principally oxidative metabolism but contain both a high level of oxidative enzymes and glycogen. They contract rapidly but are also fatigue resistant. Type IIB fibers are found in small mammals and are the most fatigable but fastest-contracting fiber types. They also are the largest in diameter. They utilize anaerobic glycolysis primarily and contain a large amount of gly-

cogen but relatively few oxidative enzymes. Human laryngeal muscles generally contain a mixture of type I, IIA, and IIX fibers, with the proportion of each varying from muscle to muscle. The fiber composition of laryngeal muscles differs from that of most larger skeletal muscles. Elsewhere, muscle fiber diameters are fairly constant, ranging between 60 and 80 microns. In laryngeal muscles, there is considerably more variability,[53,54] and fiber diameters vary between 10 and 100 microns, with an average diameter of 40–50 microns. The TA and lateral CT muscles are designed for rapid contraction. Laryngeal muscles have a higher proportion of type IIA fibers than most other muscles, which makes them particularly well suited to rapid contraction with fatigue resistance.[55] In addition, many laryngeal motor units have multiple neural innervations. There appear to be approximately 20 to 30 muscle fibers per motor unit in a human CT muscle,[56] suggesting that the motor unit size of this laryngeal muscle is similar to that of extraocular and facial muscles.[57] In the human TA muscle, 70%–80% of muscle fibers have 2 or more nerve endplates and some fibers have as many as 5 nerve endplates.[58] Only 50% of CT and LCA muscle fibers have multiple endplates, and multiple endplates are even less common in the PCA muscle (5%). It is still not known whether one muscle fiber can be part of more than one motor unit (receive endplates from different motor neurons), or whether all of the endplates on each muscle are associated with the same motor neuron.[55]

Recent research has provided additional interesting observations in laryngeal muscles. Wu et al found that human PCA and TA muscles express 3 types of myosin heavy-chain (MyHC) isoforms, including slow type I, fast type 2A, and fast type 2X.[59] Single-fiber analysis has demonstrated regional differences, and the common occurrence of hybrid fibers.[59] Recent research by Malmgren and coworkers has also demonstrated that laryngeal muscles remain capable of spontaneous regeneration over a lifetime and that the proportion of regenerating fibers (identified immunohistochemically by the presence of the developmental myosin isoforms) increases as the TA muscle ages.[60] Malmgren et al also speculate that the increase in regenerating fibers may be a compensatory response to an age-related increase in muscle fiber injury or death. These new findings are consistent with clinical observations that many "aging changes" of the voice can be reversed through voice therapy.[61]

Larynx: Innervation

The recurrent and superior laryngeal nerves are branches of the 10th cranial nerves, or the vagus nerves, which are the longest of the cranial nerves. The vagus nerves originate from 8 to 10 rootlets in a groove in the brainstem between the olive and inferior cerebellar peduncles, in close association with the origins of the 9th and 11th cranial nerves. The rootlets attach to the medulla oblongata in the brainstem, and course below the cerebellar flocculus, where they unite to form the 10th cranial nerve, which exits the cranium through the jugular foramen with the spinal accessory nerve, the glossopharyngeal nerve, and the jugular vein. The hypoglossal nerve exits the skull through the hypoglossal canal, which is adjacent to the jugular foramen and separated from it by a septum. The first ganglion of the vagus nerve is the jugular ganglion, which is located in the jugular foramen, and is known also as the superior ganglion of the vagus nerve. The nodose ganglion (inferior ganglion) is the second ganglion of the vagus nerve and is located in the neck,

slightly inferior to the jugular foramen. The vagus nerve contains branchial motor fibers, somatic sensory fibers (from the posterior external auditory canal, from skin adjacent to the ear in some people, and from the tympanic membrane and pharynx), special sensory fibers (taste), visceral motor fibers, and visceral afferent fibers (from the upper respiratory tract, esophagus, stomach, pancreas, abdominal viscera, aortic bodies, aortic arch, and heart). Cells for the visceral, special sensory afferent, and somatic sensory afferent fibers originate in the jugular ganglion and the nodose ganglion. Visceral afferent fibers have cell bodies in the inferior vagal ganglion. Their axons ascend to the medulla oblongata, then descend in the tractus solitarius from which they enter the caudal aspect of the nucleus of the tractus solitarius, also called the nucleus solitarius. Sensory afferent fibers from the larynx and pharynx travel with the visceral afferent fibers via the recurrent and superior laryngeal nerves to their cell bodies in the inferior ganglion.

The nucleus ambiguus is the branchial motor nucleus for the external branch of the superior laryngeal nerve, the recurrent laryngeal nerve, and the pharyngeal nerve and its plexus. Bilateral corticobulbar fibers from the motor cortexes descend through the internal capsule to synapse with the nucleus ambiguus. This bilateral innervation is important in maintaining coordinated, voluntary control of the laryngeal muscles. The motor neurons of the CT muscle are situated rostrally in the nucleus ambiguus, just caudal to the nucleus of the facial nerve. More rostrally, the motor neurons of the TA, LCA, and PCA muscles are located in overlapping pools.[62,63] The LCA, TA, and IA motor neurons are located in close association to each other (partially overlapping) and are separate from the CT motor neurons, which are more rostrally co-located with pharyngeal and palatal motor neurons.[64] Davis and Nail[62] have shown that there are larger motor neurons associated with the TA and LCA muscles (fast-acting muscles used to constrict and protect the airway) than with the PCA and CT muscle (slower-acting muscles that dilate the airway for respiration). Many other neuromotor regions of importance to phonation are beyond the scope of this chapter (mouth, tongue, palate, pharynx, chest, abdomen) but should be considered part of the anatomy of the voice.

Premotor neurons, or interneurons, control motor neurons; motor neurons with multiple functions may be controlled by more than 1 premotor neuron. For example, for phonation, the premotor neuron controlling the TA muscle is associated with the nucleus retroambiguus, located caudally in the medulla. However, for swallowing functions, the TA muscle can be driven by premotor neurons elsewhere in the medulla and pons.[65]

The periaqueductal gray (PAG) matter is a central area of particular interest to voice specialists and has been studied elegantly by several investigators, especially Pamela Davis, PhD, in Sydney, Australia. The PAG is a region of gray matter, composed of neuronal cell bodies, surrounding the cerebral aqueduct. It is contiguous with gray matter surrounding the third ventricle in the hypothalamus and thalamus rostrally and with gray matter surrounding the pontine portion of the fourth ventricle caudally. Stimulation of the PAG, or of other regions that stimulate the PAG (such as the hypothalamus),[66] produces vocalization; destruction of the PAG produces mutism.[67-70] The neurons in the PAG form longitudinal columns and are essential to emotional expression.[71] The lateral column of neurons in the PAG is responsible for vocalization, increases in blood pressure and heart rate associated with the fight-or-flight response, alterations in bodily blood flow, and nonopioid analgesia.[72-75] PAG neurons control vocalization by anastomosing with cells in the nucleus retroambiguus, the origin of premotor neurons discussed above. In addition to stimulating motor neurons in the nucleus ambiguus associated with the larynx, the nucleus retroambiguus stimulates motor neurons associated with chewing; movements of the tongue, palate, face, and pharynx; and motor activity in the chest and abdomen.[62] The PAG region receives numerous connections from the cortex,[76] and it may be involved in emotional expression associated with the voice in speech and song. It clearly plays an important role in spontaneous emotional voicing in animals, newborns, and adult humans.[77] The PAG matter is also involved in muscle control during respiration,[72,78,79] a function linked closely with phonation. Interestingly, Davis and coworkers have shown that vocalization activated by the PAG is also associated with laryngeal and vagal afferent input, suggesting that the duration of vocalization is controlled, not just by stimulation of vocalization (including emotional content), but also by the amount of air available in the lungs.[80] Ambalavanar demonstrated that afferents from the internal branch of the superior laryngeal nerve travel to the portions of the PAG involved in vocalization, which may be the pathway associated with coordinating such reflex control.[81] Interestingly, the Lombard effect, which is so important to speakers and singers (the tendency to speak more loudly in the presence of background noise), is also represented in the PAG.[82]

Bandler et al have suggested that the PAG may not activate and deactivate laryngeal, respiratory, and orofacial motoneurons directly, but rather may establish "emotional and vocal readiness," with activation actually being dependent on higher brain structures.[75] They suggest that this may explain why damage to the PAG and/or the anterior cingulate cortex produces mutism, even when other components of the voluntary vocal motor system are intact, and why motor cortex injury does not cause mutism when the lateral PAG remains intact to produce emotional vocalization.

Broca area and the sensory-motor regions of the lateral cerebral cortex are involved in control for vocalization. In 1959, Penfield and Roberts published classic descriptions of the function of the primary motor cortex based on cortical stimulation performed in patients with epilepsy.[83] Vocalization was localized in the lowest portion of the cortical strip. Stimulation of this region produced activity not only in laryngeal muscles, but also in those of the jaw, lips, and tongue. The premotor cortex (Brodmann area 6) is located close to the primary voice motor cortex, as is the supplementary motor region, which is involved in initiation of speech. Adjacent subcortical areas are also important for speech, but their functions are not understood completely. Most axons in the cerebral cortex cross the midline. So, functions such as motor control from the left hemisphere may affect primarily the right side of the body. However, some functions, including those controlled by cranial nerves (ie, facial and laryngeal muscle function), may be ipsilateral and/or contralateral.

Studies utilizing dynamic imaging techniques such as positron emission tomography (PET) have begun to improve our understanding of function in these areas of the brain. Perry et al used PET to study singing.[84] They found hyperperfusion during singing in various areas associated with the motor cortex, including the anterior cingulate cortex, precentral gyri, anterior insula, supplementary motor area, and the cerebellum. The central nervous system specializations that enable processing of acoustically complex voice signals are not understood fully, although it is likely that there are "voice cells" in the brain. Using functional magnetic resonance imaging (fMRI), in 2011 Perrodin et al identified "voice cells" analogous to "face cells" in the brains of monkeys.[85] Unlike face cells, they found that voice clusters contain moderate proportions of voice cells that exhibit high stimulus selectivity. Looking at a broader prospective of the brain's management of speech production, Simonyan and Horwitz published a review of laryngeal motor cortical control during speech and other laryngeal activities.[86] They suggested that the location of the laryngeal motor cortex is in the primary motor cortex and its direct connections with the brainstem laryngeal motor neurons in humans, as opposed to its location in the premotor cortex with only indirect connections to the laryngeal motor neurons in nonhuman primates. They suggested that this major evolutionary development in humans is associated with the human ability to speak and vocalize voluntarily. In addition to dynamic imaging (cerebral blood flow) fMRI studies, a variety of other methods can be used to study neurophysiology of brain function, including neuropsychological testing, dichotic listening, dichaptic touching, split-field tachistoscopic viewing, electroencephalography with evoked potential testing, and other techniques. Some of these approaches have been used to study cerebral dominance and its relationship to musical faculty. It is popularly believed that music and art are associated with the type of thinking performed primarily in the right brain of a right-handed individual, while language is represented primarily by processes in the left brain. At present, it is unclear whether these traditional models are valid; it seems probable that complex interactions involving numerous cortical and subcortical areas of both sides of the brain are involved in complicated activities such as emotional expression through speech or song. In a particularly interesting study, Kleber et al examined the brains of expert opera singers, conservatory-level voice students, and laymen during singing of an Italian aria, using fMRI.[87] The researchers were interested in evaluating effects of motor-skill training. Their experiments revealed that voice training is associated with increased functional activation bilaterally of the primary somatosensory cortex representing articulators in the larynx. There was additional activation in the right primary sensory motor cortex, the inferior parietal lobe, and the dorsolateral prefrontal cortex bilaterally. Expert singers also showed subcortical changes including increased activation in the basal ganglia, thalamus, and cerebellum. Increased vocal training also correlated with increased activity of a cortical network for enhanced kinesthetic motor control and sensory motor guidance, as well as increased involvement of motor memory areas at the cerebellar and subcortical levels. Further research into these observations should provide interesting information that might be applied to voice training, diagnosis, and rehabilitation. Although other areas of the brain are beyond the scope of this chapter, it should be noted that there are many brain activities of interest and importance to voice patients and clinicians. For example, hearing is essential to optimal voice and speech production, so understanding auditory brain function also is important for voice care, as is understanding areas involved in emotion and many other functions.

The superior laryngeal nerve branches off the vagus nerve high in the neck at the inferior end of the nodose ganglion. It travels between the internal and external carotid arteries, dividing into an internal and external branch near the posterior aspect of the hyoid bone. The external branch courses inferiorly with the superior thyroid artery and vein over the constrictor muscle and through the posterior cricothyroid membrane into the larynx (see Figure 2–8B). Chuang et al studied the anatomic positions of the external branch of the superior laryngeal nerve in Chinese adults. They noted that the inferior corner of the thyroid cartilage was a reliable landmark for identifying the external branch but that there were variations in the position of the nerve.[88] Using the Cernea classification,[89] after investigating 86 nerves in 43 cadavers they identified Cernea type 1 position in 16.2% (nerve crossing the superior thyroid vessels more than 1 cm above the horizontal plane passing through the upper border of the superior pole of the thyroid gland), type 2a anatomy in 39.5% (nerve crossing the vessels less than 1 cm above the horizontal plane), and type 2b in 38.3% (nerve crossing the superior thyroid vessels below the horizontal plane). They concluded that 77.8% of the superior laryngeal nerve external branches studied were in positions of high risk for injury during thyroid surgery. These findings are similar to those of other authors.[90,91] The authors recommended identifying the nerve inferiorly at the inferior cornu of the thyroid cartilage and reported a nerve identification rate significantly better than that reported by authors who identify the nerve distally at the inferior constrictor-cricothyroid junction[92] but different from those of Cernea[89] and others.[93–95] While it is possible that there may be racial differences (the Chuang study was performed off Chinese adults), Furlan studied the question and found no statistically significant different between ethnic groups, but they reported variations in the external branches superior laryngeal nerve related to individual stature and thyroid volumes.[94] The external branch supplies the CT muscle. An extension of the external branch may also supply motor and sensory innervation to the vocal folds. Wu et al have identified this extension of the external branch of the superior laryngeal nerve as the human communicating nerve.[96] This neural connection was found in 12 (44%) of 27 specimens. When present, it exited the medial surface of the cricothyroid muscle and entered the lateral surface of the thyroarytenoid muscle. The communicating nerve was composed of an intramuscular branch, which combined with the recurrent laryngeal nerve or terminated within the thyroarytenoid muscle directly, and an extramuscular branch that passed through the thyroarytenoid muscle and terminated in the subglottic mucosa in the region of the cricoarytenoid joint. The communicating nerves contain an average of 2510 myelinated axons, of which 31% were motor neurons. Wu et al believe that when the communicating nerve is present, it supplies a second source of motor innervation to the thyroarytenoid muscle and extensive sensory innervation to the subglottic area and cricoarytenoid joint.

The internal branch of the superior laryngeal nerve is responsible primarily for sensation in the mucosa at and above the level of the vocal fold, but it may be responsible for some motor innervations of laryngeal muscles, as well. The internal branch of the superior laryngeal nerves is divided into 3 divisions.[97] The superior division supplies the mucosa on the laryngeal surface of the epiglottis. The middle division supplies portions of the true vocal folds, false vocal folds, and the aryepiglottic folds. The inferior division supplies the mucosa of the arytenoids, the portion of the subglottis not supplied by the recurrent laryngeal nerve, the upper esophageal sphincter, and the anterior wall of the hypopharynx. The internal branch of the superior laryngeal nerves also supplies the thyroepiglottic and cricoarytenoid joints.

Terminal sensory nuclei also are involved in reflex pathways associated with the reticular formation. The distributions of the sensory nerves within the larynx in humans remain somewhat speculative, being inferred primarily from research performed in cats.[98] Yoshida and coworkers found that the internal branch at the superior laryngeal nerve supplies the ipsilateral side of the epiglottis, aryepiglottic fold, arytenoid eminence, rostral aspect of the vocal fold, vestibule, and mucosa overlying the PCA muscle. The posterior branch of the recurrent laryngeal nerve divides into two branches, one of which goes to Galen anastomosis. The other sensory branch provides bilateral supply with ipsilateral dominance to the caudal aspect of the vocal fold and the subglottic region. Some fibers from the internal branch of the superior laryngeal nerve join with fibers from the posterior branch of the recurrent laryngeal nerve to share innervation of the posterior wall of the glottis and the medial aspect of the arytenoids bilaterally with ipsilateral predominance.[99] The cell bodies of the sensory fibers arise primarily in the nodose ganglion and project to the ipsilateral nucleus solitarius. Special sensory fibers for taste from the epiglottis and the larynx course with the vagus nerve to the tractus solitarius and its nucleus.

The recurrent laryngeal nerves branch off the vagus in the chest. On the left, the nerve usually loops around the aortic arch from anterior to posterior and passes lateral to the ligamentum arteriosum behind the arch to enter the tracheoesophageal groove. Occasionally, the nerve is not "recurrent" and does not loop around the aortic arch. Instead it branches directly off the vagus nerve in the neck and courses directly to the larynx. On the right, it usually loops around the brachiocephalic or subclavian artery. This anatomic relationship is usually, but not always, present; and nonrecurrent recurrent nerves occur, probably in less than 1% of people. Nonrecurrent right "recurrent" laryngeal nerves are seen most commonly when the right subclavian artery arises from the descending aorta. In such cases, the "recurrent" nerve arises in the neck and travels directly to the larynx. The recurrent nerves travel superiorly in the tracheoesophageal grooves, entering the larynx between the esophagus and tracheopharyngeus muscle. As they course toward the larynx, the recurrent nerves give off branches to the heart, esophagus, trachea, pharynx, and larynx. The recurrent nerves run perpendicularly between the first 2 branches of the inferior thyroid artery and are attached closely to the posterior, medial aspect of the thyroid lobe. They enter the larynx coursing just below or under the inferior constrictor muscle and communicate with the ansa Galeni, a connection between the posterior branch of the recurrent laryngeal nerve and the internal branch of the superior laryngeal nerve, which is described in more detail in the next paragraph below. Interestingly, it has been found that the myelinated fibers in the left recurrent laryngeal nerve are larger in diameter than those on the right.[100] This led Malmgren and Gacek to speculate that differences in fiber size may allow the simultaneous activation of laryngeal muscles via faster transmission rates on the left, despite the fact that the right recurrent laryngeal nerve is shorter than the left[101] and thus should otherwise transmit faster causing signal activation sooner. More recently, Jotz et al reexamined the question of histological asymmetry of the RLN.[102] They found that the intraperineural area and perimeter of fibers of the right RLN were statistically

larger than those of the left RLN. They speculated that the morphological differences were related to the different time of arrival of the stimulus to the laryngeal muscles.

Within the larynx, the recurrent laryngeal nerve crosses from posterior to anterior usually at a level slightly below the cricoarytenoid joint. Usually, the recurrent nerve passes approximately 4 to 5 mm posterior to the cricothyroid joint, but in up to about 15% of adults, the nerve may split around the joint, or it may pass anterior to it. These landmarks may be particularly important during surgical procedures in which identification of the cricothyroid joint is necessary. As the recurrent nerve enters the region of the cricothyroid joint, it divides into branches to each of the intrinsic muscles to which it provides motor innervation. It appears that the first branch usually goes to the PCA muscle. This posterior branch also innervates the IA muscles. An anterior branch courses toward the LCA muscle and supplies the TA muscle, as well. Detailed studies of the courses and variations on the terminal branches of the recurrent laryngeal nerves have not yet been published. Research is currently underway to address this deficiency in knowledge, which has become relevant clinically because of surgical procedures such as thyroarytenoid neurectomy. Consequently, the thyroarytenoid branch was studied first.[103] In this study, we determined that the median distance from the inferior tubercle of the thyroid cartilage to the thyroarytenoid branch of the recurrent laryngeal nerve was 3.75 mm. Fifty-four percent of the nerves traveled in a horizontal direction within the larynx, but vertical and oblique orientations were observed. The thyroarytenoid division of the recurrent laryngeal nerve branched in approximately 20% of specimens. From this study, we concluded that surgeons performing thyroarytenoid neurectomy can identify the likely position of the thyroarytenoid nerve by measuring approximately 4 mm from the inferior tubercle along a perpendicular line. In most specimens, the nerve was encountered within 1 to 4 mm from the inferior tubercle. In 2007, the author (RTS) and colleagues performed similar studies on the innervation of the posterior cricoarytenoid muscle, in an effort to explore the practicality of PCA nerve section for abductor spasmodic dysphonia.[104] Microscopic dissection allowed the identification and measurement of the branches from the recurrent laryngeal nerves (RLNs) to the PCA in the 43 human cadaver larynges. The cricothyroid (CT) joint was the primary landmark for measurement. All of the PCA muscles received innervation from the anterior division of the RLN. The number of direct branches from the RLN ranged from 1 to 5 (average 2.3). More than 70% of PCA muscles also received 1–3 branches off of the branch to the interarytenoid (IA) muscle. Less than half of PCA muscles received any kind of nerve branches from the posterior division of the RLN. Branches to the PCA most commonly departed the main RLN in its vertical segment, and all entered the muscle from its deep surface. Branches departed the RLN within an average of 9.5 mm from the CT joint; the branch to the IA occurred distal to this point. The innervation to the PCA is complex and redundant, and the segment of the RLN supplying those branches is difficult to expose safely. For these reasons, selective denervation or reinnervation procedures limited to the PCA nerve branches may be difficult technically. When needing only to denervate the PCA, this can be accomplished by removing a portion of the PCA and the underlying nerve supply, maximizing efforts to avoid injury to the branches to the IA muscle. In addition to motor innervation, the recurrent laryngeal nerves are also responsible for sensory innervation primarily below the level of the true vocal folds, and of the spindles of the intrinsic muscles,[105] although they may supply portions of the vocal folds as noted above. There are interconnections between the superior and recurrent laryngeal nerves, particularly in the region of the IA muscles. The IA muscles are also the only laryngeal muscles that receive bilateral innervation (both recurrent laryngeal nerves).

Sympathetic innervation of the larynx is from the superior cervical ganglion. Parasympathetic innervation from the dorsal motor nucleus travels to the supraglottic larynx with the internal branch of the superior laryngeal nerves and to the subglottic larynx with the recurrent laryngeal nerves. The larynx also contains other important structures not discussed in detail in this chapter, including chemoreceptors, taste buds, and various mechanoreceptors, Meissner corpuscles, free nerve endings, and Merkel cells. The superior and recurrent laryngeal nerves are also connected through the ramus communicans, also called the ansa Galeni or nerve of Galen, which supplies motor innervation to the tracheal and the esophageal mucosa and the smooth muscle of the trachea. It also supplies the chemoreceptors and baroreceptors of the aortic arch. The laryngeal chemoreflex is an interesting phenomenon that produces cardiovascular changes and central apnea in response to chemical stimulation of the larynx.[106,107] The laryngeal chemoreflex may be triggered by stimuli such as gastric acid and can produce responses including laryngeal adduction, bronchoconstriction, hypotension, bradycardia, apnea, and possibly sudden infant death syndrome.[108] Like sudden infant death syndrome, the laryngeal chemoreflex is seen usually only in infants under the age of 1. It differs from the glottic closure reflex in response to swallowing and from laryngospasm, which involves glottic closure without central apnea or cardiovascular changes. There is also a laryngeal reflex that results in glottic closure in response to gentle supraglottic tactile stimulation.

The larynx also contains low-threshold, rapidly adapting proprioceptors and low-threshold slowly adapting proprioceptors. The low-threshold, rapidly adapting proprioceptors are found in laryngeal joint capsules and control laryngeal muscle tone during joint movement (such as during singing or speech). Low-threshold, slowly adapting proprioceptors are found in the laryngeal muscles and help to fine-tune laryngeal muscle tone during activities such as phonation. The laryngeal proprioceptors are associated with 2 interesting polysynaptic reflex arcs that were identified in 1966.[109] When stimulated, the facilitatory reflex arc increases the rate of motor unit firing in the TA and CT muscles. When the inhibitory reflex arch is stimulated, motor unit firing is decreased in the TA, CT, and sternothyroid muscles. Proprioceptors are probably also important in control of laryngeal muscle tone during respiration.[110]

Larynx: Extrinsic Muscles

Extrinsic laryngeal musculature maintains the position of the larynx in the neck. This group of muscles includes primarily the strap muscles. Because raising or lowering the larynx may alter the tension or angle between laryngeal cartilages, thereby changing the resting lengths of the intrinsic muscles, the extrinsic muscles are critical in maintaining a stable laryngeal skeleton that permits effective movement of the delicate intrinsic musculature. In the Western classically trained singer, the extrinsic muscles maintain the larynx in a relatively constant vertical position throughout the pitch range. Such training of the intrinsic musculature

results in vibratory symmetry of the vocal folds, producing regular periodicity of vocal fold vibration. This contributes to what the listener perceives as a "trained" voice.

The extrinsic muscles may be divided into those below the hyoid bone (infrahyoid muscles) and those above the hyoid bone (suprahyoid muscles). The infrahyoid muscles include the thyrohyoid, sternothyroid, sternohyoid, and omohyoid muscles (Figure 2–9). As a group, the infrahyoid muscles are laryngeal depressors. The thyrohyoid muscle originates obliquely from the thyroid lamina and inserts into the lower border of the greater cornu of the hyoid bone. Contraction brings the thyroid cartilage and the hyoid bone closer together, especially anteriorly. The sternothyroid muscle originates from the first costal cartilage and the posterior aspect of the manubrium of the sternum, and it inserts obliquely on the thyroid cartilage. Contraction lowers the thyroid cartilage. The sternohyoid muscle originates from the clavicle and posterior surface of the manubrium of the sternum, inserting into the lower edge of the body of the hyoid bone. Contraction lowers the hyoid bone. The inferior belly of the omohyoid originates from the upper surface of the scapula and inserts into the intermediate tendon of the omohyoid muscle low in the lateral neck. The superior belly originates from the intermediate tendon and inserts into the greater cornu of the hyoid bone. The omohyoid muscle pulls the hyoid bone down, lowering it.

The suprahyoid muscles include the digastric, mylohyoid, geniohyoid, and stylohyoid muscles. As a group, the suprahyoid muscles are laryngeal "elevators." The posterior belly of the digastric muscle originates from the mastoid process of the temporal bone and inserts into the intermediate tendon of the digastric, which connects to the hyoid bone. The anterior belly originates

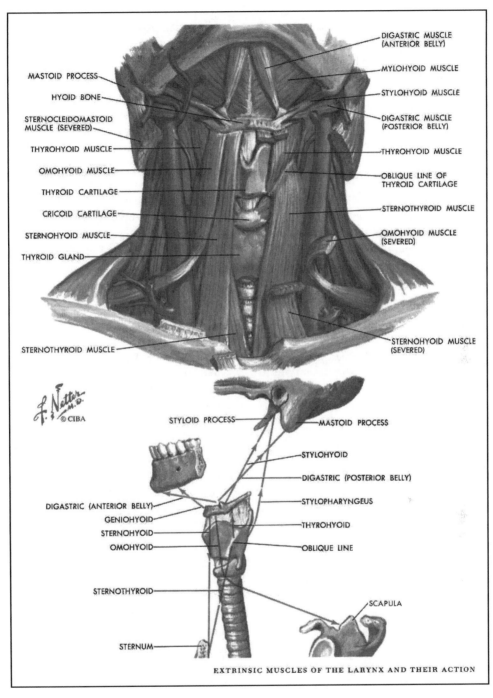

Figure 2–9. Extrinsic muscles of the larynx and their actions. (From *The Larynx. Clinical Symposia.* New Jersey: CIBA Pharmaceutical Company; 1964;16[3]: Plate 4. Copyright 1964. Icon Learning Systems, LLC, a subsidiary of MediMedia USA Inc. Reprinted with permission from Icon Learning Systems, LLC, illustrated by Frank H. Netter, MD. All rights reserved.)

from the inferior aspect of the mandible near the symphysis and inserts into the digastric intermediate tendon. The anterior belly pulls the hyoid bone anteriorly and raises it. The posterior belly pulls the hyoid bone posteriorly and also raises it. The mylohyoid muscle originates from the inner aspect of the body of the mandible (mylohyoid line) and inserts into a midline raphe on the hyoid, connecting with fibers from the opposite side. It raises the hyoid bone and pulls it anteriorly. The geniohyoid muscle originates from the spine at the mental symphysis of the mandible and inserts on the anterior surface of the body of the hyoid bone. It raises the hyoid bone and pulls it anteriorly. The stylohyoid muscle originates from the styloid process and inserts into the body of the hyoid bone. It raises the hyoid bone and pulls it posteriorly. Coordinated interaction among the extrinsic laryngeal muscles is needed to control the vertical position of the larynx, as well as other positions such as laryngeal tilt.

The Supraglottic Vocal Tract

The supraglottic larynx, tongue, lips, palate, pharynx, nasal cavity (see Figure 2–3A), oral cavity, and possibly the sinuses shape the sound quality produced by the vocal folds by acting as resonators. Minor alterations in the configuration of these structures may produce substantial changes in voice quality. The hypernasal speech typically associated with a cleft palate and/or the hyponasal speech characteristic of severe adenoid hypertrophy are obvious. However, mild edema from an upper respiratory tract infection, pharyngeal scarring, or changes in muscle tension produce less obvious sound alterations. These are immediately recognizable to a trained vocalist or astute critic, but they often elude the laryngologist.

The Tracheobronchial Tree, Lungs, Thorax, Abdomen, and Back

The lungs supply a constant stream of air that passes between the vocal folds and provides power for voice production, which is especially important in singing (Figure 2–10). Singers often are thought of as having "big chests." Actually, the primary respiratory difference between trained and untrained singers is not increased total lung capacity, as popularly assumed. Rather, the trained singer learns to use a higher proportion of the air in his or her lungs, thereby decreasing his or her residual volume and increasing respiratory efficiency.[111]

The abdominal musculature is the so-called "support" of the singing voice, although singers generally refer to their support mechanism as their "diaphragm." The function of the diaphragm muscle in singing is complex, and somewhat variable from singer to singer (or actor to actor). The diaphragm primarily generates inspiratory force. Although the abdomen can also perform this function in some situations,[112] it is primarily an expiratory-force generator. Interestingly, the diaphragm is coactivated by some performers during singing and appears to play an important part in the fine regulation of singing.[113] Actually, the anatomy and physiology of support for phonation are quite complicated and not understood completely. Both the lungs and rib cage generate passive expiratory forces under many common circumstances; however, passive inspiratory forces also occur. The active respiratory muscles working in concert with passive forces include the intercostal, abdominal, back, and diaphragm muscles. The principal muscles of inspiration are the diaphragm and external intercostal muscles. Accessory muscles of inspiration include the pectoralis major; pectoralis

The Respiratory System

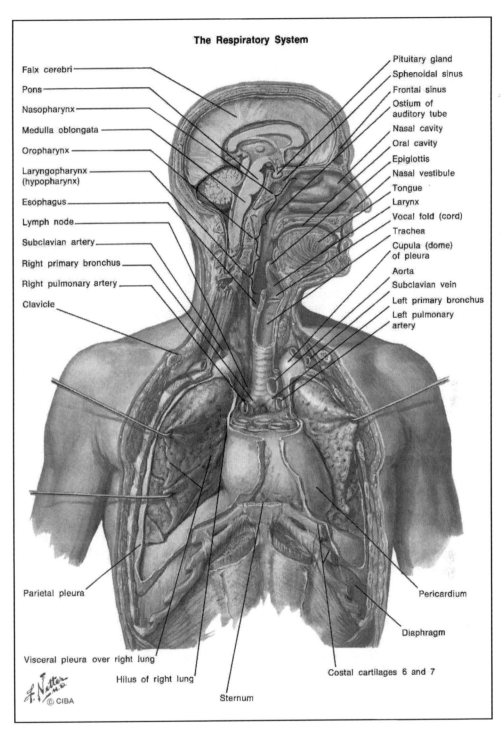

Falx cerebri
Pons
Nasopharynx
Medulla oblongata
Oropharynx
Laryngopharynx (hypopharynx)
Esophagus
Lymph node
Subclavian artery
Right primary bronchus
Right pulmonary artery
Clavicle

Pituitary gland
Sphenoidal sinus
Frontal sinus
Ostium of auditory tube
Nasal cavity
Oral cavity
Epiglottis
Nasal vestibule
Tongue
Larynx
Vocal fold (cord)
Trachea
Cupula (dome) of pleura
Aorta
Subclavian vein
Left primary bronchus
Left pulmonary artery

Parietal pleura

Visceral pleura over right lung
Hilus of right lung
Sternum

Pericardium

Diaphragm

Costal cartilages 6 and 7

Figure 2–10. The respiratory system, showing the relationship of supraglottic structures. The line marking the vocal fold actually stops on the false vocal fold. The level of the true vocal fold is slightly lower. The diaphragm is also visible in relation to the lungs, ribs, and abdomen muscles. (From The Development of the Lower Respiratory System. *Clinical Symposia.* New Jersey: CIBA Pharmaceutical Company; 1975;27[4]: Plate 1. Copyright 1964. Icon Learning Systems, LLC, a subsidiary of MediMedia USA Inc. Reprinted with permission from Icon Learning Systems, LLC, illustrated by Frank H. Netter, MD. All rights reserved.)

47

minor; serratus anterior; subclavius; sterno-cleidomastoid; anterior, medial, and posterior scalenus, serratus posterior and superior; latissimus dorsi; and levatores costarum muscles. During quiet respiration, expiration is largely passive. Many of the muscle used for active expiration (forcing air out of the lungs) are also employed in "support" for singing and acting voice tasks, including abdominal, back, and chest muscles.

Muscles of active expiration either raise the intraabdominal pressure forcing the diaphragm upward or decrease the diameter of the ribs or sternum to decrease the volume dimension of the thorax, or both. They include the internal intercostals, which stiffen the rib interspaces and pull the ribs down; the transversus thoracis, the subcostal muscles, and the serratus posterior inferior muscles, all of which pull the ribs down; and the quadratus lumborum, which depresses the lowest rib. In addition, the latissimus dorsi, which may also act as a muscle of inspiration, is capable of compressing the lower portion of the rib cage and can act as a muscle of expiration as well. The above muscles all participate in active expiration and support. However, the primary muscles of active expiration are the abdominal muscles. They include the external oblique, internal oblique, rectus abdominus, and transversus abdominus muscles. The external oblique is a flat broad muscle located on the side and front of the lower chest and abdomen. Upon contraction, it pulls the lower ribs down and raises the abdominal pressure by displacing abdominal contents inward. It should be noted that this muscle is strengthened by leg lifting and lowering and other exercises but is not developed effectively by traditional trunk curls or sit-ups. Appropriate strengthening exercises of the external oblique muscles are often neglected in voice training. The internal oblique is a flat muscle in the side and

front walls of the abdomen. It lies deep to the external oblique. When contracted, the internal oblique drives the abdominal wall inward and lowers the lower ribs. The rectus abdominis runs parallel to the midline of the abdomen, originating from the xiphoid process of the sternum and the fifth, sixth, and seventh costal (rib) cartilages. It inserts into the pubic bone. It is encased in the fibrous abdominal aponeurosis. Contraction of the rectus abdominis also forces the abdominal contents inward and lowers the sternum and ribs. The transversus abdominis is a broad muscle located under the internal oblique on the side and front of the abdomen. Its fibers run horizontally around the abdomen. Contraction of the transverse abdominis compresses the abdominal contents, elevating intraabdominal pressure. Back (especially lower back) and other muscles (eg, iliocostalis dorsi, iliocostalis lumborum, longissimus dorsi) are also extremely important to power source "support" function, and especially to support for projected speech and singing.

The abdominal and back musculatures receive considerable attention in vocal training. The purpose of support is to maintain an efficient, constant power source and inspiratory-expiratory mechanism. There is disagreement among voice teachers as to the best model for teaching support technique. Some experts describe positioning the abdominal musculature under the rib cage; others advocate distension of the abdomen. Either method may result in vocal problems if used incorrectly, but distending the abdomen (the inverse pressure approach) is especially dangerous, because it tends to focus the singer's muscular effort in a downward and outward direction, which is ineffective. Thus, the singer may exert considerable effort, believing he or she is practicing good support technique, without obtaining the desired effect. Proper abdominal muscle training is essential to good singing and speaking, and the physician must consider abdominal function when evaluating vocal dysfunction.

The Musculoskeletal System

Musculoskeletal conditioning and position throughout the body (posture) affect the vocal mechanism and may produce tension or impairment of function, resulting in voice dysfunction or injury. Stance deviation, such as from standing to supine, produces obvious changes in respiratory function. However, lesser changes, such as distributing one's weight over the calcaneus rather than forward over the metatarsal heads (a more athletic position), alter the configuration of the abdominal and back muscle function enough to influence the voice. Tensing arm and shoulder muscles promote cervical muscle strain, which can adversely affect laryngeal function. Careful control of muscle tension is fundamental to good vocal technique. In fact, some teaching methods use musculoskeletal conditioning and relaxation as the primary focus of voice training.

The Psychoneurological System

The psychological constitution of the singer or professional voice user impacts directly on the vocal mechanism. Psychological phenomena are reflected through the autonomic nervous system, which controls mucosal secretions and other functions critical to voice production. The nervous system is also important for its mediation of fine muscle control. This fact is worthy of emphasis, because minimal voice disturbances may occasionally be the first sign of serious neurologic disease.

Physiology

The physiology of voice production is exceedingly complex and will be summarized only briefly in this chapter. Greater detail may be found elsewhere in this book. For more information, the reader is advised to consult subsequent chapters and other literature, including publications listed in the bibliographies of other chapters and in the Suggested Readings list near the end of this book. Respiratory physiology is included in some detail below.

Overview of Phonatory Physiology

Volitional voice production begins in the cerebral cortex. Complex interactions among the centers for speech, musical, and artistic expression establish the commands for vocalization. The "idea" of the planned vocalization is conveyed to the precentral gyrus in the motor cortex, which transmits another set of instructions to motor nuclei in the brainstem and spinal cord (Figure 2–11). These areas transmit the complicated messages necessary for coordinated activity of the laryngeal, thoracic, and abdominal musculature and of the vocal tract articulators and resonators. Additional refinement of motor activity is provided by the extrapyramidal (cerebral cortex, cerebellum, and basal ganglion) and the autonomic nervous systems. These impulses combine to produce a sound that is transmitted not only to the ears of listeners but also to those of the speaker or singer. Auditory feedback is transmitted from the ear to the cerebral cortex via the brainstem, and adjustments are made to permit the vocalist to match the sound produced with the intended sound. There is also tactile feedback from the throat

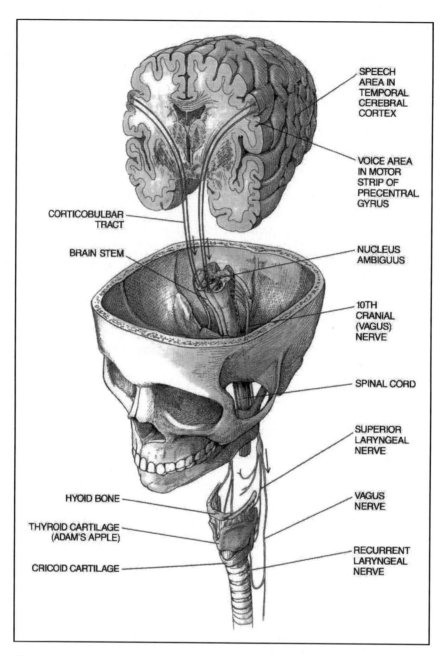

Figure 2–11. How the voice is produced. The production of speech or song, or even just a vocal sound, entails a complex orchestration of mental and physical actions. The idea for making a sound originates in the cerebral cortex of the brain—for example, in the speech area. The movement of the larynx is controlled from the voice area and is transmitted to the larynx by various nerves. As a result, the vocal folds vibrate, generating a buzzing sound. It is the resonation of that sound throughout the area of the vocal tract above the glottis—an area that includes the pharynx, tongue, palate, oral cavity, and nose—that gives the sound the qualities perceived by a listener. Auditory feedback and tactile feedback enable the speaker or singer to achieve fine-tuning of the vocal output. (Reproduced with permission from Sataloff.[12])

and other muscles involved in phonation that undoubtedly help in fine-tuning vocal output, although the mechanism and role of tactile feedback are not fully understood. In many trained singers, the ability to use tactile feedback effectively is cultivated as a result of frequent interference with auditory feedback by ancillary noise in the concert environment (eg, an orchestra or band).

The voice requires interactions among the power source, the oscillator, and the resonator. The power source compresses air and forces it toward the larynx. The vocal folds close and open, permitting small bursts of air to escape between them. Numerous factors affect the sound produced at the glottal level, as discussed in greater detail in a subsequent chapter. Several of these factors include the pressure that builds up below the vocal folds (subglottal pressure), the amount of resistance to opening the glottis (glottal impedance), volume velocity of airflow at the glottis, and supraglottal pressure. The vocal folds do not vibrate like the strings on a violin. Rather, they separate and collide somewhat like buzzing lips.

The number of times they do so in any given second (ie, their frequency) determines the number of air puffs that escape. The frequency of glottal closing and opening is a factor in pitch determination. Other factors affect loudness, such as subglottal pressure, glottal resistance, and amplitude of vocal fold displacement from the midline during each vibratory cycle. The sound created at the vocal fold level is a buzz, similar to the sound produced when blowing between 2 blades of grass. This sound contains a complete set of harmonic partials and is responsible in part for the acoustic characteristics of the voice. However, complex and sophisticated interactions in the supraglottic vocal tract may accentuate or attenuate harmonic partials, acting as resonators (Figure 2–12). This portion of the vocal tract is largely responsible for the beauty and variety of the sound produced.

Interactions among the various components of the vocal tract ultimately are responsible for all the vocal characteristics produced. Many aspects of the voice still lack complete understanding and classification.

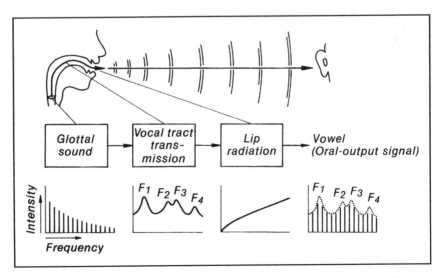

Figure 2–12. Some of the factors determining the spectrum of a vowel. (Reproduced with permission from Hirano.[13(p67)])

Vocal range is reasonably well understood, and broad categories of voice classifications are generally accepted (Figure 2–13). Other characteristics, such as vocal register, are controversial. Registers are expressed as quality changes within an individual voice. From low to high, they may include vocal fry, chest, middle, head voice, falsetto, and whistle, although not everyone agrees that all categories exist. The term *modal register*, used most frequently in speech terms, refers to the voice quality generally used by healthy speakers, as opposed to a low, gravelly vocal fry, or high falsetto.

Vibrato is a rhythmic variation in frequency and intensity. Its exact source remains uncertain, and its desirable characteristics depend on voice range and the type of music sung. It appears most likely that the frequency (pitch) modulations are controlled primarily by intrinsic laryngeal muscles, especially the cricothyroid and adductor muscles. However, extrinsic laryngeal muscles and muscles of the supraglottic vocal tract may also play a role. Intensity (loudness) variations may be caused by variations in subglottal pressure, glottal adjustments that affect subglottal pressure, secondary effects of the frequency variation because of changes in the distance between the fundamental frequency and closest formant, or rhythmic changes in vocal tract shape that cause fluctuations in formant frequencies. When evaluating vibrato, it is helpful to consider the waveform of the vibrato signal, its regularity, extent, and rate. The waveform is usually fairly sinusoidal, but considerable variation may occur. The regularity, or similarity of each vibrato event compared to previous and subsequent vibrato events, is greater in trained singers than in untrained voice users. This regularity appears to be one of the characteristics perceived as a "trained sound." Vibratory extent refers to deviation from the standard

frequency (not intensity variation) and can be less than ±0.1 semitone in some styles of solo and choral singing, such as some Renaissance music. For most well-trained Western operatic singing, the usual vibrato extent at comfortable loudness is ±0.5 to 1 semitone for singers in most voice classifications. Vibrato rate (the number of modulations per second) is generally 5 to 7. Rate may also vary greatly from singer to singer and in the same singer. Vibrato rate can increase with increased emotional content of the material, and rate tends to decrease with older age (although the age at which this change occurs is highly variable). When variations from the central frequency become too wide, a "wobble" in the voice is perceived; this is generally referred to as tremolo. It is not generally considered a good musical sound, and it is unclear whether it is produced by the same mechanisms responsible for normal vibrato. Ongoing research should answer many of the remaining questions.

Respiration

Basic functions of the nose, larynx, and elemental concepts of inspiration and expiration are discussed elsewhere in this book. However, a brief review of selected aspects of pulmonary function is included here to assist readers in understanding the processes that underlie "support," as well as in understanding pulmonary disorders and their assessment.

Starting from the mouth, the respiratory system consists of progressively smaller airway structures. The trachea branches at the carina into mainstem bronchi, which then branch into progressively smaller bronchial passages and terminate in alveoli. Gas exchange (oxygen and carbon dioxide,

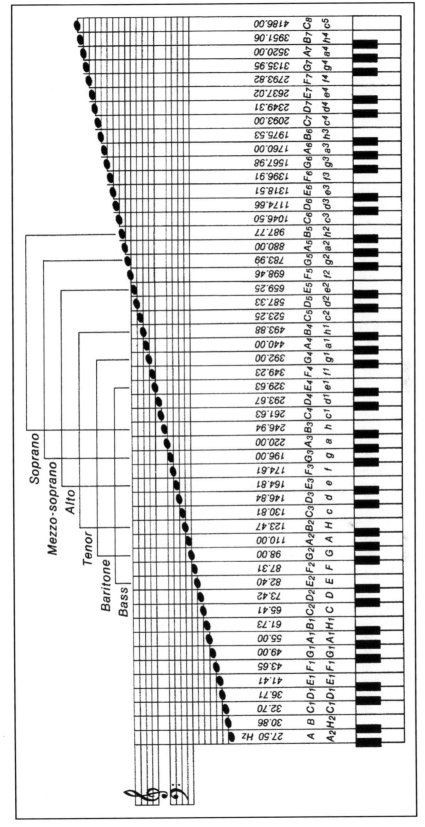

Figure 2–13. Correlation between a piano keyboard, pitch names (the lower in capital letters is used in music and voice research, and in this book), frequency, musical notation, and usual voice range. (Reproduced with permission from Hirano.[13(p89)])

primarily) between the lungs and the bloodstream occurs at the alveolar level. Air moves in and out of the alveoli in order to permit this exchange of gases. Air is forced out of the alveoli to create the airstream through which phonation is produced. Hence, ultimately alveolar pressure is the primary power source for phonation and is responsible for the creation of the subglottal pressure involved in vocal fold opening and closing. Alveolar pressure is actually greater than subglottal pressure during phonation and expiration, because some pressure is lost due to airway resistance between alveoli and the larynx. As the air passes the alveoli, it enters first the bronchioles, which are small, collapsible airways surrounded by smooth muscle but devoid of cartilage. From the bronchioles, air passes to progressively larger components of the bronchial tree and eventually to the trachea. These structures are supported by cartilage and are not fully collapsible, but they are compressible and respond to changes in external pressure during expiration and inspiration. During expiration, the pressure in the respiratory system is greatest in the alveolus (alveolar pressure) and least at the opening of the mouth where pressure is theoretically equal to atmospheric pressure. Thus, theoretically, all pressure is dissipated between the alveolus and the mouth during expiration due to airway resistance between these structures. Expiration pressure is the total of the elastic recoil combined with active forces created by muscular compression of the airway. The active pressure is distributed throughout all the components of the airway, although it may exert greater effect on the alveoli and bronchioles because they are fully collapsible. When the airway is opened, the air pressure in the alveoli (alveolar pressure) is equal to the atmospheric pressure in the room. In order to fill the alveoli, the alveolar pressure must be decreased to less than

atmosphere pressure, creating a vacuum, which sucks air into the lungs. In order to breathe out, alveolar pressure must be greater than atmospheric pressure. As discussed above, there are passive and active forces operative during the inspiratory/expiratory process.

To clarify the mechanisms involved, the alveoli may be thought of as tiny balloons. If a balloon is filled with air, and the filling spout is opened, the elastic properties of the balloon will allow most of the air to rush out. This is analogous to passive expiration, which relies on the elastic properties of the respiratory system. Alternatively, we may wrap our hands around the balloon and squeeze the air out. This may allow us to get the air out faster and more forcefully, and it will allow us to get more of the air out of the balloon than is expelled through the passive process alone. This is analogous to active expiration, which involves the abdominal, chest, and back muscles. If we partially pinch the filling spout of the balloon, air comes out more slowly because the outflow tract is partially blocked. The air also tends to whistle as it exits the balloon. This is analogous to obstructive pulmonary disease, and its commonly associated wheeze. If we try to blow up the balloon while our hands are wrapped around it, the balloon is more difficult to inflate and cannot be inflated fully, because it is restricted physically by our hands. This is somewhat analogous to restrictive lung disease. Under these circumstances, it may also take more pressure to fill the balloon, because the filling process must overcome the restricting forces. Under any of these circumstances, the more we fill the alveolar "balloon," the greater the pressure, as long as the balloon is not ruptured. When the pressure is greater, the increased elastic recoil results in more rapid and forceful air escape when the air is released. The pressure inside the balloon can be increased even above its maximal elastic recoil level simply by squeezing the outside of the balloon. This analogy is helpful in understanding the forces involved in breathing (especially expiration) and in generating support for phonation.

Although inspiration is extremely important, this discussion will concentrate primarily on expiration, which is linked so closely to "support" for speech and singing. The elastic component of expiratory pressure (specifically, alveolar pressure) depends on lung volume and the elastic forces exerted by the chest and the lungs. The lung is never totally deflated. At rest, it is inflated to about 40% of total lung capacity (TLC). The amount of air in the lungs at rest is the functional residual capacity (FRC). At FRC, the thorax is at a volume much less than its rest (or a neutral) posture, which is actually closer to 75% of TLC. Hence, at FRC the thorax has a passive tendency to expand, as happens during inspiration. Conversely, at FRC the lung is greater than its neutral position and would collapse if it were not acted upon by other forces. The collapsing elastic forces of the lung are balanced by the expanding elastic forces of the thorax. The lung and thorax interact closely, and their relative positions of contact vary constantly. This is facilitated by the anatomy of the boundary zone. The inner surface of the thorax is covered by a membrane called the parietal pleura, and the lung is covered by a similar membrane called the visceral pleura. A thin layer of pleural fluid exists between them. Hydrostatic forces hold these surfaces together while allowing them to slide freely. Under pathologic circumstances (eg, following surgery or radiation) these surfaces may stick together, impairing lung function and affecting support for phonation adversely.

Thoracic and lung elastic behavior can be measured. The basic principle for doing so involves applying pressure and noting the volume changes caused by the pressure. This creates a pressure/volume (P/V) curve. The slope with the P/V curve for the thorax reflects its compliance (cCW), and the slope of the P/V curve for the lung represents its compliance (CL). When pressure is applied to the entire system, a difference P/V curve is created and its slope reflects the compliance of the entire respiratory system (CRS). Starting from FRC, if air is expelled the volume of the system is dropped below FRC, and an expanding force is created. It is increased as the volume decreases. Conversely, during inspiration above FRC, collapsing forces increase with increasing volume.

To phonate, we inspire, increasing volumes well above FRC. If we wish simply to expire, we relax and the passive elastic recoil forces air out of the alveoli, because inflating them has created an alveolar pressure that is greater than atmospheric pressure (and is predictable using the pressure-volume curve). The deeper the inspiration, the greater is the elastic recoil, hence the greater the expiratory air pressure. Inspiration from FRC is an active process, primarily. Thoracic muscles elevate the ribs and increase the diameter of the thorax. The external intercostal muscles are important to this process. Inspiration also involves contraction of the diaphragm muscle, which flattens and also increases thoracic volume, and accessory muscles discussed above.

Expiration is created by forces that decrease thoracic volume. If the entire thoracic and pulmonary complex is thought of as a balloon, this process is easy to understand. If one wishes to increase the pressure in a balloon to force the air out, one simply squeezes the balloon. When the container (balloon or thorax) containing a volume of gas (air) is decreased, the pressure in the gas increases. Expiration is achieved by muscles that pull the ribs down or compress the abdominal contents and push them up, making the volume of the thorax smaller. The principal muscles involved are the internal intercostal muscles, which decrease intercostal space and pull the ribs down, abdominal, back, and other muscles, as reviewed earlier in this chapter.

For projected phonations such as singing or acting, support involves (essentially, is) active expiration. After inspiration, elastic recoil and external forces created by expiratory muscles determine alveolar pressure, which is substantially greater than atmospheric pressure. The combination of passive (elastic) and active (muscular) forces pushes air out against airway resistance. As the pressure decreases on the path from alveolar (maximal to mouth atmospheric) pressure, there is a point at which the pressure inside the airway equals the active expiratory pressure (without the elastic recoil component), which is called the *equal pressure point* (EPP). As expiration continues toward the mouth, pressure drops below the EPP. As airway pressure diminishes below the active expiratory pressure, the airways begin to collapse. This physiologic collapse of the airways increases airway resistance by decreasing the diameter of the airways. The greater the active expiratory forces, the greater is the airway compression after the EPP has been passed. Expiratory pressure and airway compression are important to the control of expiratory airflow rate and are influenced by EPP.

Under normal circumstances, the EPP is reached in the cartilaginous airways, which do not collapse completely ordinarily, even during very forceful expiration or phonation. This is part of the physiological mechanism that allows us to continue to sing even as we are running out of air. However, under pathologic circumstance, the location of the EPP may be shifted. Asthma is the classic example. During bronchospasm or bronchoconstriction, the diameter of the

bronchioles is narrowed by smooth muscle contraction, and airway resistance in the bronchioles is increased. Hence, as the air moves from the alveoli into the bronchioles, airway pressure diminishes much more quickly than normal, and EPP may be reached closer to the alveoli and bronchioles, in smaller airways that collapse more easily and more completely. In severe circumstances, the distal airways may collapse fully causing hyperinflation of the lungs and trapping air in the alveoli. Expiratory airflow rate is lowered substantially by the increased resistance in the distal airways, resulting in a lower-than-normal subglottic pressure. This can have profoundly adverse effects on phonation.

Other lung dysfunction also can impair subglottal pressure even if airway resistance is normal. The classic example is emphysema, which occurs commonly in smokers. This condition results in damage to the alveoli. Consequently, because elastic recoil pressures are lower, alveolar pressure is decreased compared to normal. Even if the active expiratory forces are normal, if passive (elastic) expiratory forces are decreased, the normal airway resistance acting against diminished alveolar pressure will shift the EPP distally toward or into collapsible airways. Even when active expiratory efforts are increased under these circumstances, they do not help because they collapse the distal airways trapping air in the alveoli, and diminishing subglottal pressure.

Although this overview is oversimplified and highlights only some of the more important components of lower respiratory physiology, it is important for laryngologists to bear these principles in mind in order to understand the importance of diagnosis and treatment of respiratory dysfunction in voice professionals. In patients with Olympic voice demands, even slight changes from optimal physiology may have profound consequences on phonatory function, and they are responsible commonly for compensatory efforts that are diagnosed (correctly) as hyperfunctional voice use (muscle tension dysphonia). If we treat voice hyperfunction as if it were the primary problem, failing to recognize that it is secondary to an underlying, organic, pulmonary disorder, then treatment will not be successful in the long term, and preventable voice dysfunction and vocal fold injury may ensue.

Other Considerations

In addition to the obvious clinical implications of a thorough understanding of laryngeal anatomy, newer technology offers interesting potential for study and teaching of laryngeal anatomy. For example, Hunter and Titze[114] presented an elegant report on more than 1500 measurements from 37 subjects. They suggested that, using a database of individual subject laryngeal dimensions, it should be possible to design a laryngeal model that could be changed from one subject to the next, predicting subject-specific laryngeal function. They also speculated that such work could lead to computer modeling of patient-specific laryngeal disorders and prediction of therapeutic outcomes. Although this elegant research was published more than a decade ago, its potential has not been realized, yet.

Newer technologies also have been applied to teaching laryngeal anatomy. The time-honored method of teaching human anatomy is through cadaver dissection; however, this traditional method has fallen out of favor in contemporary medical school curricula in the United States,[115] United Kingdom,[116] Australia,[117] and Holland.[118] Computer-aided instruction has risen in popularity, and the Association of American Medical Colleges (AAMC) recognizes the ubiquitous nature of these new educational technologies as being mainstream and integral to the medical school curriculum.[119] Hu et al has created a 3-dimensional, educational computer model of the larynx to teach laryngeal anatomy to medical students and residents.[120] Cadaveric necks were imaged with computed tomography and magnetic resonance imaging, and segmentation software was used to render the 3-dimensional images. This computer program has been received warmly by students.[120] Prospective randomized controlled trials have shown that this computer program is as efficacious as standard written lecture notes in teaching laryngeal anatomy.[121–123]

Conclusion

This chapter and those that follow provide only enough information on the terminology, components, and workings of the voice to permit an understanding of practical, everyday clinical problems and their solutions. The otolaryngologist, speech-language pathologist, singing or acting teacher, singer, actor, or other voice professional would benefit greatly from more extensive study of voice science.

Acknowledgment. The author is grateful to Mary Hawkshaw for her assistance in reviewing this chapter.

References

1. Pernkopf E. *Atlas of Topographical and Applied Human Anatomy.* Munich, Germany: Urban & Schwarzenberg; 1963.
2. Hatley W, Samuel E, Evison G. The pattern of ossification in the laryngeal cartilages:

a radiological study. *Br J Radiol.* 1965;38: 585–591.

3. Hamdan AL, Husseini ST, Halawi A, Sibai A. Arytenoid asymmetry in relation to vocal symptoms in singers. *J Voice.* 2011; 25(2):241–244.

4. Husseini ST, Ashkar J, Halawi A, Sibai A, Hamdan AL. Arytenoid asymmetry in relation to posture, neck tension and glottal attack in singers. *J Voice.* 2011;63(5): 264–268.

5. Bonilha HS, O'Sields M, Gerlach TT, Deliyski DD. Arytenoid adduction asymmetries in persons with and without voice disorders. *Logoped Phoniatr Vocol.* 2009; 34(3):128–134.

6. Adams J, Gross N, Riddle S, Andersen P, Cohen JI. An external landmark for the anterior commissure. *Laryngoscope.* 1999; 109:1134–1136.

7. Storck C, Gehrer R, Fischer C, et al. The role of the cricothyroid joint anatomy in cricothyroid approximation surgery. *J Voice.* 2011;25(5):632–637.

8. Randestad Å, Lindholm CE, Fabian P. Dimensions of the cricoid cartilage and the trachea. *Laryngoscope.* 2000;110:1957–1961.

9. Jotz GP, Stefani MA, Pereira da Costa Filho O, Malysz T, Soster PR, Leão HZ. A morphometric study of the larynx. *J Voice.* 2014;28(6):668–672.

10. Goyal N, Yoo F, Setabutr D, Goldenberg D. Surgical anatomy of the supraglottic larynx using the da Vinci robot. *Head Neck.* 2014;36(8):1126–1131.

11. Thompson AC, Griffin NR. Langerhan cells in normal and pathological vocal cord mucosa. *Acta Otolaryngol* (Stockh). 1995; 115:830–832.

12. Sataloff RT. The human voice. *Sci Am.* 1992;267:108–115.

13. Hirano M. *Clinical Examination of Voice.* New York, NY: Springer-Verlag; 1981.

14. Gray S, Hirano M, Sato K. Molecular and cellular structure of vocal fold tissue. In: Titze IR, ed. *Vocal Fold Physiology.* San Diego, CA: Singular Publishing Group; 1993:4.

15. Hirano M. Structure and vibratory pattern of the vocal folds. In: Sawashima M, Cooper FS, eds. *Dynamic Aspects of the Speech Production.* Tokyo, Japan: University of Tokyo Press; 1977:13–27.

16. Gray SD, Pignatari SS, Harding P. Morphologic ultrastructure of anchoring fibers in normal vocal fold basement zone. *J Voice.* 1994;8:48–52.

17. Hammond TH, Zhou R, Hammond EH, Pawlak A, Gray SD. The intermediate layer: a morphologic study of the elastin and hyaluronic acid constituents of normal vocal folds. *J Voice.* 1997;11:59–66.

18. Hammond TH, Gray SD, Butler J, Zhou R, Hamond E. Age and gender-related elastin distribution changes in human vocal folds. *Otolaryngol Head Neck Surg.* 1998; 119:314–322.

19. Catten M, Gray SD, Hammond TH, Zhou R, Hammond E. Analysis of cellular location and concentration in vocal fold lamina propria. *Otolaryngol Head Neck Surg.* 1998; 118:663–667.

20. Gray SD, Hammond E, Hanson DF. Benign pathologic responses of the larynx. *Ann Otol Rhinol Laryngol.* 1995;104:13–18.

21. Madruga de Melo EC, Lemos M, Aragão Ximenes Filho J, Sennes LU, Nascimento Saldiva PH, Tsuji DH. Distribution of collagen in the lamina propria of the human vocal fold. *Laryngoscope.* 2003;113(12): 2187–2191.

22. Prades JM, Dumollard JM, Duband S, et al. Lamina propria of the human vocal fold: histomorphometric study of collagen fibers. *Surg Radiol Anat.* 2010;32(4):377–382.

23. Hirano M, Kurita S, Nakashima T. Growth, development of aging of human vocal folds. In: Bless DM, Abbs JH, eds. *Vocal Fold Physiology.* San Diego, CA: College Hill Press; 1983:22–43.

24. Hirano M, Nakashima T. Vascular network of the vocal fold. In: Stevens KN, Hirano M, eds. *Vocal Fold Physiology.* Tokyo, Japan: University of Tokyo Press; 1981:45–59.

25. Sato K. Functional fine structures of human vocal fold mucosa. In: Rubin JS,

Sataloff RT, Korovin G, eds. *Diagnosis and Treatment of Voice Disorders.* 2nd ed. Albany, NY: Singular Thomson Learning; 2003:41–48.

26. Kurita S, Nagata K, Hirano M. Comparative histology of mammalian vocal folds. In: Kirchner JA, ed. *Vocal Fold Histopathology: A Symposium.* San Diego, CA: College Hill Press; 1986:1–10.

27. Stiblar-Martincic D. Histology of laryngeal mucosa. *Acta Otolaryngol Suppl* (Stockh). 1997;527:138–141.

28. Friedrich G, Kainz J, Freidl W. Zur funktionellen Struktur der menschlichen Stimmlippe. *Laryngorhinootologie.* 1993;72(5):215–224.

29. Tucker JA, Tucker ST. Posterior commissure of the human larynx revisited. *J Voice.* 2010;24(3):252–259.

30. Hirano M, Kurita S, Kiyokawa K, Kiminori S. Posterior glottis. Morphological study in excised human larynges. *Ann Otol Rhinol Laryngol.* 1986;95:576–581.

31. Hirano M. Surgical anatomy and physiology of the vocal folds. In: Gould WJ, Sataloff RT, Spiegel JR, eds. *Voice Surgery.* St. Louis, MO: Mosby; 1993:135–258.

32. Sato K, Hirano M, Nakashima T. Stellate cells in the human vocal fold. *Ann Otol Rhinol Laryngol.* 2001;110:319–325.

33. Sato K, Hirano M, Nakashima T. Vitamin A—storing stellate cells in the human vocal fold. *Acta Otolaryngol.* 2003;123:106–110.

34. Sato K, Hirano M, Nakashima T. 3D structure of the macula flava in the human vocal fold. *Acta Otolaryngol.* 2003;123:269–273.

35. Sato K, Hirano M, Nakashima T. Age-related changes of collagenous fibers in the human vocal fold mucosa. *Ann Otol Rhinol Laryngol.* 2003;111:15–20.

36. Sato K, Hirano M. Age-related changes of elastic fibers in the superficial layer of the lamina propria of the vocal folds. *Ann Otol Rhinol Laryngol.* 1997;106:44–48.

37. Hirano M, Kurita S, Sakaguchi S. Ageing of the vibratory tissue of the human vocal folds. *Acta Otolaryngol* (Stockh). 1989;107:428–433.

38. Sato K, Sakaguchi S, Kurita S, Hirano M. A morphological study of aged larynges. *Larynx Jpn.* 1992;4:84–94.

39. Sato K, Shirouzu H, Nakashima T. Irradiated macula flava in the human vocal fold mucosa. *Am J Otolaryngol.* 2008;29(5):312–318.

40. Fuja TJ, Probst-Fuja MN, Titze IR. Transdifferentiation of vocal-fold stellate cells and all-trans retinol-induced deactivation. *Cell Tissue Res.* 2005;322(3):417–424.

41. Hirano M, Yoshida T, Kurita S, et al. Anatomy and behavior of the vocal process. In: Baer T, Sasaki C, Harris K, eds. *Laryngeal Function in Phonation and Respiration.* Boston, MA: College-Hill Press; 1987:1–13.

42. Gray S. Basement membrane zone injury in vocal nodules. In: Gauffin J, Hammarberg B, eds. *Vocal Fold Physiology: Acoustic, Perceptual and Physiologic Aspects of Voice Mechanics.* San Diego, CA: Singular Publishing Group; 1991:21–27.

43. Sundberg J. The acoustics of the singing voice. *Sci Am.* 1977;236(3):82–91.

44. Franz P, Aharinejad S. The microvascular of the larynx: a scanning electron microscopy study. *Scanning Microsc.* 1994;5:257–263.

45. Nakai Y, Masutani H, Moriguchi M, Matsunaga K, Sugita M. Microvascular structure of the larynx. *Acta Otolaryngol Suppl* (Stockh). 1991;486:254–263.

46. Hochman I, Sataloff RT, Hillman RE, Zeitels SM. Ectasias and varices of the vocal fold: clearing the striking zone. *Ann Otol Rhinol Laryngol.* 1999;108:10–16.

47. De Biase NG, Pontes PA. Blood vessels of vocal folds: a videolaryngoscopic study. *Arch Otolaryngol Head Neck Surg.* 2008;134(7):720–724.

48. Frenzel H, Kleinsasser O. Ultrastructural study on the small blood vessels of human vocal cords. *Arch Otorhinolaryngol.* 1982;236:147–160.

49. Sanders I. Microanatomy of the vocal fold musculature. In: Rubin JS, Sataloff RT, Korovin GS, eds. *Diagnosis and Treatment of Voice Disorders.* 2nd ed. Albany, NY: Delmar Thomson Learning; 2003:49–68.

50. de Campos D, do Nascimento PS, Ellwanger JH, et al. Histological organization is similar in human vocal muscle and tongue—a study of muscles and nerves. *J Voice*. 2012;26(6):811,e19–26.

51. Brandon CA, Rosen C, Georgelis G, Horton MJ, Mooney MP, Sciote JJ. Staining of human thyroarytenoid muscle with myosin antibodies reveals some unique extrafusal fibers, but no muscle spindles. *J Voice*. 2003;17(2):245–254.

52. Asanau A, Timoshenko AP, Prades JM, Galusca B, Martin C, Féasson L. Posterior cricoarytenoid bellies: relationship between their function and histology. *J Voice*. 2011;25(2):e67–73.

53. Brooke MH, Engle WK. The histographic analysis of human muscle biopsies with regard to fibre types. 1. Adult male and female. *Neurology*. 1969;19:221–233.

54. Sadeh M, Kronenberg J, Gaton E. Histochemistry of human laryngeal muscles. *Cell Mol Biol*. 1981;27:643–648.

55. Lindestad P. *Electromyographic and Laryngoscopic Studies of Normal and Disturbed Vocal Function*, Stockholm, Sweden: Suddinge University;1994:1–12,

56. English DT, Blevins CE. Motor units of laryngeal muscles. *Arch Otolaryngol*. 1969; 89:778–784.

57. Faaborg-Andersen K. Electromyographic investigation of intrinsic laryngeal muscles in humans. *Acta Physiol Scand Suppl*. 1957; 41(suppl 140):1–149.

58. Rossi G, Cortesina G. Morphological study of the laryngeal muscles in man: insertions and courses of the muscle fibers, motor end-plates and proprioceptors. *Acta Otolaryngol* (Stockh). 1965;59:575–592.

59. Wu YZ, Crumley RL, Armstrong WB, Caiozzzo VJ. New perspectives about human laryngeal muscle: single fiber analyses and interspecies comparisons. *Arch Otolaryngol Head Neck Surg*. 2000;126:857–864.

60. Malmgren LT, Lovice DB, Kaufman MR. Age-related changes in muscle fiber regeneration in the human thyroarytenoid muscle. *Arch Otolaryngol Head Neck Surg*. 2000;126:851–856.

61. Sataloff RT. Vocal aging. *Curr Opin Otolaryngol Head Neck Surg*. 1998;6:421–428.

62. Davis PJ, Nail BS. On the location and size of laryngeal motoneurons in the cat and rabbit. *J Comp Neurol*. 1984;230:13–22.

63. Yoshida Y, Miyazaki O, Hirano M, et al. Arrangement of motoneurons innervating the intrinsic laryngeal muscles of cats as demonstrated by horseradish peroxidase. *Acta Otolaryngol*. 1982;94:329–334.

64. Yoshida Y, Miyazaki T, Hirano M, Kanaseki T. Localization of the laryngeal motoneurons in the brain stem and myotopical representation of the motoneurons in the nucleus ambiguus of cats—an HRP study. In: Titze I, Scherer R, eds. *Vocal Fold Physiology: Biomechanics, Acoustics and Phonatory Control*. Denver, CO: Denver Center for the Performing Arts; 1983:75–90.

65. Zhang SP, Bandler R, Davis P. Integration of vocalization: the medullary nucleus retroambigualis. *J Neurophysiol*. 1995;74: 2500–2512.

66. Bandler R. Induction of "rage" following microinjections of glutamate into midbrain but not hypothalamus of cats. *Neurosci Lett*. 1982;30:183–188.

67. Kelly AH, Beaton LE, Magoun HW. A midbrain mechanism for facio-vocal activity. *J Neurophysiol*. 1946;9:181–189.

68. Adametz J, O'Leary JL. Experimental mutism resulting from periaqueductal lesions in cats. *Neurology*. 1959; 9;636–642.

69. Skultety FM. Experimental mutism in dogs. *Arch Neurol*. 1962;6:235–241.

70. Esposito A, Demeurisse G, Alberti B, Fabbro F. Complete mutism after midbrain periaqueductal gray lesion. *Neuroreport*. 1999;10:681–685.

71. Bandler R, Shipley MT. Columnar organization in the midbrain periaqueductal gray: modules for emotional expression? *Trends Neurosci*. 1994;17:379–389.

72. Zhang SP, Davis PJ, Bandler R, Carrive P. Brain stem integration of vocalization: role of the midbrain periaqueductal gray. *J Neurophysiol*. 1994;72:1337–1356.

73. Bandler R, Carrive P. Integrated defence reaction elicited by excitatory amino acid

microinjection in the midbrain periaqueductal grey region of the unrestrained cat. *Brain Res.* 1988;439:95–106.

74. Bandler R, Depaulis A. Midbrain periaqueductal gray control of defensive behavior in the cat and the rat. In: Depaulis A, Bandler R, eds. *The Midbrain Periaqueductal Gray Matter: Functional, Anatomical and Immunohistochemical Organization.* New York, NY: Plenum Press; 1991:175–198.

75. Bandler R, Keay K, Vaughan C, Shipley MT. Columnar organization of PAG neurons regulating emotional and vocal expression. In: Fletcher N, Davis P, eds. *Vocal Fold Physiology: Controlling Complexity and Chaos.* San Diego, CA: Singular Publishing Group; 1996:137–153.

76. Shipley MT, Ennis M, Rizvi TA, Behbehani MM. Topographical specificity of forebrain inputs to the midbrain periaqueductal gray: evidence for discrete longitudinally organized input columns. In: Depaulis A, Bandler R, eds. *The Midbrain Periaqueductal Gray Matter: Functional, Anatomical and Immunohistochemical Organization.* New York, NY: Plenum Press; 1991:417–448.

77. Davis P, Zhang SP. What is the role of the midbrain periaqueductal gray in respiration and vocalization? In: Depaulis A, Bandler R, eds. *The Midbrain Periaqueductal Gray Matter: Functional, Anatomical and Immunohistochemical Organization.* New York, NY: Plenum Press; 1991:57–66.

78. Davis P, Zhang SP, Winkworth A, Bandler R. The neural control of vocalization: respiratory and emotional influences. *J Voice.* 1996;10:23–38.

79. Davis PJ, Zhang SP, Bandler R. Midbrain and medullary control of respiration and vocalization. *Prog Brain Res.* 1996;107: 315–325.

80. Davis PJ, Zhang SP, Bandler R. Pulmonary and upper airway afferent influences on the motor pattern of vocalization evoked by excitation of the midbrain periaqueductal gray of the cat. *Brain Res.* 1993;607:61–80.

81. Ambalavanar R, Tanaka Y, Damirjian M, Ludlow CL. Laryngeal afferent stimulation enhances Fos immunoreactivity in periaq-

ueductal gray in the cat. *J Comp Neurol.* 1999;409(3):411–423.

82. Nonaka S, Takahashi R, Enomoto K, Katada A, Unno T. Lombard reflex during PAG-induced vocalization in decerebrate cats. *Neurosci Res.* 1997;29:283–289.

83. Penfield W, Roberts L. *Speech and Brain Mechanisms.* Princeton, NJ: Princeton University Press; 1959.

84. Perry DW, Zatorre RJ, Petrides M, Alivisatos B, Meyer E, Evans AC. Localization of cerebral activity during simple singing. *Neuroreport.* 1999;10:3979–3984.

85. Perrodin C, Kayser C, Logothetis NK, Petkov CI. Voice cells in the primate temporal lobe. *Current Biology: CB.* 2011;21(16): 1408–1415.

86. Simonyan K, Horwitz B. Laryngeal motor cortex and control of speech in humans. *Neuroscientist.* 2011;17(2):197–208.

87. Kleber B, Veit R, Birbaumer N, Gruzelier J, Lotze M. The brain of opera singers: experience-dependent changes in functional activation. *Cereb Cortex.* 2010; 20(5):1144–1152.

88. Chuang FJ, Chen JY, Shyu JF, et al. Surgical anatomy of the external branch of the superior laryngeal nerve in Chinese adults and its clinical applications. *Head Neck.* 2010; 32(1):53–57.

89. Cernea CR, Ferraz AR, Nishio S, et al. Surgical anatomy of the external branch of the superior laryngeal nerve. *Head Neck.* 1992; 14:380–383.

90. Aina EN, Hisham AN. External laryngeal nerve in thyroid surgery: recognition and surgical implications. *ANZ J Surg.* 2001;71: 212–214.

91. Hurtado-Lopez LM, Zaldivar-Ramirez FR. Risk of injury to the external branch of the superior laryngeal nerve in thyroidectomy. *Laryngoscope.* 2002;112:626–629.

92. Friedman M, Losalvio P, Ibrahim H, et al. Superior laryngeal nerve identification and preservation in thyroidectomy. *Arch Otolaryngol Head Neck Surg.* 2002;128: 296–303.

93. Kierner A, Ainger M, Burian M. The external branch of the superior laryngeal nerve:

its topographical anatomy as related to surgery of the neck. *Arch Otolaryngol Head Neck Surg.* 1998;124:301–303.

94. Furlan JC, Cordeiro AC, Brandao LG. Study of some "intrinsic risk factors" that can enhance an iatrogenic injury of the external branch of the superior laryngeal nerve. *Otolaryngol Head Neck Surg.* 2003; 128:396–400.

95. Bellantone R, Boscherini M, Lombardi CP, et al. Is the identification of the external branch of the superior laryngeal nerve mandatory in thyroid operation? Results of a prospective randomized study. *Surgery.* 2001;130:1055–1059.

96. Wu BL, Sanders I, Mu L, Biller HF. The human communicating nerve: an extension of the external superior laryngeal nerve that innervates the vocal cord. *Arch Otolaryngol.* 1994;120(12):1321–1328.

97. Sanders I, Mu L. Anatomy of human internal superior laryngeal nerve. *Anat Rec.* 1998;252:646–656.

98. Yoshida Y, Tanaka Y, Mitsumasu T, Hirano M, Kanaseki T. Peripheral course and intramucosal distribution of the laryngeal sensory nerve fibers of cats. *Brain Res Bull.* 1986;17(1):95–105.

99. Yoshida Y, Tanaka Y, Hirano M, Nakashima T. Sensory innervation of the pharynx and larynx. *Am J Med.* 2000; 108(suppl 4a): 51S–61S.

100. Harrison D. Fibre size frequency in the recurrent laryngeal nerves of men and giraffe. *Acta Otolaryngol.* 1981;91:383–389.

101. Malmgren L, Gacek R. Peripheral motor innervation of the larynx. In: Blitzer A, Brin MF, Sasaki CT, Fahn S, Harris KS, eds. *Neurologic Disorders of the Larynx.* New York, NY: Thieme Medical Publishers; 1992:36–44.

102. Jotz GR, de Campos D, Rodrigues MF, Xavier LL. Histological asymmetry of the human recurrent laryngeal nerve. *J Voice.* 2011;25(1):8–14.

103. Scheid SC, Nadeau DP, Friedman O, Sataloff RT. Anatomy of the thyroarytenoid branch of the recurrent laryngeal nerve. *J Voice.* 2004;8(3):279–284.

104. Eller RL, Miller M, Weinstein J, Sataloff RT. The innervations of the posterior cricoarytenoid muscle: exploring clinical possibilities. *J Voice.* 2009;23(2):229–234.

105. Sato K, Hirano M. Fine three-dimensional structure of pericytes in the vocal fold mucosa. *Ann Otol Rhinol Laryngol.* 1997; 106:490–494.

106. Heman-Ackah YD, Goding GS Jr. Laryngeal chemoreflex severity and end-apnea PaO_2, and $PaCO_2$. *Otolaryngol Head Neck Surg.* 2000;123(3):157–163.

107. Heman-Ackah YD, Goding GS Jr. The effects of intralaryngeal carbon dioxide and acetazolamide on the laryngeal chemoreflex. *Ann Otol Rhinol Laryngol.* 2000; 109(10):921–928.

108. Heman-Ackah YD, Rimell F. Current progress in understanding sudden infant death syndrome. *Curr Opin Otolaryngol Head Neck Surg.* 1999;7(6):320–327.

109. Abo-el-Enein M. Laryngeal myotactic reflexes. *Nature.* 1966;209:682–685.

110. Tomori Z, Widdicomb J. Muscular bronchomotor and cardiovascular reflexes elicited by mechanical stimulation of the respiratory tract. *J Physiol.* 1969;200:25–49.

111. Gould WJ, Okamura H. Static lung volumes in singers. *Ann Otol Rhinol Laryngol.* 1973;82:89–95.

112. Hixon TJ, Hoffman C. Chest wall shape during singing. In: Lawrence V, ed. *Transcripts of the Seventh Annual Symposium, Care of the Professional Voice.* New York, NY: The Voice Foundation; 1978;9–10.

113. Sundberg J, Leanderson R, von Euler C. Activity relationship between diaphragm and cricothyroid muscles. *J Voice.* 1989; 3(3):225–232.

114. Hunter EJ, Titze IR. Individual subject laryngeal dimensions of multiple mammalian species for biomedical models. *Ann Otol Rhinol Laryngol.* 2005;114(10):809–818.

115. Scott TM. How we teach anatomy efficiently and effectively. *Med Teach.* 1993;15: 67–75.

116. McLachlan JC, Bligh J, Bradley P, et al. Teaching anatomy without cadavers. *Med Educ.* 2004;38:418–424.

117. Parker LM. What's wrong with the dead body? Use of the human cadaver in medical education. *Med J Aust.* 2002;176(2):74–76.

118. Prince KJAH, Mameren H van, Hylkema N, et al. Does problem-based learning lead to deficiencies in basic science knowledge? An empirical case on anatomy. *Med Educ.* 2003;37:15–21.

119. American Association of Medical Colleges Institute for Improving Medical Education. *Effective Use of Educational Technology in Medical Education.* Washington, DC: Association of American Medical Colleges; 2007:3.

120. Hu A, Wilson T, Ladak H, et al. Three-dimensional educational computer model of the larynx: voicing a new direction. *Arch Otolaryngol Head Neck Surg.* 2009;135(7): 677–682.

121. Hu A, Wilson T, Ladak H, Haase P, Doyle P, Fung K. Evaluation of a three-dimensional educational computer model of the larynx: voicing a new direction. *J Otolaryngol Head Neck Surg.* 2010;39(3):315–322.

122. Fritz D, Hu A, Wilson T, Ladak H, Haase P, Fung K. Long-term retention of a three dimensional educational computer model of the larynx. *Arch Otolaryngol Head Neck Surg.* 2011;137(6):598–603.

123. Tan S, Hu A, Wilson T, Ladak H, Haase P, Fung K. Role of computer generated 3D-visualization in laryngeal anatomy teaching for advanced learners. *J Laryngol Otol.* 2012;126(4):395–401.

3

Patient History[*]

Robert Thayer Sataloff

A comprehensive history and physical examination usually reveal the cause of voice dysfunction. Effective history taking and physical examination depend on a practical understanding of the anatomy and physiology of voice production.[1-3] Because dysfunction in virtually any body system may affect phonation, medical inquiry must be comprehensive. The current standard of care for all voice patients evolved from advances inspired by medical problems of voice professionals such as singers and actors. Even minor problems may be particularly symptomatic in singers and actors, because of the extreme demands they place on their voices. However, a great many other patients are voice professionals. They include teachers, salespeople, attorneys, clergy, physicians, politicians, telephone receptionists, and anyone else whose ability to earn a living is impaired in the presence of voice dysfunction. Because good voice quality is so important in our society, the majority of our patients are voice professionals, and all patients should be treated as such.

The scope of inquiry and examination for most patients is similar to that required for singers and actors, except that performing voice professionals have unique needs, which require additional history and examination. Questions must be added regarding performance commitments, professional status and voice goals, the amount and nature of voice training, the performance environment, rehearsal practices, abusive habits during speech and singing, and many other matters. Such supplementary information is essential to proper treatment selection and patient counseling in singers and actors. However, analogous factors must also be taken into account for stockbrokers, factory shop foremen, elementary school teachers, homemakers with several noisy children, and many others. Physicians familiar with the management of these challenging patients are well equipped to evaluate all patients with voice complaints.

Patient History

Obtaining extensive historical background information is necessary for thorough evaluation of the voice patient, and the

---

[*]Reprinted with permission from Rubin J, Sataloff R, Korovin G. *Diagnosis and Treatment of Voice Disorders*, 4th ed. San Diego, CA: Plural Publishing; 2014.

otolaryngologist who sees voice patients (especially singers) only occasionally cannot reasonably be expected to remember all the pertinent questions. Although some laryngologists consider a lengthy inquisition helpful in establishing rapport, many of us who see a substantial number of voice patients each day within a busy practice need a thorough but less time-consuming alternative. A history questionnaire can be extremely helpful in documenting all the necessary information, helping the patient sort out and articulate his or her problems, and saving the clinician time recording information. The author has developed a questionnaire[4] that has proven helpful (Appendix 3–A). The patient is asked to complete the relevant portions of the form at home prior to his or her office visit or in the waiting room before seeing the doctor. A similar form has been developed for voice patients who are not singers.

No history questionnaire is a substitute for direct, penetrating questioning by the physician. However, the direction of most useful inquiry can be determined from a glance at the questionnaire, obviating the need for extensive writing, which permits the physician greater eye contact with the patient and facilitates rapid establishment of the close rapport and confidence that are so important in treating voice patients. The physician is also able to supplement initial impressions and historical information from the questionnaire with seemingly leisurely conversation during the physical examination. The use of the history questionnaire has added substantially to the efficiency, consistent thoroughness, and ease of managing these delightful, but often complex, patients. A similar set of questions is also used by the speech-language pathologist with new patients and by many enlightened singing teachers when assessing new students.

How Old Are You?

Serious vocal endeavor may start in childhood and continue throughout a lifetime. As the vocal mechanism undergoes normal maturation, the voice changes. The optimal time to begin serious vocal training is controversial. For many years, most singing teachers advocated delay of vocal training and serious singing until near puberty in the female and after puberty and voice stabilization in the male. However, in a child with earnest vocal aspirations and potential, starting specialized training early in childhood is reasonable. Initial instruction should teach the child to vocalize without straining and to avoid all forms of voice abuse. It should not permit premature indulgence in operatic bravado. Most experts agree that taxing voice use and singing during puberty should be minimized or avoided altogether, particularly by the male. Voice maturation (attainment of stable adult vocal quality) may occur at any age from the early teenage years to the fourth decade of life. The dangerous tendency for young singers to attempt to sound older than their vocal years frequently causes vocal dysfunction.

All components of voice production are subject to normal aging. Abdominal and general muscular tone frequently decrease, lungs lose elasticity, the thorax loses its distensibility, the mucosa of the vocal tract atrophies, mucous secretions change character and quantity, nerve endings are reduced in number, and psychoneurologic functions change. Moreover, the larynx itself loses muscle tone and bulk and may show depletion of submucosal ground substance in the vocal folds. The laryngeal cartilages ossify, and the joints may become arthritic and stiff. Hormonal influence is altered. Vocal range, intensity, and quality all may be modified. Vocal fold atrophy may be the most striking alteration. The clinical effects of aging seem more pronounced in female singers, although vocal fold histologic changes may be more prominent in males. Excellent male singers occasionally extend their careers into their 70s or beyond.[5,6] However, some degree of breathiness, decreased range, and other evidence of aging should be expected in elderly voices. Nevertheless, many of the changes we typically associate with elderly singers (wobble, flat pitch) are due to lack of conditioning, rather than inevitable changes of biological aging. These aesthetically undesirable concomitants of aging can often be reversed.

What Is Your Voice Problem?

Careful questioning as to the onset of vocal problems is needed to separate acute from chronic dysfunction. Often an upper respiratory tract infection will send a patient to the physician's office, but penetrating inquiry, especially in singers and actors, may reveal a chronic vocal problem that is the patient's real concern. Identifying acute and chronic problems before beginning therapy is important so that both patient and physician may have realistic expectations and make optimal therapeutic selections.

The specific nature of the vocal complaint can provide a great deal of information. Just as dizzy patients rarely walk into the physician's office complaining of "rotary vertigo," voice patients may be unable to articulate their symptoms without guidance. They may use the term *hoarseness* to describe a variety of conditions that the physician must separate. Hoarseness is a coarse or scratchy sound that is most often associated with abnormalities of the leading edge of the vocal folds such as laryngitis or mass lesions. Breathiness is a vocal quality characterized by excessive loss of air during vocalization. In some cases, it is due to improper technique. However, any condition that prevents full approximation of the vocal folds can be responsible. Possible causes include vocal fold paralysis, a mass lesion separating the leading edges of the vocal folds, arthritis of the cricoarytenoid joint, arytenoid dislocation, scarring of the vibratory margin, senile vocal fold atrophy (presbyphonia), psychogenic dysphonia, malingering, and other conditions.

Fatigue of the voice is inability to continue to speak or sing for extended periods without change in vocal quality and/or control. The voice may show fatigue by becoming hoarse, losing range, changing timbre, breaking into different registers, or exhibiting other uncontrolled aberrations. A well-trained singer should be able to sing for several hours without vocal fatigue.

Voice fatigue may occur through more than one mechanism. Most of the time, it is assumed to be due to muscle fatigue. This is often the case in patients who have voice fatigue associated with muscle tension dysphonia. The mechanism is most likely to be peripheral muscle fatigue and due to chemical changes (or depletion) in the muscle fibers. "Muscle fatigue" may also occur on a central (neurologic) basis. This mechanism is common in certain neuropathic disorders, such as some patients with multiple sclerosis; may occur with myasthenia gravis (actually neuromuscular junction pathology); or may be associated with paresis from various causes. However, the voice may also fatigue due to changes in the vibratory margin of the vocal fold. This phenomenon may be described as "lamina propria" fatigue (our descriptive, not universally used). It, too, may be related to chemical or fluid changes in the lamina propria or cellular damage associated with conditions such as phonotrauma and dehydration. Excessive voice use, suboptimal tissue environment (eg, dehydration, effects of pollution, etc), lack of sufficient time of recovery between phonatory stresses, and genetic or structural tissue weaknesses that predispose to injury or delayed recovery from trauma all may be associated with lamina propria fatigue.

Although it has not been proven, this author (RTS) suspects that fatigue may also be related to the linearity of vocal fold vibrations. However, briefly, voices have linear and nonlinear (chaotic) characteristics. As the voice becomes more trained, vibrations become more symmetrical, and the system becomes more linear. In many pathologic voices, the nonlinear components appear to become more prominent. If a voice is highly linear, slight changes in the vibratory margin may have little effect on the output of the system. However, if the system has substantial nonlinearity due to vocal fold pathology, poor tissue environment, or other causes, slight changes in the tissue (slight swelling, drying, surface cell damage) may cause substantial changes in the acoustic output of the system (the butterfly effect), causing vocal quality changes and fatigue much more quickly with much smaller changes in initial condition in more linear vocal systems.

Fatigue is often caused by misuse of abdominal and neck musculature or oversinging, singing too loudly, or too long. However, we must remember that vocal fatigue also may be a sign not only of general tiredness or vocal abuse (sometimes secondary to structural lesions or glottal closure problems) but also of serious illnesses such as myasthenia gravis. So, the importance of this complaint should not be understated.

Volume disturbance may manifest as inability to sing loudly or inability to sing softly. Each voice has its own dynamic range. Within the course of training, singers learn to sing more loudly by singing more efficiently. They also learn to sing softly, a

more difficult task, through years of laborious practice. Actors and other trained speakers go through similar training. Most volume problems are secondary to intrinsic limitations of the voice or technical errors in voice use, although hormonal changes, aging, and neurologic disease are other causes. Superior laryngeal nerve paralysis impairs the ability to speak or sing loudly. This is a frequently unrecognized consequence of herpes infection (cold sores) and Lyme disease and may be precipitated by any viral upper respiratory tract infection.

Most highly trained singers require only about 10 minutes to half an hour to "warm up the voice." Prolonged warm-up time, especially in the morning, is most often caused by reflux laryngitis. Tickling or choking during singing is most often a symptom of an abnormality of the vocal fold's leading edge. The symptom of tickling or choking should contraindicate singing until the vocal folds have been examined. Pain while singing can indicate vocal fold lesions, laryngeal joint arthritis, infection, or gastric acid reflux irritation of the arytenoid region. However, pain is much more commonly caused by voice abuse with excessive muscular activity in the neck rather than an acute abnormality on the leading edge of a vocal fold. In the absence of other symptoms, these patients do not generally require immediate cessation of singing pending medical examination. However, sudden onset of pain (usually sharp pain) while singing may be associated with a mucosal tear or a vocal fold hemorrhage and warrants voice conservation pending laryngeal examination.

Do You Have Any Pressing Voice Commitments?

If a singer or professional speaker (eg, actor, politician) seeks treatment at the end of a busy performance season and has no pressing engagements, management of the voice problem should be relatively conservative and designed to ensure long-term protection of the larynx, the most delicate part of the vocal mechanism. However, the physician and patient rarely have this luxury. Most often, the voice professional needs treatment within a week of an important engagement and sometimes within less than a day. Younger singers fall ill shortly before performances, not because of hypochondria or coincidence, but rather because of the immense physical and emotional stress of the preperformance period. The singer is frequently working harder and singing longer hours than usual. Moreover, he or she may be under particular pressure to learn new material and to perform well for a new audience. The singer may also be sleeping less than usual because of additional time spent rehearsing or because of the discomforts of a strange city. Seasoned professionals make their living by performing regularly, sometimes several times a week. Consequently, any time they get sick is likely to precede a performance. Caring for voice complaints in these situations requires highly skilled judgment and bold management.

Tell Me About Your Vocal Career, Long-Term Goals, and the Importance of Your Voice Quality and Upcoming Commitments

To choose a treatment program, the physician must understand the importance of the patient's voice and his or her long-term career plans, the importance of the upcoming vocal commitment, and the consequences of canceling the engagement. Injudicious prescription of voice rest can

be almost as damaging to a vocal career as injudicious performance. For example, although a singer's voice is usually his or her most important commodity, other factors distinguish the few successful artists from the multitude of less successful singers with equally good voices. These include musicianship, reliability, and "professionalism." Canceling a concert at the last minute may seriously damage a performer's reputation. Reliability is especially critical early in a singer's career. Moreover, an expert singer often can modify a performance to decrease the strain on his or her voice. No singer should be allowed to perform in a manner that will permit serious injury to the vocal folds, but in the frequent borderline cases, the condition of the larynx must be weighed against other factors affecting the singer as an artist.

How Much Voice Training Have You Had?

Establishing how long a singer or actor has been performing seriously is important, especially if his or her active performance career predates the beginning of vocal training. Active untrained singers and actors frequently develop undesirable techniques that are difficult to modify. Extensive voice use without training or premature training with inappropriate repertoire may underlie persistent vocal difficulties later in life. The number of years a performer has been training his or her voice may be a fair index of vocal proficiency. A person who has studied voice for 1 or 2 years is somewhat more likely to have gross technical difficulties than is someone who has been studying for 20 years. However, if training has been intermittent or discontinued, technical problems are common, especially among singers. In addition, methods of technical voice use vary among voice teachers. Hence, a student who has had many teachers in a relatively brief period of time commonly has numerous technical insecurities or deficiencies that may be responsible for vocal dysfunction. This is especially true if the singer has changed to a new teacher within the preceding year. The physician must be careful not to criticize the patient's current voice teacher in such circumstances. It often takes years of expert instruction to correct bad habits.

All people speak more often than they sing, yet most singers report little speech training. Even if a singer uses the voice flawlessly while practicing and performing, voice abuse at other times can cause damage that affects singing.

Under What Kinds of Conditions Do You Use Your Voice?

The Lombard effect is the tendency to increase vocal intensity in response to increased background noise. A well-trained singer learns to compensate for this tendency and to avoid singing at unsafe volumes. Singers of classical music usually have such training and frequently perform with only a piano, a situation in which the balance can be controlled well. However, singers performing in large halls, with orchestras, or in operas early in their careers tend to oversing and strain their voices. Similar problems occur during outdoor concerts because of the lack of auditory feedback. This phenomenon is seen even more among "pop" singers. Pop singers are in a uniquely difficult position; often, despite little vocal training, they enjoy great artistic and financial success and endure extremely stressful demands on their time and voices. They are required to sing in large halls or outdoor arenas not designed for musical per-

formance, amid smoke and other environmental irritants, accompanied by extremely loud background music. One frequently neglected key to survival for these singers is the proper use of monitor speakers. These direct the sound of the singer's voice toward the singer on the stage and provide auditory feedback. Determining whether the pop singer uses monitor speakers and whether they are loud enough for the singer to hear is important.

Amateur singers are often no less serious about their music than are professionals, but generally they have less ability to compensate technically for illness or other physical impairment. Rarely does an amateur suffer a great loss from postponing a performance or permitting someone to sing in his or her place. In most cases, the amateur singer's best interest is served through conservative management directed at long-term maintenance of good vocal health.

A great many of the singers who seek physicians' advice are primarily choral singers. They often are enthusiastic amateurs, untrained but dedicated to their musical recreation. They should be handled as amateur solo singers, educated specifically about the Lombard effect, and cautioned to avoid the excessive volume so common in a choral environment. One good way for a singer to monitor loudness is to cup a hand to his or her ear. This adds about 6 dB[7] to the singer's perception of his or her own voice and can be a very helpful guide in noisy surroundings. Young professional singers are often hired to augment amateur choruses. Feeling that the professional quartet has been hired to "lead" the rest of the choir, they often make the mistake of trying to accomplish that goal by singing louder than others in their sections. These singers should be advised to lead their section by singing each line as if they were soloists giving a voice lesson to the people standing next to them and as if there were a microphone in front of them recording their choral performance for their voice teacher. This approach usually not only preserves the voice but also produces a better choral sound.

How Much Do You Practice and Exercise Your Voice? How, When, and Where Do You Use Your Voice?

Vocal exercise is as essential to the vocalist as exercise and conditioning of other muscle systems is to the athlete. Proper vocal practice incorporates scales and specific exercises designed to maintain and develop the vocal apparatus. Simply acting or singing songs or giving performances without routine studious concentration on vocal technique is not adequate for the vocal performer. The physician should know whether the vocalist practices daily, whether he or she practices at the same time daily, and how long the practice lasts. Actors generally practice and warm up their voices for 10 to 30 minutes daily, although more time is recommended. Most serious singers practice for at least 1 to 2 hours per day. If a singer routinely practices in the late afternoon or evening but frequently performs in the morning (religious services, school classes, teaching voice, choir rehearsals, etc), one should inquire into the warm-up procedures preceding such performances as well as cool-down procedures after voice use. Singing "cold," especially early in the morning, may result in the use of minor muscular alterations to compensate for vocal insecurity produced by inadequate preparation. Such crutches can result in voice dysfunction. Similar problems may result from instances of voice use other than formal singing. School teachers, telephone receptionists, salespeople, and oth-

ers who speak extensively also often derive great benefit from 5 or 10 minutes of vocalization of scales first thing in the morning. Although singers rarely practice their scales too long, they frequently perform or rehearse excessively. This is especially true immediately before a major concert or audition, when physicians are most likely to see acute problems. When a singer has hoarseness and vocal fatigue and has been practicing a new role for 14 hours a day for the last 3 weeks, no simple prescription will solve the problem. However, a treatment regimen can usually be designed to carry the performer safely through his or her musical obligations.

The physician should be aware of common habits and environments that are often associated with abusive voice behavior and should ask about them routinely. Screaming at sports events and at children is among the most common. Extensive voice use in noisy environments also tends to be abusive. These include noisy rooms, cars, airplanes, sports facilities, and other locations where background noise or acoustic design impairs auditory feedback. Dry, dusty surroundings may alter vocal fold secretions through dehydration or contact irritation, altering voice function. Activities such as cheerleading, teaching, choral conducting, amateur singing, and frequent communication with hearing-impaired persons are likely to be associated with voice abuse, as is extensive professional voice use without formal training. The physician should inquire into the patient's routine voice use and should specifically ask about any activities that frequently lead to voice change such as hoarseness or discomfort in the neck or throat. Laryngologists should ask specifically about other activities that may be abusive to the vocal folds such as weight lifting, aerobics, and the playing of some wind instruments.

Are You Aware of Misusing or Abusing Your Voice During Singing?

A detailed discussion of vocal technique in singing is beyond the scope of this chapter but is discussed in other chapters. The most common technical errors involve excessive muscle tension in the tongue, neck, and larynx; inadequate abdominal support; and excessive volume. Inadequate preparation can be a devastating source of voice abuse and may result from limited practice, limited rehearsal of a difficult piece, or limited vocal training for a given role. The latter error is common. In some situations, voice teachers are at fault; both the singer and teacher must resist the impulse to "show off" the voice in works that are either too difficult for the singer's level of training or simply not suited to the singer's voice. Singers are habitually unhappy with the limitations of their voices. At some time or another, most baritones wish they were tenors and walk around proving they can sing high Cs in "Vesti la giubba." Singers with other vocal ranges have similar fantasies. Attempts to make the voice something that it is not, or at least that it is not yet, frequently are harmful.

Are You Aware of Misusing or Abusing Your Voice During Speaking?

Common patterns of voice abuse and misuse will not be discussed in detail in this chapter. Voice abuse and/or misuse should be suspected particularly in patients who complain of voice fatigue associated with voice use, whose voices are worse at the end of a working day or week, and in any patient who is chronically hoarse. Technical errors in voice use may be the primary etiology of a voice complaint, or it may develop secondarily due to a patient's effort to compensate for voice disturbance from another cause.

Dissociation of one's speaking and singing voices is probably the most common cause of voice abuse problems in excellent singers. Too frequently, all the expert training in support, muscle control, and projection is not applied to a singers' speaking voice. Unfortunately, the resultant voice strain affects the singing voice as well as the speaking voice. Such damage is especially likely to occur in noisy rooms and in cars, where the background noise is louder than it seems. Backstage greetings after a lengthy performance can be particularly devastating. The singer usually is exhausted and distracted; the environment is often dusty and dry, and generally a noisy crowd is present. Similar conditions prevail at postperformance parties, where smoking and alcohol worsen matters. These situations should be avoided by any singer with vocal problems and should be controlled through awareness at other times.

Three particularly abusive and potentially damaging vocal activities are worthy of note. *Cheerleading* requires extensive screaming under the worst possible physical and environmental circumstances. It is a highly undesirable activity for anyone considering serious vocal endeavor. This is a common conflict in younger singers because the teenager who is the high school choir soloist often is also student council president, yearbook editor, captain of the cheerleaders, and so on.

Conducting, particularly choral conducting, can also be deleterious. An enthusiastic conductor, especially of an amateur group, frequently sings all 4 parts intermittently, at volumes louder than the entire choir, during lengthy rehearsals. Conducting is a common avocation among singers but must be done with expert technique and special precautions to prevent voice injury. Hoarseness or loss of soft voice control after conducting a rehearsal or concert suggests voice abuse during conducting. The patient should be instructed to record his or her voice throughout the vocal range singing long notes at dynamics from soft to loud to soft. Recordings should be made prior to rehearsal and following rehearsal. If the voice has lost range, control, or quality during the rehearsal, voice abuse has occurred. A similar test can be used for patients who sing in choirs, teach voice, or perform other potentially abusive vocal activities. Such problems in conductors can generally be managed by additional training in conducting techniques and by voice training, including warm-up and cool-down exercises.

Teaching singing may also be hazardous to vocal health. It can be done safely but requires skill and thought. Most teachers teach while seated at the piano. Late in a long, hard day, this posture is not conducive to maintenance of optimal abdominal and back support. Usually, teachers work with students continually positioned to the right or left of the keyboard. This may require the teacher to turn his or her neck at a particularly sharp angle, especially when teaching at an upright piano. Teachers also often demonstrate vocal works in their students' vocal ranges rather than their own, illustrating bad as well as good technique. If a singing teacher is hoarse or has neck discomfort, or his or her soft singing control deteriorates at the end of a teaching day (assuming that the teacher warms up before beginning to teach voice lessons), voice abuse should be suspected. Helpful modifications include teaching with a grand piano, sitting slightly sideways on the piano bench, or alternating student position to the right and left of the piano to facilitate better neck alignment. Retaining an accompanist so that the teacher can stand rather than teach from sitting behind a piano, and many other helpful modifications, are possible.

Do You Have Pain When You Talk or Sing?

Odynophonia, or pain caused by phonation, can be a disturbing symptom. It is not uncommon, but relatively little has been written or discussed on this subject. A detailed review of odynophonia is beyond the scope of this publication. However, laryngologists should be familiar with the diagnosis and treatment of at least a few of the most common causes, at least, as discussed elsewhere in this book.

What Kind of Physical Condition Are You In?

Phonation is an athletic activity that requires good conditioning and coordinated interaction of numerous physical functions. Maladies of any part of the body may be reflected in the voice. Failure to maintain good abdominal muscle tone and respiratory endurance through exercise is particularly harmful because deficiencies in these areas undermine the power source of the voice. Patients generally attempt to compensate for such weaknesses by using inappropriate muscle groups, particularly in the neck, causing vocal dysfunction. Similar problems may occur in the well-conditioned vocalist in states of fatigue. These are compounded by mucosal changes that accompany excessively long hours of hard work. Such problems may be seen even in the best singers shortly before important performances in the height of the concert season.

A popular but untrue myth holds that great opera singers must be obese. However, the vivacious, gregarious personality that often distinguishes the great performer seems to be accompanied frequently by a propensity for excess, especially culinary excess. This excess is as undesirable in the vocalist as it is in most other athletic artists, and it should be prevented from the start of one's vocal career. Appropriate and attractive body weight has always been valued in the pop music world and is becoming particularly important in the opera world as this formerly theater-based art form moves to television and film media. However, attempts at weight reduction in an established speaker or singer are a different matter. The vocal mechanism is a finely tuned, complex instrument and is exquisitely sensitive to minor changes. Substantial fluctuations in weight frequently cause deleterious alterations of the voice, although these are usually temporary. Weight reduction programs for people concerned about their voices must be monitored carefully and designed to reduce weight in small increments over long periods. A history of sudden recent weight change may be responsible for almost any vocal complaint.

How Is Your Hearing?

Hearing loss can cause substantial problems for singers and other professional voice users. This may be true especially when the voice patient is unaware that he or she has hearing loss. Consequently, not only should voice patients be asked about hearing loss, tinnitus, vertigo, and family history of hearing loss, but it is also helpful to inquire of spouses, partners, friends, or others who may have accompanied the patient to the office whether they have suspected a hearing impairment in the patient.

Have You Noted Voice or Bodily Weakness, Tremor, Fatigue, or Loss of Control?

Even minor neurologic disorders may be extremely disruptive to vocal function. Specific questions should be asked to rule out neuromuscular and neurologic diseases such as myasthenia gravis, Parkinson disease, tremors, other movement disorders, spasmodic dysphonia, multiple sclerosis, central nervous system neoplasm, and other serious maladies that may be present with voice complaints.

Do You Have Allergy or Cold Symptoms?

Acute upper respiratory tract infection causes inflammation of the mucosa, alters mucosal secretions, and makes the mucosa more vulnerable to injury. Coughing and throat clearing are particularly traumatic vocal activities and may worsen or provoke hoarseness associated with a cold. Postnasal drip and allergy may produce the same response. Infectious sinusitis is associated with discharge and diffuse mucosal inflammation, resulting in similar problems, and may actually alter the sound of a voice, especially the patient's own perception of his or her voice. Futile attempts to compensate for disease of the supraglottic vocal tract in an effort to return the sound to normal frequently result in laryngeal strain. The expert singer or speaker should compensate by monitoring technique by tactile rather than by auditory feedback, or singing "by feel" rather than "by ear."

Do You Have Breathing Problems, Especially After Exercise?

Voice patients usually volunteer information about upper respiratory tract infections and postnasal drip, but the relevance of other maladies may not be obvious to them. Consequently, the physician must seek out pertinent history.

Respiratory problems are especially important in voice patients. Even mild respiratory dysfunction may adversely affect the power source of the voice.[8] Occult asthma may be particularly troublesome.[9] A complete respiratory history should be obtained in most patients with voice complaints, and pulmonary function testing is often advisable.

Have You Been Exposed to Environmental Irritants?

Any mucosal irritant can disrupt the delicate vocal mechanism. Allergies to dust and mold are aggravated commonly during rehearsals and performances in concert halls, especially older theaters and concert halls, because of numerous curtains, backstage trappings, and dressing room facilities that are rarely cleaned thoroughly. Nasal obstruction and erythematous conjunctivae suggest generalized mucosal irritation. The drying effects of cold air and dry heat may also affect mucosal secretions, leading to decreased lubrication, a "scratchy" voice, and tickling cough. These symptoms may be minimized by nasal breathing, which allows inspired air to be filtered, warmed, and humidified. Nasal breathing, whenever possible, rather than mouth breathing, is proper vocal technique. While the performer is backstage between appearances or during rehearsals, inhalation of dust and other irritants may be controlled by wearing a protective mask, such as those used by carpenters, or a surgical mask that does not contain fiberglass. This is especially helpful when sets are being constructed in the rehearsal area.

A history of recent travel suggests other sources of mucosal irritation. The air in airplanes is extremely dry, and airplanes are noisy.[10] One must be careful to avoid talking loudly and to maintain good hydration and nasal breathing during air travel. Environmental changes can also be disruptive. Las Vegas is infamous for the mucosal irritation caused by its dry atmosphere and smoke-filled rooms. In fact, the resultant complex of hoarseness, vocal "tickle," and fatigue is referred to as "Las Vegas voice." A history of recent travel should also suggest jet lag and generalized fatigue, which may be potent detriments to good vocal function.

Environmental pollution is responsible for the presence of toxic substances and conditions encountered daily. Inhalation of toxic pollutants may affect the voice adversely by direct laryngeal injury, by causing pulmonary dysfunction that results in voice maladies, or through impairments elsewhere in the vocal tract. Ingested substances, especially those that have neurolaryngologic effects, may also adversely affect the voice. Nonchemical environmental pollutants such as noise can cause voice abnormalities, as well. Laryngologists should be familiar with the laryngologic effects of the numerous potentially irritating substances and conditions found in the environment. We must also be familiar with special pollution problems encountered by performers. Numerous materials used by artists to create sculptures, drawings, and theatrical sets are toxic and have adverse voice effects. In addition, performers are exposed routinely to chemicals encountered through stage smoke and pyrotechnic effects. Although it is clear that some of the "special effects" may result in serious laryngologic consequences, much additional study is needed to clarify the nature and scope of these occupational problems.

Do You Smoke, Live With a Smoker, or Work Around Smoke?

The effects of smoking on voice performance were reviewed recently in the *Journal of Singing*,[11] and that review is recapitulated here. Smoking tobacco is the number one cause of preventable death in the United States as well as the leading cause of heart disease, stroke, emphysema, and cancer. The Centers for Disease Control and Prevention (CDC) attributes approximately 442,000 premature (shortened life expectancy) deaths annually in the United States to smoking, which is more than the combined incidence of deaths caused by highway accidents, fires, murders, illegal drugs, suicides, and AIDS.[12] Approximately 4 million deaths per year worldwide result from smoking, and if this trend continues, by 2030, this figure will increase to about 10 million deaths globally.[13] In addition to causing life-threatening diseases, smoking impairs a great many body systems, including the vocal tract. Harmful consequences of smoking or being exposed to smoke influence voice performance adversely.

Singers need good vocal health to perform well. Smoking tobacco can irritate the mucosal covering of the vocal folds, causing redness and chronic inflammation, and can have the same effect on the mucosal lining of the lungs, trachea, nasopharynx (behind the nose and throat), and mouth. In other words, the components of voice production—the generator, the oscillator, the resonator, and the articulator—all can be compromised by the harmful effects of tobacco use. The onset of effects from smoking may be immediate or delayed.

Individuals who have allergies and/or asthma are usually more sensitive to cigarette smoke with potential for an immediate adverse reaction involving the lungs, larynx, nasal cavities, and/or eyes. Chronic use of tobacco, or exposure to it, causes the toxic chemicals in tobacco to accumulate in the body, damaging the delicate linings of the vocal tract, as well as the lungs, heart, and circulatory system.

The lungs are critical components of the power source of the vocal tract. They help generate an airstream that is directed superiorly through the trachea toward the undersurface of the vocal folds. The vocal folds respond to the increase in subglottic pressure by producing sounds of variable intensities and frequencies. The number of times per second the vocal fold vibrate influences the pitch, and the amplitude of the mucosal wave influences the loudness of the sound. The sound produced by the vibration (oscillation) of the vocal folds passes upward through the oral cavity and nasopharynx where it resonates, giving the voice its richness and timbre, and eventually it is articulated by the mouth, teeth, lips, and tongue into speech or song.

Any condition that adversely affects lung function such as chronic exposure to smoke or uncontrolled asthma can contribute to dysphonia by impairing the strength, endurance, and consistency of the airsteam responsible for establishing vocal fold oscillation. Any lesion that compromises vocal fold vibration and glottic closure can cause hoarseness and breathiness. Inflammation of the cover layer of the vocal folds and/or the mucosal lining of the nose, sinuses, and oral nasopharyngeal cavities can affect the quality and clarity of the voice.

Tobacco smoke can damage the lungs' parenchyma and the exchange of air through respiration. Cigarette manufacturers add hundreds of ingredients to their tobacco products to improve taste, to make smoking seem milder and easier to inhale, and to prolong burning and shelf life.[14] More than 3000 chemical compounds have been identified in tobacco smoke, and more than 60 of these compounds are carcinogens.[15] The tobacco plant, *Nicotiana tabacum*, is grown for its leaves, which can be smoked, chewed, or sniffed with various effects. The nicotine in tobacco is the addictive component and rivals crack cocaine in its ability to enslave its users. Most smokers want to stop, yet only a small percentage are successful in quitting cigarettes; the majority who quit relapse into smoking once again.[16] Tar and carbon monoxide are among the disease-causing components in tobacco products. The tar in cigarettes exposes the individual to a greater risk of bronchitis, emphysema, and lung cancer. These chemicals affect the entire vocal tract as well as the cardiovascular system (Table 3–1).

Cigarette smoke in the lungs can lead also to increased vascularity, edema, and excess mucous production, as well as epithelial tissue and cellular changes. The toxic agents in cigarette smoke have been associated with an increase in the number and severity of asthma attacks, chronic bronchitis, emphysema, and lung cancer, all of which can interfere with the lungs' ability to generate the stream of air needed for voice production.

Chronic bronchitis due to smoking has been associated with an increase in the number of goblet (mucous) cells, an increase in the size (hyperplasia) of the mucosal secreting glands, and a decrease in the number of ciliated cells, the cells used to clean the lungs. Chronic cough and sputum production are also seen more commonly in smokers compared with nonsmokers. Also, the heat and chemicals of unfiltered cigarette and marijuana smoke are especially irritating to the lungs and larynx.

An important component of voice quality is the symmetrical, unencumbered vibration of the true vocal folds. Anything that prevents the epithelium covering the vocal folds from vibrating or affects the loose connective tissue under the epithelium (in the superficial layer of the lamina propria known as the Reinke's space) can cause dysphonia. Cigarette smoking can cause the epithelium of the true vocal folds to become red and swollen, develop whitish discolorations (leukoplakia), undergo chronic inflammatory changes, or develop squamous metaplasia or dysplasia (tissue changes from normal to a potentially malignant state). In chronic smokers, the voice may become husky due to the accumulation of fluid in the Reinke's space (Reinke's edema). These alterations in structure can interfere with voice production by changing the biomechanics of the vocal folds and their vibratory characteristics. In severe cases, cancer can deform and paralyze the vocal folds.

Vocal misuse often follows in an attempt to compensate for dysphonia and an alerted self-perception of one's voice. The voice may feel weak, breathy, raspy, or strained. There may be a loss of range, vocal breaks, long warm-up time, and fatigue. The throat may feel raw, achy, or tight. As the voice becomes unreliable, bad habits increase as the individual struggles harder and harder to compensate vocally. As selected sound waves move upward, from the larynx toward and through the pharynx, nasopharynx, mouth, and nose (the resonators), sounds gain a unique richness and timbre. Exposing the pharynx to cigarette smoke aggravates the

Table 3–1. Chemical Additives Found in Tobacco and Commercial Products

Tobacco Chemical Additives	Also Found In
Acetic acid	Vinegar, hair dye
Acetone	Nail polish remover
Ammonia	Floor cleaner, toilet cleaner
Arsenic	Poison
Benzene	A leukemia-producing agent in rubber cement
Butane	Cigarette lighter fluid
Cadmium	Batteries, some oil paints
Carbon monoxide	Car exhaust
DDT	Insecticides
Ethanol	Alcohol
Formaldehyde	Embalming fluid, fabric, laboratory animals
Hexamine	Barbecue lighter
Hydrazine	Jet fuel, rocket fuel
Hydrogen cyanide	Gas chamber poison
Methane	Swamp gas
Methanol	Rocket fuel
Naphthalene	Explosives, mothballs, paints
Nickel	Electroplating
Nicotine	Insecticides
Nitrobenzene	Gasoline additive
Nitrous oxide phenols	Disinfectant
Phenol	Disinfectants, plastics
Polonium-210	A radioactive substance
Stearic acid	Candle wax
Styrene	Insulation materials
Toluene	Industrial solvent, embalmer's glue
Vinyl chloride	Plastic manufacturing, garbage bags

linings of the oropharynx, mouth, nasopharynx, sinuses, and nasal cavities. The resulting erythema, swelling, and inflammation predispose one to nasal congestion and impaired mucosal function; there may be predisposition to sinusitis and pharyngitis, in which the voice may become hypo-nasal, the sinus achy, and the throat painful.

Although relatively rare in the United States, cancer of the nasopharynx has been associated with cigarette smoking,[17] and one of the presenting symptoms is unilateral hearing loss due to fluid in the middle ear caused by eustachian tube obstruction from the cancer. Smoking-induced cancers of the oral cavity, pharynx, larynx, and lung are common throughout the world, including in the United States.

The palate, tongue, cheeks, lips, and teeth articulate the sound modified by the resonators into speech. Cigarettes, cigar, or pipe smoking may cause a "black hairy tongue," precancerous oral lesions (leuko-plakia), and/or cancer of the tongue and lips.[18] Any irritation that causes burning or inflammation of the oral mucosa can affect phonation, and all tobacco products are capable of causing these effects.

Smokeless "spit" tobacco is highly addictive, and users who dip 8 to 10 times a day may get the same nicotine exposure as those who smoke 1½ to 2 packs of cigarettes per day.[19] Smokeless tobacco has been associated with gingivitis, cheek carcinoma, and cancer of the larynx and hypopharynx.

Exposure to environmental tobacco smoke (ETS), also called secondhand smoke, sidestream smoke, or passive smoke, accounts for an estimated 3000 lung cancer deaths and approximately 35 000 deaths in the United States from heart disease in non-smoking adults.[20]

Secondhand smoke is the "passive" inhalation of tobacco smoke from environmental sources such as smoke given off by pipes, cigars, cigarettes (sidestream), or the smoke exhaled from the lungs of smokers and inhaled by other people (mainstream). This passive smoke contains a mixture of thousands of chemicals, some of which are known to cause cancer. The National Institutes of Health (NIH) lists ETS as a "known" carcinogen, and the more you are exposed to secondhand smoke, the greater your risk.[21]

Infants and young children are affected particularly by secondhand smoke with increased incidences of otitis media (ear infections), bronchitis, and pneumonia. If small children are exposed to secondhand smoke, the child's resulting illness can have a stressful effect on the parent who frequently catches the child's illness. Both the illness and the stress of caring for the sick child may interfere with voice performance. People who are exposed routinely to secondhand smoke are at risk for lung cancer, heart disease, respiratory infection, and an increased number of asthma attacks.[22]

There is an intricate relationship between the lungs, larynx, pharynx, nose, and mouth in the production of speech and song. Smoking can have deleterious effects on any part of the vocal tract, causing the respiratory system to lose power, damaging the vibratory margins of the vocal folds, and detracting from the richness and beauty of a voice.

The deleterious effects of tobacco smoke on mucosa are indisputable. Anyone concerned about the health of his or her voice should not smoke. Smoking causes erythema, mild edema, and generalized inflammation throughout the vocal tract. Both smoke itself and the heat of the cigarette appear to be important. Marijuana produces a particularly irritating, unfiltered smoke that is inhaled directly, causing considerable mucosal response. Voice patients who refuse to stop smoking marijuana should at least be advised to use a water pipe to cool and partially filter the smoke. Some vocalists are required to perform in smoke-filled environments and may suffer the same effects as the smokers themselves. In some theaters, it is possible to place fans upstage or direct the ventilation system so as to create a gentle draft toward the audience, clearing the smoke away from the stage. "Smoke eaters" installed in some theaters are also helpful.

Do Any Foods Seem to Affect Your Voice?

Various foods are said to affect the voice. Traditionally, singers avoid milk and ice cream before performances. In many people, these foods seem to increase the amount and viscosity of mucosal secretions. Allergy and casein have been implicated, but no satisfactory explanation has been established. In some cases, restriction of these foods from the diet before a voice performance may be helpful. Chocolate may have the same effect and should be viewed similarly. Chocolate also contains caffeine, which may aggravate reflux or cause tremor. Voice patients should be asked about eating nuts. This is important not only because some people experience effects similar to those produced by milk products and chocolate but also because they are extremely irritating if aspirated. The irritation produced by aspiration of even a small organic foreign body may be severe and impossible to correct rapidly enough to permit performance. Highly spiced foods may also cause mucosal irritation. In addition, they seem to aggravate reflux laryngitis. Coffee and other beverages containing caffeine also aggravate gastric reflux and may promote dehydration and/ or alter secretions and necessitate frequent throat clearing in some people. Fad diets, especially rapid weight-reducing diets, are notorious for causing voice problems. Eating a full meal before a speaking or singing engagement may interfere with abdominal support or may aggravate upright reflux of gastric juice during abdominal muscle contraction. Lemon juice and herbal teas are considered beneficial to the voice. Both may act as demulcents, thinning secretions, and may very well be helpful.

Do You Have Morning Hoarseness, Bad Breath, Excessive Phlegm, a Lump in Your Throat, or Heartburn?

Reflux laryngitis is especially common among singers and trained speakers because of the high intraabdominal pressure associated with proper support and because of lifestyle. Singers frequently perform at night. Many vocalists refrain from eating before performances because a full stomach can compromise effective abdominal support. They typically compensate by eating heartily at postperformance gatherings late at night and then go to bed with a full stomach.

Chronic irritation of arytenoid and vocal fold mucosa by reflux of gastric secretions may occasionally be associated with dyspepsia or pyrosis. However, the key features of this malady are bitter taste and halitosis on awakening in the morning, a dry or "coated" mouth, often a scratchy sore throat or a feeling of a "lump in the throat," hoarseness, and the need for prolonged vocal warm-up. The physician must be alert to these symptoms and ask about them routinely; otherwise, the diagnosis will often be overlooked, because people who have had this problem for many years or a lifetime do not even realize it is abnormal.

Do You Have Trouble With Your Bowels or Belly?

Any condition that alters abdominal function, such as muscle spasm, constipation, or diarrhea, interferes with support and may result in a voice complaint. These symptoms may accompany infection, anxiety, various gastroenterological diseases, and other maladies.

Are You Under Particular Stress or in Therapy?

The human voice is an exquisitely sensitive messenger of emotion. Highly trained voice professionals learn to control the effects of anxiety and other emotional stress on their voices under ordinary circumstances. However, in some instances, this training may break down or a performer may be inadequately prepared to control the voice under specific stressful conditions. Preperformance anxiety is the most common example, but insecurity, depression, and other emotional disturbances are also generally reflected in the voice. Anxiety reactions are mediated in part through the autonomic nervous system and result in a dry mouth, cold clammy skin, and thick secretions. These reactions are normal, and good vocal training coupled with assurance that no abnormality or disease is present generally overcomes them. However, long-term, poorly compensated emotional stress and exogenous stress (from agents, producers, teachers, parents, etc) may cause substantial vocal dysfunction and may result in permanent limitations of the vocal apparatus. These conditions must be diagnosed and treated expertly. Hypochondriasis is uncommon among professional singers, despite popular opinion to the contrary.

Recent publications have highlighted the complexity and importance of psychological factors associated with voice disorders.[23] A comprehensive discussion of this subject is also presented elsewhere in this book. It is important for the physician to recognize that psychological problems may not only cause voice disorders but also delay recovery from voice disorders that were entirely organic in etiology. Professional voice users, especially singers, have enormous psychological investment and personality identifications associated with their voices. A condition that causes voice loss or permanent injury often evokes the same powerful psychological responses seen following death of a loved one. This process may be initiated even when physical recovery is complete if an incident (injury or surgery) has made the vocalist realize that voice loss is possible. Such a "brush with death" can have profound emotional consequences in some patients. It is essential for laryngologists to be aware of these powerful factors and manage them properly if optimal therapeutic results are to be achieved expeditiously.

Do You Have Problems Controlling Your Weight? Are You Excessively Tired? Are You Cold When Other People Are Warm?

Endocrine problems warrant special attention. The human voice is extremely sensitive to endocrinologic changes. Many of these are reflected in alterations of fluid content of the lamina propria just beneath the laryngeal mucosa. This causes alterations in the bulk and shape of the vocal folds and results in voice change. Hypothyroidism[24–28] is a well-recognized cause of such voice disorders, although the mechanism is not fully understood. Hoarseness, vocal fatigue, muffling of the voice, loss of range, and a sensation of a lump in the throat may be present even with mild hypothyroidism. Even when thyroid function tests results are within the low normal range, this diagnosis should be entertained, especially if thyroid-stimulating hormone levels are in the high normal range or are elevated. Thyrotoxicosis may result in similar voice disturbances.[25]

Do You Have Menstrual Irregularity, Cyclical Voice Changes Associated With Menses, Recent Menopause, or Other Hormonal Changes or Problems?

Voice changes associated with sex hormones are encountered commonly in clinical practice and have been investigated more thoroughly than have other hormonal changes.[29,30] Although a correlation appears to exist between sex hormone levels and depth of male voices (higher testosterone and lower estradiol levels in basses than in tenors),[29] the most important hormonal considerations in males occur during or related to puberty.[31,32] Voice problems related to sex hormones are more common in female singers.[33–49]

Do You Have Jaw Joint or Other Dental Problems?

Dental disease, especially temporomandibular joint (TMJ) dysfunction, introduces muscle tension in the head and neck, which is transmitted to the larynx directly through the muscular attachments between the mandible and the hyoid bone and indirectly as generalized increased muscle tension. These problems often result in decreased range, vocal fatigue, and change in the quality or placement of a voice. Such tension often is accompanied by excess tongue muscle activity, especially pulling of the tongue posteriorly. This hyperfunctional behavior acts through hyoid attachments to disrupt the balance between the intrinsic and extrinsic

laryngeal musculature. TMJ problems are also problematic for wind instrumentalists and some string players, including violinists. In some cases, the problems may actually be caused by instrumental technique. The history should always include information about musical activities, including instruments other than the voice.

Do You or Your Blood Relatives Have Hearing Loss?

Hearing loss is often overlooked as a source of vocal problems. Auditory feedback is fundamental to speaking and singing. Interference with this control mechanism may result in altered vocal production, particularly if the person is unaware of the hearing loss. Distortion, particularly pitch distortion (diplacusis), may also pose serious problems for the singer. This appears to be due not only to aesthetic difficulties in matching pitch but also to vocal strain that accompanies pitch shifts.[50]

In addition to determining whether the patient has hearing loss, inquiry should also be made about hearing impairment occurring in family members, roommates, and other close associates. Speaking loudly to people who are hard of hearing can cause substantial, chronic vocal strain. This possibility should be investigated routinely when evaluating voice patients.

Have You Suffered Whiplash or Other Bodily Injury?

Various bodily injuries outside the confines of the vocal tract may have profound effects on the voice. Whiplash, for example, commonly causes changes in technique, with consequent voice fatigue, loss of range, difficulty singing softly, and other problems. These problems derive from the neck muscle spasm, abnormal neck posturing secondary to pain, and consequent hyperfunctional voice use. Lumbar, abdominal, head, chest, supraglottic, and extremity injuries may also affect vocal technique and be responsible for the dysphonia that prompted the voice patient to seek medical attention.

Did You Undergo Any Surgery Prior to the Onset of Your Voice Problems?

A history of laryngeal surgery in a voice patient is a matter of great concern. It is important to establish exactly why the surgery was done, by whom it was done, whether intubation was necessary, and whether voice therapy was instituted preor postoperatively if the lesion was associated with voice abuse (vocal nodules). If the vocal dysfunction that sent the patient to the physician's office dates from the immediate postoperative period, surgical trauma must be suspected.

Otolaryngologists frequently are asked about the effects of tonsillectomy on the voice. Singers especially may consult the physician after tonsillectomy and complain of vocal dysfunction. Certainly removal of tonsils can alter the voice.[51,52] Tonsillectomy changes the configuration of the supraglottic vocal tract. In addition, scarring alters pharyngeal muscle function, which is trained meticulously in the professional singer. Singers must be warned that they may have permanent voice changes after tonsillectomy; however, these can be minimized by dissecting in the proper plane to lessen scarring. The singer's voice generally requires 3 to 6 months to stabilize or return to normal after surgery, although it is generally safe to begin limited singing within 2 to 4 weeks following surgery. As with any procedure for which general anesthesia may be needed, the anesthesiologist should be advised preoperatively that the patient is a professional singer. Intubation and extubation should be performed with great care, and the use of nonirritating plastic rather than rubber or ribbed metal endotracheal tubes is preferred. Use of a laryngeal mask may be advisable for selected procedures for mechanical reasons, but this device is often not ideal for tonsillectomy, and it can cause laryngeal injury such as arytenoid dislocation.

Surgery of the neck, such as thyroidectomy, may result in permanent alterations in the vocal mechanism through scarring of the extrinsic laryngeal musculature. The cervical (strap) muscles are important in maintaining laryngeal position and stability of the laryngeal skeleton, and they should be retracted rather than divided whenever possible. A history of recurrent or superior laryngeal nerve injury may explain a hoarse, breathy, or weak voice. However, in rare cases, even a singer can compensate for recurrent laryngeal nerve paralysis and have a nearly normal voice.

Thoracic and abdominal surgery interferes with respiratory and abdominal support. After these procedures, singing and projected speaking should be prohibited until pain has subsided and healing has occurred sufficiently to allow normal support. Abdominal exercises should be instituted before resumption of vocalizing. Singing and speaking without proper support are often worse for the voice than not using the voice for performance at all.

Other surgical procedures may be important factors if they necessitate intubation or if they affect the musculoskeletal system so that the person has to change stance or balance. For example, balancing on one foot after leg surgery may decrease the effectiveness of the support mechanism.

What Medications and Other Substances Do You Use?

A history of alcohol abuse suggests the probability of poor vocal technique. Intoxication results in incoordination and decreased awareness, which undermine vocal discipline designed to optimize and protect the voice. The effect of small amounts of alcohol is controversial. Although many experts oppose its use because of its vasodilatory effect and consequent mucosal alteration, many people do not seem to be adversely affected by small amounts of alcohol such as a glass of wine with a meal. However, some people have mild sensitivities to certain wines or beers. Patients who develop nasal congestion and rhinorrhea after drinking beer, for example, should be made aware that they probably have a mild allergy to that particular beverage and should avoid it before voice commitments.

Patients frequently acquire antihistamines to help control "postnasal drip" or other symptoms. The drying effect of antihistamines may result in decreased vocal fold lubrication, increased throat clearing, and irritability leading to frequent coughing. Antihistamines may be helpful to some voice patients, but they must be used with caution.

When a voice patient seeking the attention of a physician is already taking antibiotics, it is important to find out the dose and the prescribing physician, if any, as well as whether the patient frequently treats himself or herself with inadequate courses of antibiotics often supplied by colleagues. Singers, actors, and other speakers sometimes have a "sore throat" shortly before important vocal presentations and start themselves on inappropriate antibiotic therapy, which they generally discontinue after their performance.

Diuretics are also popular among some performers. They are often prescribed by gynecologists at the vocalist's request to help deplete excess water in the premenstrual period. They are not effective in this scenario, because they cannot diurese the protein-bound water in the laryngeal ground substance. Unsupervised use of these drugs may cause dehydration and consequent mucosal dryness.

Hormone use, especially use of oral contraceptives, must be mentioned specifically during the physician's inquiry. Women frequently do not mention them routinely when asked whether they are taking any medication. Vitamins are also frequently not mentioned. Most vitamin therapy seems to have little effect on the voice. However, high-dose vitamin C (5 to 6 g/d), which some people use to prevent upper respiratory tract infections, seems to act as a mild diuretic and may lead to dehydration and xerophonia.[53]

Cocaine use is common, especially among pop musicians. This drug can be extremely irritating to the nasal mucosa, causes marked vasoconstriction, and may alter the sensorium, resulting in decreased voice control and a tendency toward vocal abuse.

Many pain medications (including aspirin and ibuprofen), psychotropic medications, and others may be responsible for a voice complaint. So far, no adverse vocal effects have been reported with selective COX-2 inhibiting anti-inflammatory medications (which do not promote bleeding, as do other nonsteroidal anti-inflammatory medicines and aspirin) such as celecoxib (Celebrex; Pfizer, Inc, New York, New York) and valecoxib (Bextra; Pharmacia Corp, New York, New York). However this group of drugs has been demonstrated to have other side effects, and should in our view only be taken under the care of a physician.[54] The effects of other new medications such as sildenafil citrate (Viagra; Pfizer, Inc) and medications used to induce abortion remain unstudied and unknown, but it seems plausible that such medication may affect voice function, at least temporarily. Laryngologists should be familiar with the laryngologic effects of the many substances ingested medically and recreationally.

References

1. Sataloff RT. Professional singers: the science and art of clinical care. *Am J Otolaryngol.* 1981;2:251–266.
2. Sataloff RT. The human voice. *Sci Am.* 1992; 267:108–115.
3. Sundberg J. *The Science of the Singing Voice.* DeKalb, IL: Northern Illinois University Press; 1987.
4. Sataloff RT. Efficient history taking in professional singers. *Laryngoscope.* 1984;94: 1111–1114.
5. Ackerman R, Pfan W. Gerontology studies on the susceptibility to voice disorders in professional speakers. *Folia Phoniatr (Basel).* 1974;26:95–99.
6. von Leden H. Speech and hearing problems in the geriatric patient. *J Am Geriatr Soc.* 1977;25:422–426.
7. Schiff M. *Comment.* Presented at: Seventh Symposium on Care of the Professional Voice; June 15–16, 1978; The Juilliard School, New York, NY.
8. Spiegel JR, Cohn JR, Sataloff RT, et al. Respiratory function in singers: medical assessment, diagnoses, treatments. *J Voice.* 1988;2:40–50.
9. Cohn JR, Sataloff RT, Spiegel JR, et al. Airway reactivity-induced asthma in singers (ARIAS). *J Voice.* 1991;5:332–337.
10. Feder RJ. The professional voice and airline flight. *Otolaryngol Head Neck Surg.* 1984;92: 251–254.
11. Anticaglia A, Hawkshaw M, Sataloff RT. The effects of smoking on voice performance. *J Singing.* 2004;60:161–167.
12. Centers for Disease Control and Prevention (CDC). Annual smoking-attributable, mortality, years of potential life lost, and economic costs, United States—1995–1999. *MMWR Morb Mortal Wkly Rep.* 2002;51(14): 300–303.
13. World Health Organization. *World Health Report 1999.* Geneva, Switzerland: World Health Organization; 1999.
14. United States Department of Health Services (USDHHS). *Tobacco Products Fact Sheet.* Washington, DC: Government Printing Office; 2000.
15. National Cancer Institute. Environmental tobacco smoke. *Fact sheet* 3.9;1999. http// cis.nci.nih.gov/fact/3_9htm
16. Centers for Disease Control and Prevention. Cigarette smoking among adults—United States, 1993. *MMWR Morb Mortal Wkly Rep.* 1994;3:925–929.
17. Chow WH, McLaughlin JK, Hrubec Z, et al. Tobacco use and nasopharyngeal carcinoma in a cohort of US veterans. *Int J Cancer.* 1993;55(4):538–540.
18. Casiglia J, Woo, SB. A comprehensive view of oral cancer. *Gen Dent.* 2001;49(1):72–82.
19. Centers for Disease Control and Prevention. Determination of nicotine pH and moisture content of six U.S. commercial moist snuff products. *MMWR Morb Mortal Wkly Rep.* 1999;48(19):398.
20. American Cancer Society. *Cancer Facts and Figures 2002.* Atlanta, GA: American Cancer Society; 2002.
21. National Toxicology Program (NTP). *Report on Carcinogens.* 10th ed. Research Triangle Park, NC: U.S. Department Health and Human Services, Public Health Service, National Toxicology Program; 2002. http:// ehp.niehs.nih.gov/roc/toc10.html
22. Academy of Pediatrics, Committee on Environmental Health. Environmental tobacco smoke; a hazard to children. *Pediatrics.* 1997;99(4):639–642.

23. Rosen DC, Sataloff RT. *Psychology of Voice Disorders*. San Diego, CA: Singular Publishing Group; 1997.

24. Gupta OP, Bhatia PL, Agarwal MK, et al. Nasal pharyngeal and laryngeal manifestations of hypothyroidism. *Ear Nose Throat J.* 1997;56:10–21.

25. Malinsky M, Chevrie-Muller, Cerceau N. Etude clinique et electrophysiologique des alterations de la voix au cours des thyrotoxioses. *Ann Endocrinol (Paris).* 1997;38: 171–172.

26. Michelsson K, Sirvio P. Cry analysis in congenital hypothyroidism. *Folia Phoniatr (Basel).* 1976;28:40–47.

27. Ritter FN. The effect of hypothyroidism on the larynx of the rat. *Ann Otol Rhinol Laryngol.* 1964;67:404–416.

28. Ritter FN. Endocrinology. In: Paparella M, Shumrick D, eds. *Otolaryngology*. Vol. I. Philadelphia, PA: Saunders; 1973:727–734.

29. Meuser W, Nieschlag E. Sex hormones and depth of voice in the male [in German]. *Dtsch Med Wochenschr.* 1977:102:261–264.

30. Schiff M. The influence of estrogens on connective tissue. In: Asboe-Hansen G, ed. *Hormones and Connective Tissue*. Copenhagen, Denmark: Munksgaard Press; 1967: 282–341.

31. Brodnitz F. The age of the castrato voice. *J Speech Hear Disord.* 1975;40:291–295.

32. Brodnitz F. Hormones and the human voice. *Bull NY Acad Med.* 1971;47:183–191.

33. Carroll C. Personal communication with Dr. Hans von Leden; 1992; Arizona State University at Tempe.

34. von Gelder L. Psychosomatic aspects of endocrine disorders of the voice. *J Commun Disord.* 1974;7:257–262.

35. Lacina O. Der Einfluss der Menstruation auf die Stimme der Sangerinnen. *Folia Phoniatr (Basel).* 1968;20:13–24.

36. Wendler J. The influence of menstruation on the voice of the female singer. *Folia Phoniatr (Basel).* 1972;24:259–277.

37. Brodnitz F. Medical care preventive therapy (panel). In: Lawrence VL, ed. *Transcripts of the Seventh Annual Symposium, Care of the Professional Voice*. Vol. 3. New York, NY: The Voice Foundation; 1978:86.

38. Dordain M. Etude Statistique de l'influence des contraceptifs hormonaux sur la voix. *Folia Phoniatr (Basel).* 1972;24:86–96.

39. Pahn J, Goretzlehner G. Voice changes following the use of oral contraceptives [in German]. *Zentralbl Gynakol.* 1978;100:341–346.

40. Schiff M. "The pill" in otolaryngology. *Trans Am Acad Ophthalmol Otolaryngol.* 1968;72: 76–84.

41. von Deuster CV. Irreversible vocal changes in pregnancy [in German]. *HNO.* 1977;25: 430–432.

42. Flach M, Schwickardi H, Simen R. Welchen Einfluss haben Menstruation und Schwangerschaft auf die augsgebildete Gesangsstimme? *Folia Phoniatr (Basel).* 1968;21: 199–210.

43. Arndt HJ. Stimmstorungen nach Behandlung mit Androgenen und anabolen Hormonen. *Munch Med Wochenschr.* 1974;116: 1715–1720.

44. Bourdial J. Les troubles de la voix provoques par la therapeutique hormonale androgene. *Ann Otolaryngol Chir Cervicofac.* 1970;87: 725–734.

45. Damste PH. Virilization of the voice due to anabolic steroids [in Dutch]. *Ned Tijdschr Geneeskd.* 1963;107:891–892.

46. Damste PH. Voice changes in adult women caused by virilizing agents. *J Speech Hear Disord.* 1967;32:126–132.

47. Saez S, Francoise S. Recepteurs d'androgenes: mise en evidence dans la fraction cytosolique de muqueuse normale et d'epitheliomas phryngolarynges humains. *C R Acad Sci Hebd Seances Acad Sci D.* 1975;280:935–938.

48. Vuorenkoski V, Lenko HL, Tjernlund P, et al. Fundamental voice frequency during normal and abnormal growth, and after androgen treatment. *Arch Dis Child.* 1978;53: 201–209.

49. Imre V. Hormonell bedingte Stimmstorungen. *Folia Phoniatr (Basel).* 1968;20:394–404.

50. Sundberg J, Prame E, Iwarsson J. Replicability and accuracy of pitch patterns in professional singers. In: Davis PJ, Fletcher NH,

eds. *Vocal Fold Physiology: Controlling Chaos and Complexity.* San Diego, CA: Singular Publishing Group; 1996:291–306.

51. Gould WJ, Alberti PW, Brodnitz F, Hirano M. Medical care preventive therapy [Panel]. In: Lawrence VL, ed. *Transcripts of the Seventh Annual Symposium, Care of the Professional Voice.* Vol. 3. New York, NY: The Voice Foundation; 1978:74–76.

52. Wallner LJ, Hill BJ, Waldrop W, Monroe C. Voice changes following adenotonsillectomy. *Laryngoscope.* 1968;78:1410–1418.

53. Lawrence VL. Medical care for professional voice (panel). In: Lawrence VL, ed. *Transcripts from the Annual Symposium, Care of the Professional Voice.* Vol. 3. New York, NY: The Voice Foundation; 1978:17–18.

54. Cannon CP. COX-2 inhibitors and cardiovascular risk. *Science.* 2012;336(6087): 1386–1387.

APPENDIX 3–A

Patient History Form for Professional Voice Users

Name _____ Age _____ Sex _____ Race _____

Height _____ Weight _____ Date _____

How long have you had your present voice problem?

   Who noticed it?

   Do you know what caused it?   Yes   No

   If so, what?

   Did it come on slowly or suddenly?   Slowly   Suddenly

   Is it getting: Worse   Better   Same?

Which symptoms do you have? (Please check all that apply.)

   Hoarseness (coarse or scratchy sound)

   Fatigue (voice tires or changes quality after speaking for a short period of time)

   Volume disturbance (trouble speaking) softly, loudly

   Loss of range: high, low

   Prolonged warm-up time (over ½ hour to warm up)

   Breathiness

   Tickling or choking sensation while speaking

   Pain in throat while speaking

   Other (Please specify):

Have you ever had training for your singing voice?

   Yes   No

Have there been periods of months or years without lessons in that time?

   Yes   No

How long have you studied with your present teacher?

   Teacher's name:

   Teacher's address:

   Teacher's telephone number:

Please list previous teachers and years during which you studied with them:

In what capacity do you use your voice professionally?

    Actor

    Announcer (television/radio/sports arena)

    Attorney

    Clergy

    Politician

    Salesperson

    Teacher

    Telephone operator or receptionist

    Other (Please specify):

Do you have an important performance soon?

    Yes   No

    Date(s):

Do you do regular voice exercises?

    Yes   No

    If yes, describe:

Do you play a musical instrument?

    Yes   No

    If yes, please check all that apply:

        Keyboard (Piano, Organ, Harpsichord, Other _____)

        Violin, Viola, Cello

        Bass

        Plucked Strings (Guitar, Harp, Other _____)

        Brass

        Wind with single reed

        Wind with double reed

        Flute, Piccolo

        Percussion

        Bagpipe

        Accordion

        Other (Please specify):

Do you warm up your voice before practice or performance?

   Yes   No

Do you cool down after using it?

   Yes   No

How much are you speaking at present (average hours per day)?

   Rehearsal   Performance   Other

Please check all that apply to you:

   Voice worse in the morning

   Voice worse later in the day, after it has been used

   Sing performances or rehearsals in the morning

   Speak extensively (teacher, clergy, attorney, telephone, work, etc)

   Cheerleader

   Speak extensively backstage or at postperformance parties

   Choral conductor

   Frequently clear your throat

   Frequent sore throat

   Jaw joint problems

   Bitter or acid taste; bad breath or hoarseness first thing in the morning

   Frequent "heartburn" or hiatal hernia

   Frequent yelling or loud talking

   Frequent whispering

   Chronic fatigue (insomnia)

   Work around extreme dryness

   Frequent exercise (weight lifting, aerobics, etc)

   Frequently thirsty, dehydrated

   Hoarseness first thing in the morning

   Chest cough

   Eat late at night

   Ever use antacids

   Under particular stress at present (personal or professional)

   Frequent bad breath

   Live, work, or perform around smoke and fumes

Traveled recently:

When:

Where:

Your family doctor's name, address, and telephone number:

Your laryngologist's name, address, and telephone number:

Recent cold?

Yes   No

Current cold?

Yes   No

Have you been evaluated by an allergist?

Yes   No

If yes, what allergies do you have?

[none, dust, mold, trees, cats, dogs, foods, other]

If yes, give name and address of allergist:

Are you allergic to any medications?   Yes   No

If yes, please list:

How many packs of cigarettes do you smoke per day?

Smoking history:

Never

Quit. When?

Smoked about _____ packs per day for _____ years.

Smoke _____ packs per day. Have smoked for _____ years.

Do you work in a smoky environment?

Yes   No

How much alcohol do you drink?

none   rarely   a few times per week   daily

If daily, or a few times per week, on the average, how much do you consume?

1   2   3   4   5   6   7   8   9   10 more   glasses per   day   week of   beer   wine   liquor

Did you drink more heavily in the past?

Yes   No

How many cups of coffee, tea, cola, or other caffeine-containing drinks do you drink per day?

List other recreational drugs you use:

marijuana   amphetamines   barbiturates   heroin   other _____

Have you noticed any of the following? (Check all that apply.)

Hypersensitivity to heat or cold

Excessive sweating

Change in weight: gained/lost _____ lb. in _____ weeks/_____ months

Change in your voice

Change in skin or hair

Palpitation (fluttering) of the heart

Emotional lability (swings of mood)

Double vision

Numbness of the face or extremities

Tingling around the mouth or face

Blurred vision or blindness

Weakness or paralysis of the face

Clumsiness in arms or legs

Confusion or loss of consciousness

Difficulty with speech

Difficulty with swallowing

Seizure (epileptic fit)

Pain in the neck or shoulder

Shaking or tremors

Memory change

Personality change

For females:

    Are you pregnant?   Yes   No

    Are your menstrual periods regular?   Yes   No

    Have you undergone hysterectomy?   Yes   No

    Were your ovaries removed?   Yes   No

    At what age did you reach puberty?

    Have you gone through menopause?   Yes   No

Have you ever consulted a psychologist or psychiatrist?

    Yes   No

Are you currently under treatment?

    Yes   No

Have you injured your head or neck (whiplash, etc)?

    Yes   No

Describe any serious accidents related to this visit:

Are you involved in legal action involving problems with your voice?

    Yes   No

List names of spouse and children:

Brief summary of ENT problems, some of which may not be related to your present complaint.

Hearing loss	Nosebleeds
Ear pain	Mouth sores
Ear noises	Trouble swallowing
Facial pain	Trouble breathing
Lump in face or head	Eye problem
Lump in neck	Excess eye skin
Dizziness	Excessive facial skin
Stiff neck	Jaw joint problem
Facial paralysis	Other (please specify):
Nasal obstruction	
Nasal deformity	

Do you have or have you ever had:

Diabetes	Heart attack
Seizures	Angina
Hypoglycemia	Irregular heartbeat
Psychological therapy or counseling	Rheumatic fever
Thyroid problems	Other heart problems
Frequent bad headaches	Unexplained weight loss
Syphilis	Cancer of _____
Ulcers	Other tumor _____
Gonorrhea	Blood transfusions
Herpes	Hepatitis
Urinary problems	Tuberculosis
Cold sores (fever blisters)	AIDS
Arthritis or skeletal	Glaucoma
High blood pressure problems	Meningitis
Severe low blood pressure	Multiple sclerosis
Cleft palate	Other illnesses (Please specify):
Intravenous antibiotics or diuretics	
Asthma, lung or breathing problems	

Do any blood relatives have:
   Diabetes
   Hypoglycemia
   Cancer
   Heart disease

Other major medical problems such as those listed above.
   Please specify:

Describe serious accident unless directly related to your doctor's visit here.
   None
   Occurred with head injury, loss of consciousness, or whiplash
   Occurred without head injury, loss of consciousness, or whiplash
   Describe:

List all current medications and doses (include birth control pills and vitamins).

    None

    Aspirin

    Codeine

    Medication for allergies

    Novocaine

    Penicillin

    Sulfamides

    Tetracycline

    Erythromycin

    Keflex/Ceclor/Ceftin

    Iodine

    X-ray dyes

    Adhesive tape

    Other (Please specify):

List operations:

    Tonsillectomy (age _____)

    Adenoidectomy (age _____)

    Appendectomy (age _____)

    Heart surgery (age _____)

    Other (Please specify):

List toxic drugs or chemicals to which you have been exposed:

    Streptomycin, Neomycin, Kanamycin

    Lead

    Mercury

    Other (Please list):

Have you had x-ray treatments to your head or neck (including treatments for acne or ear problems as a child), treatments for cancer, etc?

    Yes   No

    Describe serious health problems of your spouse or children:

4

Physical Examination*

Robert Thayer Sataloff

Physical Examination

A detailed history frequently reveals the cause of a voice problem even before a physical examination is performed. However, a comprehensive physical examination, often including objective assessment of voice function, also is essential.[1-3] In response to feedback from readers of the previous editions, this chapter has been expanded to include a brief overview of objective voice assessment, and other subjects covered more comprehensively in subsequent chapters. This overview is provided here for the reader's convenience.

Physical examination must include a thorough ear, nose, and throat evaluation and assessment of general physical condition. A patient who is extremely obese or appears fatigued, agitated, emotionally stressed, or otherwise generally ill has increased potential for voice dysfunction. This could be due to any number of factors: altered abdominal support, loss of fine motor control of laryngeal muscles, decreased bulk of the submucosal vocal fold ground substance, change in the character of mucosal secretions, or other similar mechanisms. Any physical condition that impairs the normal function of the abdominal musculature is suspect as cause for dysphonia. Some conditions, such as pregnancy, are obvious; however, a sprained ankle or broken leg that requires the singer to balance in an unaccustomed posture may distract him or her from maintaining good abdominal support and thereby result in voice dysfunction. A tremorous neurologic disorder, endocrine disturbances such as thyroid dysfunction or menopause, the aging process, and other systemic conditions also may alter the voice. The physician must remember that maladies of almost any body system may result in voice dysfunction, and the doctor must remain alert for conditions outside the head and neck. If the patient uses his or her voice professionally for singing, acting, or other vocally demanding professions, physical examination should also include assessment of the patient during typical professional vocal tasks. For example, a singer should be asked to sing.

---

*Reprinted with permission from Rubin J, Sataloff R, Korovin G. *Diagnosis and Treatment of Voice Disorders*. 4th ed. San Diego, CA: Plural Publishing; 2014.

Complete Ear, Nose, and Throat Examination

Examination of the ears must include assessment of hearing acuity. Even a relatively slight hearing loss may result in voice strain as a singer tries to balance his or her vocal intensity with that of associate performers. Similar effects are encountered among speakers, but they are less prominent in the early stages of hearing loss. This is especially true of hearing losses acquired after vocal training has been completed. The effect is most pronounced with sensorineural hearing loss. Diplacusis, distortion of pitch perception, makes vocal strain even worse. With conductive hearing loss, singers tend to sing more softly than appropriate rather than too loudly, and this is less harmful.

During an ear, nose, and throat examination, the conjunctivae and sclerae should be observed routinely for erythema that suggests allergy or irritation, for pallor that suggests anemia, and for other abnormalities such as jaundice. These observations may reveal the problem reflected in the vocal tract even before the larynx is visualized. Hearing loss in a spouse may be problematic as well if the voice professional strains vocally to communicate.

The nose should be assessed for patency of the nasal airway, character of the nasal mucosa, and nature of secretions, if any. A patient who is unable to breathe through the nose because of anatomic obstruction is forced to breathe unfiltered, unhumidified air through the mouth. Pale gray allergic mucosa or swollen infected mucosa in the nose suggests abnormal mucosa elsewhere in the respiratory tract.

Examination of the oral cavity should include careful attention to the tonsils and lymphoid tissue in the posterior pharyngeal wall, as well as to the mucosa. Diffuse lymphoid hypertrophy associated with a complaint of "scratchy" voice and irritative cough may indicate infection. The amount and viscosity of mucosal and salivary secretions also should be noted. Xerostomia is particularly important. The presence of scalloping of the lateral aspects of the tongue should be noted. This finding is caused commonly by tongue thrust and may be associated with inappropriate tongue tension and muscle tension dysphonia. Dental examination should focus not only on oral hygiene but also on the presence of wear facets suggestive of bruxism. Bruxism is a clue to excessive tension and may be associated with dysfunction of the temporomandibular joints, which should also be assessed routinely. Thinning of the enamel of the central incisors in a normal or underweight patient may be a clue to bulimia. However, it may also result from excessive ingestion of lemons, which some singers eat to help thin their secretions.

The neck should be examined for masses, restriction of movement, excess muscle tension and/or spasm, and scars from prior neck surgery or trauma. Laryngeal vertical mobility is also important. For example, tilting of the larynx produced by partial fixation of cervical muscles cut during previous surgery may produce voice dysfunction, as may fixation of the trachea to overlying neck skin. Particular attention should be paid to the thyroid gland. Examination of posterior neck muscles and range of motion should not be neglected. The cranial nerves should also be examined. Diminished fifth nerve sensation, diminished gag reflex, palatal deviation, or other mild cranial nerve deficits may indicate cranial polyneuropathy. Postviral, infectious neuropathies may involve the superior laryngeal nerve(s) and cause weakness of the vocal fold muscle secondary to decreased neural input, fatigability, and loss of range and projection in the voice. The recurrent laryngeal nerve is also affected in some cases. More serious neurologic disease may also be associated with such symptoms and signs.

Laryngeal Examination

Examination of the larynx begins when the singer or other voice patient enters the physician's office. The range, ease, volume, and quality of the speaking voice should be noted. If the examination is not being conducted in the patient's native language, the physician should be sure to listen to a sample of the patient's mother tongue, as well. Voice use is often different under the strain or habits of foreign language use. Rating scales of the speaking voice may be helpful.[4,5] The classification proposed by the Japanese Society of Logopedics and Phoniatrics is one of the most widely used. It is known commonly as the GRBAS Voice Rating Scale and is discussed below in the section on psychoacoustic evaluation.[6]

Physicians are not usually experts in voice classification. However, the physicians should at least be able to discriminate substantial differences in range and timbre, such as between bass and tenor, or alto and soprano. Although the correlation between speaking and singing voices is not perfect, a speaker with a low, comfortable bass voice who reports that he is a tenor may be misclassified and singing inappropriate roles with consequent voice strain. This judgment should be deferred to an expert, but the observation should lead the physician to make the appropriate referral. Excessive volume or obvious strain during speaking clearly indicates that voice abuse is present and may be contributing to the patient's singing complaint. The speaking voice can be evaluated more consistently and accurately using standardized reading passages, and such assessments are performed

routinely by speech-language pathologists, by phoniatricians, and sometimes by laryngologists.

The definition of "register" or "registration" is controversial, and many different terms are used by musicians and scientists. Often, the definitions are unclear. Terms to describe register include chest, creek, falsetto, head, heavy, light, little, low, middle, modal, normal, pulse, upper, vocal fry, voce di petto, voce di mista, voce di testa, and whistle (also called flageolet and flute register). A register is a range of frequencies that has a consistent quality or timbre. The break between registers is an area of instability called the passaggio. During vocal training, singers are taught to integrate qualities of their various registers and to smooth and obscure the transition between registers. Registers occur not only in voices but also in some instruments, notably the organ. Vocal register changes are associated with changes in laryngeal musculature and in vocal fold shape. For example, in chest register, contraction of the thyroarytenoid muscles causes thickening of the vocal folds, with a square-shaped glottis and large vibratory margin contact area. In falsetto in men and head voice in women, cricothyroid muscle contraction is dominant, vocal folds are elongated, and the contact area is much thinner and more triangular than in chest voice. Vertical phase differences are diminished in head voice in comparison with chest voice. Controversy remains on the use of traditional terms in males such as chest, middle, head and falsetto register, or chest and head register in females. Voice scientists commonly prefer terms such as modal register. In any case, health care professionals should understand that there is a difference between the terms *register* and *range*. For example, if a singer complains of inability to sing high notes, this should be described as a loss of upper range, not a loss of upper register. Register and range difficulties should be noted.

Vibrato is a fluctuation of the fundamental frequency of a note. It is produced by the vocal mechanism under neural control and is present naturally in adult voices. The primary components of vibrato include rate (the number of frequency fluctuations per second), extent (number of Hertz of fluctuation above and below the center frequency), regularity (consistency of frequency variations from one cycle to the next), and wave form. Rate and extent have been studied most extensively and are arguably the most important components in determining how the vibrato is perceived. Natural vibrato generally is about 6 Hz. Vibrato rate is slower in males than in females, and vocal pitch and effort do not have a substantial influence on vibrato. However, singers are able to alter vibrato rate and pitch oscillation voluntarily for stylistic purposes. The athletic choice of vibrato rate varies over time. For example, vibrato rates of 6 to 7 Hz were popular in classical Western (operatic) singing in the early 20th century, but a vibrato rate of 5.5 to 6 Hz was considered more attractive by the end of the 20th century. In general, pitch fluctuation covers about 1 semitone (half a semitone above and half a semitone below the center frequency) at present. A prominent wobble, as may be heard in some elderly singers who are not in ideal physical and vocal condition generally, is referred to as a tremolo. The excessive pitch (and sometimes intensity) fluctuations are caused by muscle activity, sometimes with a respiratory component, and are superimposed on the individual's vibrato in most cases, rather than actually being a widened, distorted vibrato. The true source of natural vibrato is uncertain, although the larynx, pharynx, tongue, and other components of the vocal tract may move in concert with vibrato, as well as with tremolo.

Vibrato is thought not to be due primarily to phonatary structural activity rather than to respiratory source. The pressure of vibrato abnormalities or tremolo should be documented.

Any patient with a voice complaint should be examined by indirect laryngoscopy at least (Figure 4–1A). It is not possible to judge voice range, quality, or other vocal attributes by inspection of the vocal folds. However, the presence or absence of nodules, mass lesions, contact ulcers, hemorrhage, erythema, paralysis, arytenoid erythema (reflux), and other anatomic abnormalities must be established. Erythema and edema of the laryngeal surface of the epiglottis is seen often in association with muscle tension dysphonia and with frequent coughing or clearing of the throat. It is caused by direct trauma from the arytenoids during these maneuvers. The mirror or a laryngeal telescope often provides a better view of the posterior portion of the endolarynx than is obtained with flexible endoscopy. Stroboscopic examination adds substantially to diagnostic abilities (Figure 4–1B), as discussed below. Another occasionally helpful adjunct is the operating microscope. Magnification allows visualization of small mucosal disruptions and hemorrhages that may be significant but overlooked otherwise. This technique also allows photography of the larynx with a microscope camera. Magnification may also be achieved through magnifying laryngeal mirrors or by wearing loupes. Loupes usually provide a clearer image than do most of the magnifying mirrors available.

A laryngeal telescope may be combined with a stroboscope to provide excellent visualization of the vocal folds and related structures. The author usually uses a 70-degree laryngeal telescope, although 90-degree telescopes are required for some patients. The combination of a telescope

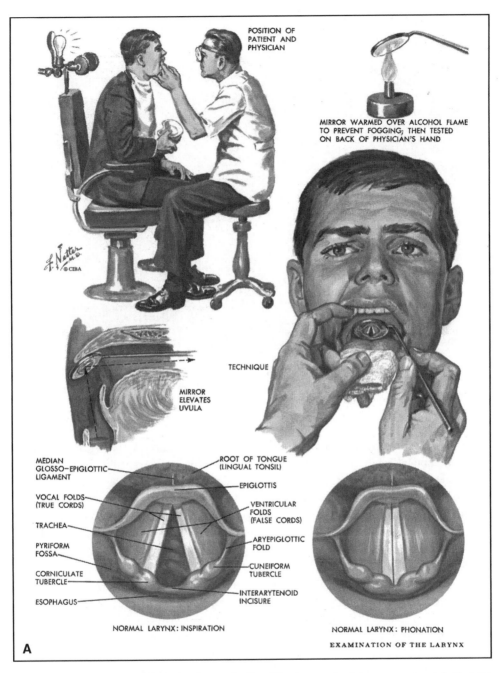

POSITION OF PATIENT AND PHYSICIAN

MIRROR WARMED OVER ALCOHOL FLAME TO PREVENT FOGGING; THEN TESTED ON BACK OF PHYSICIAN'S HAND

TECHNIQUE

MIRROR ELEVATES UVULA

MEDIAN GLOSSO–EPIGLOTTIC LIGAMENT

ROOT OF TONGUE (LINGUAL TONSIL)

EPIGLOTTIS

VOCAL FOLDS (TRUE CORDS)

VENTRICULAR FOLDS (FALSE CORDS)

TRACHEA

PYRIFORM FOSSA

ARYEPIGLOTTIC FOLD

CORNICULATE TUBERCLE

CUNEIFORM TUBERCLE

ESOPHAGUS

INTERARYTENOID INCISURE

NORMAL LARYNX: INSPIRATION

NORMAL LARYNX: PHONATION

A

EXAMINATION OF THE LARYNX

Figure 4–1. A. Traditional laryngeal examination. The laryngologist uses a warmed mirror to visualize the vocal fold indirectly. The tongue is grasped between the thumb and third finger. The thumb is placed as far posteriorly as possible in the middle third of the tongue (farther back than illustrated). The grip optimizes tongue depression and rotation. If the third finger is held firmly against the lower teeth and used to pivot rather than pull, discomfort along the frenulum can be avoided. The mirror is placed against the soft palate while the patient phonates on the vowel /i/. Placing the mirror during the phonation decreases the tendency to gag, and the vowel /i/ puts the larynx in the best position for visualization. (From the Larynx, *Clinical Symposia*, New Jersey: CIBA Pharmaceutical Company, 1964;16[3]: Plate VI. Copyright 1964. Icon Learning Systems, LLC, a subsidiary of MediMedia USA Inc. Reprinted with permission from Icon Learning Systems, LLC, illustrated by Frank H. Netter, MD. All rights reserved.) *(continues)*

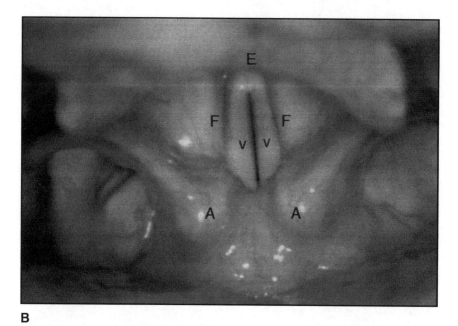

B

Figure 4–1. *(continued)* **B.** Normal larynx showing the true vocal folds (V), false vocal folds (F), arytenoids (A), and epiglottis (E).

and stroboscope provides optimal magnification and optical quality for assessment of vocal fold vibration. However, it is generally performed with the tongue in a fixed position, and the nature of the examination does not permit assessment of the larynx during normal phonatory gestures.

Flexible fiberoptic laryngoscopy can be performed as an office procedure and allows inspection of the vocal folds in patients whose vocal folds are difficult to visualize indirectly. In addition, it permits observation of the vocal mechanism in a more natural posture than does indirect laryngoscopy, permitting sophisticated dynamic voice assessment. In the hands of an experienced endoscopist, this method may provide a great deal of information about both speaking and singing techniques. The combination of a fiberoptic laryngoscope with a laryngeal stroboscope may be especially useful. This system permits magnification, photography, and detailed inspection of

vocal fold motion. Sophisticated systems that permit flexible or rigid fiberoptic strobovideolaryngoscopy are currently available commercially. They are invaluable assets for routine clinical use. The video system also provides a permanent record, permitting reassessment, comparison over time, and easy consultation. A refinement not currently available commercially is stereoscopic fiberoptic laryngoscopy, accomplished by placing a laryngoscope through each nostril, fastening the 2 together in the pharynx, and observing the larynx through the eyepieces.[7] This method allows visualization of laryngeal motion in 3 dimensions. However, it is used primarily in a research setting.

Rigid endoscopy under general anesthesia may be reserved for the rare patient whose vocal folds cannot be assessed adequately by other means or for patients who need surgical procedures to remove or biopsy laryngeal lesions. In some cases, this may be done with local anesthesia, avoiding the need for intubation and the traumatic coughing and vomiting that may occur even after general anesthesia administered by mask. Coughing after general anesthesia may be minimized by using topical anesthesia in the larynx and trachea. However, topical anesthetics may act as severe mucosal irritants in a small number of patients. They may also predispose the patient to aspiration in the postoperative period. If a patient has had difficulty with a topical anesthetic administered in the office, it should not be used in the operating room. When used in general anesthesia cases, topical anesthetics should usually be applied at the end of the procedure. Thus, if inflammation occurs, it will not interfere with performance of microsurgery. Postoperative duration of anesthesia is also optimized. The author has had the least difficulty with 4% Xylocaine.

Objective Tests

Reliable, valid, objective analysis of the voice is extremely important and is an essential part of a comprehensive physical examination.[2] It is as valuable to the laryngologist as audiometry is to the otologist.[8,9] Familiarity with some of the measures and technological advances currently available is helpful. This information is covered in greater detail elsewhere in this book but is included here as a brief overview for the convenience of the reader.

Strobovideolaryngoscopy

Integrity of the vibratory margin of the vocal fold is essential for the complex motion required to produce good vocal quality. Under continuous light, the vocal folds vibrate approximately 250 times per second while phonating at middle C. Naturally, the human eye cannot discern the necessary details during such rapid motion. The vibratory margin may be assessed through high-speed photography, strobovideolaryngoscopy, high-speed video, videokymography, electroglottography (EGG), or photoglottography. Strobovideolaryngoscopy provides the necessary clinical information in a practical fashion. Stroboscopic light allows routine slow-motion evaluation of the mucosal cover layer of the leading edge of the vocal fold. This state-of-the-art physical examination permits detection of vibratory asymmetries, structural abnormalities, small masses, submucosal scars, and other conditions that are invisible under ordinary light.[10,11] Documentation of the procedure by coupling stroboscopic light with the video camera allows later reevaluation by the laryngologist or other health care providers.

Stroboscopy does not provide a true slow-motion image, as obtained through high-speed photography (Figure 4–2). The stroboscope actually illuminates different points on consecutive vocal fold waves, each of which is retained on the retina for 0.2 seconds. The stroboscopically lighted portions of the successive waves are fused visually, and thus the examiner is actually evaluating simulated cycles of phonation. The slow-motion effect is created by having the stroboscopic light desynchronized with the frequency of vocal fold vibration by approximately 2 Hz. When vocal fold vibration and the stroboscope are synchronized exactly, the vocal folds appear to stand still, rather than move in slow motion (Figure 4–3). In most instances, this approximation of slow motion provides all the clinical information necessary. Our routine stroboscopy protocol is described elsewhere.[11] We use a modification of the standardized method of subjective assessment of strobovideolaryngoscopic images, as proposed by Bless

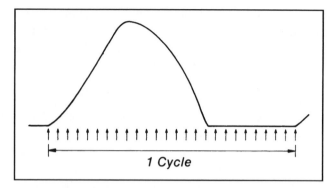

Figure 4–2. The principle of ultrahigh-speed photography. Numerous images are taken during each vibratory cycle. This technique is a true slow-motion representation of each vocal fold vibration.

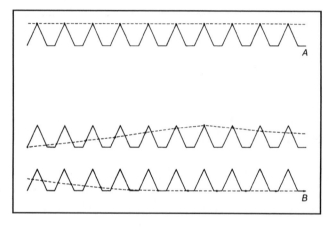

Figure 4–3. The principle of stroboscopy. The stroboscopic light illuminates portions of successive cycles. The eye fuses the illuminated points into an illusion of slow motion. **A.** If the stroboscope is synchronized with vocal fold vibration, a similar point is illuminated on each successive cycle and the vocal fold appears to stand still. **B.** If the stroboscope is slightly desynchronized, each cycle is illuminated at a slightly different point, and the slow motion effect is created.

et al[12] and Hirano.[13] Characteristics evaluated include the fundamental frequency, the symmetry of movements, periodicity, glottic closure, the amplitude of vibration, the mucosal wave, the presence of nonvibrating portions of the vocal fold, and other unusual findings. With practice, perceptual judgments of stroboscopic images provide a great deal of information. However, it is easy for the inexperienced observer to draw unwarranted conclusions because of normal variations in vibration. Vibrations depend on fundamental frequency, intensity, and vocal register. For example, failure of glottic closure occurs normally in falsetto phonation. Consequently, it is important to note these characteristics and to examine each voice under a variety of conditions.

Other Techniques to Examine Vocal Fold Vibration

Other techniques to examine vocal fold vibration include ultrahigh-speed photography, electroglottography (EGG), photoelectroglottography and ultrasound glottography, and most recently videokymography[14] and high-speed video (digital or analog). Ultrahigh-speed photography provides images that are in true slow motion, rather than simulated. High-speed video offers similar advantages without most of the disadvantages of high-speed motion pictures. Videokymography offers high-speed imaging of a single line along the vocal fold. EGG uses 2 electrodes placed on the skin of the neck above the thyroid laminae. It traces the opening and closing of the glottis and can be compared with stroboscopic images.[15] EGG allows objective determination of the presence or absence of glottal vibrations and easy determination of the fundamental period of vibration and is reproducible. It reflects the glottal condition more accurately during its closed phase. Photo electroglottography and ultrasound glottography are less useful clinically.[16]

Measures of Phonatory Ability

Objective measures of phonatory ability are easy to use, readily available to the laryngologist, helpful in the treatment of professional vocalists with specific voice disorders, and quite useful in assessing the results of surgical therapies. Maximum phonation time is measured with a stopwatch. The patient is instructed to sustain the vowel /a/ for as long as possible after deep inspiration,

vocalizing at a comfortable frequency and intensity. The frequency and intensity may be determined and controlled by an inexpensive frequency analyzer and sound level meter. The test is repeated 3 times, and the greatest value is recorded. Normal values have been determined.[16] Frequency range of phonation is recorded in semitones and documents the vocal range from the lowest note in the modal register (excluding vocal fry) to the highest falsetto note. This is the physiologic frequency range of phonation and disregards quality. The musical frequency range of phonation measures lowest to highest notes of musically acceptable quality. Tests for maximum phonation time, frequency ranges, and many of the other parameters discussed later (including spectrographic analysis) may be preserved on a tape recorder or digitized and stored for analysis at a convenient future time and used for pre- and posttreatment comparisons. Recordings should be made in a standardized, consistent fashion.

Frequency limits of vocal register also may be measured. The registers are (from low to high) vocal fry, chest, mid, head, and falsetto. However, classification of registers is controversial, and many other classifications are used. Although the classification listed above is common among musicians, at present, most voice scientists prefer to classify registers as pulse, modal, and loft. Overlap of frequency among registers occurs routinely.

Testing the speaking fundamental frequency often reveals excessively low pitch, an abnormality associated with chronic voice abuse and development of vocal nodules. This parameter may be followed objectively throughout a course of voice therapy. Intensity range of phonation (IRP) has proven a less useful measure than frequency range. It varies with fundamental frequency (which should be recorded) and is greatest in the middle frequency range. It is recorded in sound pressure level (SPL) (re 0.0002 microbar). For healthy adults who are not professional vocalists, measuring at a single fundamental frequency, IRP averages 54.8 dB for males and 51 dB for females.[17] Alterations of intensity are common in voice disorders, although IRP is not the most sensitive test to detect them. Information from these tests may be combined in a fundamental frequency-intensity profile,[16] also called a *phonetogram.*

Glottal efficiency (ratio of the acoustic power at the level of the glottis to subglottal power) provides useful information but is not clinically practical because measuring acoustic power at the level of the glottis is difficult. Subglottic power is the product of subglottal pressure and airflow rate. These can be determined clinically. Various alternative measures of glottic efficiency have been proposed, including the ratio of radiated acoustic power to subglottal power,[18] airflow intensity profile,[19] and ratio of the root mean square value of the AC component to the mean volume velocity (DC component).[20] Although glottal efficiency is of great interest, none of these tests is particularly helpful under routine clinical circumstances.

Aerodynamic Measures

Traditional pulmonary function testing provides the most readily accessible measure of respiratory function. The most common parameters measured include (1) tidal volume, the volume of air that enters the lungs during inspiration and leaves during expiration in normal breathing; (2) functional residual capacity, the volume of air remaining in the lungs at the end of inspiration during normal breathing, which can be divided into expiratory reserve volume (maximal additional volume that can be exhaled) and residual volume (the volume of air remaining in the lungs at the end of maximal exhalation); (3) inspiratory capacity, the maximal volume of air that can be inhaled starting at the functional residual capacity; (4) total lung capacity, the volume of air in the lungs following maximal inspiration; (5) vital capacity, the maximal volume of air that can be exhaled from the lungs following maximal inspiration; (6) forced vital capacity, the rate of air flow with rapid, forceful expiration from total lung capacity to residual volume; (7) FEV_1, the forced expiratory volume in 1 second; (8) FEV_3, the forced expiratory volume in 3 seconds; and (9) maximal mid-expiratory flow, the mean rate of airflow over the middle half of the forced vital capacity (between 25% and 75% of the forced vital capacity).

For singers and professional speakers with an abnormality caused by voice abuse, abnormal pulmonary function tests may confirm deficiencies in aerobic conditioning or reveal previously unrecognized asthma.[21] Flow glottography with computer inverse filtering is also a practical and valuable diagnostic for assessing flow at the vocal fold level, evaluating the voice source, and imaging the results of the balance between adductory forces and subglottal pressure.[22] It also has therapeutic value as a biofeedback tool.

The spirometer, readily available for pulmonary function testing, can also be used for measuring airflow during phonation. However, the spirometer does not allow simultaneous display of acoustic signals, and its frequency response is poor. A pneumotachograph consists of a laminar air resistor, a differential pressure transducer, and an amplifying and recording system. It allows measurement of airflow and simultaneous recording of other signals when coupled with a polygraph. A hot-wire anemometer allows determination of airflow velocity by measuring the electrical drop across the hot wire. Modern hot-wire anemometers containing electrical feedback circuitry that maintains the temperature of the hot wire provide a flat response up to 1 kHz and are useful clinically.

The 4 parameters traditionally measured in the aerodynamic performance of a voice are subglottal pressure (P_{sub}), supraglottal pressure (P_{sup}), glottal impedance, and the volume velocity of airflow at the glottis. These parameters and their rapid variations can be measured under laboratory circumstances. However, clinically their mean value is usually determined as follows:

$$P_{sub} - P_{sup} = MFR \times GR$$

where *MFR* is the mean (root mean square) flow rate and *GR* is the mean (root mean square) glottal resistance. When vocalizing the open vowel /a/, the supraglottic pressure equals the atmospheric pressure, reducing the equation to

$$P_{sub} = MFR \times GR$$

The mean flow rate is a useful clinical measure. While the patient vocalizes the vowel /a/, the mean flow rate is calculated by dividing the total volume of air used during phonation by the duration of phonation. The subject phonates at a comfortable pitch and loudness either over a determined period of time or for a maximum sustained period of phonation.

Air volume is measured by the use of a mask fitted tightly over the face or by phonating into a mouthpiece while wearing a nose clamp. Measurements may be made using a spirometer, pneumotachograph, or hot-wire anemometer. The normal values for mean flow rate under habitual phonation, with changes in intensity or register, and under various pathologic circumstances,

were determined in the 1970s.[16] Normal values are available for both adults and children. Mean flow rate also can be measured and is a clinically useful parameter to follow during treatment for vocal nodules, recurrent laryngeal nerve paralysis, spasmodic dysphonia, and other conditions.

Glottal resistance cannot be measured directly, but it may be calculated from the mean flow rate and mean subglottal pressure. Normal glottal resistance is 20 to 100 dyne seconds/cm^5 at low and medium pitches and 150 dyne seconds/cm^5 at high pitches.[18] The normal values for subglottal pressure under various healthy and pathologic voice conditions have also been determined by numerous investigators.[16] The phonation quotient is the vital capacity divided by the maximum phonation time. It has been shown to correlate closely with maximum flow rate[23] and is a more convenient measure. Normative data determined by various authors have been published.[16] The phonation quotient provides an objective measure of the effects of treatment and is particularly useful in cases of recurrent laryngeal nerve paralysis and mass lesions of the vocal folds, including nodules.

Acoustic Analysis

Acoustic analysis equipment can determine frequency, intensity, harmonic spectrum, cycle-to-cycle perturbations in frequency (jitter), cycle-to-cycle perturbations in amplitude (shimmer), harmonics/noise ratios, breathiness index, and many other parameters. The DSP Sona-Graph Sound Analyzer Model 5500 (Kay Elemetrics, Lincoln Park, New Jersey) is an integrated voice analysis system. It is equipped for sound spectrography capabilities. Spectrography provides a visual record of the voice. The acoustic signal is depicted using time (*x*-axis), frequency (y-axis), and intensity (z-axis), shading of light vs dark. Using the bandpass filters, generalizations about quality, pitch, and loudness can be made. These observations are used in formulating the voice therapy treatment plan. Formant structure and strength can be determined using the narrow-band filters, of which a variety of configurations are possible. In clinical settings in which singers and other professional voice users are evaluated and treated routinely, this feature is extremely valuable. A sophisticated voice analysis program (an optional program) may be combined with the Sona-Graph and is an especially valuable addition to the clinical laboratory. The voice analysis program (Computer Speech Lab; Kay Elemetrics) measures speaking fundamental frequency, frequency perturbation (jitter), amplitude perturbation (shimmer), and harmonics-to-noise ratio and provides many other useful values. An electroglottograph may be used in conjunction with the Sona-Graph to provide some of these voicing parameters. Examining the EGG waveform alone is possible with this setup, but its clinical usefulness has not yet been established. An important feature of the Sona-Graph is the long-term average (LTA) spectral capability, which permits analysis of longer voice samples (30–90 seconds). The LTA analyzes only voiced speech segments and may be useful in screening for hoarse or breathy voices. In addition, computer interface capabilities (also an optional program) have solved many data storage and file maintenance problems.

In analyzing acoustic signals, the microphone may be placed at the level of the mouth or positioned in or over the trachea, although intratracheal recordings are used for research purposes only. The position should be standardized in each office or laboratory.[24] Various techniques are being developed to improve the usefulness of acoustic analysis. Because of the enormous amount of information carried in the acoustic signal, further refinements in objective acoustic analysis should prove particularly valuable to the clinician.

Laryngeal Electromyography

Electromyography (EMG) requires an electrode system, an amplifier, an oscilloscope, a loudspeaker, and a recording system.[25] Electrodes are placed transcutaneously into laryngeal muscles. EMG can be extremely valuable in confirming cases of vocal fold paresis, in differentiating paralysis from arytenoid dislocation, distinguishing recurrent laryngeal nerve paralysis from combined recurrent and superior nerve paralysis, diagnosing other more subtle neurolaryngologic pathology, and documenting functional voice disorders and malingering. It is also recommended for needle localization when using botulinum toxin for treatment of spasmodic dysphonia and other conditions.

Psychoacoustic Evaluation

Because the human ear and brain are the most sensitive and complex analyzers of sound currently available, many researchers have tried to standardize and quantify psychoacoustic evaluation. Unfortunately, even definitions of basic terms such as hoarseness and breathiness are still controversial. Psychoacoustic evaluation protocols and interpretations are not standardized. Consequently, although subjective psychoacoustic analysis of voice is of great value to the individual skilled clinician, it remains generally unsatisfactory for comparing research among laboratories or for reporting clinical results.

The GRBAS scale[6] helps standardize perceptual analysis for clinical purposes. It rates the voice from a scale from 0 to 3, with regrading to grade, roughness, breathiness, asthenia, and strain. Grade 0 is normal, 1 is slightly abnormal, 2 is moderately abnormal, and 3 is extremely abnormal. Grade refers to the degree of hoarseness or voice abnormality. Roughness refers to the acoustic/auditory impression of irregularity of vibration and corresponds with gear and shimmer. Breathiness refers to the acoustic/auditory impression of air leakage and corresponds to turbulence. Asthenic evaluation assesses weakness or lack of power and corresponds to vocal intensity and energy in higher harmonics. Strain refers to the acoustic/auditory impression of hyperfunction and may be related to fundamental frequency, noise in the high-frequency range, and energy in higher harmonics. For example, a patient's voice might be graded as G2, R2, B1, A1, S2.

Outcomes Assessment

Measuring the impact of a voice disorder has always been challenging. However, recent advances have begun to address this problem. Validated instruments such as the Voice Handicap Index (VHI)[26] are currently in clinical use and are likely to be used widely in future years.

Voice Impairment and Disability

Quantifying voice impairment and assigning a disability rating (percentage of whole person) remain controversial. This subject is still not addressed comprehensively even in the most recent editions (2008, 6th edi-tion) of the American Medical Association's *Guidelines for the Evaluation of Impairment and Disability* (The Guides). The Guides still do not take into account the person's profession when calculating disability. Alternative approaches have been proposed,[27] and advances in this complex arena are anticipated over the next few years.

Evaluation of the Singing Voice

The physician must be careful not to exceed the limits of his or her expertise, especially in caring for singers. However, if voice abuse or technical error is suspected, or if a difficult judgment must be reached on whether to allow a sick singer to perform, a brief observation of the patient's singing may provide invaluable information. This is accomplished best by asking the singer to stand and sing scales either in the examining room or in the soundproof audiology booth. Similar maneuvers may be used for professional speakers, including actors (who can vocalize and recite lines), clergy and politicians (who can deliver sermons and speeches), and virtually all other voice patients. The singer's stance should be balanced, with the weight slightly forward. The knees should be bent slightly and the shoulders, torso, and neck should be relaxed. The singer should inhale through the nose whenever possible allowing filtration, warming, and humidification of inspired air. In general, the chest should be expanded, but most of the active breathing is abdominal. The chest should not rise substantially with each inspiration, and the supraclavicular musculature should not be involved obviously in inspiration. Shoulders and neck muscles should not be tensed even with deep inspiration. Abdominal musculature should be contracted shortly before the initiation of the tone. This may be evaluated visually or by palpation (Figure 4–4). Muscles of the neck and face should be relaxed. Economy is a basic principle of all art forms. Wasted energy and motion and muscle tension are incorrect and usually deleterious.

The singer should be instructed to sing a scale (a 5-note scale is usually sufficient) on the vowel /a/, beginning on any comfortable note. Technical errors are usually most obvious as contraction of muscles in the neck and chin, retraction of the lower lip, retraction of the tongue, or tightening of the muscles of mastication. The singer's mouth should be open widely but comfortably. When singing /a/, the singer's tongue should

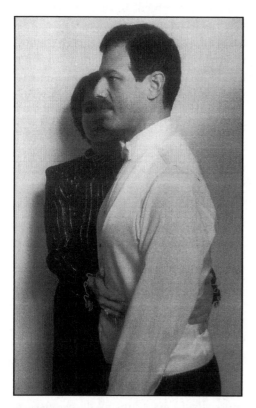

Figure 4–4. Bimanual palpation of the support mechanism. The singer should expand posteriorly and anteriorly with inspiration. Muscles should tighten prior to onset of sung tone.

rest in a neutral position with the tip of the tongue lying against the back of the singer's mandibular incisors. If the tongue pulls back or demonstrates obvious muscular activity as the singer performs the scales, improper voice use can be confirmed on the basis of positive evidence (Figure 4–5). The position of the larynx should not vary substantially with pitch changes. Rising of the larynx with ascending pitch is evidence of technical dysfunction. This examination also gives the physician an opportunity to observe any dramatic differences between the qualities and ranges of the patient's speaking voice and the singing voice. A physical examination summary form has proven helpful in organization and documentation.[3]

Remembering the admonition not to exceed his or her expertise, the physician who examines many singers can often glean valuable information from a brief attempt to modify an obvious technical error. For example, deciding whether to allow a singer with mild or moderate laryngitis to perform is often difficult. On one hand, an expert singer has technical skills that allow him or her to compensate safely. On the other hand, if a singer does not sing with correct technique and does not have the discipline to modify volume, technique, and repertoire as necessary, the risk of vocal injury may be increased substantially even by mild inflammation of the vocal folds. In borderline circumstances, observation of the singer's technique may greatly help the physician in making a judgment.

If the singer's technique appears flawless, the physician may feel somewhat more secure in allowing the singer to proceed with performance commitments. More commonly, even good singers demonstrate technical errors when experiencing voice difficulties. In a vain effort to compensate for dysfunction at the vocal fold level, singers often modify their technique in the neck and

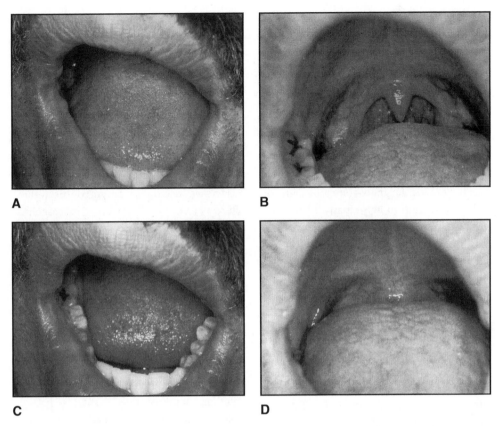

Figure 4–5. Proper relaxed position of the anterior (**A**) and posterior (**B**) portions of the tongue. Common improper use of the tongue pulled back from the teeth (**C**) and raised posteriorly (**D**).

supraglottic vocal tract. In the good singer, this usually means going from good technique to bad technique. The most common error involves pulling back the tongue and tightening the cervical muscles. Although this increased muscular activity gives the singer the illusion of making the voice more secure, this technical maladjustment undermines vocal efficiency and increases vocal strain. The physician may ask the singer to hold the top note of a 5-note scale; while the note is being held, the singer may simply be told, "Relax your tongue." At the same time, the physician points to the singer's abdominal musculature. Most good singers immediately correct to good technique. If they do, and if upcoming performances are particularly important, the singer may be able to perform with a reminder that meticulous technique is essential. The singer should be advised to "sing by feel rather than by ear," consult his or her voice teacher, and conserve the voice except when it is absolutely necessary to use it. If a singer is unable to correct from bad technique to good technique promptly, especially if he or she uses excessive muscle tension in the neck and ineffective abdominal support, it is generally safer not to perform with even a mild vocal fold abnormality. With increased experience and training, the laryngologist may make other observations that aid in providing appropriate treatment recommendations for singer patients. Once these skills have been mastered for the care of singers, applying them to other patients is relatively easy, so long as the laryngologist takes the time to understand the demands of the individual's professional, avocational, and recreational vocal activities.

If treatment is to be instituted, making at least a tape recording of the voice is advisable in most cases and essential before any surgical intervention. The author routinely uses strobovideolaryngoscopy for diagnosis and documentation in virtually all cases as well as many of the objective measures discussed. Pretreatment testing is extremely helpful clinically and medicolegally.

Additional Examinations

A general physical examination should be performed whenever the patient's systemic health is questionable. Debilitating conditions such as mononucleosis may be noticed first by the singer as vocal fatigue. A neurologic assessment may be particularly revealing. The physician must be careful not to overlook dysarthrias and dysphonias, which are characteristic of movement disorders and of serious neurologic disease. Dysarthria is a defect in rhythm, enunciation, and articulation that usually results from neuromuscular impairment or weakness such as may occur after a stroke. It may be seen with oral deformities or illness, as well. Dysphonia is an abnormality of vocalization usually caused by problems at the laryngeal level.

Physicians should be familiar with the 6 types of dysarthria, their symptoms, and their importance.[28,29] Flaccid dysarthria occurs in lower motor neuron or primary muscle disorders such as myasthenia gravis and tumors or strokes involving the brainstem nuclei. Spastic dysarthria occurs in upper motor neuron disorders (pseudobulbar palsy) such as multiple strokes and cerebral palsy. Ataxic dysarthria is seen with cerebellar disease, alcohol intoxication, and multiple sclerosis. Hypokinetic dysarthria accompanies Parkinson disease. Hyperkinetic dysarthria may be spasmodic, as in the Gilles de la Tourette disease, or dystonic, as in chorea and cerebral palsy. Mixed dysarthria occurs in amyotrophic lateral sclerosis (ALS) or Lou Gehrig disease. The preceding classification actually combines dysphonic and dysarthric characteristics but is very useful clinically. The value of a comprehensive neurolaryngologic evaluation[30] cannot be overstated. More specific details of voice changes associated with neurologic dysfunction and their localizing value are available elsewhere.[2,31]

It is extremely valuable for the laryngologist to assemble an arts-medicine team that includes not only a speech-language pathologist, singing voice specialist, acting voice specialist, and voice scientist but also medical colleagues in other disciplines. Collaboration with an expert neurologist, pulmonologist, endocrinologist, psychologist, psychiatrist, internist, physiatrist, and others with special knowledge of, and interest in, voice disorders is invaluable in caring for patients with voice disorders. Such interdisciplinary teams have not only changed the standard of care in voice evaluation and treatment but are also largely responsible for the rapid and productive growth of voice as a subspecialty.

References

1. Sataloff RT. Professional singers: the science and art of clinical care. *Am J Otolaryngol.* 1981;2:251–266.

2. Rubin JS, Sataloff RT, Korovin GS. *Diagnosis and Treatment of Voice Disorders*. 3rd ed. San Diego, CA: Plural Publishing; 2006.

3. Sataloff RT. The professional voice: part II, physical examination. *J Voice*. 1987;1:91–201.

4. Fuazawa T, Blaugrund SM, El-Assuooty A, Gould WJ. Acoustic analysis of hoarse voice: a preliminary report. *J Voice*. 1988;2(2):127–131.

5. Gelfer M. Perceptual attributes of voice: development and use of rating scales. *J Voice*. 1988;2(4):320–326.

6. Hirano M. *Clinical Examination of the Voice*. New York, NY: Springer-Verlag; 1981:83–84.

7. Fujimura O. Stereo-fiberoptic laryngeal observation. *J Acoust Soc Am*. 1979;65:70–72.

8. Sataloff RT, Spiegel JR, Carroll LM, Darby KS, Hawkshaw MJ, Rulnick RK. The clinical voice laboratory: practical design and clinical application. *J Voice*. 1990;4:264–279.

9. Sataloff RT, Heuer RH, Hoover C, Baroody MM. Laboratory assessment of voice. In: Gould WJ, Sataloff RT, Spiegel JR. *Voice Surgery*. St. Louis, MO: Mosby; 1993:203–216.

10. Sataloff RT, Spiegel JR, Carroll LM, Schiebel BR, Darby KS, Rulnick RK. Strobovideolaryngoscopy in professional voice users: results and clinical value. *J Voice*. 1986;1:359–364.

11. Sataloff RT, Spiegel JR, Hawkshaw MJ. Strobovideolaryngoscopy: results and clinical value. *Ann Otol Rhinol Laryngol*. 1991;100:725–727.

12. Bless D, Hirano M, Feder RJ. Video stroboscopic evaluation of the larynx. *Ear Nose Throat J*. 1987;66:289–296.

13. Hirano M. Phonosurgery: basic and clinical investigations. *Otologia (Fukuoka)*. 1975;21:239–442.

14. Svec J, Shutte H. Videokymography: high-speed line scanning of vocal fold vibration. *J Voice*. 1996;10:201–205.

15. Leclure FLE, Brocaar ME, Verscheeure J. Electroglottography and its relation to glottal activity. *Folia Phoniatr (Basel)*. 1975;27:215–224.

16. Hirano M. *Clinical Examination of the Voice*. New York, NY: Springer-Verlag; 1981:25–27, 85–98.

17. Coleman RJ, Mabis JH, Hinson JK. Fundamental frequency sound pressure level profiles of adult male and female voices. *J Speech Hear Res*. 1977;20:197–204.

18. Isshiki N. Regulatory mechanism of voice intensity variation. *J Speech Hear Res*. 1964;7:17–29.

19. Saito S. Phonosurgery: basic study on the mechanisms of phonation and endolaryngeal microsurgery. *Otologia (Fukuoka)*. 1977;23:171–384.

20. Isshiki N. Functional surgery of the larynx. *Report of the 78th Annual Convention of the Oto-Rhino-Laryngological Society of Japan*. Fukuoka, Japan: Kyoto University; 1977.

21. Cohn JR, Sataloff RT, Spiegel JR, Fish JE, Kennedy K. Airway reactivity-induced asthma in singers (ARIAS). *J Voice*. 1991;5:332–337.

22. Sundberg J. *The Science of the Singing Voice*. Dekalb, IL: Northern Illinois University Press; 1987:11, 66, 77–89.

23. Hirano M, Koike Y, von Leden H. Maximum phonation time and air usage during phonation. *Folia Phoniatr (Basel)*. 1968;20:185–201.

24. Price DB, Sataloff RT. A simple technique for consistent microphone placement in voice recording. *J Voice*. 1988;2:206–207.

25. Sataloff RT, Mandel S, Ma.on-Espaillat R, et al. *Laryngeal Electromyography*. 2nd ed. San Diego, CA: Plural Publishing; 2006.

26. Benninger MS, Gardner GM, Jacobson BH. New dimensions in measuring voice treatment outcomes. In: Sataloff RT. *Professional Voice: The Science and Art of Clinical Care*. 3rd ed. San Diego, CA: Plural Publishing; 2005:471–478.

27. Sataloff RT. Voice and speech impairment and disability. In: Sataloff RT. *Professional Voice: The Science and Art of Clinical Care*. 3rd ed. San Diego, CA: Plural Publishing; 2005:1427–1432.

28. Darley FL, Aronson AE, Brown JR. Differential diagnostic of patterns of dysarthria. *J Speech Hear Res*. 1969;12(2):246–249.

29. Darley FL, Aronson AE, Brown JR. Clusters of deviant speech dimensions in the dysarthrias. *J Speech Hear Res*. 1969;12(3):462–496.

30. Rosenfield DB. Neurolaryngology. *Ear Nose Throat J.* 1987;66:323–326.

31. Raphael BN, Sataloff RT. Increasing vocal effectiveness. In: Sataloff RT. *Professional Voice: Science and Art of Clinical Care.* 3rd ed. San Diego, CA: Plural Publishing; 2005: 993–1004.

5

Obesity, Body Size, and Voice

Abdul-Latif Hamdan, Robert Thayer Sataloff, and Mary J. Hawkshaw

The question whether voice is a good predictor of body size is a subject of thorough debate in the literature with no clear consensus. The assumption that listeners can predict body size stems from 2 facts: one is the isometric development of the vocal tract and body,[1] and the second is the hormone-induced laryngeal growth in parallel with the musculoskeletal system.[2–4] Numerous studies indicate that sex hormones have a direct effect on the larynx and body distribution of fat and muscle mass.[2–6] The exposure of the larynx to circulating endogenous sex hormones at puberty results in enlargement of its structures with subsequent increase in the vocal folds' mass and length. As these 2 factors are the main determinants of vocal fundamental frequency, there is consequent decrease in the rate of vibration of the vocal folds, more so in men than in women.[5] Similarly, it is also known that sex hormones play a key role in body metabolism and fat distribution. Androgens play a key role in the metabolic profile of men and women and are considered major determinants of body characteristics.[6]

Despite the fact that hormonal activity at pubescence causes both laryngeal and body growth, there is no consensus on the correlation between vocal and body characteristics. The notion that one's hormonal profile defines both vocal print and body traits is challenged, among other issues, by the constrained descent of the larynx, which is more pronounced in men compared with women.[5,7] Consequently, voice-based body size estimation derived from the hormone-induced laryngeal growth is confounded by the vocal tract descent and elongation, and there are conflicting reports about whether listeners can or cannot predict the speaker's size, with no clear understanding of which acoustic parameters are used in the prediction process. Based on the study by Lass and Davis[8] in 1976, the average probability of guessing correctly the weight in female and male speakers was 65% and 48%, respectively. In that study, the listeners used a multiple-choice response task to make their judgments. Overall, the results indicated that the probability of correct identification of height was significantly different from chance for both male and female speakers, and the probability of making the correct judgment for weight was significantly different from chance in male speakers. The prediction of both weight and height was based on the presence of vocal cues, namely,

115

breathiness, loudness, and pitch. However, the influence of pitch on the judgments made by the 30 judges in that study was not consistent or directional, meaning that although listeners used pitch to estimate the speaker's body characteristics, there was no obvious trend. Some listeners interpreted high vocal pitch as a cue for heavy weight, whereas others used it for light weight.[8] A year later in 1977, the same authors, Lass et al,[9] investigated the ability of listeners to make the same estimation by listening to recorded speech samples. The results indicated that they could identify the weights and heights of the speakers accurately. These findings have led other investigators to try to determine which acoustic cues influence the decision-making process of listeners. Several vocal indices have been examined in relation to voice production-related anatomy with emphasis on the fundamental frequency (F0) as a cue to laryngeal size and formant frequencies as cues to vocal tract shape and length.[10-17] Bachorowski and Owren[10] demonstrated that combining F0 and vocal tract length provides a strong acoustic cue in identifying talker's sex and less so for identifying speaker's identity. The analysis was performed on short vowel segments extracted from natural, running speech of 125 subjects. Similarly, Smith and Patterson[11] highlighted the predictive role of glottal pulse rate and vocal tract length, individually and in combination, in judging speaker size, sex, and age.

Considering the findings above, this chapter reviews the literature on 2 main acoustic cues that have been investigated thoroughly as predictors of body size and shape: F0 and formant frequencies. It is helpful to understand the association between vocal tract dimensions and body characteristics when contemplating the relationship between obesity and voice.

Fundamental Frequency in Relation to Body Size

The correlation between body size and fundamental frequency (F0) is controversial. Many authors reported lack of or poor correlation between F0 and body weight and height,[12-16] whereas others reported an association between male body traits and vocal pitch.[17] Four decades ago, Lass[15] investigated the correlation between F0 and body characteristics. The study was conducted on 15 males and 15 females who were asked to read the "Rainbow Passage" while the fundamental frequency indicator was used to extract the mean speaking F0 from the readings. The body characteristics used were height, weight, and body surface area. The results showed a nonsignificant negative correlation in females and a nonsignificant positive correlation in males between mean speaking F0 and body characteristics. Hence the assumption that "direction of influence of vocal pitch would be in an inverse manner to the perceived size of the speaker" was not substantiated by the authors.[15(p1219)] Similarly, Lass et al[18] in 1980 reported that although speakers' characteristics could be estimated accurately by listening to voiced and whispered speech, pitch was not key in this identification process. That same year, Cohen et al[19] in their critic report refuted altogether the assertion that voice is a reliable carrier of information that listeners can use to estimate body characteristics. This conclusion was supported 2 years later by Gunter and Manning[20] who reported "significant differences between actual and estimates of weights and heights of 20 individual speakers." The study was based on 40 listeners who were asked to estimate both height and weight by listening to filtered and nonfiltered signals of 4 steady vowels produced by 20 speakers.[20] Künzel[12] in 1989 shed further light on the controversial relationship between F0 and body characteristics. In his investigation of 183 subjects, the author reported no significant correlation between average F0 and body height and weight. He concluded that F0 is not an acoustic cue to these constitutional characteristics and that speech does not contain information on weight and height. The author asserted that F0 cannot be used to predict body measures, especially in forensic speaker identification. This conclusion was consistent with the author's experience in criminal case investigation.[12] Similarly, van Dommelen[13] in 1993 reevaluated the data presented by Lass et al and refuted the claim that listeners can estimate speaker's height and weight. The author reported no correlation between estimated body size and actual body size. Two years later, he investigated further the correlation between several acoustic measures and body characteristics using both isolated words and reading text paragraphs as material for analysis. Using regression analysis, no significant correlation was found between any of the acoustic measures (including F0) and body weight or height.[14] Similarly, in 2005 Rendall et al[21] showed that F0 variation failed to track body size variation within sexes. Though F0 was lower in males compared to females, it did not correlate significantly with body size. Going a step further, Hamdan et al[16] in 2011 investigated the correlation between body weight, mass composition, and F0 in 40 adult males. The authors attempted to answer 2 questions: Is there a correlation between body weight and F0 and, if so, does F0 correlate with fat mass, muscle mass, or both? The results indicated lack of correlation between F0 and body weight or body composition variables. The fat weight in the group of subjects investi-gated ranged between 3 and 25 kg with a higher concentration being reported in the extremities and trunk (61.84% and 16.20%, respectively). Although the authors anticipated that subjects with android type of obesity had lower F0 given that the concentration of androgen receptors is higher in visceral adipose tissue, the results indicated no such findings. However, there was a weak correlation ($r = 0.328$) between trunk fat and cycle-to-cycle variation in intensity. This finding was in keeping with the results of Damrose[22] in his report on the impact of androgen therapy on voice in a 33-year-old biological female who underwent gender reassignment. The authors demonstrated an increase in shimmer after 3 months of androgen treatment.

To corroborate the aforementioned reports, de Souza et al[23] in 2014 investigated the correlation between F0 and obesity in a group of 74 subjects, 30 as controls and 44 with a body mass index (BMI) higher than 35 kg/m^2. The results showed no significant difference in F0 between the obese group and the control group, although the prevalence of vocal complaints was significantly higher in the former. Close to 70% of obese subjects had phonatory symptoms, namely vocal fatigue and/or the need to exert more effort to talk. The authors attributed these symptoms to the increase in airway resistance secondary to excess fat deposition in the vocal tract, excessive tension within extrinsic laryngeal muscles, and impaired respiratory function.[23] Also in 2014, Pisanski et al[24] conducted a meta-analysis looking at vocal indicators in relation to body size. The authors demonstrated that F0 explains no more than 2% of the variance in body size. The study was conducted on 39 samples taken across 5 different continents where various vocal indices were examined. Two years later, the same authors investigated the relationship between 8 body indices that included weight and 19 voice parameters. The authors found that mean fundamental frequency was more useful in explaining variance in body shape rather than predicting height and weight.[25]

Contrary to all the aforementioned reports that substantiate no role or a confounding role for F0 in reliably predicting body weight, there are numerous studies that indicate the presence of perceptual, acoustic, and aerodynamic differences between obese and nonobese subjects.[17,26–28] Evans et al[17] in 2006 reported a significant negative correlation between F0 and weight ($r = -.34$, $p = .02$), shoulder circumference ($r = -0.29$, $p = .04$), and chest circumference ($r = -.28$, $p = .04$) in a group of 50 heterosexual males. However, there was no correlation between F0 and body height or the remaining body shape measures. Same year, Da Cunha et al[27] studied the vocal features in a group of 45 adults with a body mass index that exceeded 35 kg/m^2 in comparison to a control group matched by age and gender. The voice was evaluated subjectively and objectively using acoustic and airflow measurements. The presence or absence of vocal fry or strangulation at the end of a vocal emission was reported also. Although F0 was not examined in this study, the authors reported perceptual vocal alterations in obese subjects compared with controls. These vocal alterations included hoarseness, "murmuring," and phonatory instability in 62%, 27%, and 44% of the cases, respectively. These findings were explained on the basis of shorter maximum phonation time (MPT) in obese subjects in comparison to controls (8 seconds vs 14 seconds in men, respectively, and 7 seconds vs 14 seconds in women, respectively). Similarly, there was a significantly higher prevalence of strangulation in the obese group compared with

the control group ($p = .001$). This latter was attributed by the authors to "stress phonation."[27] In parallel with these perceptual vocal alterations, there was also an increase in the perturbation parameters, jitter, and shimmer, in addition to noise. The authors related these acoustic changes to several factors: one, to breathing impairment secondary to excessive weight and "the influence of obese individual's thoracic plethora on the respiratory phenomenon"[27(p344)]; two, to the fat deposition along the laryngopharyngeal complex and in particular the palate, uvula, and posterolateral pharyngeal wall; and last but not least, to the high prevalence of laryngopharyngeal reflux disease in obese subjects.[27]

In 2013, Barsties et al[28] investigated the possible changes in audio-perceptual, acoustic, and aerodynamic measures in relation to weight and body fat volume. The study was conducted on 29 subjects who were stratified as morbidly obese, normal weight, and underweight. Out of 25 outcome measures used (which included the speaking fundamental frequency and sound pressure level [SPL] at comfortable speech), 10 measures differed among the groups. Morbidly obese subjects had higher minimum intensity, maximum intensity, and sound pressure level compared to the normal and underweight groups.[28] These findings were hypothetically attributed to a larger diaphragmatic muscle in obese compared to nonobese subjects. The large diaphragmatic muscle could hypothetically generate greater muscle strength and motion, thus leading to higher subglottal pressure and vocal intensity level.[29] Another speculated reason for the high habitual intensity of speech in obese subjects is narrowing of the pharyngeal lumen with subsequent increase in supralaryngeal resistance. This high resistance results in a higher supraglottal and hence subglottal pressure, which in turn leads to higher vocal intensity. There were also significantly lower shimmer values in the obese group compared to the underweight group, for which the authors had no clear explanation. On the other hand, there was no significant difference in the speaking fundamental frequency in the obese group compared with the normal-weight and underweight groups. Furthermore, the lowest fundamental frequency in the underweight group was significantly higher in comparison to the normal group, though there was no statistically significant difference in the fundamental frequency between the obese and overweight groups. One explanation offered by the authors is the hypothetical decrease in vocal fold mass, a hypothesis that is not in keeping with the report of Titze,[30] which asserts that vocal fold length and tension are more important determinants of vocal pitch than vocal fold mass. With respect to aerodynamic measures, the obese group had greater vital capacity but lower maximum phonation time compared with normal-weight subjects. However, there was a significantly reduced vital capacity in the underweight group compared to the normal-weight group. The reduced vital capacity and maximum phonation time were attributed to the reduced strength and performance of the diaphragm in underweight subjects compared to normal-weight subjects.[29,31] Pisanski et al[32] in 2014, in their investigation on the role of vocal pitch in listeners' size assessment, demonstrated that F0 facilitates body size assessment when combined with formant measures. Despite the lack of relationship between body height and vocal pitch, the authors demonstrated that vocal pitch "provides a carrier signal for vocal tract resonances."[32] Acurio et al[33] investigated the association between several acoustic param-

eters that included F0 and salivary interleukin-6 in obese and nonobese school teachers who were stratified according to weight. Because of the interplay between proinflammatory cytokines, vocal loading, and obesity, the authors questioned whether vocal loading affects acoustic parameters and the concentration of interleukin-6 in a differential manner with respect to weight. The results showed that following vocal loading, there is an elevation in F0 and an increase in salivary interleukin-6 in obese teachers, with significant correlation between the salivary interleukin-6 and harmonic-to-noise ratio (HNR) in this group of subjects. The authors concluded that obesity has an effect on certain acoustic parameters and that HNR correlated with salivary interleukin-6 in overweight subjects.[33] However, it is important to note that there was no significant correlation between BMI and any of the acoustic parameters, including F0.

In all the aforementioned reports, there is a clear inclination that F0 is not a reliable indicator of body weight and height. This is not surprising if we consider the disproportionate differences in speaking F0 and body size in male and female adults. In the study by Rendall et al[21] on the role of vocalizer body size and voice acoustics, the difference in F0 between males and females was not commensurate with the body size differences among the 2 genders. The F0 dimorphism of 1.81 was only partially attributed to the dimorphism in vocal fold length and volume. Three possible explanations for the lack of correlation between F0 and body size are suggested: one is the dissonance or allometric (ie, out of phase) growth of the vocal folds and rest of the body. The independent growth of the laryngeal framework can be attributed to the unconstrained position of the larynx in the neck in relation to the base of skull and chest. Unlike other animal species, the human larynx is allowed to expand freely and thus enjoys a flexibility in growth independent of its contiguous structures.[21] The second possible explanation for the mismatch between body size and F0 is the "body size exaggeration hypothesis," whereby a speaker modulates his or her F0 in attempt to project a false image of his or her body size.[1,34,35] Third is the psychological element in alignment with the hormonal profile of the speaker. To that end, dishonest variations in F0 might be signaling sexual physiology rather than true body measurements, meaning to say a given sex hormone status.[21]

In conclusion, there are not enough data to support the role of F0 in predicting body weight despite its added value when combined with other acoustic parameters that relate to vocal tract length.[12,36] Though the glottal pulse rate depends on the size of the vocal folds, it is not a valid sensory cue to the speaker's size. Nevertheless, it is important to note that obesity does affect other perturbation parameters of the glottal source in addition to many upper and lower aerodynamic measures. Further research on the correlation between BMI, F0, and vocal fold mass, length, and volume is warranted.

Body Size and Formant Frequencies

The association between obesity and formant frequencies with emphasis on vocal tract variations in relation to body size (height and weight) warrants understanding. The topic can be considered in 3 subdivisions: formants position and distribution in relation to vocal tract morphology, variations in vocal tract morphology in relation to body size, and the role of formant profiles in predicting body size.

Formant Profiles and Vocal Tract Morphology

As a multidimensional signal, human speech not only conveys the phonetics essential for communication but also a myriad of nonlinguistic cues of speaker identity. The vocal parameters most commonly examined as acoustic cues to vocal tract morphology are formant frequencies derived from vowel sounds that offer salient cues to vocal tract anatomical variations. According to the source-filter theory discussed by Titze[37] in 1994, the vocal signal emitted by the vocal folds is filtered in the vocal tract into various harmonics. The position of these harmonic frequencies is related to the configuration of the vocal tract, which in turn is determined by articulation and growth-related morphologic features.[1,37–42] Indeed, the disparity in formant profiles across gender is attributed partially to the dimorphic growth of the vocal tract at pubescence. In that regard, Roers et al[40] reported the female to male ratio of vocal tract length as 0.89, a figure comparable to the ratio of 0.93 reported by Fitch and Giedd[1] in 1999 (150 mm in females vs 161 mm in males). An elongated vocal tract in males correlates with lower formants that are narrowly interspaced, whereas a short vocal tract in females correlates with higher formants that are widely interspaced.[37] Bennett[42] in 1981 reported lower formants in males compared to females with a range of 3% for F1 of /i/ to about 16% for F1 of /ae/. The author inferred that these differences in vowel formants were related to differences in vocal tract dimensions and variations in articulatory behavior between males and females. Her findings were in accordance with the longitudinal cephalometric study by King,[38] which revealed longer pharyngeal cavities in boys in comparison to girls, and also in accordance with the morphologic study of

Fant[39] in 1973, which attributed differences in formant frequencies to different measures in pharyngeal cavities across gender.

The strong link between formant profiles and vocal tract dimensions has also been demonstrated within same sex.[40,43,44] Subjects with different voice classifications have been reported to have different vocal tract morphology. Cleveland[43] in 1977 reported differences in formant-frequency percentage between tenors and basses, and he alluded to the potential role of oral and pharyngeal lengths in voice classification. Similarly, Dmitriev and Kiselev[44] in 1979 demonstrated a correlation between the integrated spectra of different singing voices and the buccopharyngeal tract length, which is fixed for every voice type. The authors reported that the buccopharyngeal length decreases from bass singers to baritone, tenor, mezzo-soprano, and soprano. Roers et al[40] in 2009 also investigated the correlation between vocal tract length and voice classification in a large group of singers. Using radiologic images, the vocal tract length was computed by adding 3 sections, the pharyngeal section that extended from the most "anterior point of the laryngeal prominence to the lowermost anterior edge,"[40] the velor section that extended from the latter point to the most anterior part of the third molar in the maxilla, and the oral section, which started from this last point to the lowermost point of the upper incisor contour. The results indicated that vocal tract length differed significantly among most voice classifications except "the mezzosopranos who did not differ significantly from sopranos or altos, and for the altos who did not differ significantly from baritones."[40(p506)] In particular, the pharyngeal length was most influential among the various vocal tract measurements.[40]

In keeping with all the aforementioned studies substantiating the strong relationship between vocal tract morphology and vocal characteristics in the context of sexual dimorphism and voice classification, many imaging studies of the vocal tract during vocalized vowels and consonants have corroborated the role of vocal tract agility in phonation.[45,46] Lakshminaryanan et al[47] in 1991 used magnetic resonance imaging to visualize the vocal tract during the production of 5 sustained vowels. Images taken from the region extending from the glottis to the lips were used to build an acoustic tube model. The formant frequencies measured from the reconstructed acoustic tube were comparable to those obtained from the subjects' speech analysis. The authors emphasized the added value of magnetic resonance imaging in understanding speech production and simulation of sustained vowels.[47] That same year, Baer et al[45] examined vocal tract shape and dimensions during the vocalization of 4 different vowels in two male speakers. Midsagittal and cross-sectional images were used to measure the width and functional areas of the vocal tract. The area functions obtained were commensurate with the expected patterns of narrowing and/or widening of the oral cavity and pharynx across all studied vowels. Despite the differences between the formant frequencies uttered by the subjects and the computed resonances, the vowel waveforms were comparable to the original utterances as perceived by skilled and unskilled listeners.[45] Story et al[46] reported a 3-dimensional catalogue of functional areas of the vocal tract with 18 air space shapes drawn during vocalization. These 3-dimensional images were used to reconstruct the vocal tract from which formants location were extracted. A comparison of these simulated formants with those produced naturally by the subject revealed fair similarity.

All the aforementioned reports support the known correlation between formant profiles and vocal tract morphology. Formants profiles play an important role in signaling vocal tract shape and dimension. However, what remains unanswered is their role as vocal indices to body size. In the below 2 subdivisions, 2 main questions are addressed: First, are there any distinctive variations or alterations in the vocal tract of obese subjects? Second, what are the acoustic implications of these variations or alterations?

Variations in Vocal Tract Morphology in Relation to Body Size

In considering the literature on vocal tract morphologic features in obese subjects in comparison to nonobese subjects, it is useful to focus on vocal tract shape and length, with emphasis on the pharynx as a major division of the vocal tract.

Vocal Tract Shape in Relation to Body Weight

Most of the information on vocal tract shape in obese subjects is derived from studies on the pathogenic role of obesity in patients with obstructive sleep apnea (OSA). In 1989, Horner et al[48] examined the size and distribution of fat along the vocal tract in obese subjects with and without OSA. Their radiologic investigation revealed excessive fat deposits at various sites of the vocal tract in most subjects, more so in those with OSA in comparison with weight-matched subjects. Though no fat deposit was found within oropharyngeal tissues, fat was identified in the palate-pharyngeal area and anterior to the laryngopharyngeal space in all subjects. Moreover, fat was found within the tongue in 40% to 50% of the cases and

in the palate in two-thirds of obese patients with OSA. Refer to Figures 5–1, 5–2, and 5–3. The distribution of fat at the various sites has been implicated in the pathogenesis of OSA, with various mechanisms being

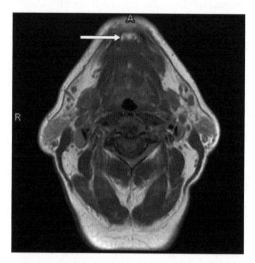

Figure 5–1. Axial TW1_TSE MRI image showing submental fat distribution (*arrow*) in a 65-year-old man with a weight of 103 kg (body mass index 34.87 kg/m²).

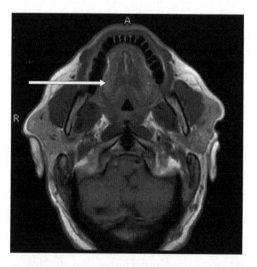

Figure 5–2. Axial TW1_TSE MRI image showing base of tongue (*arrow*) fat distribution in a 65-year-old man with a weight of 103 kg (body mass index 34.87 kg/m²).

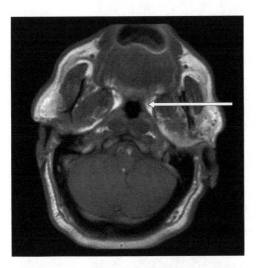

Figure 5–3. Axial TW1_TSE MRI image showing and palate-pharyngeal (*arrow*) fat distribution in a 65-year-old man with a weight of 103 kg (body mass index 34.87 kg/m^2).

suggested. The palate-pharyngeal fat, for instance, was considered as a predisposing factor for narrowing of the retropalatal space either by direct mechanical pressure or by impairing the inherent elasticity of the pharyngeal wall. The authors concluded that this functional impairment, in addition to the fat deposit in the palate, might lead to collapse of the retropalatal space. Although the discussion in the manuscript by Horner et al[48] was geared toward better understanding the pathogenesis of OSA, the results of their investigation provided invaluable information on the anatomical variations of the vocal tract in obese subjects. Similarly, in 1993, Shelton et al[49] investigated the role of adipose tissue in the pathogenesis of obstructive sleep apnea with emphasis on the area adjacent to the pharyngeal airway. This radiologic study using magnetic resonance imaging was conducted on 30 subjects with and without OSA, 2 of whom were examined before and after weight loss. The interesting finding was that all subjects had pharyngeal adipose tissue that corre-

lated with the apnea-hypopnea index, and most importantly that the concentration of that adipose tissue decreased with weight loss. This change in the volume of pharyngeal adipose tissue in relation to body weight accentuates the dynamic interaction between body weight and vocal tract configuration, which further suggests a possible relationship between vocal tract variations and vocal changes in obese subjects.[49] Mortimore et al[50] in 1998 investigated fat deposition and distribution in the upper airway in obese vs nonobese patients with sleep apnea/hypopnea syndrome (SAHS) and in comparison with controls matched by age. The results indicated that the difference in neck tissue volume in obese patients with SAHS vs controls was greater than the difference in neck tissue volume in nonobese patients with SAHS vs controls (28% vs 10%). The percentage of neck tissue volume attributed to fat was greater in both obese groups with and without SAHS in comparison with controls (67% and 27%, respectively). Refer to Figures 5–4 and 5–5. The fat was found primarily anterolateral to the upper airway, resulting in narrowing of the retropalatal and retroglossal cross-sectional areas.[50]

In addition to the presence of soft tissue changes in the vocal tract of obese subjects compared with nonobese subjects, there are also bony and structural differences that might further accentuate variations in vocal tract shape in relation to obesity. In 1999, Sakakibara et al[51] investigated the cephalometric measures in obese and nonobese patients with obstructive sleep apnea in comparison with controls. The authors demonstrated a correlation between BMI, soft tissues abnormalities, and cephalometric measures. With respect to upper airway soft tissue abnormalities, obese subjects had longer and larger base of tongue measures, narrowing of the airway width and

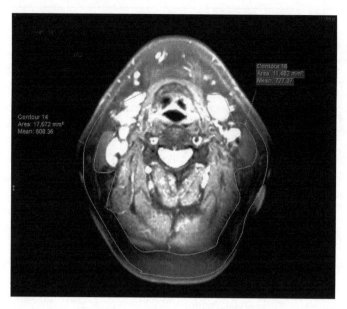

Figure 5–4. Magnetic resonance imaging (T1) illustrating the distribution and concentration of adipose tissue in the neck of a 65-year-old man weighing 103 kg (body mass index 34.87 kg/m^2). The total cross-sectional area is 17,672 mm^2 and subcutaneous fat covers an area of 6190 mm^2 (17,672 mm^2 – 11,482 mm^2). Subcutaneous fat tissue is 35.02% of total cross-sectional area.

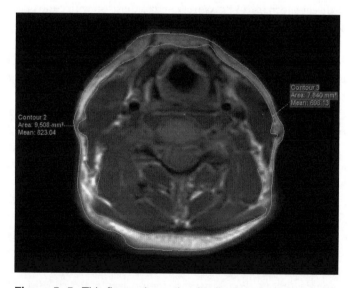

Figure 5–5. This figure shows the distribution of subcutaneous fat tissue in the neck of a 53-year-old female weighing 50.5 kg. The total cross-sectional area is 9508 mm^2 and subcutaneous fat covers an area of 1668 mm^2 (9508 mm^2 – 7840 mm^2). Subcutaneous fat tissue is 17.54% of total cross-sectional area.

oropharyngeal space, and thickening of soft tissues in the nasopharynx[51] (Figure 5–6). With respect to craniofacial bony structures, obese patients with OSA had inferiorly and anteriorly displaced hyoid bones, narrowing of the bony oropharynx (PNS-AA), and decrease in the anteroposterior distances between base of skull and anterior jaw measures.

It is clear that there are variations in the shape and configuration of the vocal tract in obese subjects compared to nonobese. These variations are secondary to excess fat deposition at various sites of the upper airway.

Vocal Tract Length in Relation to Body Size

There are many reports suggesting that not only vocal tract shape varies with weight but also vocal tract length. Most of the information on that topic is derived from studies on the correlation between body size and vocal tract length.[1,42,52] The presence of

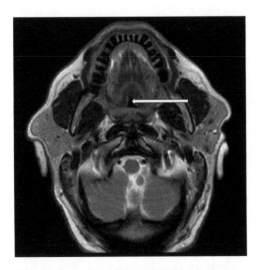

Figure 5–6. Axial T2W MRI images at the level of base of tongue in a 65-year-old male weighing 103 kg showing narrowing at the level of the retroglossal area.

variations in vocal tract length in relation to body size leads to the premise that subjects with large body size (either tall or obese) probably have a longer vocal tract and subsequently different acoustic properties than subjects with normal body weight or subjects who are underweight. Bennett[42] in 1981 estimated vocal tract length based on weight, height, and neck circumference in a group of preadolescent males and females. She reported multiple negative correlations (ranging between −0.506 and −0.866) between the aforementioned body indices and formant frequencies. Her findings supported the inference that boys who were 7 cm taller and 4 kg heavier than girls of the same age had longer vocal tracts.[42] In 1999, Fitch and Giedd[1] investigated the relationship between vocal tract length and body size using magnetic resonance imaging of the vocal tract in 129 subjects between the ages of 20 and 25 years. There was a positive correlation between body size and vocal tract length, which was measured from the lips to the glottis and stratified into 5 segments that included lips, anterior two-thirds of tongue, tongue dorsum, velum, and pharynx. However, the authors alluded to the obscuring role of weight variation, which might have weakened that correlation. Subject's position, lip position, and potential movement of the hyolaryngeal complex during imaging may have also affected the measurement of the vocal tract length. These results corroborated those of a study by the same author in 1997 conducted on 23 rhesus macaques of different ages (1–9 years) and different sizes (2.6–15.6 kg). Vocal tract length was measured using radiographic techniques, namely tracings of x-ray images, and acoustic signals were extracted from threat vocalizations such as "pant-threats" and "pant-barks" with the lips in a nonprotrusive position. The results indicated a strong correlation between vocal tract length, body weight and height, and skull size.[52] Consistent with these findings, Shen et al[53] in 2002 reported a strong correlation between nasopharyngeal tract length measured from nostrils to the vocal folds, and body height and weight ($r = 0.83$ and $r = 0.81$, respectively). The lengths analyzed were retrieved from fiberoptic endoscopic measurements of 413 infants. Moreover, in a study by Roers et al[40] in 2009 conducted on 34 students, the authors reported a significant correlation between body weight and vocal tract length in the entire group but not within the female or male groups alone (ie, within the same gender).

In summary, there is enough evidence to support the presence of a correlation between vocal tract length and body size. The growth of the vocal tract and body in parallel is based on the anatomical constraints of the vocal tract related to its contiguous structures, namely, skull and neck.[1] Other important physiologic constraints to the hyolaryngeal descent are the muscles of deglutition. Physiologic restrictions imposed by swallowing may also present one of the spatial constraints to the downward migration of the laryngopharyngeal structures.[7]

The Predictive Role of Formant Profiles in Estimating Body Size

Given the strong correlation between body size and vocal tract length, and the strong correlation between vocal tract length and formant profiles,[37,41] one might suspect that formant position and distribution should be reliable acoustic cues to the speaker's size, namely weight and height. However, based on a thorough review of the literature, the question whether formant profiles predict body weight reliably and whether

obese subjects have distinctive vocal features in comparison to nonobese remains unanswered. In 1995, van Dommelen and Moxness[14] reexamined the argument presented by Lass and Davis in 1976,[8] namely, that listeners can judge speaker's height and weight by listening to speech samples, and reported a significant correlation between estimated weight/height and actual weight/height only in male speakers. The study was conducted on both male and female speakers who were asked to read isolated words and text paragraphs, while male and female listeners were asked to estimate the speaker height and weight. Although there was consistency in the speakers' weight and height estimates given by listeners, neither men nor women listeners were able to predict the weight and height of female speakers accurately. Moreover, using specific speech signal parameters that included the mean frequency of the second formant during sustained vowel /a/, the investigators also failed to demonstrate a correlation between any of the speech signal parameters and speaker body dimensions, except for speech rate, which correlated significantly with the male speaker weight. Male subjects with reduced tempo were perceived as heavier. However, it is important to note that this observation was based on having subjects read a text rather than talk spontaneously. In 2000, Collins[54] also investigated the correlation between male body characteristics and vocal characteristics, and the role of these latter as cues to physical appearance. The study was conducted on 34 males with a mean age of 22.41 years who were asked to sustain 5 vowels at a comfortable pitch and loudness. The judges consisted of 54 Dutch women who were asked to score the attractiveness of men whose voices had been recorded, as well as to estimate their weight and age. Some of the judges also were asked to estimate other body characteristics such as height, body type, and chest hair. The main acoustic measures included harmonic peaks, overall peak, harmonic spacing, and the peak frequency of the first 3 to 5 harmonics. Although weight was reliably estimated from the male voice, there was no correlation between any of the aforementioned acoustic measures and body characteristics.[54] In judging acoustic characteristics, women were consistently more attracted to voices with lower formants and narrower interspaces. These men who were judged to be more attractive were estimated to be more muscular and hairy (on the chest). The authors alluded to the possibility that women used the formant frequency characteristics as an acoustic cue to certain body characteristic such as wide musculoskeletal structure, which in turn implies high testosterone level. The interesting finding in this study is the lack of correlation between body size and harmonics despite the fact that the harmonics component (low frequency and closely interspaced) was an honest cue to the listeners and a good predictor of estimated weight.[54] Similarly, González[55] in 2004 investigated the relationship between body size and formant frequencies within the same-sex gender. The study was based on 2 experiments: sustained phonation of 5 Spanish vowels recorded from 82 speakers and reading of a paragraph by 91 speakers. In the first experiment, the fundamental frequency and first 4 formant center frequencies were computed, and in the second experiment, the long-term average spectrum analysis of connected speech was used to derive vocal tract resonance characteristics. The results indicated a weak relationship between these acoustic parameters and body attributes, namely weight and height.[55] Based on the aforementioned, the author refuted the

assumption that formant frequencies and dispersion are acoustic cues to body size, despite the correlation between vocal tract length and formant distribution according to the source-filter theory.[37]

Contrary to all the aforementioned studies and in agreement with Fitch's hypothesis on the parallel growth of the vocal tract and body, other authors reported the presence of a correlation between formant profile and body measures. In 2005, Rendall et al[21] investigated the formant profiles of human vowels and their role in predicting body size. A total of 68 students were asked to produce isolated vowels, a list of single-syllable words, and 4 short sentences. The speech material contained a total of 23 different vowel sounds that were analyzed. The authors demonstrated that formants do reflect body size and that the gender difference in formants profile is consistent with body size dimorphism to a given extent. Moreover, the authors reported a correlation between formant variation and height in males but not in females. The inconsistent results in regard to gender were explained on the increasingly important role of voice cuing in men compared to women in a social context, in which, although we believe that this explanation must be viewed with critical skepticism, men assume a higher competitive role.[21] Along the same line, Evans et al[17] in 2006 investigated the relationship between body size, body shape, and various vocal measures that included formant dispersion. The study was conducted on 50 heterosexual males with a mean age of 29.08 years who were asked to sustain the vowels /a/, /i/, /aːi/, and /o/. The results indicated a significant correlation between weight, height, and formant dispersion ($r = -.43$ and $r = -.32$, respectively) despite the lack of any relationship with the remaining body size measures, which included body mass index.[17] There was also a negative correlation between formant dispersion and body shape measures such as neck, shoulder, chest and waist circumference, and shoulder/hip ratio. Subjects who were tall, were heavy, and had large shoulder, neck, and chest circumference had smaller formant dispersion.

A large meta-analysis conducted by Pisanski et al[24] in 2014 looking at the vocal indicators of body size showed that 11 out of 12 vocal tract length estimates predicted weight variance up to 10%. Moreover, "ninety-three percent of the derived mean weighted correlations between formants and body size reached statistical significance."[24] The authors concluded that formants are a cue to body size in humans similar to other vertebrates. In a large study by the same authors in 2016 conducted on 700 men and women, the authors confirmed the results of their previous meta-analysis in 2014. The results indicated that vocal tract resonance predicts height and weight and thus can explain most of the variances in these characteristics. However, perturbation parameters and harmonics-to-noise ratio correlated with other components of body shape such as hip circumferences, waist-to-hip ratio, and chest-to-hip ratio.[25]

In summary, there are conflicting reports on the correlation between formant profiles and body weight and height. Although formants correlate more reliably with body size than F0, still there is not enough evidence to support a correlation between formant position and distribution and body weight across and within genders. Nevertheless, it is important to note that the hypothesis that listeners can estimate body weight accurately, more so in males, has been proven by some authors. What remains unknown are the acoustic cues used in the estimation process. Future research is needed to clarify the predictive role of formants and other accurate cues in estimating body weight.

References

1. Fitch WT, Giedd J. Morphology and development of the human vocal tract: a study using magnetic resonance imaging. *J Acoust Soc Am*. 1999;106(3):1511–1522.
2. Newman SR, Butler J, Hammond EH, Gray SD. Preliminary report on hormone receptors in the human vocal fold. *J Voice*. 2000; 14(1):72–81.
3. Voelter Ch, Kleinsasser N, Joa P, et al. Detection of hormone receptor in the human vocal fold. *Eur Arch Otorhinolaryngol*. 2008; 265(10):1239–1244.
4. Rios OA, Duprat Ade C, Santos AR. Immunohistochemical searching for estrogen and progesterone receptors in women vocal fold epithelia. *Braz J Otorhinolaringol*. 2008; 74(4):487–493.
5. Sataloff RT. Clinical anatomy and physiology of the voice. In: Sataloff RT, ed. *Professional Voice: The Science and Art of Clinical Care*. 4th ed. San Diego, CA: Plural Publishing; 2017:157–195.
6. Blouin K, Boivin A, Tchernof A. Androgens and body fat distribution. *J Steroid Biochem Mol Biol*. 2008;108(3–5):272–280.
7. Lieberman DE, McCarthy RC, Hiiemae KM, Palmer JB. Ontogeny of postnatal hyoid and larynx descent in humans. *Arch Oral Biol*. 2001;46(2):117–128.
8. Lass NJ, Davis M. An investigation of speaker height and weight identification. *J Acoust Soc Am*. 1976;60(3):700–703.
9. Lass NJ, Beverly AS, Nicosia DK, Simpson LA. An investigation of speaker height and weight identification: II. direct estimations. *J Acoust Soc Am*. 1977;61(suppl 1):S70.
10. Bachorowski JA, Owren MJ. Acoustic correlates of talker sex and individual talker identity are present in a short vowel segment

produced in running speech. *J Acoust Soc Am.* 1999;106(2):1054–1063.

11. Smith DR, Patterson RD. The interaction of glottal-pulse rate and vocal-tract length in judgements of speaker size, sex, and age. *J Acoust Soc Am.* 2005;118(5):3177–3186.

12. Künzel HJ. How well does average fundamental frequency correlate with speaker height and weight? *Phonetica.* 1989;46(1–3):117–125.

13. van Dommelen WA. Speaker height and weight identification: a re-evaluation of some old data. *J Phon.* 1993;21(3):337–341.

14. van Dommelen WA, Moxness BH. Acoustic parameters in speaker height and weight identification: sex-specific behavior. *Lang Speech.* 1995;38(pt 3):267–287.

15. Lass NJ. Correlational study of speakers' heights, weights, body surface areas, and speaking fundamental frequencies. *J Acoust Soc Am.* 1978;63(4):1218–1220.

16. Hamdan AL, Al-Barazi R, Tabri D, et al. Relationship between acoustic parameters and body mass analysis in young males. *J Voice.* 2012;26(2):144–147.

17. Evans S, Neave N, Wakelin D. Relationships between vocal characteristics and body size and shape in human males: an evolutionary explanation for a deep male voice. *Biol Psychol.* 2006;72(2):160–163.

18. Lass NJ, Kelley DT, Cunningham CM, Sheridan KJ. A comparative study of speaker height and weight identification from voiced and whispered speech. *J Phon.* 1980;8(2):195–204.

19. Cohen JR, Crystal TH, House AS, Neuburg EP. Weighty voices and shaky evidence: a critique. *J Acoust Soc Am.* 1980;68(6):1884–1886.

20. Gunter CD, Manning WH. Listener estimations of speaker height and weight in unfiltered and filtered conditions. *J Phon.* 1982;10(3):251–257.

21. Rendall D, Kollias S, Ney C, Lloyd P. Pitch (F 0) and formant profiles of human vowels and vowel-like baboon grunts: the role of vocalizer body size and voice-acoustic allometry. *J Acoust Soc Am.* 2005;117(2):944–955.

22. Damrose EJ. Quantifying the impact of androgen therapy on the female larynx. *Auris Nasus Larynx.* 2009;36(1):110–112.

23. de Souza LB, Pereira RM, dos Santos MM, de Almeida Godoy CM. Fundamental frequency, phonation maximum time and vocal complaints in morbidly obese women. *Arq Bras Cir Dig.* 2014;27(1):43–46.

24. Pisanski K, Fraccaro PJ, Tigue CC, et al. Vocal indicators of body size in men and women: a meta-analysis. *Animal Behav.* 2014;95:89–99.

25. Pisanski K, Jones BC, Fink B, et al. Voice parameters predict sex-specific body morphology in men and women. *Animal Behav.* 2016;112:13–22.

26. Collins LC, Hoberty PD, Walker JF, Fletcher EC, Peiris AN. The effect of body fat distribution on pulmonary function tests. *Chest.* 1995;107(5):1298–1302.

27. Da Cunha MG, Passerotti GH, Weber R, Zilberstein B, Cecconello I. Voice feature characteristic in morbid obese population. *Obes Surg.* 2011;21(3):340–344.

28. Barsties B, Verfaillie R, Roy N, Maryn Y. Do body mass index and fat volume influence vocal quality, phonatory range, and aerodynamics in females? *Codas.* 2013;23(4):310–318.

29. Kantarci F, Mihmanli I, Demirel MK, et al. Normal diaphragmatic motion and the effects of body composition: determination with M-mode sonography. *J Ultrasound Med.* 2004;23(2):255–260.

30. Titze IR. Vocal fold mass is not a useful quantity for describing F0 in vocalization. *J Speech Lang Hear Res.* 2011;54(2):520–522.

31. Lan CC, Su CP, Chou LL, Yang MC, Lim CS, Wu YK. Association of body mass index with exercise cardiopulmonary responses in lung function-matched patients with chronic obstructive pulmonary disease. *Heart Lung.* 2012;41(4):374–381.

32. Pisanski K, Fraccaro PJ, Tigue CC, O'Connor JJ, Feinberg DR. Return to Oz: voice pitch facilitates assessments of men's body size. *J Exp Psychol Hum Percept Perform.* 2014; 40(4):1316–1331.

33. Acurio J, Celis C, Perez J, Escudero C. Acoustic parameters and salivary IL-6 levels in overweight and obese teachers. *J Voice.* 2014;28(5):574–581.

34. Morton ES. On the occurrence and significance of motivation-structural rules in some bird and mammal sounds. *Am Nat.* 1977; 111(981):855–869.

35. Fitch WT. The evolution of speech: a comparative review. *Trends Cogn Sci.* 2000;4(7): 258–267.

36. Smith DR, Walters TC, Patterson RD. Discrimination of speaker sex and size when glottal-pulse rate and vocal-tract length are controlled. *J Acoust Soc Am.* 2007;122(6): 3628–3639.

37. Titze IR. *Principles of Vocal Production.* Englewood Cliffs, NJ: Prentice Hall; 1994.

38. King EW. A roentgenographic study of pharyngeal growth. *Angle Orthod.* 1952;22(1): 23–37.

39. Fant G. *Speech Sounds and Features.* Cambridge, MA: The MIT Press; 1973.

40. Roers F, Mürbe D, Sundberg J. Voice classification and vocal tract of singers: a study of x-ray images and morphology. *J Acoust Soc Am.* 2009;125(1):503–512.

41. Sataloff RT. Vocal tract resonance. In Sataloff RT, ed. *Professional Voice: The Science and Art of Clinical Care.* 4th ed. San Diego, CA: Plural Publishing; 2017:309–328.

42. Bennett S. Vowel formant frequency characteristics of preadolescent males and females. *J Acoust Soc Am.* 1981;69(1):231–238.

43. Cleveland TF. Acoustic properties of voice timbre types and their influence on voice classification. *J Acoust Soc Am.* 1977;61(6): 1622–1629.

44. Dmitriev L, Kiselev A. Relationship between the formant structure of different types of singing voices and the dimensions of supraglottic cavities. *Folia Phoniatr.* 1979;31(4): 238–241.

45. Baer T, Gore JC, Gracco LC, Nye PW. Analysis of vocal tract shape and dimensions using magnetic resonance imaging: vowels. *J Acoust Soc Am.* 1991;90(2):799–828.

46. Story BH, Titze IR, Hoffman EA. Vocal tract area functions from magnetic resonance imaging. *J Acoust Soc Am.* 1996;100(1):537–554.

47. Lakshminarayanan AV, Lee S, McCutcheon MJ. MR imaging of the vocal tract during vowel production. *J Magn Reson Imaging.* 1991;1(1):71–76.

48. Horner RL, Mohiaddin RH, Lowell DG, et al. Sites and sizes of fat deposits around the pharynx in obese patients with obstructive sleep apnoea and weight matched controls. *Eur Respir J.* 1989;2(7):613–622.

49. Shelton KE, Woodson H, Gay S, Suratt PM. Pharyngeal fat in obstructive sleep apnea. *Am Rev Respir Dis.* 1993;148(2):462–466.

50. Mortimore IL, Marshall I, Wraith PK, Sellar RJ, Douglas NJ. Neck and total body fat deposition in nonobese and obese patients with sleep apnea compared with that in control subjects. *Am J Respir Crit Care Med.* 1998;157(1):280–283.

51. Sakakibara H, Tong M, Matsushita K, Hirata M, Konishi Y, Suetsugu S. Cephalometric abnormalities in non-obese and obese patients with obstructive sleep apnoea. *Eur Respir J.* 1999;13(2):403–410.

52. Fitch WT. Vocal tract length and formant frequency dispersion correlate with body size in rhesus macaques. *J Acoust Soc Am.* 1997;102(2):1213–1222.

53. Shen CM, Soong WJ, Jeng MJ, Lee YS, Cheng CY, Sun J, Hwang B. Nasopharyngeal tract length measurement in infants. *Acta Paediatr Taiwan.* 2002;43(2):82–85.

54. Collins SA. Men's voices and women's choices. *Anim Behav.* 2000;60(6):773–780.

55. González J. Formant frequencies and body size of speaker: a weak relationship in adult humans. *J Phon.* 2004;32(2):277–287.

6

Obesity, Sex Hormones, and Voice

Abdul-Latif Hamdan, Robert Thayer Sataloff, and Mary J. Hawkshaw

Sex hormones play a major role in energy utilization and weight accumulation. Numerous investigations have highlighted their impact on adipose tissue distribution and their modulating effect on cardiometabolic health in both genders.[1-4] Women have high body fat content and accrue fat subcutaneously, while men have low body fat content and grow adipose tissue in the visceral region. The deposition of fat subcutaneously in women and centrally in men has been attributed partially to the differential activity of lipoprotein lipase, a major fat-based enzymatic activity influenced markedly by sex hormones, mainly testosterone.[2,3] Obesity also is known to temper sex hormone concentration in both genders. The effect of adiposity on energy homeostasis through secretions of various hormones and molecules has been documented.[5] Adipose tissue is a source of estrogen and a site for estrone biosynthesis from androgens derivatives via cytochrome P450.

Amid this congruence between obesity and sex hormones, various systems in the body are affected, including the phonatory system. The effect of sex hormones on laryngeal structures through hormonal receptors has been reported in numerous studies.[6-8]

Newman et al[6] described vocal folds' cytoplasmic and nuclear receptors and reported an association between androgen receptor staining and gender stratification. Similarly, Voelter et al,[9] using monoclonal antibodies, reported the presence of sex hormones receptors in 104 patients with different vocal fold pathologies. It appears that both testosterone and estrogen play major roles in voice maturation at puberty. Obesity also has been reported to affect voice. de Souza et al[10] in 2014 reported significantly higher prevalence of vocal complaints in obese subjects in comparison to subjects with normal body weight. Da Cunha et al[11] also reported perceptual vocal alterations in subjects with body mass index (BMI) greater than 35 kg/m^2. These alterations were described as hoarseness and phonatory instability in 62% and 44% of cases, respectively. Similarly, Barsties et al,[12] in their investigation on acoustic and aerodynamic measures in obese vs normal-weight subjects, reported higher minimum intensity and maximum intensity sound pressure levels in the obese group. These acoustic alterations were attributed to anatomical variations in the vocal tract and diaphragm muscle.

Given the interrelationship between sex hormones and obesity, on one hand, and sex hormones and voice, on the other, it is logical to infer that obesity-induced hormonal variations can impact voice. It is important to understand the interplay between variations in sex hormones, adiposity, and vocal characteristics.

Sex Hormones and Obesity

Estrogen and Obesity

The interplay between obesity and sex hormones is well known. Numerous reports indicate reduced levels of testosterone and increased levels of estradiol (E2) and estrone (E1) in obese men and women in comparison with normal-weight subjects.[13–20] The increase in estrogen level is attributed partially to increased conversion of androstenedione and testosterone in the adipose tissue. This conversion is catalyzed by 2 important enzymes, active aromatase and 17 beta-hydroxysteroid dehydrogenase, the concentrations of which depend on the number and size of adipose cells.[21] Estrogen also affects fat concentration and distribution. By selective alteration in sympathetic nervous system stimulation to adipose tissue, there is differential fat deposition subcutaneously in women and viscerally in men. The gynoid type of obesity characterized by the pear shape with fat accumulation in the thighs, hips, and buttocks is seen predominantly in premenopausal women, whereas the android type characterized by the apple shape with visceral fat deposition is seen more commonly in men and postmenopausal women.[1]

The mode of action of estrogen on adiposity is both peripheral and central.[22–25] At the cellular level, several mechanisms have been suggested: one is alteration in blood supply to the adipose tissues leading to overexpression of vascular endothelial growth factor with hyperplasia of adipocytes, and another is an increase in the metabolic rate, leading to a higher level of mitochondrial activity or "browning" of adipose tissue with subsequent increase in estrogen levels; a third possible mechanism is activation and suppression of estrogen receptors, namely estrogen receptor alpha and estrogen receptor beta. By controlling lipolysis/lipogenesis, these antagonist receptors modulate fat content and distribution in the subcutaneous and visceral reserves differentially.[25] Another mechanism by which estrogen may act on adiposity is centrally. Similar to gonadal hormones and stress, sex hormones, and estrogen in particular, modulate the activity of the limbic-pituitary-adrenal axis.[26,27] To that end, estrogen has been shown to suppress appetite and enhance energy expenditure. High levels of estrogen present during the follicular and periovulatory phases of the menstrual cycle decrease appetite while high levels of progestin during the luteal phase increase eating. The suppression of appetite is affected by the activity of other mediators such as leptin, brain-derived neurotrophic factors, and cholecystokinin.[28–29] Moreover, a rise in estrogen has been reported to increase energy expenditure. This effect is seen mostly in postmenopausal women in whom the decrease in estrogen results in a parallel decrease in energy expenditure. As such, estrogen is considered as a protective hormone against obesity in women, the loss of which after menopause results in adiposity and increase in metabolic diseases. This latter problem may be mitigated by the intake of hormone replacement therapy.[30,31]

In summary, the synergy between adiposity and estrogen highlights the vital role of estrogen in fat deposition, distribution, and energy homeostasis.

Androgen and Obesity: Association Between Testosterone Level and Obesity in Adults

There are many reports on the negative correlation between obesity and testosterone in adults.[32–41] In the study by Abate et al[40] on 33 patients with type 2 diabetes, the authors reported an inverse relationship between sex hormones binding globulin (SHBG) and obesity, and they concluded that the plasma concentration of testosterone can predict the extent of and variations in fat deposition. Though the correlation between androgen and obesity is well established, the temporal relation between the two is still an issue of debate. Whether obesity precedes the drop in total and free testosterone levels, or whether the decrease in these sex hormones precipitates obesity, is controversial. What favors the first hypothesis is that adipose tissue is a depot for the conversion of testosterone to estradiol.[5] However, there is mounting evidence in the literature indicating that bioavailable testosterone enhances lipolysis, and thus a decrease in testosterone can lead to excessive adiposity.[42,43] Katznelson et al[44] in 1996 reported a 14% decrease in total fat measures following administration of testosterone. Similarly, Woodhouse et al[45] demonstrated a testosterone dose-dependent change in total body fat in a group of 54 men following induction of hypogonadism. A subphysiologic level of testosterone was associated with an increase in abdominal and visceral fat.[45] Suggested mechanisms for the sex hormone-induced fat reduction include inhibition of the differentiation of mesenchymal multipotent cells into adipogenic cells and their inhibition into the adipogenic lineage.[46,47]

Though both subcutaneous and visceral fat affect sex hormones levels negatively, visceral fat is more influential. There is increasing evidence to support that men with similar BMI but different body fat distribution have different levels of testosterone.[48] In 1990, Seidell et al[49] reported an association between testosterone level and visceral adipose tissue in a group of 23 men. Similarly, Khaw and Barrett-Connor,[50] in their study on 511 men, demonstrated an inverse relationship between SHBG, testosterone, and central obesity. The authors alluded to the predictive role of endogenous androgens in relation to central obesity.[50] In 1993, Haffner et al investigated the relationship between sex hormones and body indices in 178 men. The authors demonstrated a significant negative correlation between waist-to-hip ratio, with conicity defined as "abdominal circumference divided by 0.109 multiplied by the square root of weight/height,"[51(p643)] and free testosterone and dehydroepiandrosterone sulphate (DHEA-SO4).[51] Tsai et al,[52] in their longitudinal study on 110 men over the course of 7.5 years, reported an association between intra-abdominal fat (IAF) measured using computerized tomography and testosterone level. Four years later, Svartberg et al[41] also noted the correlation between sex hormones and central obesity in their study on 1584 men. Interestingly, the association between total testosterone and waist circumference ($r = -0.34$) remained even after adjusting for age, lifestyle factors, and BMI. The authors concluded that waist circumference is a good anthropometric predictive measure of testosterone level. Last, Derby et al[53] in their study on 942 men also showed a negative correlation between free testosterone, total testosterone, and 3 body indices. Their findings corroborated those of Haffner et al[51] and were in partial agreement with the results of Svartberg et al.[41]

In summary, we can conclude that androgens are important determinants of not only total body fat percentage but also body composition and contour.

Association Between Testosterone Level and Obesity in Prepubertal Subjects and Elderly

Although both small and large study groups agree that adult men with high BMI have consistently lower free and total testosterone levels in comparison with men with normal weight, and that body indices are good predictors of androgen levels, the relationship between obesity and sexual maturation remains controversial.[54-62] The study by Wang[62] conducted on a group of 1520 boys showed that high BMI is associated with late maturity, whereas the study by He and Karlberg[56] conducted on 3650 Swedish children revealed that heavier boys and girls had earlier onset of puberty. The disparities in the results were attributed to limitations in diagnosing puberty in boys and to the use of BMI as an index of obesity. Similarly, the association between obesity and sex hormones levels in the prepubertal and adolescent years is inconclusive with conflicting reports on the level of serum testosterone in relation to body mass index. Vandewalle et al[63] reported comparable levels of free testosterone in 90 obese boys between the ages of 10 and 19 years compared with 90 age-matched controls, whereas other investigators such as Reinehr et al reported higher levels of testosterone and DHEAS in obese prepubertal children compared to normal-weight children.[64] When the levels of total and free testosterone are lower, the decrease

is invariably associated with a lower level of SHBG, which in turn has been related to the high insulin level in affected subjects.[65]

Obesity also has been shown to accentuate the natural decline in testosterone that occurs with aging. Having a body weight of more than 120% of ideal as reported by the Massachusetts male aging study is associated with a 25% lower total testosterone level in comparison with nonobese age-matched subjects.[66] A longitudinal study conducted by Travison et al[67] on the impact of aging and lifestyle on testosterone level showed that gaining weight over the years may simulate the effect of aging. Similarly, a study by Ponholzer et al[68] on 375 men between the ages of 45 and 85 years revealed a negative correlation between BMI and testosterone level. The authors noted the negative impact of lifestyle factors on serum androgen levels, in addition to chronological aging.

In summary, there is no consensus on the negative correlation between testosterone level and obesity in prepubertal subjects. However, obesity may mimic aging by lowering total and free testosterone levels.

Interplay Between Sex Hormones, Obesity, and Voice

How does all the aforementioned relate to voice? The phonatory apparatus is intimately linked to our body morphology and sexual identity. Laryngeal exposure to sex hormones at puberty results in marked alteration in vocal characteristics. Estrogen induces subtle growth of the vocal folds with thinning and lubrication of the overlying mucus, whereas testosterone and its metabolic derivatives result in greater changes of laryngeal cartilaginous, muscular, and soft tissue structures. Based on animal studies, the growth is dose dependent and affects mostly the thyroid cartilage.[69] The development of the thyroid cartilage anteroposteriorly and vertically leads to elongation of the vocal folds, resulting in an estimated membranous vocal fold length of 15.1 ± 2.31 mm in adult men and 10.4 ± 1.9 mm in adult women.[70] There is also enlargement of the vocal folds almost twice in men compared to women, 63% vs 34%, respectively.[71] These morphologic changes, in addition to differentiation of the vocal fold ligament as reported by Hirano et al,[72] lead to vocal dimorphism among genders. As the vocal pitch is determined by vocal folds' length, tension, and mass per cross-sectional area, the hormone-induced increase in vocal fold size results in lowering of the fundamental frequency, more in men than in women. In parallel with vocal folds' morphologic changes, there is elongation of the vocal tract. Fitch and Giedd[73] in their magnetic resonance imaging study reported changes in the proportions of the oral and pharyngeal cavities. As a result to these alterations to the vocal tract, there is lowering of the formants and narrowing of their interspace, leading to further deepening of the voice.

After puberty, sex hormones may also exert cyclic effects on voice that are more noticeable in women as well as acute effects. During women's reproductive years, estrogen induces a cyclic increase in capillary permeability and an increase in supraglottic and subglottic glandular secretions.[74,75] Its proliferative effect, most pronounced on the 21st day of the menstrual cycle, leads to polymerization of the vocal folds' mucopolysaccharides. Progesterone reduces capillary permeability and leads to vocal folds' congestion. At the mucosal level, there is desquamation and dryness with thickening of the secretions. In parallel with these secretary changes, a constellation of phonatory changes initially described as "laryngo-

pathia premenstrualis"[76] and now referred to as "premenstrual vocal syndrome" may emerge. In a study on 104 singers, Davis and Davis[77] reported the prevalence of 3 premenstrual vocal symptoms on average per singer. Similar to the effect of sex hormones on voice in women in their reproductive years, the drop in estrogen and progesterone at menopause may lead to an array of vocal symptoms in up to 77% of cases.[78] The most commonly reported symptoms are throat clearing, oropharyngeal dryness, voice fatigue, and loss of high notes. These vocal complaints have been attributed to vocal fold atrophic changes in addition to reduction in laryngeal glandular secretions as reported by Abitbol et al.[78] Other authors have concurred with these findings in similar reports on phonatory disturbances and acoustic changes, particularly in singers and professional voice users.[79] Of clinical interest is the reversibility of these acoustic changes and regression of these vocal symptoms following the initiation of hormonal replacement. The intake of estrogen/progesterone has been proven to mitigate the aforementioned phonatory alterations. The studies by D'haeseleer et al[80–82] clearly indicate that menopausal women have lower habitual pitch than nonmenopausal women and that menopausal women on hormonal therapy have higher habitual pitch than those not on therapy.

In keeping with the impact of sex hormones on voice discussed above, there are numerous reports on the predictive value of vocal pitch in sex hormone variations.[83,84] Meuser and Nieschlag[85] in 1977 reported higher testosterone/estradiol ratio in bass singers compared to baritones and tenors. The study on the correlation between depth of male voice and sex hormones level was conducted on 102 singers. A decade later, Pedersen et al[86] concurred the relation between testosterone and vocal pitch in a group of 48 boys between the ages of 8 and 20 years. Total testosterone, dihydrotestosterone, and free testosterone negatively correlated with the fundamental frequency in continuous speech ($r = -0.73$, $r = -0.68$, and $r = -0.76$, respectively). Similarly, in 1999, Dabbs and Mallinger[84] confirmed the strong interplay between salivary testosterone level and vocal pitch using radioimmune assay. The negative correlation ($r = -0.26$) was present only in men ($n = 61$) and not in women ($n = 88$). The authors discussed the importance of psychological factors or vocal style on lowering the pitch, in addition to the physiologic changes at the level of the vocal folds. These results were supported further by Evans et al[83] on 40 healthy males between the ages of 18 and 45 years. The authors reported a negative correlation between salivary testosterone level and fundamental frequency. Testosterone levels were measured using salivary samples taken 3 times per day.

In addition to physiologic hormone changes, voice can be affected by acute changes in sex hormones. This topic is discussed well in transgender literature, and in literature on voice change associated with androgens consumed for medical reasons or for body building as referenced below.[87]

In summary, given that the larynx is a hormonal target markedly influenced by sex hormones, and given the strong interplay between sex hormones and obesity as discussed in the first section of this chapter, one can speculate that adiposity-induced hormonal changes will affect voice. There are no studies in the current literature on the impact of obesity on voice in the context of variations in sex hormones. There are no data on acoustic changes as a result of obesity-induced hormonal variations, specifically decrease in total and free testosterone in men, and the increase in estradiol in men and women. Although there are a few studies on vocal changes in obese subjects in comparison to normal-weight subjects,[10-12] the causal relationship between these changes and obesity-induced hormonal variations has not been proven. It is known that hypogonadism impedes voice maturation at puberty[88] and that the intake of exogenous androgens deepens the adult female's voice and induces myogenesis in men with androgen deficiency.[89-91] However, there is no consensus on the impact of decreased testosterone on the adult male voice. Gugatschka et al[92] reported no significant difference in the vocal characteristics of eugonade vs hypogonade patients. In their study cohort of 63 men, there was no relation between androgen level and voice parameters. However, other authors reported higher fundamental frequency in patients with hypogonadism in comparison with controls.[93,94] Akcam et al[93] reported a decrease in mean fundamental frequency following androgen therapy in a group of patients with isolated hypogonadotropic hypogonadism. Similarly, Hamdan et al[94] reported higher habitual pitch in patients with prostatic cancer who underwent androgen ablation therapy. Along the same line of thinking, there is little evidence in the literature to substantiate the association between fat-induced estrogen variations and voice. In women, the effect of increased estrogen is more pronounced at menopause and less so during the reproductive years. Studies have shown that menopausal women with high body mass index tend to have higher fundamental frequency than those with low body mass index.[80-82] The fat-induced estrogen excess described in the "Rubenesque" type of women as reported by Abitbol et al[78] is likely to compensate for the loss of ovarian estrogen and to compensate for the ovarian-derived androgens after menopause. To that end, BMI is an important variable to consider in the interpretation of phonatory changes and acoustic findings in menopausal women. However, there are no studies on the correlation between estrogen level, vocal changes, and weight variations. Similarly, there is scant information on vocal characteristics in men with variation in estrogen level. In the study by Gugatschka et al,[92] higher fundamental frequency was reported in male subjects with lower estrogen levels. The impact of fat-induced high estrogen level on voice in adult men has not been reported.

In summary, there are no data to substantiate an association between vocal characteristics and obesity-induced hormonal changes in obese vs normal-weight subjects. Moreover, there is no consensus that the decrease in free and total testosterone level reported in obese men has an effect on voice. However, the high level of estrogen in women with elevated BMI plays an important role in mitigating the menopausal syndrome, which includes phonatory changes. Future studies are needed to document the causality between the vocal characteristics and sex hormonal variations induced by excessive weight.

References

1. Davis KD, Neinast M, Sun KM, et al. The sexually dimorphic role of adipose and adipocyte estrogen receptors in modulating adipose tissue expansion, inflammation, and fibrosis. *Mol Metab.* 2013;2(3):227–242.
2. Arner P, Lithell H, Wahrenberg H, Brönnegard M. Expression of lipoprotein lipase in different human subcutaneous adipose tissue regions. *J Lipid Res.* 1991;32(3):423–429.
3. Ramirez ME, McMurry MP, Wiebke GA, et al. Evidence for sex steroid inhibition of lipoprotein lipase in men: comparison of abdominal and femoral adipose tissue. *Metabolism.* 1997;46(2):179–185.
4. Clegg D, Hevener AL, Moreau KL, et al. Sex hormones and cardiometabolic health: role of estrogen and estrogen receptors. *Endocrinology.* 2017;158(5):1095–1105.
5. Kim JH, Cho HT, Kim YJ. The role of estrogen in adipose tissue metabolism: insights into glucose homeostasis regulation. *Endocr J.* 2014;61(11):1055–1067.
6. Newman SR, Butler J, Hammond EH, Gray SD. Preliminary report on hormone receptors in the human vocal fold. *J Voice.* 2000; 14(1):72–81.
7. Toral I, Ciliv G, Gürsel B, Ozdem C. Androgen receptors in laryngeal carcinoma. *Eur Arch Otorhinolaryngol.* 1990;247(4):244–246.
8. Aufdemorte TB, Sheridan PJ, Holt GR. Autoradiographic evidence of sex steroid receptors in laryngeal tissues of the baboon. *Laryngoscope.* 1983;93(12):1607–1611.
9. Voelter Ch, Kleinsasser N, Joa P, et al. Detection of hormone receptors in the human vocal fold. *Eur Arch Otorhinolaryngol.* 2008; 265(10):1239–1244.
10. de Souza LB, Pereira RM, dos Santos MM, Godoy CMA. Fundamental frequency, phonation maximum time and vocal complaints in morbidly obese women. *Arq Bras Circ Dig.* 2014;27(1):43–46.
11. Da Cunha MG, Passerotti GH, Weber R, Zilberstein B, Cecconello I. Voice feature characteristic in morbid obese population. *Obes Surg.* 2011;21(3):340–344.
12. Barsties B, Verfaillie R, Roy N, Maryn Y. Do body mass index and fat volume influence vocal quality, phonatory range, and aerodynamics in females? *Codas.* 2013;25(4): 310–318.
13. Barbato AL, Landau RL. Testosterone deficiency of morbid obesity. *Clin Res.* 1974;22: 647.
14. Glass AR, Swerdloff RS, Bray GA, Dahms WT, Atkinson RL. Low serum testosterone and sex-hormone-binding-globulin in massively obese men. *J Clin Endocrinol Metab.* 1977;45(6):1211–1219.
15. Amatruda JM, Harman SM, Pourmotabbed G, Lockwood DH. Depressed plasma testosterone and fractional binding of testosterone

in obese males. *J Clin Endocrinol Metab.* 1978;47(2):268–271.

16. Schneider G, Kirschner MA, Berkowitz R, Ertel NH. Increased estrogen production in obese men. *J Clin Endocrinol Metab.* 1979; 48(4):663–668.

17. Kley HK, Solbach HG, McKinnan JC, Kruskemper HL. Testosterone decrease and oestrogen increase in male patients with obesity. *Eur J Endocrinol.* 1979;91:553–563.

18. Bernasconi D, Del Monte P, Meozzi M, et al. The impact of obesity on hormonal parameters in hirsute and nonhirsute women. *Metabolism.* 1996;45(1):72–75.

19. Grenman S, Rönnemaa T, Irjala K, Kaihola HL, Grönroos M. Sex steroid, gonadotropin, cortisol and prolactin levels in healthy, massively obese women: correlation with abdominal fat cell size and effect of weight reduction. *J Clin Endocrinol Metab.* 1986; 63(6):1257–1261.

20. Pasquali R, Antenucci D, Casimirri F, et al. Clinical and hormonal characteristics of obese amenorrheic hyperandrogenic women before and after weight loss. *J Clin Endocrinol Metab.* 1989;68(1):173–179.

21. Deslypere JP, Verdonck L, Vermeulen A. Fat tissue: a steroid reservoir and site of steroid metabolism. *J Clin Endocrinol Metab.* 1985;61(3):564–570.

22. López M, Tena-Sempere M. Estradiol and brown fat. *Best Pract Res Clin Endocrinol Metab.* 2016;30(4):527–536.

23. Gealekman O1, Guseva N, Hartigan C, et al. Depot-specific differences and insufficient subcutaneous adipose tissue angiogenesis in human obesity. *Circulation.* 2011;123(2): 186–194.

24. Nookaew I, Svensson PA, Jacobson P, et al. Adipose tissue resting energy expenditure and expression of genes involved in mitochondrial function are higher in women than in men. *J Clin Endocrinol Metab.* 2013; 98(2):E370–E378.

25. Luglio HF. Estrogen and body weight regulation in women: the role of estrogen receptor alpha (ER-α) on adipocyte lipolysis. *Acta Med Indones.* 2014;46(4):333–338.

26. Michopoulos V. Stress-induced alterations in estradiol sensitivity increase risk for obesity in women. *Physiol Behav.* 2016;166:56–64.

27. Clegg DJ, Brown LM, Woods SC, Benoit SC. Gonadal hormones determine sensitivity to central leptin and insulin. *Diabetes.* 2006; 55(4):978–987.

28. Geary N. Estradiol, CCK and satiation. *Peptides.* 2001;22(8):1251–1263.

29. Messina MM, Boersma G, Overton JM, Eckel LA. Estradiol decreases the orexigenic effect of melanin-concentrating hormone in ovariectomized rats. *Physiol Behav.* 2006; 88(4–5):523–528.

30. Gambacciani M, Ciaponi M, Cappagli B, et al. Body weight, body fat distribution, and hormonal replacement therapy in early postmenopausal women. *J Clin Endocrinol Metab.* 1997;82(2):414–417.

31. Palmer BF, Clegg DJ. The sexual dimorphism of obesity. *Mol Cell Endocrinol.* 2015; 402:113–119.

32. Couillard C, Gagnon J, Bergeron J, et al. Contribution of body fatness and adipose tissue distribution to the age variation in plasma steroid hormone concentrations in men: the HERITAGE Family Study. *J Clin Endocrinol Metab.* 2000;85(3):1026–1031.

33. Ferrini RL, Barrett-Connor E. Sex hormones and age: a cross-sectional study of testosterone and estradiol and their bioavailable fractions in community dwelling men. *Am J Epidemiol.* 1998;147(8):750–754.

34. Harman SM, Metter EJ, Tobin JD, et al. Longitudinal effects of aging on serum total and free testosterone levels in healthy men. Baltimore Longitudinal Study of Aging. *J Clin Endocrinol Metab.* 2001;86(2):724–731.

35. Phillips GB, Jing T, Heymsfield SB. Relationships in men of sex hormones, insulin, adiposity, and risk factors for myocardial infarction. *Metabolism.* 2003;52(6):784–790.

36. Seidell JC, Bjorntorp P, Sjostrom L, Kvist H, Sannertedt R. Visceral fat accumulation in men is positively associated with insulin, glucose, and C-peptide levels, but negatively with testosterone levels. *Metabolism.* 1990; 39(9):897–901.

37. Simon D, Preziosi P, Barrett-Connor E, et al. The influence of aging on plasma sex hormones in men: the Telecom Study. *Am J Epidemiol.* 1992;135(7):783–791.

38. Svartberg J, Midtby M, Bonaa KH, Sundsfjord J, Joakimsen RM, Jorde R. The associations of age, lifestyle factors and chronic disease with testosterone in men: the Tromso Study. *Eur J Endocrinol.* 2003;149(2):145–152.

39. Zumoff B, Strain GW, Miller LK, et al. Plasma free and non-sex-hormone-binding-globulin-bound testosterone are decreased in obese men in proportion to their degree of obesity. *J Clin Endocrinol Metab.* 1990;71(4):929–931.

40. Abate N, Haffner SM, Garg A, Peshock RM, Grundy SM. Sex steroid hormones, upper body obesity, and insulin resistance. *J Clin Endocrinol Metab.* 2002;87(10):4522–4527.

41. Svartberg J, von Mühlen D, Sundsfjord J, Jorde R. Waist circumference and testosterone levels in community dwelling men. The Tromsø study. *Eur J Epidemiol.* 2004;19(7):657–663.

42. Blouin K, Boivin A, Tchernof A. Androgens and body fat distribution. *J Steroid Biochem Mol Biol.* 2008;108(3–5):272–280.

43. Sattler FR, Castaneda-Sceppa C, Binder EF, et al. Testosterone and growth hormone improve body composition and muscle performance in older men. *J Clin Endocrinol Metab.* 2009;94(6):1991–2001.

44. Katznelson L, Finkelstein JS, Schoenfeld DA, Rosenthal DI, Anderson EJ, Klibanski A. Increase in bone density and lean body mass during testosterone administration in men with acquired hypogonadism. *J Clin Endocrinol Metab.* 1996;81(12):4358–4365.

45. Woodhouse LJ, Gupta N, Bhasin M et al. Dose-dependent effects of testosterone on regional adipose tissue distribution in healthy young men. *J Clin Endocrinol Metab.* 2004;89(2):718–726.

46. Singh R, Artaza JN, Taylor WE, et al. Testosterone inhibits adipogenic differentiation in 3T3-L1 cells: nuclear translocation of androgen receptor complex with beta-catenin and T-cell factor 4 may bypass canonical Wnt signaling to down-regulate adipogenic transcription factors. *Endocrinology.* 2006;147(1):141–154.

47. Bhasin S, Taylor WE, Singh R et al. The mechanisms of androgen effects on body composition: mesenchymal pluripotent cell as the target of androgen action. *J Gerontol A Biol Sci Med Sci.* 2003;58(12):M1103–M1110.

48. Segal KR, Dunaif A, Gutin B, Albu J, Nyman A, Pi-Sunyer FX. Body composition, not body weight, is related to cardiovascular disease risk factors and sex hormone levels in men. *J Clin Invest.* 1987;80(4):1050–1055.

49. Seidell JC, Bjorntorp P, Sjostrom L, Kvist H, Sannerstedt R. Visceral fat accumulation in men is positively associated with insulin, glucose, and C-peptide levels, but negatively with testosterone levels. *Metabolism.* 1990;39(9):897–901.

50. Khaw KT, Barrett-Connor E. Lower endogenous androgens predict central adiposity in men. *Ann Epidemiol.* 1992;2(5):675–682.

51. Haffner SM, Valdez RA, Stern MP, Katz MS. Obesity, body fat distribution and sex hormones in men. *Int J Obes Relat Metab Disord.* 1993;17(11):643–649.

52. Tsai EC, Boyko EJ, Leonetti DL, Fujimoto WY. Low serum testosterone level as a predictor of increased visceral fat in Japanese-American men. *Int J Obes Relat Metab Disord.* 2000;24(4):485–491.

53. Derby CA, Zilber S, Brambilla D, Morales KH, McKinlay JB. Body mass index, waist circumference and waist to hip ratio and change in sex steroid hormones: the Massachusetts Male Aging Study. *Clin Endocrinol (Oxf).* 2006;65(1):125–131.

54. Vandewalle S, De Schepper J, Kaufman JM. Androgens and obesity in male adolescents. *Curr Opin Endocrinol Diabetes Obes.* 2015;22(3):230–237.

55. Allan CA, McLachlan RI. Androgens and obesity. *Curr Opin Endocrinol Diabetes Obes.* 2010;17(3):224–232.

56. He Q, Karlberg J. BMI in childhood and its association with height gain, timing of puberty, and final height. *Pediatr Res.* 2001;49(2):244–251.

57. Aksglaede L, Juul A, Olsen LW, Sørensen TIA. Age at puberty and the emerging obesity epidemic. *PLoS One.* 2009;4(12):e8450.

58. Vignolo M, Naselli A, Di Battista E, Mostert M, Aicardi G. Growth and development in simple obesity. *Eur J Pediatr.* 1988;147(3): 242–244.

59. Juul A, Magnusdottir S, Scheike T, et al. Age at voice break in Danish boys: effects of pre-pubertal body mass index and secular trend. *Int J Androl.* 2007;30(6):537–542.

60. Denzer C, Weibel A, Muche R, Karges B, Sorgo W, Wabitsch M. Pubertal development in obese children and adolescents. *Int J Obes (Lond).* 2007;31(10):1509–1519.

61. Laron Z. Is obesity associated with early sexual maturation? *Pediatrics.* 2004;113(1, pt 1):171–172.

62. Wang Y. Is obesity associated with early sexual maturation? A comparison of the association in American boys versus girls. *Pediatrics.* 2002;110(5):903–910.

63. Vandewalle S, Taes Y, Fiers T, et al. Sex steroids in relation to sexual and skeletal maturation in obese male adolescents. *J Clin Endocrinol Metab.* 2014;99(8):2977–2985.

64. Reinehr T, de Sousa G, Roth CL, Andler W. Androgens before and after weight loss in obese children. *J Clin Endocrinol Metab.* 2005;90(10):5588–5595.

65. Gascón F, Valle M, Martos R, et al. Sex hormone-binding globulin as a marker for hyperinsulinemia and/or insulin resistance in obese children. *Eur J Endocrinol.* 2000; 143(1):85–89.

66. Gray A, Feldman HA, McKinlay JB, Longcope C. Age, disease, and changing sex hormone levels in middle-aged men: results of the Massachusetts Male Aging Study. *J Clin Endocrinol Metab.* 1991;73(5):1016–1025.

67. Travison TG, Araujo AB, Kupelian V, O'Donnell AB, McKinlay JB. The relative contributions of aging, health, and lifestyle factors to serum testosterone decline in men. *J Clin Endocrinol Metab.* 2007;92(2): 549–555.

68. Ponholzer A, Plas E, Schatzl G, et al. Relationship between testosterone serum levels and lifestyle in aging men. *Aging Male.* 2005; 8(3–4):190–193.

69. Beckford NS, Rood SR, Schaid D, Schanbacher B. Androgen stimulation and laryngeal development. *Ann Otol Rhinol Laryngol.* 1985;94(6, pt 1):634–640.

70. Mobashir MK, Mohamed AERS, Quriba AS, Anany AM, Hassan EM. Linear measurements of vocal folds and laryngeal dimensions in freshly excised human larynges. *J Voice.* 2018;32(5):525–528.

71. Kahane JC. Growth of the human prepubertal and pubertal larynx. *J Speech Hear Res.* 1982;25(3):446–455.

72. Hirano M, Kurita S, Nakashima T. The structure of the vocal folds. In: Stevens KN, Hirano M, eds. *Vocal Fold Physiology.* Tokyo, Japan: University of Tokyo Press; 1981:33–41.

73. Fitch WT, Giedd J. Morphology and development of the human vocal tract: a study using magnetic resonance imaging. *J Acoust Soc Am.* 1999;106(3, pt 1):1511–1522.

74. Abitbol J, de Brux J, Millot G, et al. Does a hormonal vocal cord cycle exist in women? Study of vocal premenstrual syndrome in voice performers by videostroboscopy-glottography and cytology on 38 women. *J Voice.* 1989;3(2):157–162.

75. Sataloff RT. Endocrine function. In: Sataloff RT, ed. *Professional Voice: The Science and Art of Clinical Care.* 4th ed. San Diego, CA: Plural Publishing; 2017:655–669.

76. Van Gelder L. Psychosomatic aspects of endocrine disorders of the voice. *J Commun Disord.* 1974;7(3):257–262.

77. Davis CB, Davis ML. The effects of premenstrual syndrome (PMS) on the female singer. *J Voice.* 1993;7(4):337–353.

78. Abitbol J, Abitbol P, Abitbol B. Sex hormones and the female voice. *J Voice.* 1999; 13(3):424–446.

79. Raj A, Gupta B, Chowdhury A, Chadha S. A study of voice changes in various phases of menstrual cycle and in postmenopausal women. *J Voice.* 2010;24(3):363–368.

80. D'haeseleer E, Depypere H, Claeys S, Van Lierde KM. The relation between body mass index and speaking fundamental frequency

in premenopausal and postmenopausal women. *Menopause*. 2011;18(7):754–758.

81. D'haeseleer E, Van Lierde K, Claeys S, Depypere H. The impact of menopause and hormone therapy on voice and nasal resonance. *Facts Views Vis Obgyn*. 2012;4(1):38–41.

82. D'haeseleer E, Depypere H, Van Lierde K. Comparison of speaking fundamental frequency between premenopausal women and postmenopausal women with and without hormone therapy. *Folia Phoniatr Logop*. 2013;65(2):78–83.

83. Evans S, Neave N, Wakelin D, Hamilton C. The relationship between testosterone and vocal frequencies in human males. *Physiol Behav*. 2008;93(4–5):783–788.

84. Dabbs JM, Mallinger A. High testosterone levels predict low voice pitch among men. *Pers Indiv Dif*. 1999;27(4):801–804.

85. Meuser W, Nieschlag. Sex hormones and depth of voice in the male (author's transl.). *Dtsch Med Wochenschr*. 1977;102(8):261–264.

86. Pedersen MF, Møller S, Krabbe S, Bennett P. Fundamental voice frequency measured by electroglottography during continuous speech: a new exact secondary sex characteristic in boys in puberty. *Int J Pediatr Otorhinolaryngol*. 1986;11(1):21–27.

87. Sataloff RT. Management of gender reassignment patients. In: Sataloff RT, ed. *Professional Voice: The Science and Art of Clinical Care*. 4th ed. San Diego, CA: Plural Publishing; 2017:1649–1658.

88. van Durme CM, Kisters JM, van Paassen P, van Etten RW, Tervaert JW. Multiple endocrine abnormalities. *Lancet*. 2011;378(9790):540.

89. Bermon S, Vilain E, Fenichel P, Ritzen M. Women with hyperandrogenism in elite sports: scientific and ethical rationales for regulating. *J Clin Endocrinol Metab*. 2015;100(3):828–830.

90. Griggs RC, Kingston W, Jozefowicz RF, Herr BE, Forbes G, Halliday D. Effect of testosterone on muscle mass and muscle protein synthesis. *J Appl Physiol*. 1989;66(1):498–503.

91. Sassoon D, Segil N, Kelley D. Androgen-induced myogenesis and chondrogenesis in the larynx of *Xenopus laevis*. *Dev Biol*. 1986;113(1):135–140.

92. Gugatschka M, Kiesler K, Obermayer-Pietsch B, et al. Sex hormones and the elderly male voice. *J Voice*. 2010;24(3):369–373.

93. Akcam T, Bolu E, Merati AL, Durmus C, Gerek M, Ozkaptan Y. Voice changes after androgen therapy for hypogonadotrophic hypogonadism. *Laryngoscope*. 2004;114(9):1587–1591.

94. Hamdan AL, Jabbour J, Saadeh R, Kazan I, Nassar J, Bulbul M. Vocal changes in patients with prostate cancer following androgen ablation. *J Voice*. 2012;26(6):812.e11-5.

7

Respiratory Dysfunction

Robert Thayer Sataloff, John R. Cohn, and Mary J. Hawkshaw

Anyone who works with singers and actors has encountered the term "support." Although the laryngologist, speech-language pathologist, voice scientist, singing teacher, acting teacher, and performer may have slightly different understandings of the word, virtually everyone agrees that support is essential to efficient, healthy, professional voice production. Although singers and actors frequently use the term *diaphragm* synonymously with support, it is actually a combination of rib cage, thoracic, back, and abdominal muscle function. This support mechanism constitutes the power source of the voice and should generate a vector of force in the direction of the air column passing between the vocal folds. The diaphragm is an inspiratory muscle, of course, and represents only a portion of the support mechanism. Practitioners in all fields recognize that proper training of the thoracic and abdominal support mechanism is essential. Deficiencies in anatomy or technique, or diseases undermining the effectiveness of the abdominal musculature and respiratory system, often result not only in unacceptable vocal quality and projection, but also in abusive compensatory vocal behavior and laryngeal injury.

To optimize diagnosis and treatment of respiratory dysfunction in voice profession-

als, it is helpful to understand fundamental concepts in respiratory physiology. Physiology of respiration is reviewed elsewhere in this book, particularly in Chapter 2. Breathing is a complex process. Voice scientists have struggled for years to break it down into component parts in order to study breathing more effectively. Basic research has provided insight into optimal methods of inspiration, prephonatory positioning of the chest and abdomen, and expiration. The knowledge acquired through scientific research has helped guide the speech-language pathologist, singing teacher, and acting teacher in modifying vocal behavior. It has helped reinforce some traditional practices and explained why others have often failed and should be abandoned.

Respiratory problems are especially problematic to singers and other voice professionals, and special considerations for medical evaluation have been stressed since the 1980s.[1] They also cause similar problems for wind instrumentalists, also by interfering with support. The effects of severe respiratory infection are obvious and will be discussed only briefly in this chapter. Restrictive lung disease such as that associated with obesity may impair support by decreasing lung volume and respiratory efficiency. Even mild obstructive lung disease can impair support enough to result in increased neck and tongue muscle tension and abusive voice use capable of producing vocal nodules. This scenario occurs with unrecognized asthma. This may be difficult to diagnose unless suspected, because such cases of asthma may be performance induced, analogous to exercise-induced asthma from forms of exercise other than singing. Performance is a form of exercise. The singer will deny perception of shortness of breath at baseline and may even have normal pulmonary function tests at rest. He or she will also usually support well and sing with good technique during the first portion of a performance. However, as performance exercise continues, obstruction occurs. It is theorized that hyperventilation and airway drying lead to impairment of pulmonary function, as occurs with exercise asthma. Air trapping or other problems related to small airway bronchoconstriction may lead to early fatigue. This effectively impairs support and results in compensatory abusive technique. When suspected, this entity can be confirmed through a methacholine challenge test. Treatment of the underlying airway hyperreactivity is essential to resolving the vocal problem.

Treating asthma is rendered more difficult in professional voice users because of the need in some patients to avoid not only inhalers, but also drugs that produce even a mild tremor, which may be audible during soft singing. A skilled pulmonologist or allergist can usually tailor a satisfactory regimen.

Assessment

The respiratory system consists of the nose, nasopharynx, oropharynx, larynx, trachea, lungs, musculoskeletal thorax, and abdominal musculature. Its function is influenced by the overall health and fitness of the individual. Assessment and care of the entire respiratory system are essential.

Assessment of a professional voice user's respiratory complaints begins with a complete history and physical examination and is followed by appropriate laboratory testing. It is particularly important to identify the correct diagnosis in a singer, since empiric trials of "shotgun" treatments may have deleterious effects on the voice (ie, laryngeal inflammation encountered with some inhaled steroids, drying effects of antihistamines, etc) and may affect performance adversely.

History

Evaluation begins with a complete history, emphasizing questions related to each portion of the respiratory tract. Symptoms may be constant or intermittent, have seasonal variation, be brought on or relieved by environmental changes (ie, exposure to animals, plants, dusty environments, chemicals, perfumes, etc), be relieved by medication, or be associated with other symptoms. Many singers and actors are symptomatic only when they perform outdoors or in dusty buildings. Further confounding management, performers may spend long periods of time in performance venues and hotels in which they have little control over the environment.

Questions regarding respiratory complaints begin with the nose. Has the patient noted obstruction, congestion, epistaxis, rhinorrhea, or postnasal drip? Does he or she have a history of nasal trauma? Trauma that leads to nasal obstruction may not involve a significantly displaced nasal fracture. Minor nasal trauma, especially in early life, can lead to severe intranasal deformities as facial growth progresses.

Throat dryness and pain during performance may be noted by singers with nasal obstruction. Complaints of swelling in the throat, dysphagia, odynophagia, otalgia, and hyponasality are found with obstructing lesions. Such complaints may also be due to causes other than primary pathology in the respiratory system such as gastroesophageal reflux.

Laryngeal complaints may be due to either primary lesions that obstruct breathing or dysfunction of the lower respiratory tract. Mass lesions can cause stridor, hoarseness, breathiness, diplophonia, or pain with use of the singing or speaking voice. Symptoms such as loss of vocal range or vocal fatigue may be due to either primary laryngeal lesions or inadequate airflow being produced by the lungs. Singers and actors may complain of stiffness or pain in the neck during or after rehearsal and performance. These symptoms are usually secondary to tension and may result from changes in technique to compensate for inadequate respiratory function. A history of a neck mass may indicate infection, laryngocele, neoplasm, pharyngocele, or other serious pathology. However, occasionally the "mass" will turn out to be severe spasm of neck muscles. This is especially common after trauma such as whiplash and often is associated with severe vocal dysfunction. Questions regarding breathing strength, support, and control are critical. Does the vocalist feel short of breath, and, if so, is this symptom related to performance? Is there wheezing or chest tightness related to dyspnea? Is there a cough, and is this cough productive? Is there hemoptysis? Chest pain can be related to dyspnea, hard coughing, improper vocal technique, reflux, or other causes. Singers, like more conventional athletes may recognize difficulty only with performing.

The history also investigates the patient's overall health. Nutritional status is evaluated, remembering that the presence of obesity or anorexia can affect the bellows action of the chest. Allergies and asthma are especially important, because of their direct effect on breathing. A history of abdominal hernias, symptoms of gastroesophageal reflux (throat clearing, thick mucus, intermittent hoarseness, halitosis, prolonged warm-up time, dyspepsia), neurologic weaknesses, paresthesia, and lesions of the extremities may lead the physician to the cause of the voice complaint. In patients known to have reflux or suspected of having reflux, the physician should inquire as to whether reflux precautions have been followed consistently. Laryngopharyngeal reflux is discussed at length elsewhere in this book, but it is worth noting that matters as simple as elevating the head of the bed can be helpful in controlling respiratory and allergic symptoms that can be triggered or aggravated by reflux.[2]

The past medical history is evaluated first for previous pulmonary diseases including tuberculosis (especially in recent immigrants, immunosuppressed patients, and the inner-city population), pneumonia, and environmental exposure to pulmonary irritants such as asbestos. Cardiac disease can influence respiratory function directly or can have indirect effects when it leads to exercise intolerance. Thyroid disease can have effects on both the general health of the patient and local compressive effects on the trachea.

The patient must be questioned about any drugs he or she is taking, including over-the-counter preparations and herbal medicines. Noncardioselective beta-blockers such as propranalol, used by some performers to reduce anxiety, can exacerbate an underlying asthmatic condition.[3] Long-term antibiotic use can cause secondary infections with opportunistic organisms. Antihistamines and decongestants produce drying of the upper airway that can alter respiratory function.

Alcohol and tobacco use and dietary and sleeping habits also give an indication of the patient's general and respiratory health status. Cigarette smoking is the leading cause of respiratory disease in the United States and should be avoided by all professional voice users. Cigarette smoking by family members or in the workplace may also cause symptoms. Smoking marijuana and cocaine may be especially deleterious.

Specific questions about vocal training and technique are helpful in determining the diagnosis and the most appropriate treatment for the professional voice user.[4] The history and current level of vocal training, experience, and career goals provide an assessment of the patient's professional skill and needs. It is important to determine the date of the next critical performance or audition. Physicians who care for singers should also be aware of the basics of technique in both the singing and speaking voice.

Physical Examination

The patient is evaluated for obesity or lack of appropriate muscle mass. Affect is assessed for signs of anxiety or depression, which may affect breathing patterns.

A complete head and neck examination is required. The nose is examined during forceful inspiration for collapse of the critical nasal "valve" area, as well as for deformities that can lead to nasal obstruction. Mucosal inflammation, mass lesions, and the presence and quality of nasal secretions are noted.

Examination of the oral cavity reveals the level of dental hygiene, moisture of the mucosal surfaces, and motion of the tongue and soft palate. Mass lesions that can cause upper airway obstruction are noted. Patients with a history of adenoidectomy

are evaluated for nasopharyngeal stenosis from excessive scar formation and for velopharyngeal incompetence.

The larynx is examined by indirect laryngoscopy, flexible laryngoscopy, and/or strobovideolaryngoscopy as the situation demands. Large obstructive mass lesions, severe mucosal edema, and recurrent nerve paralysis usually can be detected by laryngoscopy in the office. Examination of the larynx in a singer is not complete without examination of the singing voice.[4] Posture during singing or acting, abdominal support, breath control, and the development of dyspnea while performing are assessed, and the voice is evaluated for range, hoarseness, breathiness, and fatigue. Assessment of voice technique and efficiency often reveals the etiology of the performer's complaints.

The chest is examined to evaluate rales, wheezes, rhonchi, and areas of hyper- and hypoaeration. Auscultation of the chest with forced expiration may accentuate wheezing not apparent during quiet breathing. Most singers who complain of voice issues, primarily, will not have obvious abnormal findings. Auscultation of the heart is performed to determine rate, rhythm, the presence of murmurs, or a pericardial friction rub. The abdomen is examined for masses, hernias, and muscle tone. Extremities are evaluated for weakness, level of sensation, and deformities. The neurologic examination must be complete. Cranial nerve problems can affect the upper airway, whereas generalized problems of muscle weakness and loss of coordination can affect severely the thoracic and abdominal respiratory musculature.

Laboratory Tests

Rhinomanometry is considered the most useful test for quantifying nasal airflow before and after treatment.[5,6] However, variability among tests limits its clinical usefulness.[7,8] Additional research is needed to develop a more valid, reliable technique for assessing nasal function.

Airflow Rate Testing

Airflow rate testing determines the flow of air across the larynx during phonation. It is usually measured with a spirometer but can be evaluated with a pneumotachograph or hot-wire anemometer. The mean flow rate is defined as the total volume of air expired during phonation divided by the duration of the phonation. The average is 89 to 141 mL/s and the normal range is 72 to 200 mL/s.[9] There is no significant difference noted between males and females or between older children and adults.[10] The phonation quotient is defined as the vital capacity of the patient divided by the maximum time of phonation. The average for this test is 120 to 190 mL/s with an upper limit of 200 to 300 mL/s.[8] Both these determinates are used to evaluate laryngeal lesions that affect upper respiratory function. Lesions that cause glottic incompetence, reducing laryngeal efficiency (ie, vocal nodules, vocal fold paralysis), will lead to increased flow rates. Airflow testing is also useful for documenting the results of treatment for lesions such as nodules, a problem found frequently in professional voice users.[10,11]

Pulmonary Function Testing

The cornerstone of pulmonary function testing is spirometry. Spirometry is based on the measurement of the forced vital capacity (FVC) and its components (Figure 7–1).

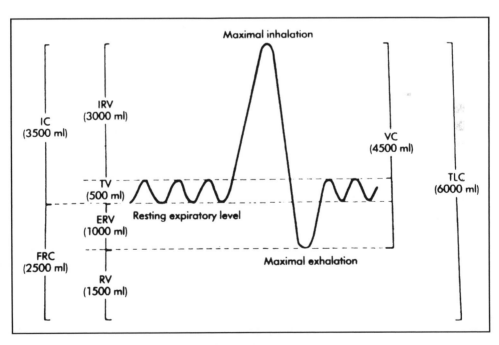

Figure 7–1. Lung volumes (normal adult averages). (*ERV* = expiratory reserve volume; *FRC* = functional reserve capacity; *IC* = inspiratory capacity; *IRV* = inspiratory reserve volume; *RV* = reserve volume; *TLC* = total lung capacity; *TV* = tidal volume; *VC* = vital capacity.)

The FVC is the quantity of air that is exhaled after the lungs are maximally filled (to total lung capacity [TLC]) and then forcefully emptied. This is classically plotted as a volume vs time curve, but newer computer-driven analysis has made flow-volume loops readily available. From this curve, the vital capacity (VC), forced expiratory volume in 1 s (FEV1), and maximal midexpiratory flow rate (MMEFR, FEF 25%–75%) can be determined (Figure 7–2), although with modern equipment this is usually a calculated value performed through the spirometer's processor. The MMEFR is the volume of air expired between the 25% point of the FVC (FEV25%) and the 75% point of the FVC (FEV75%) divided by the time it takes to expire that volume. This measurement, also known as the FEF 25%–75% is the most sensitive value in diagnosing obstructive pulmonary disease that can be measured with standard office-based equipment.[12]

The peak expiratory flow rate correlates well with normal functional limitations, but it is dependent on effort, and needs to be done correctly to get valid and reliable results. The ratio of FEV1/FVC may help quantitate the degree of airflow obstruction, but that also can be effort dependent, with accuracy limited by a shorter-than-appropriate expiratory time. The skill of the technician performing the test, and the patient's understanding and effort are critical in interpretation of results, along with adherence to published guidelines.[13]

The computer-generated flow vs volume loop has become popular as a more sensitive means of evaluating ventilatory impairment. The computer measures the instantaneous flow at multiple points during a forced expiration followed by a forced inspiration and plots the instantaneous flow against the volume expired or inspired at each point on a continuous graph (Figure 7–3). This "loop"

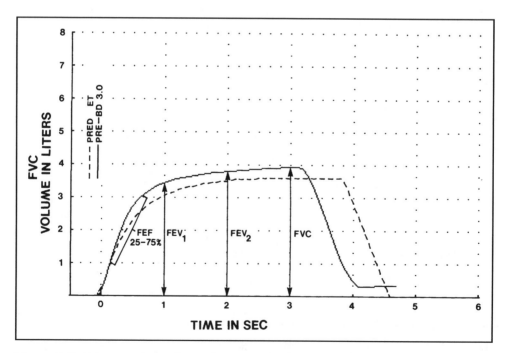

Figure 7–2. Volume vs time spirometric tracing. (*FEF*25%–75%; *FEV*1, *FEV*3 = forced expiratory volume in 1 and 3 s, respectively; *FVC* = forced vital capacity; *RV* = reserve volume.)

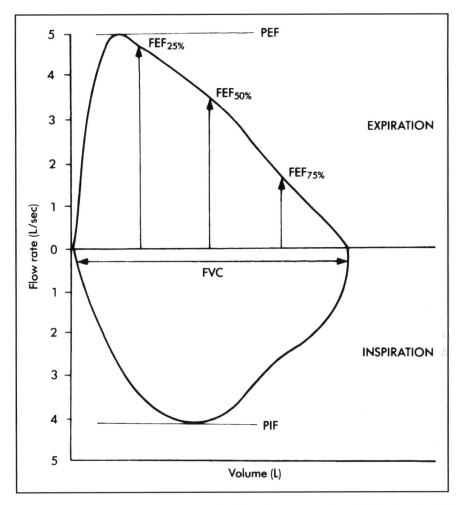

Figure 7–3. Flow vs volume loop. (*FEF* = forced expiratory flow; *FVC* = forced vital capacity; *PEF* = peak expiratory flow; *PIF* = peak inspiratory flow.)

has a characteristic shape that can be useful in detecting and characterizing pulmonary and laryngeal pathology.[14]

Spirometry is performed with the nose occluded and the patient making forceful expirations into the spirometer. The patient should complete 3 FVC trials with less than 5% variability in FEV1 and FVC in order to consider a test acceptable. Predicted normal values are determined from the height, weight, and gender of the patient. African Americans tend to have smaller lung volumes, so adjusted predicted values should

be used. Normal values for the test subject are considered to be anything greater than or equal to 80%, or within 1.64 standard deviations of these predicted values.[15]

Patterns of pulmonary disease can be determined from both the standard spirometric plot and the flow volume loop.[16] In obstructive disease, there are decreased flows represented by decreased FEV, and a decreased FEV1/FVC ratio (Figure 7–4). A flow-volume loop initially will show increased convexity of the expiratory phase, while, with more severe obstruction, there

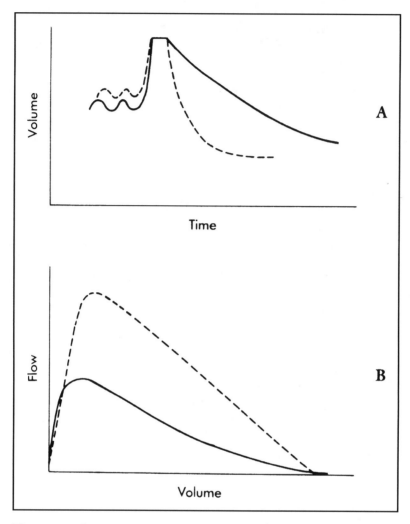

Figure 7–4. Spirometric pattern in obstructive disease. **A.** Volume vs time curve. **B.** Flow vs volume curve, expiratory phase. Normal, dotted line; abnormal, solid line.

may be loss of expiratory volume. Flattening of both or one of the inspiratory or expiratory phases may suggest large airway obstruction or laryngeal pathology. These characteristics can be variable, especially in the flow-volume loop, depending on the site and duration of the obstruction. Even when FEV1 and FEV1/FVC are normal, a decreased MMEFR can be noted in patients with asymptomatic asthma and in smokers. Patients with restrictive lung disease have decreased volumes but normal flow (Figure 7–5). Thus, the FEV1 and FVC are decreased proportionately, causing the FEV1/FVC ratio to be normal or even increased.

Determination of reversible obstructive pulmonary disease can be made if an increase of 12% is noted in the FVC and FEV, or 25% in the MMEFR after treatment with inhaled bronchodilators.[15] If the diagnosis is suspected but the test results

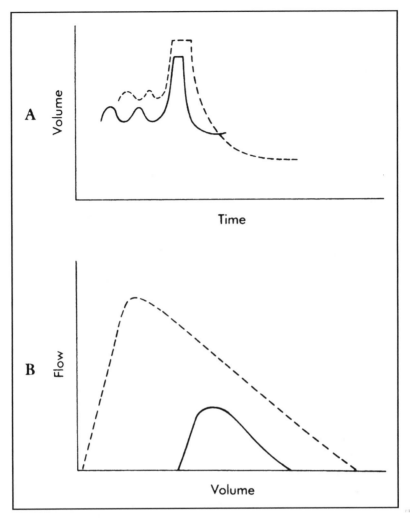

Figure 7–5. Spirometric pattern in restrictive disease. **A.** Volume vs time curve. **B.** Flow vs volume curve, expiratory phase. Normal, dotted line; abnormal, solid line.

are inconclusive or normal, a methacholine challenge may be performed using progressively greater concentrations of methacholine, with measurement of the FEV1 and MMEFR after each dose. The test is completed when the FEV1 is decreased by 20% or more.[17] This provocative dose that is measured or calculated to have caused a 20% fall in the FEV1 is called the PD20FEV1. Generally, nonasthmatic subjects will have a PD20 greater than 8 mg/mL

of methacholine.[18] This measure of relative airway reactivity is particularly important in the diagnosis of mild asthma that is symptomatic under performance conditions.[19]

Diffusing Capacity

Diffusing capacity is the relative ability of oxygen to diffuse across the arteriole-alveolar membranes in the lung, although the matching of ventilation and perfusion may be of equal or greater importance. It is tested by measuring diffusion of inhaled carbon monoxide into the blood (DL_{CO}). This determination is useful in the evaluation of patients with interstitial lung disease and correlates with oxygen desaturation during exercise.[20]

Lung Volumes

TLC is measured indirectly by first determining functional residual capacity (FRC) using an inert gas dilution technique, nitrogen washout, or body plethysmographic technique. Decreased TLC is the *sine qua non* of restrictive lung disease. Of interest, highly trained singers do not have substantially increased TLC but have improved their pulmonary efficiency by increasing VC and reducing reserve volume (RV).[21]

Radiology

A chest radiograph or chest computed tomography (CT) scan is commonly obtained on symptomatic patients with persistent pulmonary complaints to rule out infectious or neoplastic disease. Patients with more common ailments such as asthma and bronchitis generally have normal chest radiographs. When mass lesions or other significant pulmonary pathology is identified, more detailed evaluation is required. Patients with nasal obstruction and acute or chronic sinonasal symptoms may be evaluated first with plain radiographs or CT of the sinuses. If extensive disease is suspected, CT using axial and coronal sections will define this region better.

Other Tests

Arterial blood gas (ABG) analysis may be useful in the diagnosis of pulmonary dis-
ease. Appropriate stains of a sputum smear can provide important information in the diagnosis of infectious, allergic, and neoplastic pulmonary disease.

An electrocardiogram (ECG) and echocardiogram may assist in the diagnosis of dyspnea not readily explained by other studies. A complete blood count (CBC) may demonstrate anemia, which contributes to dyspnea; an increased white blood cell count, which may be a sign of infection; or eosinophilia, suggesting allergy or other systemic disease.

Allergy Testing

Allergy tests are used to confirm the diagnosis and assist in the treatment of allergic disease. The most commonly used technique is skin testing, which can be performed by prick, or intradermal technique.[22–24] Prick testing causes minimal discomfort and can be used to determine the presence of allergy to specific substances rapidly. The intradermal injection of antigens is the most sensitive test for allergy.[24] When performed properly, either test, but particularly the intradermal technique, can be used to rule out immediate and late-phase allergic responses. Proponents of skin test–based therapy argue that it is the most sensitive and least expensive way to determine the presence of allergy and plan treatment.[25]

In recent years, a blood test for antigen-specific immunoglobulin E (IgE) to both inhaled and food antigens has become available. Originally done with a radioimmunoassay technique, the radioallergosorbent test (RAST),[26] now ImmunoCAP is performed commonly as an enzyme-linked immunoabsorbent assay. These tests quantify the immunoglobulins responsible for the allergic reaction to each antigen. The proponents of blood test–based treatment, primarily otolaryngologists, contend that this precise measure of relative allergic response can be used to formulate individualized immunotherapy for the patient[27] and that RAST testing can be used to monitor the patient's response to therapy,[28] but this has not been demonstrated in controlled, randomized, blinded studies.

Endoscopy

Fiberoptic technology allows accurate visualization of the entire respiratory tract. Nasopharyngoscopy using a short, narrow fiberoptic endoscope is useful in defining internal nasal anatomy and in the diagnosis of pharyngeal and laryngeal obstruction. Mass lesions can be defined fully and their relationship to the vibrating edge of the vocal fold can be determined, especially when strobovideolaryngoscopy is also employed. Less obvious lesions such as arytenoid dislocation, vocal fold paresis, and scar are often much more apparent under stroboscopic light. Using bronchoscopy, mass lesions of the lower respiratory tract can be assessed clinically and, with the use of endobronchial biopsy, transbronchial biopsy, or brushings, can be identified pathologically, but that is well beyond the scope of this chapter.

Diagnosis and Treatment

Nasal Airway Obstruction

Obstruction of the nasal airway can be due to structural deformities, mass lesions, foreign bodies, or inflammation. Structural deformities usually involve deviation of the bony and/or cartilaginous nasal septum. Nasal deformity can be complicated also by inflammatory hypertrophy of the inferior turbinates and collapse of the external skeleton. Treatment of the obstructing nasal septum is surgical and involves resection and/or repositioning of the abnormal portions. It is suggested that the approach to surgery of the inferior turbinates be conservative in singers because long-term drying effects have occurred secondary to mucociliary disruption when extensive resection is performed.[29] Usually, mass lesions are apparent readily on examination. After adequate radiologic assessment, sometimes including arteriography, most are removed surgically.

Inflammatory nasal obstruction may be infectious or allergic. Viral rhinitis is manifested by clear or mucoid rhinorrhea, postnasal drip, associated nasal obstruction, and other symptoms such as low-grade fever, sore throat, hoarseness, cough, myalgia, and malaise. Treatment is supportive with oral decongestants and hydration. When a patient has a crucial performance within 24 to 48 hours, intramuscular or oral steroids can be used to relieve many of the obstructive symptoms.

Allergic rhinitis usually involves the common "hay fever" symptoms of sneezing, itchiness, clear rhinorrhea, nasal obstruction, and associated complaints of allergic conjunctivitis. Symptoms may be related to geographical location, exposure to specific plants or wild life, changes in diet, and the general environmental aspects and ventilation systems of lodgings and concert halls. The diagnosis is assisted by specific allergy testing. Skin tests or ImmunoCAP may be employed, but enhanced sensitivity, reduced cost, and speed make skin testing preferred for patients who do not have a contraindication. Skin testing is used almost exclusively in our evaluation of patients. When a single specific allergen can be defined, avoidance is the simplest solution. Removal of plants or pets, or taking precautions to avoid dust exposure within the home environment can yield dramatic improvement. Treatment of allergic rhinitis in a singer with multiple allergies by specific allergen immunotherapy is advisable. This initially involves weekly injections of increasing concentrations of a serum containing all the antigens to which the patient is allergic. This can provide relief from symptoms without the side effects that may be caused by oral drug preparations or nasal sprays. The success of immunotherapy is enhanced by proper selection of patients and antigens and is limited by variable patient compliance, as well as other alternative mechanisms accounting for the patient's symptoms.

Multiple pharmaceutical preparations are available to alleviate symptoms for patients who cannot avoid fully their allergic stimulus and are not candidates for immunotherapy. Topical steroid sprays (eg, flunisolide, beclomethasone, fluticasone, budesonide, triamcinolone, and mometasone) can reduce nasal symptoms, and in proper doses, these steroids are safe.[30] They are now available over the counter. Topical antihistamines azelastine and olopatadine may be useful in allergic and nonallergic rhinitis patients. Montelukast, a leukotriene receptor blocker originally used in the treatment of asthma has also been shown to be effective in treating rhinitis. Oral decongestant/antihistamine preparations can reduce most symptoms significantly, but the side effects of drying of the mucosal membranes and sedation, and the development of tolerance, limit the use of these medications in vocal performers. Parenteral and oral steroids rapidly reduce the edema associated with the allergic response without these side effects. However, they have other undesirable side effects, including laryngitis caused by inhaled steroids. In an acute obstructive phenomenon they may be necessary to maintain the airway. However, long-term use should be avoided whenever possible because of the many potential serious side effects.

Sinusitis can cause partial or total nasal obstruction and can exacerbate an asthmatic condition.[31] Major symptoms are mucopurulent rhinorrhea, postnasal drip, facial pressure, retro-orbital headache, and fever. Radiologic confirmation of chronic inflammatory changes or opacification of the paranasal sinuses and documentation of pathologic bacteria on culture of the sinus are helpful. Treatment of the acute phase of this illness includes antibiotics for 2 to 3 weeks, oral and topical decongestants, and steam inhalations. Performance usually can be permitted in most cases. In chronic conditions, long-term antibiotics and treatment of any underlying conditions such as nasal obstruction blocking a sinus ostium, dental disease, or allergy are necessary. In persistent cases, surgical therapy of the paranasal sinuses may be required.

Pharyngeal Obstruction

Most cases of pharyngeal obstruction are due to adenoid and palatine tonsil hypertrophy in the adolescent or young adult. The patient usually complains of nasal obstruction and chronic mouth breathing and may have a significant snoring history. The source of the obstruction usually is apparent on physical examination and can be confirmed with lateral neck radiographs. When the obstruction is secondary to an acute infection, it is treated with high-dose oral or parenteral antibiotics. When rapid increase in the size of adenoids and tonsils is seen, mononucleosis should be considered, especially if there is associated cervical, axillary, or inguinal adenopathy. Adenoidectomy and tonsillectomy may be indicated in patients who have chronic symptomatic hypertrophy. Detailed examination of the palate is made prior to consideration of adenoidectomy. The presence of a submucous cleft, bifid uvula, or short palate can lead to significant hypernasality postoperatively.[32]

Laryngeal Obstruction

Laryngeal lesions severe enough to cause respiratory impairment usually will cause changes in the voice. Edema secondary to infection, allergy, gastroesophageal reflux, and voice abuse can lead to partial upper airway obstruction in rare, severe cases. Anatomic defects, trauma, stenosis, neoplasm, and epiglottitis are more likely to cause airway problems. Diagnosis is made by laryngeal examination, except in cases of epiglottitis. Radiographs are helpful in some patients. The degree of respiratory dysfunction is determined by airflow testing and pulmonary function testing. Steroids may be effective in reducing edema quickly in most of these conditions and should be accompanied by treatment of the underlying problem. Lesions that alter the respiratory function of the larynx such as vocal fold paralysis/paresis, laryngeal webs, and arytenoid dislocation usually cause vocal impairment to a far greater degree than they impair respiratory function. However, some patients elect improvement of their voices through compensatory vocal techniques or surgery, which may leave them with an adequate voice and impaired respiratory function. Treatment of the respiratory problems that these lesions cause in singers is extremely difficult. Surgical intervention to reduce the upper airway obstruction often disturbs vocal quality. Optimizing pulmonary function to overcome laryngeal inefficiency is the best approach in some patients.

Most laryngeal lesions potentially capable of interfering with respiration will not persist long enough to cause severe upper airway obstruction requiring tracheotomy, because vocal impairment occurs early in their course. When a laryngeal mass is found, endoscopic removal may be necessary if the lesion is not amenable to other therapy. These masses should be removed using an operating microscope and meticulous microsurgical technique. Local anesthesia is used frequently in order to assess the surgical result during the procedure and avoid intubation, but excellent sedation by an anesthesiologist is necessary to keep the patient motionless even in cooperative patients. When general anesthesia is necessary, the laryngologist must take responsibility for protecting the larynx during intubation and extubation, avoiding intubation trauma to the lesion, and the most skilled anesthesiologist available should be used.

Pulmonary Lesions

Obstructive Conditions

The most common obstructive airway disease is asthma, affecting approximately 8 million people in the United States.[33] It is defined as reversible obstructive airway disease, in the absence of an alternative explanation such as heart failure. Classic asthma is manifested by paroxysms of dyspnea, wheezy respirations, chest tightness, and cough, although a chronic cough can be the only presenting symptom.[34] While it is usually allergic, the etiology can be nonallergic or mixed. Nonallergic groups of patients are usually older and may have symptoms associated with chronic infectious phenomena such as sinusitis or bronchitis. Symptoms can also be induced by exercise or exposure to cold air[35] or be associated with a triad including aspirin sensitivity and nasal polyps.[36] The diagnosis of asthma is made by history or by demonstrating an obstructive pattern on pulmonary function testing that is reversible with bronchodilators either acutely or with chronic treatment. Bronchoprovocation with methacholine may be necessary to demonstrate the presence of asthma in patients with normal pulmonary function. Additional testing such as chest imaging, pulse oximetry, arterial blood gasses, lung volumes, diffusion capacity, and noninvasive cardiac studies may be useful in ruling out other conditions and diagnosing the long-term sequelae of obstructive disease.

Airway reactivity-induced asthma in singers (ARIAS) is a special form of exercise-induced asthma.[37] It is postulated that airway obstruction is caused by the hyperventilation of singing performance. Decreased airflow undermines support, creating problems similar to those seen with improper abdominal muscle use. The singer may become short of breath, or may simply note voice fatigue, decreased range, and impaired volume control. As in other conditions that impair the power source of the voice, compensatory efforts are common, including increased jaw tension, tongue retraction, and strap muscle hyperfunction. Treatment of the singing-induced asthma helps restore support for the singing voice and allows the singer to resume correct singing technique. In conjunction with singing lessons (and speech training when appropriate), voice symptoms usually disappear quickly.

The treatment of asthmatic conditions in singers is somewhat different from that of the general population. One must eliminate even mild airway reactivity in order to optimize respiratory function for performance. Inhaled steroids should be avoided if at all possible in singers because of the possibility of laryngitis and dysphonia from the propellant, or steroid themselves, steroid effects on the laryngeal musculature, or from *Candida* overgrowth.[38–40] Mild asthma usually can be treated with sustained-release oral theophylline with an inhaled beta-2 agonist for acute attacks or before performing. Leukotriene antagonists (montelukast,

zafirlukast) may be variably effective in the treatment of asthma. They have the advantage of being administered orally and inhibiting inflammation, which is thought to be a key component in the pathophysiology of asthma. Appropriate allergen immunotherapy is used in the care of allergic asthma and can reduce the need for bronchodilators. In more severe cases, an oral beta-2 agonist may be necessary. Systemic steroids are effective in obtaining rapid control of asthmatic symptoms; however, they are usually reserved for severe acute exacerbations because of the side effects of prolonged use. Combination products containing a long-acting beta agonist and inhaled corticosteroid may help minimize the steroid dose.

Chronic obstructive pulmonary disease (COPD) is a general term that is applied to airway obstruction that is not fully reversible. The most common cause of COPD is cigarette smoking. It is manifested by either bronchitis or emphysema, although many patients have elements of both diseases. Patients with bronchitis have a chronic productive cough. In emphysema, there is destruction of alveolar membranes. Patients with bronchitis or emphysema may have severe obstructive changes on pulmonary function testing and an abnormal radiograph with increased lung volume due to air trapping. Exacerbations of bronchitis are treated with antibiotics. Otherwise, treatment is similar to that for asthma, but, because of the irreversibility of much of the airway disease, less response can be expected. In singers, hydration and cough suppressants reduce laryngeal trauma associated with coughing unless the pulmonary condition and need to clear secretions militate against the use of antitussives.

Another less commonly recognized cause of persistent pulmonary symptoms is gastroesophageal reflux. Vagal stimulation and chronic aspiration of gastric juice or particulate matter can result in chronic coughing, increased airway reactivity, or recurrent pneumonia.[41-46] There is evidence that reflux of gastric acid into the esophagus can increase airway reactivity even without reaching the larynx or lungs, although results of studies of the addition of antireflux measures to the treatment of asthma have been mixed. Diagnosis is made by noting arytenoid and posterior glottic inflammation on laryngeal examination, reflux during radiologic upper gastrointestinal study, by esophagoscopy, and esophageal manometric testing and 24 hour esophageal pH monitoring. Acid levels should be measured specifically during singing. Treatment includes antacids, elevation of the head of the bed, and histamine-2 antagonists and/or proton pump inhibitors. When medical treatment fails, surgical plication of the lower esophageal sphincter may be performed. Recently, laparoscopic fundoplication has decreased the morbidity of this procedure including disruption of important abdominal wall muscles. Even more recent techniques show promise and are less traumatic than even laparoscopic surgery.

Pneumonia presents special problems for the singer. It often takes longer than a singer realizes for lung function to return to normal. Singing too soon after such infections may result in vocal difficulties as attempts are made to compensate for minor deficiencies in the power source of the voice.

Restrictive Conditions

Restrictive lung disease can be divided into 2 groups. The first involves restriction of the chest bellows function. Weakness of the musculoskeletal support system is found in myasthenia gravis, Guillain-Barré syndrome, poliomyelitis, multiple sclero-

sis, spinal cord injury, and diaphragmatic paralysis. Additionally, massive obesity, kyphoscoliosis, and flail chest from thoracic trauma impair the function of the chest wall. A second group of restrictive lesions affects the pulmonary parenchyma and includes hypersensitivity pneumonitis, atelectasis, sarcoidosis, pulmonary fibrosis, pulmonary edema, pneumonia, neoplasm, drug reactions, and congestive heart failure. The diagnosis of restrictive respiratory impairment is confirmed by detailed pulmonary function testing. These patients have decreased lung volume with proportionately normal flow rates. The treatment of each of these syndromes is complex and not within the scope of this review. However, obesity is one cause of restrictive lung disease, and many singers have a significant weight problem. The effects of obesity on the voice have not been studied adequately; yet, there is no doubt that excessive weight can alter respiratory function. Restrictive pulmonary function due to excess weight has adverse effects on the endurance of a singer and probably on his or her longevity as a performer. Obesity is also related to hypertension, diabetes, and other conditions that may actually shorten the performer's life. Finally, a restrictive pattern of pulmonary function in a previously healthy singer may indicate early neurologic or neuromuscular disease, and comprehensive evaluation is warranted whenever this finding appears.

Conclusion

Most singers and actors come to the laryngologist with complaints about changes in their voices; yet, many times the problem is not in the vocal folds but rather in the production of adequate airflow to drive the voice. Mild respiratory maladies such as cough or nasal congestion may not alter the voice primarily but can cause irritation or changes in technique that can impair vocal performance. Minor alterations in respiratory function that would go barely noticed in the general population can have significant effects on a professional voice user, causing vocal fatigue, loss of range, hyperfunctional abusive compensation, and other problems. Adequate knowledge of respiratory function and its disorders is essential to comprehensive care of the professional voice.

Much additional research about breathing and support is needed although a substantial body of good literature exists. Remembering that the end point of this research is the training and maintenance of healthy, beautiful professional voices, it is essential for voice scientists, voice teachers, and physicians to work together closely in clinical and basic research. Only through concerted efforts can we define the right questions and discover the right answers.

References

1. Spiegel JR, Sataloff RT, Cohn JR, Hawkshaw M. Respiratory function in singers: medical assessment, diagnoses and treatments. *J Voice.* 1988; 2(1):40–50.
2. Cohn JR. Elevation of the head of bed to treat supraesophageal reflux: controlling the trigger and reducing the "drip." *J Allergy Clin Immunol: In Practice* 2015;3:362–364.
3. Thorn GW, Adams RD, Braunwald E, et al., eds. *Harrison's Principles of Internal Medicine.* New York, NY: McGraw-Hill; 1977:1215.
4. Sataloff RT. Professional singers: the science and art of clinical care. *Am J Otolaryngol.* 1981;2:251–266.
5. Mertz JS, McCaffrey TV, Kern EB. Objective evaluation of anterior septal surgical reconstruction. *Otolaryngol Head Neck Surg.* 1984;92:308–311.
6. Orgel HA, Meltzer EO, Kemp JP, Welch MJ. Clinical, rhinomanometric, and cytologic evaluation of seasonal allergic rhinitis treated with beclamethasone dipropionate as aqueous nasal spray or pressurized aerosol. *J Allergy Clin Immunol.* 1986;77:858–864.
7. McCaffrey TV, Kern EB. Clinical evaluation of nasal obstruction. *Arch Otolaryngol.* 1979;105:542–545.
8. Daubenspeck JA. Influence of small mechanical loads on variability of breathing pattern. *J Appl Physiol Respir Environ Exerc Physiol.* 1981;50:299–306.
9. Hirano M. *Clinical Examination of the Voice.* New York, NY: Springer-Verlag; 1981.
10. Shigemori Y. Some tests related to the air usage during phonation. *Clin Invest Otol (Fukuoka).* 1977;23:138–166.
11. Tanaka S, Gould WJ. Vocal efficiency and aerodynamic aspects in voice disorders. *Ann Otol Rhinol Laryngol.* 1985;94:29–33.
12. Segall JJ, Butterworth BA. The maximal midexpiratory flow time. *Br J Dis Chest.* 1968;62:139–145.
13. Hyatt RE, Black LF. The flow-volume curve. *Am Rev Resp Dis.* 1973;107:191–199.
14. Standardization of Spirometry—1987 Update. Official Statement of the American Thoracic Society (approved by the ATS Board of Directors), March, 1987; Reed Gardner, Ph.D. (Chairman), John L. Hankison, Ph.D., Jack L. Clausen, M.D., Robert O, Crapo, M.D., Robert L. Johnson, Jr., M.D., Gary R. Epler, M.D., *American Rev Respir Dis.* 1987;136:1285–1298.
15. Statement on spirometry: a report of the section on respiratory pathophysiology. *Chest.* 1983;83:547–550.
16. Sackner MA, ed. *Diagnostic Techniques in Pulmonary Disease.* New York, NY: Marcel Dekker; 1980.
17. Chai H, Farr RS, Froehlich LA, et al. Standardization of bronchial inhalation challenge procedures. *J Allergy Clin Immunol.* 1975;56:323–327.
18. Malo JL, Pineau L, Carter A, Martin RR. Reference values of the provocative concentrations of methacholine that cause 6% and

20% changes in forced expiratory volume in one second in a normal population. *Am Rev Resp Dis.* 1983;128:8–11.

19. Chatham M, Bleeker ER, Smith PL, et al. A comparison of histamine, methacholine, and exercise airway reactivity in normal and asthmatic subjects. *Am Rev Resp Dis.* 1982; 126:235–240.

20. Martin L. *Pulmonary Physiology in Clinical Practice.* St. Louis, MO: CV Mosby; 1987.

21. Gould WT, Okamura H. Static lung volumes in singers. *Ann Otol Rhinol Laryngol.* 1973;82:89–95.

22. Nelson HS. Diagnostic procedures in allergy. I. Allergy skin testing. *Ann Allergy.* 1983;51:411–418.

23. Practice and Standards Committee. American Academy of Allergy and Immunology position statement. *J Allergy Clin lmmunol.* 1983;72:515–517.

24. Cohn JR, Padams P, Zwillenberg J. Intradermal skin test (IDST) results correlate with atopy. *Ear Nose Throat J.* 2011 April; 90(4):E11–E16.

25. Mangi RJ. Allergy skin tests: an overview. *Otolaryngol Clin N Am.* 1985;18:719–723.

26. Nalebuff DJ. An enthusiastic view of the use of RAST in clinical allergy. *Immunol Allergy Pract.* 1981;3:77–87.

27. Fadal RG, Nalebuff DJ. A study of optimum dose immunotherapy in pharmacological treatment failures. *Arch Otolaryngol.* 1980;106:38–43.

28. Ali M. Serum concentration of allergen-specific IgG antibodies in inhalant allergy: effect of specific immunotherapy. *Am J Clin Pathol.* 1983;80:290–299.

29. Martinez SA, Nissen AJ, Stock CR, Tesmer T. Nasal turbinate resection for relief of nasal obstruction. *Laryngoscope.* 1983;93:871–875.

30. Parkin JL. Topical steroids in nasal disease. *Otolaryngol Head Neck Surg.* 1983;91: 713–714.

31. McCaurin JG. A review of the interrelationship of paranasal sinus disease and certain chest conditions, with special consideration of bronchiectasis and asthma. *Ann Otol Rhinol Laryngol.* 1935;44:344–353.

32. Croft CB, Shprintzen RJ, Ruben RJ. Hypernasal speech following adenotonsillectomy. *Otolaryngol Head Neck Surg.* 1981;88: 179–188.

33. Baum GC, Wolinsky E. *Textbook of Pulmonary Disease.* Boston, MA: Little, Brown; 1983.

34. Corraa WM, Braman SS, Irwin RS. Chronic cough as the sole presenting manifestation of bronchial asthma. *N Engl J Med.* 1979;300: 633–637.

35. Strauss RH, McFadden ER, Ingram RH, Jaeger JJ. Enhancement of exercise-induced asthma by cold air. *N Engl J Med.* 1977;297: 743–747.

36. Spector SL, Wangaard CH, Farr RS. Aspirin and concomitant idiosyncrasies in adult asthmatic patients. *J Allergy Clin Immunol.* 1979;64:500–506.

37. Cohn JR, Sataloff RT, Spiegel JR, Fish JE, Kennedy K. Airway reactivity-induced asthma in singers (ARIAS). *J Voice.* 1991; 5(4):332–337.

38. Watkins KL, Ewanowsk SJ. Effects of aerosol corticosteroids on the voice: triamcinolone acetonide and beclomethasone dipropionate. *J Speech Hearing Res.* 1985;28:301–304.

39. Toogood JH, Jennings B, Greenway RW, Chuang L. Candidiasis and dysphonia complicating beclomethasone treatment of asthma. *J Allergy Clin Immunol.* 1980;65: 145–153.

40. Williams AJ, Baghat MS, Stableforth DE, et al. Dysphonia caused by inhaled steroids: recognition of a characteristic laryngeal abnormality. *Thorax.* 1983;38:813–821.

41. Davis MV. Relationship between pulmonary disease, hiatal hernia, and gastroesophageal reflux. *NY State J Med.* 1972;72:935–938.

42. Mansfield LE, Stein MR. Gastroesophageal reflux and asthma: a possible reflex mechanism. *Ann Allergy.* 1978;41:224–226.

43. Barish CF, Wu WC, Castell DO. Respiratory complications of gastroesophageal reflux. *Arch Intern Med.* 1985;145:1882–1888.

44. Larrain A, Carrasco E, Galleguillos R, Sepulveda R, Pope CE. Medical and surgical treatment of nonallergic asthma associated with

gastroesophageal reflux. *Chest.* 1991;99(6): 1330–1335.

45. Sontag SJ, O'Connell S, Khandewal S, et al. Most asthmatics have gastroesophageal reflux with or without bronchodilator therapy. *Gastroenterology.* 1990;99(3):613–620.

46. Wesseling G, Brummer RJ, Wouters EFM, ten Velde GPM. Gastric asthma? No change in respiratory impedance during intra-esophageal acidification in adult asthmatics. *Chest.* 1993;104(6):1733–1736.

8

Obesity, Respiration, and Voice

Abdul-Latif Hamdan, Robert Thayer Sataloff,
and Mary J. Hawkshaw

Introduction

Obesity may affect voice by disturbing several systems in the body, among which is the respiratory system. This chapter discusses the current literature on the interplay between obesity, respiratory dysfunction, and dysphonia in patients with and without respiratory diseases. The authors will present 2 sections, a section on obesity and lung function in patients with no respiratory diseases and a section on obesity and lung function in patients with respiratory diseases. Understanding the pathogenesis of dysphonia in the context of obesity and respiratory dysfunction is valuable in clinical management. Respiratory dysfunction impairs the power source of the voice, and any condition that undermines the power source may lead to compensatory hyperfunction of neck and laryngeal muscles and consequent dysphonia.

Obesity and Lung Function in Patients With No Respiratory Diseases

Respiratory Symptoms and Pulmonary Function in Obese Subjects With No Pulmonary Diseases

Obese subjects are at high risk of having respiratory symptoms. In addition to the commonly reported sleep apnea symptoms, subjects with high body mass index (BMI), referred to in this chapter as greater than 25 kg/m^2 with normal BMI being less than or equal to 25 kg/m^2, often exhibit breathlessness and dyspnea even in the absence of respiratory diseases.[1] Be it at rest or during exercise, the self-reported sensation of dyspnea is often unexplained and unrelated to respiratory or cardiovascular dysfunction.

Bernhardt and Babb[2] reported that obesity can be the only clinical finding in a subject with high BMI complaining of exertion dyspnea. The study was conducted on a group of healthy obese men and women who underwent cardiopulmonary exercise testing to explore the symptom of dyspnea on exertion in the absence of confounding diseases. In another cross-sectional study on 75 subjects stratified as asthmatics, misdiagnosed asthmatics and controls, Carpio et al[3] ascertained that obesity may mimic asthma. They found that the perception of dyspnea during exercise was higher in the group of patients misdiagnosed with asthma in comparison to controls. The elevated dyspnea score in patients misdiagnosed with asthma together with the high ventilatory and metabolic demand in this group of subjects indicates that dyspnea in obese subjects may mimic asthma.[3] Sahebjami[4] in 1998 reported dyspnea (65%) in a group of 23 obese male subjects with BMI greater than 28 kg/m^2. Similarly, in 2011, Bowden et al[5] examined the predictors of breathlessness in a large population study ($n = 5331$) of adult South Australians and demonstrated that obesity among other lifestyle factors significantly affected the prevalence of breathlessness. Breathlessness occurred in 15% in subjects above the age of 50 years. Bernhardt et al[6] reported that the degree of perceived breathlessness by obese patients strongly correlates with the ratings of perceived exertion, despite its lack of association with oxygen cost of breathing. The study was conducted on 2 groups of subjects, obese subjects with low rating of breathlessness (less than or equal to 2) and obese subjects with higher rate of breathlessness (greater than or equal to 4).[6]

Obese subjects with dyspnea or breathlessness but no known respiratory diseases often exhibit abnormalities on pulmonary function tests.[7] In the cross-sectional study by Leone et al[8] that included 121 965 participants, the authors reported abdominal obesity as a strong predictor of poor lung function with an odds ratio of 1.94. Moreover, there was an association between impairment in lung function and the metabolic syndrome, which is often present in obese subjects.[8] Similarly, Littleton[9] in his review on obesity-related respiratory dysfunction reported higher respiratory rate, diminished tidal volumes, and abnormal lung compliance in obese patients in comparison to normal-weight patients. The strong correlation between abnormal pulmonary function testing (PFT) and body mass index had also been corroborated in the review of Jones and Nzekwu[10] in 2006. The authors concurred that even a mild increase in body mass index may result in reduction in functional residual capacity (FRC). Their analysis of the PFTs of 373 patients with a large range of BMI showed an exponential decrease in FRC and expiratory reserve volume (ERV) in patients with an increased body mass index. The values of FRC and ERV in markedly obese patients were 75% and 47%, respectively, of those observed in a person with a BMI less than 20 kg/m^2.[10] Other studies have reported worsening of forced expiratory volume in 1 second (FEV1), forced vital capacity (FVC), and functional residual capacity in obese compared to normal-weight subjects.[10-12] In the study by Sahebiami,[4] the reported dyspnea in obese subjects was associated with low forced expiratory flow at 75% of vital capacity and reduced maximum voluntary ventilation. In a study by Ray et al[13] of 43 massively obese subjects (mean weight: 159.4 ± 22.5 kg and mean weight/height: 0.93 ± 0.14 kg), the authors also have shown alteration in most respiratory functions. The expiratory reserve volume correlated with the degree of obesity, whereas total lung capacity and maximal voluntary ventilation were affected only in extreme cases of obesity.[13] Ofir et al[14] in their study on the relationship between breathlessness, respiratory mechanical factors, and metabolic demands reported limitations in expiratory flow during exercise and a decrease in resting end-expiratory flow volume in obese women in comparison to nonobese women.

Figures 8–1 and 8–2 illustrate the respiratory changes seen on pulmonary function testing in obese subjects with no respiratory diseases vs normal weight subjects.

The absolute value of BMI is not the only predictor of respiratory symptoms in obese subjects. Numerous reports indicate

that the distribution of fat in the body plays an equally important role in the pathogenesis of respiratory dysfunction in obese subjects.[15-18] This is not surprising given that abdominal fat has long been associated with restrictive breathing pattern. In the study by Collins et al,[15] patients with upper body fat distribution, namely with a waist to hip ratio of 0.950 or greater, had worse FVC, FEV1, and TLC than patients with lower body fat distribution. The authors emphasized the negative impact of upper body obesity on lung volumes and highlighted the association between the biceps skinfold thickness and total lung capacity. Similarly, Salome et al[19] demonstrated a significant correlation between fat distribution and functional residual capacity and expiratory reserve volume. Subjects with android pattern of fat deposition had worse lung volume/capac-

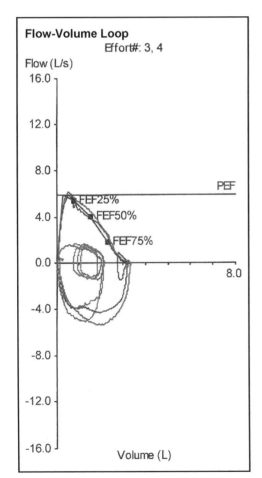

Figure 8–1. A 53-year-old woman with BMI of 22.4 showing normal flow-volume loop.

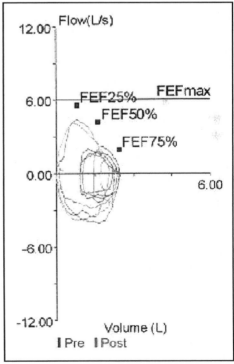

Figure 8–2. A 52-year-old woman with BMI 43.4 presenting with respiratory symptoms yet showing normal spirometry.

ity than subjects with genoid type of obesity. In a cross-sectional study of 1674 adults by Chen et al[20] in 2007, the authors reported a negative correlation between waist circumference and pulmonary function. Even an increase of 1 cm in waist circumference correlated with "a 13 mL reduction in forced vital capacity and an 11 mL reduction in forced expiratory volume in 1 s."[20] Two years later, in a study by Steele et al[17] conducted on a cohort of 320 adults with family history of type 2 diabetes, the authors found a similar association between waist circumference and lower lung volume in both genders after adjusting for physical activity energy expenditure and aerobic fitness. Another study by Sharp et al[18] found that mass loading of the lower thorax had more impact than mass loading of the upper chest on the respiratory system. Moreover, there was an alteration in the thoracic-volume pressure curve in subjects with a high mass load on the abdomen.

In summary, we can conclude that obese subjects experience dyspnea and breathlessness even in the absence of lung disease. The type of fat distribution plays a major role, with the android type of obesity being more harmful than the genoid type. The respiratory symptoms often are associated with abnormal pulmonary function testing. Forced expiratory flow is commonly affected in addition to total lung capacity and residual volume in extreme cases.

Mechanisms of the Effect of Obesity on Breathing and Pulmonary Function in Patients With No Respiratory Diseases

The cause of dyspnea and breathlessness often experienced by obese patients with no known respiratory disease is still a subject of debate in the literature. In a recent review by Dixon and Peters[7] on the asso-

ciation between lung function and obesity, the authors highlighted the clear limitations of the conventional respiratory studies in assessing the burden of obesity on breathing. Despite the ubiquity of reports on abnormal lung function in obese subjects with dyspnea, the underlying mechanistic etiology remains uncertain. There is mounting evidence to suggest that the emerging respiratory patterns clearly recognized in obese subjects are the result of complex local and systemic processes. It is helpful to understand the commonly suggested mechanisms on how obesity can affect breathing. This will be followed by a discussion on the impact of these mechanisms on voice.

Mechanical Impairment

Numerous studies have shown that obesity may affect breathing mechanically. The normal downward diaphragmatic contraction and the cephalic and forward pull of the thoracic cage are impaired in obese patients.[21] This impairment in movement secondary to excess fat deposition reduces the expansion of the diaphragm and results in its distention despite the well-reported diaphragmatic electromyographic activity during exhalation in obese subjects.[22] The ineffective diaphragmatic activity leads to abnormal respiratory function and increase in respiratory effort and ventilatory work.[23-25] Lotti et al[23] investigated the contribution of respiratory muscles to the symptom of dyspnea in obese subjects using several pulmonary function tests that included trans-diaphragmatic pressure (TDP). The authors demonstrated a correlation between TDP and the dyspnea score measured using a modified Borg scale. A review by Arena and Cahalin[26] on the cardiorespiratory fitness in obese people showed that both inspiratory and expiratory muscle functions are compromised in addition to other respiratory parameters. These impediments to breathing contribute to the limitations in cardiovascular fitness witnessed in obese subjects. Similar studies by Mafort et al[27] and other authors support the pathogenic role of mechanical impairment to breathing and the subsequent reduction in pulmonary function in morbidly obese subjects.[28]

Reduced Lung and Chest Compliance

Another suggested mechanism for pulmonary dysfunction resulting from obesity is reduced lung and/or chest compliance. A study by Pelosi et al[11] on the effect of body mass on lung volume reported an exponential decrease in total respiratory system compliance in relation to body mass index. Using the esophageal balloon technique and rapid airway occlusion technique in 8 obese and 8 morbidly obese subjects in comparison to 8 subjects with normal BMI, the authors demonstrated a reduction in respiratory compliance that was due primarily to decreased lung compliance, which can be attributed to focal atelectasis in the dependent areas of the lungs as a result of breathing pressure imbalance. The excess fat deposition and restricted motion of the diaphragm result in collapse of the small airways with subsequent increase in positive end-expiratory pressure. In addition to the reduced lung compliance, chest wall compliance may be impaired in obese patients. In a study by Naimark and Cherniack[29] on the total compliance of the respiratory system in 12 awake obese subjects vs 24 normal controls, the authors showed marked reduction in chest wall compliance that was associated with high mechanical work of breathing.

Changes in Breathing Pattern and Respiratory Neural Drive

Another suggested mechanism for pulmonary dysfunction in obese subjects is

increase in the neural respiratory drive.[30] Alteration in breathing pattern and ventilator drive have been shown to contribute to the respiratory symptoms in obese subjects. A study by Chlif et al[31] on the breathing pattern and ventilator neural drive in 34 obese subjects compared to 18 controls revealed differences between the 2 groups. The study demonstrated alteration in the breathing pattern, with lower maximal inspiratory pressure and energy cost of breathing in obese subjects. The rapid shallow breathing with changes in ventilator drive were interpreted as behavioral strategies in response to the sense of dyspnea. Obesity is considered by many as one of the restrictive lung diseases in that pulmonary imbalance in inflation and deflation imposes an additional effort to breathe that is often translated clinically as shallow pattern of breathing.[26,31]

Alteration in Airway Closing Capacity, Lung Ventilation, and Perfusion

Tidal airway closure, defined as "cyclic opening and closure of peripheral airways,"[32(p579)] is a sign of homogeneity in ventilation and gas perfusion.[32,33] When the closing volume, which is associated with the tidal airway closure, exceeds the end-expiratory lung volume (EELV), impaired ventilation and disturbances in gas exchange may occur.[32] Disorders in airway closure often are reported in patients with asthma and chronic obstructive lung disease. However, recent literature indicates that airway closure and abnormalities in ventilation/perfusion also may occur in obese subjects without these respiratory abnormalities.[33–36] Hedenstierna et al[33] investigated the airway closure and gas exchange in 10 obese subjects while breathing spontaneously and during anesthesia. The authors reported airway closure in 90% of the cases while breathing spontaneously, which could explain the hypoxemia observed in obese patients during anesthesia. Other studies suggest that closure of the small airways in the dependent areas of the lungs results in disturbances in the ventilation-perfusion ratio.[27] Rivas et al[37] reported an increase of the alveolar-arterial oxygen gradient secondary to the imbalance between perfusion and ventilation in morbidly obese patients undergoing bariatric surgery. Similarly, Dempsey et al[38] investigated the alveolar-arterial gas exchange in a group of 13 obese subjects at various levels of exercise and metabolic rates. The authors suggested that "the disorder in O2 and CO exchange in obesity was one of non-uniform ventilation distribution with reduction in the effective alveolar-capillary interface."[38(p1807)] In a study by Farebrother et al,[36] the authors reported reduced arterial oxygen pressure (PaO_2) in the supine position in 8 obese subjects. The reduction in PaO_2 improved following weight loss.[36] Similarly, in the study by Ray et al[13] on the effect of obesity on respiratory function, the authors demonstrated that the diffusing capacity for carbon monoxide (DLCO) changes in relation to degree of obesity. Saydain et al[39] reported a higher diagnosis of obesity and asthma in patients with "high single-breath diffusing capacity of the lung for carbon monoxide (DLCO)"[39(p447)] compared to those with normal DLCO.

Numerous imaging studies documented differences in regional lung ventilation in obese subjects in comparison to normal-weight subjects. Whereas ventilation is preferentially distributed to the dependent zones in nonobese people, this regional ventilation distribution is reversed in obese subjects. In a study by Holley et al,[35] regional ventilation and perfusion distribution using pulmonary function testing and radioactive technique were measured in 8 obese subjects. In 4 out of the 8 subjects, the normal tidal breath distribution was confined mainly to the upper zones and the perfusion was more prominent in the lower zones where ventilation was reduced. This pattern has been attributed to reduced diaphragmatic and chest wall movement rather than airway disease.[35,40]

The Proinflammatory State

Last but not least is the proinflammatory state induced by the release of inflammatory mediators and reactive oxygen species. The biochemical changes associated with excess adipose tissue in obese patients have been discussed extensively in the literature. Adipose tissue is considered as a source of adipokines, bioactive substances that induce oxidative stress by producing reactive oxygen species and overconsuming oxygen.[41] In parallel with the increase in oxidative stress is a reduction in antioxidants such as glutathione peroxidase, which leads to a further increase in free radicals.[42,43] Proinflammatory cytokines, namely tumor necrosis factor–alpha, interleukin-6 (IL-6), resistin, visfatin, and adinopectin, also play a major role in controlling the immune system and cell apoptosis.[44] Interleukin-6 has been shown to play a key role in controlling and regulating the degree of inflammation in addition to energy homeostasis.[45] Pedersen et al[46] have reported an association between BMI and C-reactive protein (CRP) and interleukin-6 in a study based on 2986 males. The authors concluded that adding weight during adulthood may lead to sustained, low-grade inflammation throughout midlife, whereas losing weight is advantageous.

The Pathogenic Role of Obesity-Induced Respiratory Changes in the Etiology of Dysphonia in Obese Subjects

Since the introduction of the term "vocal athlete" in 1996 to describe the distinctive respiratory abilities of well-trained singers, there is growing evidence in the literature to support the belief that breathing is an essential element in voice production.[47] Cohn et al[48] in 2001 described the "exercise-induced asthma-like" condition in which vocal athletes suffer from vocal complaints secondary to airway drying during performance causing exercise-induced asthma. The authors showed complete resolution of these symptoms following the intake of bronchodilators, in parallel with improvement in bronchial hyperactivity. Similarly, many years later, Meenan et al[49] reported poor respiratory midflows, defined as forced expiratory flow (FEF) 25% to 75% value of less than 80% of predicted, in 52.8% of 199 patients presenting with dysphonia. The high diagnostic yield of pulmonary function testing (PFT) in dysphonic patients with no prior history of pulmonary diseases led the authors to advocate routine PFT in the workup of patients with voice disorders. Despite the ubiquity of reports on the paramount importance of breathing in phonation and despite the strong link between obesity and lung function in patients with no respiratory diseases, very little has been written on how obesity, through its impact on the respiratory system, may affect voice. Aside from the aforementioned study,[49] in which the predictive value of BMI for PFT in dysphonic patients was reported as non-significant,[49] the interplay between obesity-induced respiratory changes and phonation while controlling for BMI as a variable has not been well investigated in the literature. Based on all the discussion above on the impact of excess fat on breathing, and given the extreme importance of breathing in phonation, one can fairly extrapolate that obesity-induced respiratory changes may lead to phonatory disturbances as discussed below.

The paramount role of diaphragmatic contraction in phonation is irrefutable. The interplay between diaphragmatic contrac-tion, laryngeal airflow, and laryngeal resistance during phonation is well known. The differential movement of the diaphragm during the different phases of phonation is crucial in sustaining steady subglottic pressure, which in turn is central in regulating vocal pitch, loudness, and resonance.[50-52] The dynamic MRI study conducted by Traser et al,[53] looking at the diaphragmatic contraction during the performance of various phonatory tasks at 3 different pitches and loudnesses, stresses the strong interplay between diaphragmatic behavior and phonation. The authors reported movement of the posterior and mid third of the diaphragm in parallel with reduction in intrapulmonary pressure during the beginning of phonation. All these findings lead us to extrapolate that any impairment in breathing and in particular in the function of the diaphragm, indicating obesity-induced mechanical impairment, may affect voice adversely.

Reduction in lung compliance and volume may also inadvertently affect voice. Although normal conversational speech requires only 50% of vital capacity, in professional voice users, high lung volume is essential for the initiation of musical phrases[54-56] and for projected speech. Lung volume is paramount in the control of loudness and pitch, as well as maximum phonation time. Its role in sustaining maximum phonation was investigated by Solomon et al[56] in a group of 12 subjects who were asked to perform sustained vowel and repetitive slow syllables. The contribution of vital capacity to maximum phonation duration ranged between 75% and 97%. Of equal interest was the inverse linear relationship between airway resistance and lung volume observed in 4 of the 12 subjects. The authors reported an increase in laryngeal airway resistance with a decrease in lung volume.[56]

In addition to mechanical impairment and reduced lung compliance, alteration in chest wall compliance may affect voice in obese subjects. Chest compliance is of key importance to phonation across all ages. The contribution of rib cage movement to vocalization during phonation and breathing at rest has been described by Connaghan et al[57] in children. Similarly, Huber and Spruill[58] reported the impact of chest wall compliance on phonation in elderly subjects. In their study on the effect of aging on respiratory support during speech, the authors described the usage of higher lung volume in view of the decrease in chest wall compliance. Chest wall kinematics also plays an important role in pitch control. Professional voice users often adjust the movement of abdomen-diaphragm and ribcage in their transition between the different phases of inspiration and in their transition between registers.[55] All of the aforementioned findings on the association between lung compliance, chest compliance, and phonation suggest that obesity-induced alterations in lung and or chest wall compliance may affect voice especially in professional voice users in whom optimal total lung capacity and chest wall compliance are singularly important. Future research in that domain is needed to provide evidence-based information.

Another potential cause for dysphonia in obese subjects with no respiratory diseases is the change in breathing pattern and/or respiratory neural drive. A few investigations in the literature substantiate the strong interplay between vocal changes and respiratory challenges such as high breathing rate and increase in pulmonary drive.[59,60] Sandage et al[59] investigated the impact of respiratory rate on phonation in 18 participants who were asked to perform submaximal exercise in a thermally neutral environment. The work rate was limited to 8 minutes with an average respiratory rate of 20 breaths per minute. The authors found a significant increase in phonation threshold

pressure (PTP) and a decrease in pharyngeal temperature following exercise. Similarly, Sivasankar and Erickson[60] reported on the effect of short-duration accelerated breathing pattern on voice. The investigation was carried on 12 female smokers in comparison to 12 nonsmoking controls who underwent respiratory and PTP measures before and after normal and accelerated nasal and oral breathing challenges for 3 minutes each.[60] The results indicated alteration in PTP that was not related to the route of breathing and that was partially attributed to secondary airway dehydration. These findings corroborate numerous studies by Solomon et al[62] and others on the impact of hydration on voice. Dehydration, be it local or systemic, can induce an increase in phonatory effort that is mitigated by the intake of water.[61–63] Solomon et al had previously reported a decrease in the amplitude of vocal fold vibration in 3 out of 4 men and anterior glottal gap in 2 following vocal-loading tasks. The symptoms of vocal fatigue improved following systemic hydration.[62] Similarly, Hamdan et al[63] reported vocal fatigue in 53% of 28 women during fasting with a significant decrease in maximum phonation time in comparison to nonfasting. These findings suggest that dehydration, be it systemic or local secondary to altered breathing pattern, causes phonatory changes.

The last hypothetical cause for dysphonia in obese subjects is the chronic inflammation induced and perpetuated by obesity as discussed above. Although there are no studies on the effect of this proinflammatory state on voice, there are few studies on the role of inflammation in the development of various laryngeal pathologies. An anti-inflammatory peptide ApopA-I, which carries an anti-inflammatory and antioxidant effect, has been shown to be significantly lower in patients with vocal fold polyps vs controls (1.23 vs 1.37, *p* value less than .01).[64] In patients with vocal fold paralysis or paresis, White et al[65] have recently reported elevated while blood cell count in 14.4% of patients vs 5% in the general population. The authors emphasized the importance of blood lab in patients presenting with vocal fold impaired mobility. Future studies on the correlation between inflammatory biomarkers and vocal pathology while controlling for BMI in obese vs nonobese subjects are warranted.[65]

Obesity is a major risk factor for several systemic illnesses.[66–71] Obese subjects are at increased risk for cardiovascular disorders, hypertension, stroke, renal disorders, diabetes, and respiratory disorders. Diseases such as asthma and chronic obstructive lung disease (COPD) often are masked by obesity. Understanding the interplay between asthma, COPD, and dysphonia in the context of obesity is valuable in clinical care.

Obesity, Asthma, and Voice

Obesity and Asthma: Prevalence and Control

The association between obesity and asthma prevalence has been examined in the literature.[67–71] In 2010, Hjellvik et al[68] investigated the incidence of asthma in relation to body mass index using the nationwide Norwegian prescription database over the course of 6 years. By measuring the frequency of anti-asthmatic drug usage, the authors reported a 3-fold increase in prescription rate in very

obese nonsmoker asthmatics in comparison to normal-weight nonsmoker asthmatics.[68] The study also showed that a 3-unit increase in body mass index is associated with a higher risk for asthma, more so in non-smokers compared to smokers (1.27 vs 1.14, respectively). After adjusting for comorbidities, the relative risk associated with change in body mass index remained high in smokers.[68] Similarly, the meta-analysis of prospective studies on obesity and asthma by Beuther and Sutherland[70] revealed that obesity increases the incidence of asthma. The odds ratio for asthma incidence increased in overweight and obese subjects to 1.38 and 1.92, respectively, in comparison to normal-weight subjects. In another investigation looking at predictors of persistent asthma during adolescence using a large population-based birth cohort, Guerra et al[71] reported obesity as a significant predictor of unremitting asthma in adolescence, in addition to other factors such as active sinusitis and early puberty. The mean body mass index was significantly lower in the nonwheezing group in comparison to the wheezing group. Moreover, 58% of children diagnosed with asthma or with frequent wheezing before puberty (97 out of 166), and 30% of those with infrequent wheezing before puberty had persistent wheezing episodes after puberty.

An equally important issue is the correlation between obesity and asthma control or impairment. A large investigation carried out by Schatz et al[72] on a cohort of 10 233 adults with asthma revealed a significant association between asthma control and elevated body mass index even after adjusting for confounding diseases such as gastroesophageal reflux and depression. The results indicated that overweight and obesity increased the risk of asthma exacerbations up to 40% and 57%, respectively. The relative risk for emergency department visits and asthma hospitalization in overweight and obese asthmatics was 1.4, and the relative risk for excessive usage (more than 7) of short-acting beta-agonists canisters in obese asthmatics was 1.27. In conclusion, the authors advocated weight loss as a means to control asthma.[72] Several studies confirmed the strong association between obesity and response to asthma therapy.[73-75] In an analysis of 3037 adults with various degrees of asthma, Peters-Golden et al[73] demonstrated the presence of an inverse correlation between efficacy of inhaled corticosteroids and body mass index. Similarly, a study by Boulet and Franssen[74] on 1242 asthmatic patients revealed that control of asthma was achieved less in obese patients, more so in those with BMI greater than or equal to 40. Telenga et al[75] reported a higher neutrophil count in blood and sputum samples of obese asthmatics in comparison to normal-weight asthmatics. These findings, suggestive of airway inflammation in asthmatics with increased weight, help explain the diminished response to the conventional usage of inhaled corticosteroids and the better response to montelukast.[73]

Figure 8–3 illustrates the pulmonary function testing of an obese woman with asthma.

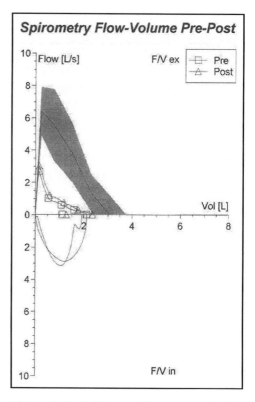

Figure 8–3. A 61-year-old woman with BMI 44.98 with severe obstructive pulmonary impairment and significant response to bronchodilator challenge.

Why the Link Between Obesity and Asthma?

The relationship between asthma and obesity is based on common systemic changes and behavioral factors. One is the high level of inflammatory mediators such as IL-6 and TNF (alpha) present in both obese and asthmatic patients.[76] As previously discussed, the adipose tissue–induced inflammation may affect the airway adversely and worsen disease control.[77] Leptin, for instance, synthesized and secreted by fat cells, induces proinflammatory reactions both systemically and within the airway via its receptors in lung tissues.[78] Another relationship between obesity and asthma is the oxidant-antioxidant imbalance partially induced by the high-fat and low-fruit and low-vegetable diet consumed by obese subjects.[79-81] Park et al[82] demonstrated the pathogenic role of increased oxidative stress in the induction and modulation of allergic airway inflammation. The upregulation of airway inflammatory cells and sputum neutrophils leads to a higher airway hyperresponsiveness and thus to a higher risk of asthma.[83] In addition to the aforementioned exacerbation of inflammatory response, obese and asthmatic patients share a common behavior, namely limited physical activity.[84,85] This carries adverse systemic effects that can be mitigated by exercise. Numerous studies have shown that increase in physical activity in the obese-asthma patient is associated with marked clinical improvement and reduction in sputum neutrophils.[86–88]

Vocal Dysfunction in Asthmatic Patients and Pathogenic Role of Obesity

It is known that asthma is a significant risk factor for dysphonia irrespective of body weight. Numerous studies confirm the increased prevalence of dysphonia in asthmatics.[89–91] The large investigation by Park and Choi[89] on more than 19,330 participants showed a higher prevalence of dysphonia in asthmatics compared to nonasthmatics (11.3% vs 5.5%, respectively) even in the absence of vocal fold pathology. The adjusted odds ratios for asthmatics who were not on asthma medications and for those who were on asthma medications were 1.62 and 1.97, respectively. Dogan et al[90] showed that 40% of asthmatics reported an elevated Voice Handicap Index in parallel with an increase in the perturbation parameters, particularly shimmer in both sexes and jitter in female patients. Similarly, in another study by Hamdan et al,[91] the authors reported a significantly higher prevalence of dysphonia in asthmatics compared to controls. Asthmatic patients had asthenic and strained voices compared to the nonasthmatic subjects.

The high prevalence of dysphonia and the abnormal vocal characteristics in obese and nonobese asthmatics is attributed to several factors. These include impairment in breathing, increased airway mucosal secretions, adverse effects of the use of inhaled corticosteroids, and the concomitant presence of allergy in many asthmatic patients.[92–97] Given the importance of breathing in phonation and the strong link between laryngeal resistance and pulmonary airway pressure and volume, any reduction in expiratory flow commonly seen in asthmatics can decrease the effectiveness of the power source and lead to change in voice quality.[50,96] Similarly, the increased thickness of mucosal secretions in asthmatics can result in cough with subsequent vocal fold edema and inflammatory changes, which in turn can lead to alteration in voice quality. Long-term use of inhaled steroids also has been shown to alter vocal quality and induce phonatory changes.[92,93] Bhalla et al[93] reported worse voice quality together with the presence of pharyngeal inflammatory changes in asthmatics on inhaled steroids compared to asthmatics not on steroids. In a retrospective review of patients with a 4-week history of dysphonia following use of corticosteroid therapy in the form of inhalers, Mirza et al[94] reported abnormal vocal fold mucosal changes in 8 of 9 patients. The authors also described reduced vibratory behavior and impaired mucosal waves. In corroboration, Lavy et al,[95] in their stroboscopic evaluation of 22 patients using inhaled steroids and complaints of dysphonia, reported mucosal changes in more than 50% of the patients in addition to apposition abnormalities in 43% of the cases. Other commonly reported laryngeal findings include dilated vessels and ectasias, mucosal plaques, and irregular vocal fold edges. Another important cause of dysphonia in asthmatic patients is allergy. Given the shared immunologic mechanisms between the upper and lower airway, allergy-induced inflammatory reaction may affect different sites of the airway equally and is not limited to one specific anatomical area.[97] This one functional unit, conceptualized as the "unified airway," emphasizes the strong association between asthma and allergy. Erbas et al[98] have reviewed the relationship between ambient exposure to pollen and asthma emergency department visits. Their meta-analysis showed a strong association between pollen concentration and asthma exacerbation, particularly in patients between the ages of 5 and 17 years. Moreover, Dhami et al[99] reported that allergen immunotherapy can lead to improvement in "short-term symptoms and medication scores" in allergic asthma patients. Their meta-analysis review on the effectiveness of allergen immunotherapy included 98 studies.

In all the aforementioned studies on dysphonia in asthmatics, the confounding effect of obesity has not been investigated. The prevalence of dysphonia in obese asthmatics in comparison to nonobese asthmatics is not known. Although obesity predisposes to asthma and asthma is a risk factor for dysphonia, the conclusion that obese asthmatics are at a higher risk of having dysphonia in comparison to nonobese asthmatics remains hypothetical. Nevertheless, we can speculate that dysphonia prevalence might be higher in obese asthmatic patients based on 2 factors: first is the compound effect of obesity and asthma regarding both physiologic and sensory response to exercise. Cortés-Télles et al[100] in 2015 showed that obese asthmatics had reduced self-reported activity levels by almost half in comparison to normal-weight asthmatics.[100] In their investigation of 14 obese asthmatics, the authors found significantly lower maximal oxygen uptake and work rate in comparison to normal-weight asthmatics. This reduced anaerobic threshold indicates a reduction in cardiorespiratory fitness. Given that vocalization is an aerobic exercise, especially in professional voice users, even a mild impairment in cardiovascular fitness might have deleterious effects on vocal performance.[50] Indeed, Welham and Maclagan[101] reported respiratory fatigue or

impairment as 1 of 5 possible causes of vocal fatigue, noting that a reduction in breathing capacity may precipitate dysphonia. Thus, it is reasonable to speculate that asthmatics with high BMI are more likely to have vocal fatigue in comparison to asthmatics with normal or low BMI.

The second factor for a possibly higher prevalence of dysphonia in obese asthmatic patients in comparison to nonobese asthmatic patients is the proinflammatory state induced by excess fat deposition. In the previous section on the link between obesity and asthma, we described the inflammatory biomarkers associated with obesity and their pathogenic role in worsening asthma. Although there are no studies on the association between these inflammatory biomarkers and dysphonia while controlling for BMI as a confounding variable, it seems likely that inflammatory biomarkers play an adverse role in obese patients with dysphonia.

In summary, although asthmatic patients are at a higher risk of having vocal dysfunction in comparison to nonasthmatics, the role of obesity in accentuating the phonatory disturbances in this subgroup of patients seems likely but has not been proven yet. Future investigation looking at the interplay between asthma, obesity, and dysphonia is needed.

Obesity, COPD and Voice

Prevalence of Obesity in COPD

The prevalence of obesity in COPD is controversial with no clear consensus.[102,103] In the study by Steuten et al,[103] obesity varied with the stage and severity of the disease. A low prevalence of obesity was reported in patients with severe disease in comparison to those with mild disease according to the Global Initiative for Chronic Obstructive Lung Disease (GOLD) staging system.[103,104] Low body weight was associated with advanced GOLD stage 4 disease, whereas high body weight was associated with GOLD stages 1 and 2.[103] The study by Montes de Oca et al[105] found that COPD is more common in normal-weight subjects, those with a BMI between 20 and 24.9 kg/m² or less than 20 kg/m². In 2013, Rutten et al[106] investigated the impact of obesity on the progression of disease over the course of 3 years in patients with COPD. In their study on 2115 COPD patients and 566 controls, the authors demonstrated that health status was affected mostly at the low and high end of obesity indices. COPD patients who had a decrease in muscle mass or had an increase in fat mass index had worsening of their health than other subjects.[106]

There is controversy not only about the prevalence of obesity in patients with COPD but also about its pathogenic role in COPD patients. The increased risk of systemic illnesses associated with obesity and COPD has confounded the association between the two. Although many studies suggest that obesity is pathogenic in COPD, several others indicate that excessive fat is advantageous to respiratory function.[106–110] Figure 8–4 shows a pulmonary function test of an obese COPD patient. Lambert et al, in their large multicenter prospective cohort study that included 3631 participants, 35% of whom were obese, reported worse quality of life, reduced 6-minute walk distance, and increased dyspnea score (greater than or equal to 2) in obese patients compared to controls.[110] Similarly, Cecere et al,[111] in their investigation on the effect of obesity on COPD health care measures, reported a higher dyspnea score measured by the Medical Research Council Dyspnea scale and poorer health-related quality of life in obese COPD patients. Similarly, the retro-

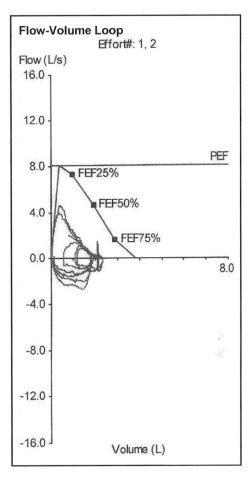

Figure 8–4. A 65-year-old man with BMI of 38.8 presenting with dyspnea. Pulmonary function testing shows obstructive pulmonary impairment with no significant response to bronchodilator challenge. Study compatible with diagnosis of COPD and obesity.

spective study by Ramachandran et al[112] on the influence of obesity on pulmonary rehabilitation in COPD patients indicated that obese COPD patients had worse baseline functional status, greater fatigue, and lower 6-minute walk performance than nonobese patients. The negative impact of obesity on health in COPD patients was later substantiated by McDonald et al.[113] In their study on the benefits of weight reduction using dietary restrictions and exercise training in 20 patients with a mean BMI of 36.3 kg/m², the authors showed that a decrease by 2.4 kg/m² was associated with a reduction in "body mass index, obstruction, dyspnea and exercise score (BODE)."[113] Contrary to the above, other investigators have shown that obesity is not a pathogenic factor in respiratory function in COPD patients. Sava et al,[114] in their investigation on the effect of obesity on COPD, reported no significant difference in the constant work-rate exercise test performance or in the St. George's Respiratory Questionnaire scores between the normal, overweight, and obese groups. However, obesity had an adverse effect on walking performance measures using the 6-minute walking test.[114] Similarly, Şahin et al[115] reported no negative effect of obesity on dyspnea and exercise tolerance, notwithstanding its adverse impact on pulmonary function tests and blood gas exchange. In their study on 218 COPD patients, the authors demonstrated "higher mean workload and walkwork figures"[115(p207)] in obese subjects vs normal-weight subjects, despite the abnormalities in PFTs and the elevated partial carbon dioxide pressure. The obese group had significantly lower vital capacity, residual volume, and expiratory reserve volume.[115] Ora et al[108] hypothesized that excessive weight carries a respiratory advantage. In their investigation on 24 COPD patients, equally divided as 12 obese and 12 normal weight, the authors reported better lung elasticity, higher intra-abdominal pressure, and less lung hyperinflation in the obese group. These findings, in addition to preserved inspiratory capacity, contributed to the report of less dyspnea and improved exercise performance.[108] O'Donnell et al[116] also studied the correlation between BMI, airway function, and static lung volumes in a cohort of 2265 subjects with chronic airway obstruction. The results indicated less lung hyperinflation and better inspiratory capac-ity and FEV1/FVC ratio with an increase in BMI. These effects were more pronounced in cases of severe airway obstruction.[116] In line with the aforementioned dichotomy in opinion on the pathogenic role of obesity in COPD, Cecere et al,[111] in their investigation on the effect of obesity on COPD, reported better lung function in the obese group despite a higher dyspnea score.

In conclusion, there is disparity in opinion on the prevalence and effect of obesity in COPD patients. The pathogenic role of obesity in COPD patients also remains inconclusive.

The Relationship Between Obesity and COPD?

The most plausible suggested mechanism for the association between obesity and COPD is the chronic inflammatory state observed in both COPD and obese patients. Several studies reported high levels of inflammatory biomarkers in association with visceral fat in patients with COPD.[117-119] These include IL-6, tumor necrosis factor–alpha, and C-reactive protein (CRP). Rutten et al,[117] in their investigation on 295 cases of moderate and severe COPD, reported an association between CRP and abdominal fat, particularly in subjects with muscle mass wasting. In an investigation carried by Agusti et al[118] on 1755 patients with COPD, 16% showed evidence of persistent systemic inflammation, which in turn was associated with poor clinical outcomes on follow-up. The inflammatory biomarkers used in their study included CRP, IL-6 and IL-8, fibrinogen, and tumor necrosis factor–alpha. Moreover, Breyer et al[119] reported that COPD patients with high BMI were more likely to have elevated CRP compared to those with normal weight. Similarly, patients with low BMI were less likely to have an elevated CRP level. The study was conducted on 628 elderly COPD patients admitted for pulmonary rehabilitation.

Vocal Dysfunction in COPD Patients and the Pathogenic Role of Obesity

The literature is scarce on phonatory disturbances in COPD patients despite the important role of breathing in phonation. There are no studies on the prevalence of phonatory changes in COPD patients with obesity. However, there are a few reports on vocal alterations and speech disorders in COPD patients vs normal subjects.[120,121] In 2011, Binazzi et al[120] highlighted the disturbances in speech in COPD patients with altered lung function. Dyspnea during speech activities reported as dyspnea score (DS) using "Speech section of the University of Cincinnati Dyspnea questionnaire" was 60% ± 23% of a maximal potential DS score. The phonatory tasks that contributed to the increase in dyspnea were raising the intensity of the voice, talking on the phone, talking in noisy places, and singing. In parallel with the aforementioned, Ryu et al[121] in 2015 reported COPD as one of many risk factors for dysphonia in elderly. Their cross-sectional study included 3759 subjects above the age of 65 years. It revealed that COPD, in addition to asthma, was associated with dysphonia even after adjusting for age, gender, and vocal fold disease as variables.

The etiology of dysphonia in COPD is multifactorial. Breathing impairment, inflammation, infectious pathogens, and drug-related causes are reported in the literature.[122-124] In 2014, Mohamed[125] reported the prevalence of dysphonia substantiated by elevated acoustic perturbation parameters in 25 of 50 patients with COPD. The grade of dysphonia, shimmer, and jitter were associated with abnormal pulmonary

function measures, namely FVC, FEV1, and MMEF5. Similarly, Hassan et al[122] in 2018 investigated further the correlation between breathing and dysphonia in a group of 60 patients with COPD vs 35 controls. All subjects underwent pulmonary function tests and a comprehensive phonatory evaluation using the GRBAS scale, acoustic analysis, and aerodynamic measures. The authors showed that 58.3% of COPD patients had dysphonia, which was perceived as strained and rough voice in the majority of cases, despite the normal laryngeal examination. In addition, the COPD group with dysphonia had higher perturbation parameters and lower maximum phonation time than those with no dysphonia and the control group. Moreover, the FVC and expiratory flow (peak and maximum mid-expiratory flow) were significantly higher in the COPD group without dysphonia as compared to those with dysphonia. In addition, there was a positive correlation between many pulmonary function measures and phonatory efficiency. The authors alluded to the pathogenic role of reduced pulmonary function in the etiology of dysphonia in COPD patients. Dysphonia in COPD patients may also be drug induced. Numerous studies indicate the adverse effect of steroid inhalers on voice secondary to thyroarytenoid myopathy, decreased tonicity of the vocal folds, inflammation, fungal infection, and/or deposition of exudate-like material on the vocal folds.[126-129]

Another less plausible suggested mechanism for dysphonia in COPD patients is laryngitis. Gilifanov et al[123] evaluated the microbial population of the larynx in 49 COPD patients at a stable stage of the diseases and reported chronic laryngitis in more than 70% of the cases. The pathogens identified most commonly were *S pyogenes* and yeast-like fungi (*C albicans*). COPD also may affect phonation through its association with laryngopharyngeal reflux disease (LPRD). Hamdan et al[124] investigated the prevalence of LPRD in a cohort of 40 patients. The authors reported a significantly higher mean of Reflux Symptom Index (RSI) in patients with COPD ($n = 27$) in comparison to controls ($n = 13$). Moreover, the frequency of positive RSI (score greater than 11) was higher in the former group (18 vs 1). The interplay between LPRD and phonation is reviewed in Chapter 9, "Reflux and Other Gastroenterologic Conditions That May Affect the Voice."[130]

In conclusion, there are no studies on vocal characteristics in COPD patients with morbid obesity in comparison to those with normal weight. Future investigation is warranted.

References

1. Parameswaran K, Todd DC, Soth M. Altered respiratory physiology in obesity. *Can Respir J.* 2006;13(4):203–210.
2. Bernhardt V, Babb TG. Exertional dyspnoea in obesity. *Eur Respir Rev.* 2016; 25(142):487–495.
3. Carpio C, Villasante C, Galera R, et al. Systemic inflammation and higher perception of dyspnea mimicking asthma in obese subjects. *J Allergy Clin Immunol.* 2016; 137(3):718–726.
4. Sahebjami H. Dyspnea in obese healthy men. *Chest.* 1998;114(5):1373–1377.
5. Bowden JA, To TH, Abernethy AP, Currow DC. Predictors of chronic breathlessness: a large population study. *BMC Public Health.* 2011;11(1):33.
6. Bernhardt V, Wood HE, Moran RB, Babb TG. Dyspnea on exertion in obese men. *Respir Physiol Neurobiol.* 2013;185(2): 241–248.
7. Dixon AE, Peters U. The effect of obesity on lung function. *Expert Rev Respir Med.* 2018;12(9):755–767.
8. Leone N, Courbon D, Thomas F, et al. Lung function impairment and metabolic syndrome: the critical role of abdominal obesity. *Am J Respir Crit Care Med.* 2009; 179(6):509–516.
9. Littleton SW. Impact of obesity on respiratory function. *Respirology.* 2012;17(1): 43–49.
10. Jones RL, Nzekwu MMU. The effects of body mass index on lung volumes. *Chest.* 2006;130(3):827–833.
11. Pelosi P, Croci M, Ravagnan I, et al. The effects of body mass on lung volumes, respiratory mechanics, and gas exchange during general anesthesia. *Anesth Analg.* 1998;87:654–660.
12. Canoy D, Luben R, Welch A, et al. Abdominal obesity and respiratory function in men and women in the EPIC-Norfolk study, United Kingdom. *Am J Epidemiol.* 2004;159(12):1140–1149.
13. Ray CS, Sue DY, Bray G, Hansen JE, Wasserman K. Effects of obesity on respiratory function. *Am Rev Respir Dis.* 1983; 128(3):501–506.
14. Ofir D, Laveneziana P, Webb KA, O'Donnell DE. Ventilatory and perceptual responses to cycle exercise in obese women. *J Appl Physiol.* 2007;102(6):2217–2226.
15. Collins LC, Hoberty PD, Walker JF, Fletcher EC, Peiris AN. The effect of body fat distribution on pulmonary function tests. *Chest.* 1995;107(5):1298–1302.
16. Lazarus R, Sparrow D, Weiss ST. Effects of obesity and fat distribution on ventilatory function: the normative aging study. *Chest.* 1997;111(4):891–898.
17. Steele RM, Finucane FM, Griffin SJ, Wareham NJ, Ekelund U. Obesity is associated with altered lung function independently of physical activity and fitness. *Obesity.* 2009;17(3):578–584.
18. Sharp JT, Henry JP, Swaeny SK, Meadows WR, Pietras RJ. Effects of mass loading the respiratory system in man. *J Appl Physiol.* 1964;19:959–966.
19. Salome CM, King GG, Berend N. Physiology of obesity and effects on lung function. *J Appl Physiol.* 2010;108(1):206–211.

20. Chen Y, Rennie D, Cormier YF, Dosman J. Waist circumference is associated with pulmonary function in normal-weight, overweight, and obese subjects. *Am J Clin Nutr.* 2007;85(1):35–39.

21. Unterborn J. Pulmonary function testing in obesity, pregnancy, and extremes of body habitus. *Clin Chest Med.* 2001;22(4):759–767.

22. Sampson MG, Grassino AE. Load compensation in obese patients during quiet tidal breathing. *J Appl Physiol.* 1983;55(4): 1269–1276.

23. Lotti P, Gigliotti F, Tesi F, et al. Respiratory muscles and dyspnea in obese nonsmoking subjects. *Lung.* 2005;183(5):311–323.

24. Kelly TM, Jensen RL, Elliott CG, Crapo RO. Maximum respiratory pressures in morbidly obese subjects. *Respiration.* 1988; 54(2):73–77.

25. Thomas PS, Milledge JS. Respiratory function in the morbidly obese before and after weight loss. *Thorax.* 1989;44:382–386.

26. Arena R, Cahalin LP. Evaluation of cardio-respiratory fitness and respiratory muscle function in the obese population. *Prog Cardiovasc Dis.* 2014;56(4):457–464.

27. Mafort TT, Rufino R, Costa CH, Lopes AJ. Obesity: systemic and pulmonary complications, biochemical abnormalities, and impairment of lung function. *Multidiscip Respir Med.* 2016;11(1):28.

28. Melo LC, da Silva MAM, Calles ACN. Obesity and lung function: a systematic review. *Einstein.* 2014;12(1):120–125.

29. Naimark A, Cherniack RM. Compliance of the respiratory system and its components in health and obesity. *J Appl Physiol.* 1960;15(3):377–382.

30. Burki NK, Baker RW. Ventilatory regulation in eucapnic morbid obesity. *Am Rev Respir Dis.* 1984;129(4):538–543.

31. Chlif M, Keochkerian D, Choquet D, Vaidie A, Ahmaidi S. Effects of obesity on breathing pattern, ventilatory neural drive and mechanics. *Respir Physiol Neurobiol.* 2009;168(3):198–202.

32. Milic-Emili J, Torchio R, D'Angelo E. Closing volume: a reappraisal (1967–2007). *Eur J Appl Physiol.* 2007;99(6):567–583.

33. Hedenstierna G, Santesson J, Norlander O. Airway closure and distribution of inspired gas in the extremely obese, breathing spontaneously and during anaesthesia with intermittent positive pressure ventilation. *Acta Anaesthesiol Scand.* 1976;20(4): 334–342.

34. Hakala K, Mustajoki P, Aittomäki J, Sovijärvi AR. Effect of weight loss and body position on pulmonary function and gas exchange abnormalities in morbid obesity. *Int J Obes Relat Metab Disord.* 1995;19(5): 343–346.

35. Holley HS, Milic-Emili J, Becklake MR, Bates DV. Regional distribution of pulmonary ventilation and perfusion in obesity. *J Clin Invest.* 1967;46(4):475–481.

36. Farebrother MJ, McHardy GJ, Munro JF. Relation between pulmonary gas exchange and closing volume before and after substantial weight loss in obese subjects. *BMJ.* 1974;3(5927):391–393.

37. Rivas E, Arismendi E, Agustí A, et al. Ventilation/perfusion distribution abnormalities in morbidly obese subjects before and after bariatric surgery. *Chest.* 2015;147(4): 1127–1134.

38. Dempsey JA, Reddan W, Rankin J, Balke B. Alveolar-arterial gas exchange during muscular work in obesity. *J Appl Physiol.* 1966;21(6):1807–1814.

39. Saydain G, Beck KC, Decker PA, Cowl CT, Scanlon PD. Clinical significance of elevated diffusion capacity. *Chest.* 2004;125(2): 446–452.

40. Fitzgerald DA. The weighty issue of obesity in paediatric respiratory medicine. *Paediatr Respir Rev.* 2017;24:4–7.

41. Fernández-Sánchez A, Madrigal-Santillán E, Bautista M, et al. Inflammation, oxidative stress, and obesity. *Int J Mol Sci.* 2011; 12(5):3117–3132.

42. Amirkhizi F, Siassi F, Minaie S, Djalali M, Rahimi A, Chamari M. Is obesity associated with increased plasma lipid peroxidation and oxidative stress in women. *ARYA Atherosclerosis.* 2007;2(4):189–192.

43. Ozata M, Mergen M, Oktenli C, et al. Increased oxidative stress and hypozincemia

in male obesity. *Clin Biochem.* 2002;35(8): 627–631.

44. Fonseca-Alaniz MH, Takada J, Alonso-Vale MI, Lima FB. Adipose tissue as an endocrine organ: from theory to practice. *J Pediatr (Rio J).* 2007;83(5):S192–S203.

45. Naugler WE, Karin M. The wolf in sheep's clothing: the role of interleukin-6 in immunity, inflammation and cancer. *Trends Mol Med.* 2008;14(3):109–119.

46. Pedersen JM, Budtz-Jørgensen E, Mortensen EL, et al. Late midlife C-reactive protein and interleukin-6 in middle-aged Danish men in relation to body size history within and across generations. *Obesity.* 2016;24(2):461–468.

47. Carroll LM, Sataloff RT, Heuer RJ, Spiegel JR, Radionoff SL, Cohn JR. Respiratory and glottal efficiency measures in normal classically trained singers. *J Voice.* 1996; 10(2):139–145.

48. Cohn JR, Sataloff RT, Branton C. Response of asthma-related voice dysfunction to allergen immunotherapy: a case report of confirmation by methacholine challenge. *J Voice.* 2001;15(4):558–560.

49. Meenan K, Catanoso L, Aoyama J, Stephan SR, Chauvin R, Sataloff RT. The utility of pulmonary function testing in patients presenting with dysphonia. *J Voice.* 2018; pii: S0892-1997(17)30513-1.

50. Sataloff RT. Clinical anatomy and physiology of the voice. In: Sataloff RT, *Professional Voice: The Science and Art of Clinical Care.* 4th ed. San Diego, CA: Plural Publishing; 2017:157–196.

51. Scherer RC. Laryngeal function during phonation. In: Sataloff RT, *Professional Voice: The Science and Art of Clinical Care.* 4th ed. San Diego, CA: Plural Publishing; 2017:281–308.

52. Sundberg J. Vocal tract resonance. In: Sataloff RT, *Professional Voice: The Science and Art of Clinical Care.* 4th ed. San Diego, CA: Plural Publishing; 2017:309–328.

53. Traser L, Özen AC, Burk F, et al. Respiratory dynamics in phonation and breathing—a real-time MRI study. *Respir Physiol Neurobiol.* 2017;236:69–77.

54. Leanderson R, Sundberg J. Breathing for singing. *J Voice.* 1988;2(1):2–12.

55. Watson PJ, Hixon TJ. Respiratory kinematics in classical (opera) singers. *J Speech Hear Res.* 1985:28(1):104–122.

56. Solomon NP, Garlitz SJ, Milbrath RL. Respiratory and laryngeal contributions to maximum phonation duration. *J Voice.* 2000;14(3):331–340.

57. Connaghan KP, Moore CA, Higashakawa M. Respiratory kinematics during vocalization and nonspeech respiration in children from 9 to 48 months. *J Speech Lang Hear Res.* 2004;47(1):70–84.

58. Huber JE, Spruill J 3rd. Age-related changes to speech breathing with increased vocal loudness. *J Speech Lang Hear Res.* 2008; 51(3):651–668.

59. Sandage MJ, Connor NP, Pascoe DD. Voice function differences following resting breathing versus submaximal exercise. *J Voice.* 2013;27(5):572–578.

60. Sivasankar M, Erickson E. Short-duration accelerated breathing challenges affect phonation. *Laryngoscope.* 2009;119(8): 1658–1663.

61. Verdolini K, Min Y, Titze IR, et al. Biological mechanisms underlying voice changes due to dehydration. *J Speech Lang Hear Res.* 2002;45(2):268–281.

62. Solomon NP, Glaze LE, Arnold RR, van Mersbergen M. Effects of a vocally fatiguing task and systemic hydration on men's voices. *J Voice.* 2003;17(1):31–46.

63. Hamdan AL, Sibai A, Rameh C. Effect of fasting on voice. *J Voice.* 2006;21:495–501.

64. Zhang HP, Zhang R. Correlations between serum apolipoprotein A-I and formation of vocal cord polyp. *J Voice.* 2017;31(3): 380-e1.

65. White M, Meenan K, Patel T, Jaworek A, Sataloff RT. Laboratory evaluation of vocal fold paralysis and paresis. *J Voice.* 2017; 31(2):168–174.

66. Kim S, Camargo CA Jr., Sex-race differences in the relationship between obesity and asthma: the behavioral risk factor surveillance system, 2000. *Ann Epidemiol.* 2003;13(10):666–673.

67. Dixon AE, Holguin F, Sood A, et al. An official American thoracic society workshop report: obesity and asthma. *Proc Am Thorac Soc.* 2010;7(5):325–335.

68. Hjellvik V, Tverdal A, Furu K. Body mass index as predictor for asthma: a cohort study of 118,723 males and females. *Eur Respir J.* 2010;35(6):1235–1242.

69. Appleton SL, Adams RJ, Wilson DH, et al. Central obesity is associated with non-atopic but not atopic asthma in a representative population sample. *J Allergy Clin Immunol.* 2006;118(6):1284–1291.

70. Beuther DA, Sutherland ER. Overweight, obesity, and incident asthma: a meta-analysis of prospective epidemiologic studies. *Am J Respir Crit Care Med.* 2007;175(7):661–666.

71. Guerra S, Wright AL, Morgan WJ, Sherrill DL, Holberg CJ, Martinez FD. Persistence of asthma symptoms during adolescence: role of obesity and age at the onset of puberty. *Am J Respir Crit Care Med.* 2004; 170(1):78–85.

72. Schatz M, Zeiger RS, Yang SJ, et al. Prospective study on the relationship of obesity to asthma impairment and risk. *J Allergy Clin Immunol Pract.* 2015;3(4):560–565.

73. Peters-Golden M, Swern A, Bird SS, Hustad CM, Grant E, Edelman JM. Influence of body mass index on the response to asthma controller agents. *Eur Respir J.* 2006;27(3):495–503.

74. Boulet LP, Franssen E. Influence of obesity on response to fluticasone with or without salmeterol in moderate asthma. *Respir Med.* 2007;101(11):2240–2247.

75. Telenga ED, Tideman SW, Kerstjens HA, et al. Obesity in asthma: more neutrophilic inflammation as a possible explanation for a reduced treatment response. *Allergy.* 2012;67(8):1060–1068.

76. Scott HA, Wood LG, Gibson PG. Role of obesity in asthma: mechanisms and management strategies. *Curr Allergy Asthma Rep.* 2017;17(8):53.

77. Scott HA, Gibson PG, Garg ML, Wood LG. Airway inflammation is augmented by obesity and fatty acids in asthma. *Eur Respir J.* 2011;38(3):594–602.

78. Bruno A, Pace E, Chanez P, et al. Leptin and leptin receptor expression in asthma. *J Allergy Clin Immunol.* 2009;124(2):230–237.

79. Wood LG, Garg ML, Gibson PG. A high-fat challenge increases airway inflammation and impairs bronchodilator recovery in asthma. *J Allergy Clin Immunol.* 2011; 127(5):1133–1140.

80. Rodríguez-Rodríguez E, Perea JM, Jiménez AI, Rodríguez-Rodríguez P, López-Sobaler AM, Ortega RM. Fat intake and asthma in Spanish schoolchildren. *Eur J Clin Nutr.* 2010;64(10):1065–1071.

81. Huang SL, Pan WH. Dietary fats and asthma in teenagers: analyses of the first Nutrition and Health Survey in Taiwan (NAHSIT). *Clin Exp Allergy.* 2001;31(12):1875–1880.

82. Park CS, Kim TB, Lee KY, et al. Increased oxidative stress in the airway and development of allergic inflammation in a mouse model of asthma. *Ann Allergy Asthma Immunol.* 2009;103(3):238–247.

83. Soutar A, Seaton A, Brown K. Bronchial reactivity and dietary antioxidants. *Thorax.* 1997;52(2):166–170.

84. Teramoto M, Moonie S. Physical activity participation among adult Nevadans with self-reported asthma. *J Asthma.* 2011;48(5): 517–522.

85. Groth SW, Rhee H, Kitzman H. Relationships among obesity, physical activity and sedentary behavior in young adolescents with and without lifetime asthma. *J Asthma.* 2016;53(1):19–24.

86. Lu KD, Billimek J, Bar-Yoseph R, Radom-Aizik S, Cooper DM, Anton-Culver H. Sex differences in the relationship between fitness and obesity on risk for asthma in adolescents. *J Pediatr.* 2016;176:36–42.

87. Garcia-Aymerich J, Varraso R, Antó JM, Camargo CA Jr. Prospective study of physical activity and risk of asthma exacerbations in older women. *Am J Respir Crit Care Med.* 2009;179(11):999–1003.

88. Bacon SL, Lemiere C, Moullec G, Ninot G, Pepin V, Lavoie KL. Association between patterns of leisure time physical activity and asthma control in adult patients. *BMJ Open Respir Res.* 2015;2(1):e000083.

89. Park B, Choi HG. Association between asthma and dysphonia: a population-based study. *J Asthma.* 2016;53(7):679–683.

90. Dogan M, Eryuksel E, Kocak I, Celikel T, Sehitoglu MA. Subjective and objective evaluation of voice quality in patients with asthma. *J Voice.* 2007;21(2):224–230.

91. Hamdan AL, Ziade G, Kasti M, Akl L, Bawab I, Kanj N. Phonatory symptoms and acoustic findings in patients with asthma: a cross-sectional controlled study. *Indian J Otolaryngol Head Neck Surg.* 2017;69(1): 42–46.

92. Ihre E, Zetterstrom O, Ihre E, Hammarberg B. Voice problems as side effects of inhaled corticosteroids patients-a prevalence study. *J Voice.* 2004;18(3):403–414.

93. Bhalla RK, Watson G, Taylor W, Jones AS, Roland NJ. Acoustic analysis in asthmatics and the influence of inhaled corticosteroid therapy. *J Voice.* 2009;23(4):505–511.

94. Mirza N, Kasper Schwartz S, Antin-Ozerkis D. Laryngeal findings in users of combination corticosteroid and bronchodilator therapy. *Laryngoscope.* 2004;114(9): 1566–1569.

95. Lavy JA, Wood G, Rubin JS, Harries M. Dysphonia associated with inhaled steroids. *J Voice.* 2000;14(4):581–588.

96. Spiegel JR, Sataloff RT, Cohn JR, Hawkshaw M. Respiratory dysfunction. In: Sataloff RT, ed. *The Professional Voice: The Science and Art of Clinical Care.* 2nd ed. San Diego, CA: Singular Publishing Group; 1997:375–386.

97. Shtraks JP, Toskala E. Manifestations of inhalant allergies beyond the nose. *Otolaryngol Clin North Am.* 2017;50(6): 1051–1064.

98. Erbas B, Jazayeri M, Lambert KA, et al. Outdoor pollen is a trigger of child and adolescent asthma emergency department presentations: a systematic review and meta-analysis. *Allergy.* 2018;73(8):1632–1641.

99. Dhami S, Kakourou A, Asamoah F, et al. Allergen immunotherapy for allergic asthma: a systematic review and meta-analysis. *Allergy.* 2017;72(12):1825–1848.

100. Cortés-Télles A, Torre-Bouscoulet L, Silva-Cerón M, et al. Combined effects of mild-to-moderate obesity and asthma on physiological and sensory responses to exercise. *Respir Med.* 2015;109(11):1397–1403.

101. Welham NV, Maclagan MA. Vocal fatigue: current knowledge and future directions. *J Voice.* 2003;17(1):21–30.

102. Vozoris NT, O'Donnell DE. Prevalence, risk factors, activity limitation and health care utilization of an obese, population-based sample with chronic obstructive pulmonary disease. *Can Respir J.* 2012;19(3): e18–e24.

103. Steuten LM, Creutzberg EC, Vrijhoef HJ, Wouters EF. COPD as a multicomponent disease: inventory of dyspnoea, underweight, obesity and fat free mass depletion in primary care. *Prim Care Respir J.* 2006; 15(2):84–91.

104. Pauwels RA, Buist S, Calverly PMA, et al. Global strategy for the diagnosis, management and prevention of chronic obstructive pulmonary disease. NHLBI/WHO global initiative for chronic obstructive lung disease (GOLD) workshop summary. *Am J Respir Crit Care Med.* 2001;163(5): 1256–1276.

105. Montes de Oca M, Tálamo C, Perez-Padilla R, et al. Chronic obstructive pulmonary disease and body mass index in five Latin America cities: the PLATINO study. *Respir Med.* 2008;102(5):642–650.

106. Rutten EP, Calverley PM, Casaburi R, et al. Changes in body composition in patients with chronic obstructive pulmonary disease: do they influence patient-related outcomes? *Ann Nutr Metab.* 2013;63(3): 239–247.

107. Ora J, Laveneziana P, Ofir D, Deesomchok A, Webb KA, O'Donnell DE. Combined effects of obesity and chronic obstructive pulmonary disease on dyspnea and exercise tolerance. *Am J Respir Crit Care Med.* 2009;180(10):964–971.

108. Ora J, Laveneziana P, Wadell K, Preston M, Webb KA, O'Donnell DE. Effect of obesity on respiratory mechanics during

rest and exercise in COPD. *J Appl Physiol.* 2011;111(1):10–19.

109. Watz H, Waschki B, Kirsten A, et al. The metabolic syndrome in patients with chronic bronchitis and COPD: frequency and associated consequences for systemic inflammation and physical inactivity. *Chest.* 2009;136(4):1039–1046.

110. Lambert AA, Putcha N, Drummond MB, et al. Obesity is associated with increased morbidity in moderate to severe COPD. *Chest.* 2017;151(1):68–77.

111. Cecere LM, Littman AJ, Slatore CG, et al. Obesity and COPD: associated symptoms, health-related quality of life, and medication use. *COPD.* 2011;8(4):275–284.

112. Ramachandran K, McCusker C, Connors M, Zuwallack R, Lahiri B. The influence of obesity on pulmonary rehabilitation outcomes in patients with COPD. *Chron Respir Dis.* 2008;5(4):205–209.

113. McDonald VM, Gibson PG, Scott HA, et al. Should we treat obesity in COPD? The effects of diet and resistance exercise training. *Respirology.* 2016;21(5):875–882.

114. Sava F, Laviolette L, Bernard S, Breton MJ, Bourbeau J, Maltais F. The impact of obesity on walking and cycling performance and response to pulmonary rehabilitation in COPD. *BMC Pulm Med.* 2010;10(1): 55.

115. Şahin H, Naz İ, Varol Y, Kömürcüoğlu B. The effect of obesity on dyspnea, exercise capacity, walk work and workload in patients with COPD. *Tuberk Toraks.* 2017; 65(3):202–209.

116. O'Donnell DE, Deesomchok A, Lam YM, et al. Effects of BMI on static lung volumes in patients with airway obstruction. *Chest.* 2011;140(2):461–468.

117. Rutten EP, Breyer MK, Spruit MA, et al. Abdominal fat mass contributes to the systemic inflammation in chronic obstructive pulmonary disease. *Clin Nutr.* 2010;29(6): 756–760.

118. Agusti A, Edwards LD, Rennard SI, et al. Persistent systemic inflammation is associated with poor clinical outcomes in COPD: a novel phenotype. *PLoS One.* 2012;7(5): e37483.

119. Breyer MK, Spruit MA, Celis AP, et al. Highly elevated C-reactive protein levels in obese patients with COPD: a fat chance? *Clin Nutr.* 2009;28(6):642–647.

120. Binazzi B, Lanini B, Romagnoli I, et al. Dyspnea during speech in chronic obstructive pulmonary disease patients: effects of pulmonary rehabilitation. *Respiration.* 2011;81(5):379–385.

121. Ryu CH, Han S, Lee MS, et al. Voice changes in elderly adults: prevalence and the effect of social, behavioral, and health status on voice quality. *J Am Geriatr Soc.* 2015;63(8):1608–1614.

122. Hassan MM, Hussein MT, Emam AM, Rashad UM, Rezk I, Awad AH. Is insufficient pulmonary air support the cause of dysphonia in chronic obstructive pulmonary disease? *Auris Nasus Larynx.* 2018; 45(4):807–814.

123. Gilifanov EA, Nevzorova VA, Artyushkin SA, Ivanets IV. The state of the larynx in the patients presenting with chronic obstructive pulmonary disease. *Vestn Otorinolaringol.* 2016;81(1):29–32.

124. Hamdan AL, Ziade G, Turfe Z, Beydoun N, Sarieddine D, Kanj N. Laryngopharyngeal symptoms in patients with chronic obstructive pulmonary disease. *Eur Arch Otorhinolaryngol.* 2016;273(4):953–958.

125. Mohamed EE. Voice changes in patients with chronic obstructive pulmonary disease. *Egypt J Chest Dis Tuberc.* 2014;63(3):561–567.

126. Williamson IJ, Matusiewicz SP, Brown PH, Greening AP, Crompton GK. Frequency of voice problems and cough in patients using pressurized aerosol inhaled steroid preparations. *Eur Respir J.* 1995;8:590–592.

127. Vogt FC. The incidence of oral candidiasis with use of inhaled corticosteroids. *Ann Allergy.* 1979;43(4):205–210.

128. Rachelefsky GS, Liao Y, Faruqi R. Impact of inhaled corticosteroid-induced oropharyngeal adverse events: results from a meta-analysis. *Ann Allergy Asthma Immunol.* 2007;98(3):225–238.

129. Kozak E, Maniecka-Aleksandrowicz B, Frank-Piskorska A, Witman D. Evaluation of the effect of chronic steroid inhalation therapy on the state of the upper airway in patients with chronic obstructive pulmonary disease. *Pneumonol Alergol Pol.* 1991; 59(9–10):33–37.

130. Sataloff RT. Reflux and other gastroenterologic conditions that may affect the voice. In: Sataloff RT, ed. *The Professional Voice: The Science and Art of Clinical Care.* 4th ed. San Diego, CA: Plural Publishing; 2017: 907–998.

9

Reflux and Other Gastroenterologic Conditions That May Affect the Voice*

Robert Thayer Sataloff, Donald O. Castell, Philip O. Katz,
Dahlia M. Sataloff, and Mary J. Hawkshaw

Laryngopharyngeal reflux (LPR) is gastro-esophageal reflux disease (GERD) that affects the pharynx and larynx. Reflux laryngitis (RL) is a component of LPR. Laryngopharyngeal reflux and reflux laryngitis are diagnoses that remain a subject for debate because their symptomatology and clinical manifestations are not the same as those of GERD (gastroesophageal reflux disease). The otolaryngology literature prior to the 1970s and 1980s is almost nonexistent. However, during the 1970s and 1980s, several reports of LPR and GERD were published.[1–15] Usually, when RL is present, symptoms and signs of more generalized LPR are also present, although they are commonly missed if not elicited by specific questions during the medical history and meticulous physical examination.

Occult chronic gastroesophageal reflux is an etiologic factor in a high percentage of patients of all ages with laryngologic (ie,

voice) complaints. In 1989, Wiener et al[16] reported the results of double-probe pH monitoring in a series of 32 otolaryngology patients with clinical LPR; 78% of them had pH-documented LPR. It has also been found to be a particularly common problem in professional voice users and singers. In 1991, Sataloff et al[17] reported reflux laryngitis in 265 of 583 consecutive professional voice users (45%), including singers and others, who sought medical care during a 12-month period. However, reflux laryngitis was often diagnosed incidentally and was not always responsible for the patient's primary voice complaint. The incidence of RL may be lower in patients with other vocations, but it is interesting to note that Koufman et al[18] found gastroesophageal reflux in 78% of patients with hoarseness and in about 50% of all patients with voice complaints. Other reports have been published on the pathogenesis of voice disorders

*Modified from Sataloff RT, Castell DO, Katz PO, Sataloff DM, and Hawkshaw MJ, Reflux and other gastroenterologic conditions that may affect the voice. In: Sataloff R.T. *Professional Voice: The Science and Art of Clinical Care, Fourth Edition*. San Diego, CA: Plural Publishing; 2017:907–997, with permission.

and other otolaryngologic manifestations of LPR and its prevalence.[19-32] Nevertheless, the prevalence of reflux laryngitis in all patients who seek evaluation for voice complaints remains unknown. Additional epidemiologic studies are needed to help clarify the clinical importance of this entity.

LPR involves multiple anatomical sites, including the sphincter between the stomach and distal esophagus; the entire length of the esophagus; the upper esophageal sphincter; the structures of the larynx, pharynx, and oral cavity; and the trachea and lungs. Consequently, it should be evident that LPR is managed best through a multidisciplinary team approach. The team includes at least a laryngologist who is uniquely qualified to diagnose disorders of the larynx, an internist or primary care physician, a gastroenterologist and his or her laboratory personnel, a speech-language pathologist, and a pulmonologist. For voice professionals, a singing voice specialist and an acting-voice specialist should be included.[33] The availability of a knowledgeable psychologist and nutritionist is highly desirable, as well.[33,34] Although it is possible for one physician to manage most or all aspects of LPR, this approach does not provide comprehensive state-of-the-art care.

Laryngeal involvement by gastroesophageal reflux disease commonly results in dysphonia for which patients attempt to compensate through hyperfunctional voice use patterns (muscular tension dysphonia). The collaboration of a speech-language pathologist and other voice team members is invaluable in eliminating compensatory behaviors and optimizing phonatory technique. Although laryngologists can certainly purchase 24-hour pH monitoring equipment and may even perform manometry, they do not generally do so with the same level of expertise as a gastroenterologist whose entire career may be devoted to disorders of the esophagus. Just as certain laryngologists subspecialize in voice care, some gastroenterologists subspecialize in the management of reflux. This group of professionals and their ancillary staff may be best equipped to diagnose gastroesophageal reflux and its consequences.

Laryngopharyngeal reflux is almost always associated with some degree of aspiration. This may be clinically insignificant, or it may cause chronic cough, reactive airway disease, difficulties controlling asthma, pneumonia, or bronchiectasis. A knowledgeable pulmonologist is essential in recognizing and treating these conditions.

There are several issues of special concern in the management of otolaryngologic patients with reflux laryngitis, especially professional voice users. First, many of these patients are young and will require prolonged or lifetime use of high doses of H2-antagonists or proton pump inhibitors. Despite being quite safe, the ultimate long-term effects of taking these medications over a long period of time are unknown, and they are expensive. The cost may be burdensome, and a financial strain often leads to poor compliance. Second, medications do not eliminate or cure reflux. They simply neutralize the refluxate and control the symptoms effectively in many patients. However, some patients may continue to aspirate pH-neutral fluid, bile salts, and other substances not appropriate for entry into the pharynx, larynx, and lungs. In professional singers and other high-performance voice users, this problem may continue to be symptomatic (throat clearing, excess phlegm, cough) even when acidity is controlled well, although no one has demonstrated that deacidified gastric acid actually causes mucosal injury.

As stated above, medications do not cure reflux; however, surgery may actually eliminate reflux. Conveniently, surgical therapy for GERD has improved dramatically with the advent of laparoscopic Nissen fundoplication and endoscopic antireflux procedures that offer alternatives to chronic medical management. An increasing percentage of patients are being referred for surgical treatment.

It is essential for otolaryngologists to be familiar with the anatomy, physiology, pathology, diagnosis, and treatment options for LPR and GERD in general. Although much of this knowledge is outside traditional otolaryngology, familiarity with the latest concepts and techniques in the management of GERD and reflux laryngitis in voice patients helps the otolaryngologist assemble an appropriate voice team, interpret information from other colleagues on the voice care team, and ensure optimal patient care.

Anatomy and Physiology of the Vocal Tract

Discussions of vocal fold physiology in previous chapters highlighted the importance of a complex, traveling mucosal wave with vertical phase differences. This complexity is necessary for normal phonation. Anything that interferes with it may result in voice dysfunction. Hence, it should be clear that gastric acid irritation of the vocal folds is capable not only of producing annoying, irritative symptoms (burning, lump in the throat), but moreover of actually interfering with phonation by causing edema of the vibratory margin and lamina propria that truly alters voice.

The anatomic and physiologic basis for many symptoms of LPR seems fairly obvious initially. Topical irritation, muscle spasm, bronchospasm in response to acidic aspiration, halitosis, sore throat, and other symptoms are easy to understand, although some have unexpectedly complex physiol-

ogy. In addition, vagal reflexes triggered by distal esophageal acid irritation may cause events and responses that affect the voice even without acid contacting the larynx. Regardless of the mechanism, the effects of reflux laryngitis on voice function often seem greater than one might anticipate based on physical findings. To understand the impact of reflux disease on phonation, it is helpful to review current concepts in anatomy and physiology of the voice, as discussed elsewhere in this book.

Anatomy and Physiology of the Esophagus and Its Sphincters

Anatomy

The human esophagus is a muscular tube that has as its major function the transport of food from the mouth to the stomach[35] (Figure 9–1). It is bounded by a tonically contracted circular muscle sphincter at each end. The median length of the esophageal body, between the 2 sphincters, is 22 centimeters (cm) in adult females and 24 cm in adult males. Individual variations in length are normally distributed in both genders[35] (Figure 9–2). The upper esophageal sphincter (UES) consists primarily of striated muscle of the cricopharyngeus muscle but is enhanced by the inferior pharyngeal constrictors and the circular muscles of the upper esophagus. The anterior attachment of the cricopharyngeus to the cricoid cartilage of the larynx results in the strongest contractile force of this sphincter occurring in the anterior-posterior direction, producing a slitlike configuration with the widest portion facing laterally.[36] The UES, like the striated musculature of the tongue, pharynx, and upper portion of the esophagus,

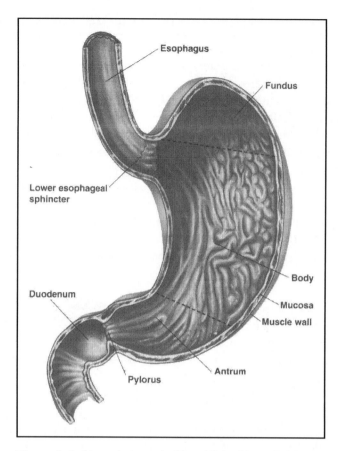

Figure 9–1. Normal stomach. (Republished from *Quick Reference to Upper GI Motility* with the permission of Janssen Pharmaceutica.)

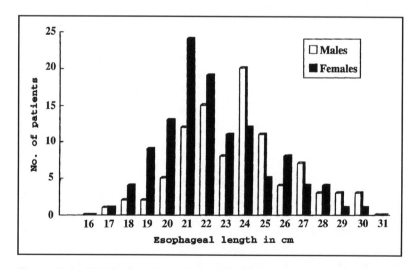

Figure 9–2. Distribution of esophageal length in 212 patients and normal volunteers. Males are shown in white, females in black. Approximation to a normal distribution is verified by similar means and medians (males: mean = 23.6 cm, median = 24 cm; females: mean = 22.4 cm, median = 22 cm).

is innervated like skeletal muscle, receiving motor input directly from the brainstem (nucleus ambiguus) to the motor endplates in the muscle. Tonicity is maintained by continuous stimulation, which is temporarily inhibited during a swallow.

The lower esophageal sphincter (LES), like most of the gastrointestinal (GI) tract, consists entirely of smooth muscle. This sphincter is much more rounded in its closure, yet still demonstrates some degree of radial asymmetry, having the higher pressures in the posterolateral direction.[37] Innervation of the LES originates from the dorsal motor nucleus of the brainstem, and the efferent fibers are carried through the vagus nerve and synapse in the myenteric plexus in the region of the LES.

The muscular wall of the esophagus is composed of an inner circular and an outer longitudinal layer, with no serosa overlying the muscle layers. The UES and the upper portion of the tubular esophagus are primarily striated muscle. Recent studies have indicated that smooth muscle occurs in the upper 4 to 5 cm of the human esophagus, although it is quite variable in different individuals and in the different muscle layers. Consistently, greater than the distal half of the human esophagus is entirely smooth muscle.[38] Like the LES, the smooth muscle portion of the tubular esophagus is innervated primarily via the vagus nerve from neurons arising in the dorsal motor nucleus connecting to the myenteric plexus.

Physiology

Swallowing, or deglutition, has 3 stages: the oral (voluntary) stage, the pharyngeal (involuntary) stage, and the esophageal stage. These 3 closely coordinated and combined processes are regulated through the swallowing center in the medulla.[39]

Oral Stage

This preparatory stage includes mechanical disruption of the food and mixing with salivary bicarbonate and enzymes (amylase, lipase). It is an essential process by which the swallowing mechanism is primed. Ingested food is voluntarily moved posteriorly by pistonlike movements of the tongue muscles, forcing the food bolus toward the pharynx and pushing it backward and upward against the palate. Once the food has been delivered to the pharynx, the process becomes involuntary. The oral, preparatory stage obviously requires proper functioning of the striated muscles of the tongue and pharynx and is the stage of swallowing that is likely to be abnormal in patients with neurologic or skeletal muscle disease. Appropriate mentation is also necessary.

Pharyngeal Stage

During this stage of swallowing, the food is passed from the pharynx, through the UES, and into the proximal esophagus. This involuntary process requires the finely tuned coordinated sequences of contraction and relaxation, resulting in transfer of the ingested material, while protecting the airway. The presence of food in the pharynx stimulates sensory receptors, which send impulses to the swallowing center in the brainstem. The central nervous system (CNS) then initiates a series of involuntary responses that include the following:

1. The soft palate is pulled upward and closes the posterior nares.
2. The palatopharyngeal folds are pulled medially, limiting the opening through the pharynx.
3. The vocal folds are closed, and the epiglottis swings backward and down to close the larynx.

4. The larynx is pulled upward and forward by the muscles attached to the hyoid bone, stretching the opening of the esophagus and UES.

5. The UES relaxes. Active relaxation of the usually tonic cricopharyngeus is essential to permit the passive opening of the UES created by the movement of the larynx.

6. Peristaltic contraction of the constrictor muscles of the pharynx produces the force that propels food into the esophagus.

This sequence is a coordinated mechanism that includes impulses carried by 5 cranial nerves. Sensory information to the swallowing center is carried along cranial nerves V, VII, IX, and X. The motor responses from the swallowing center are carried along cranial nerves V, VII, IX, X, and XII and also the ansa cervicalis (C-1 and C-2). This intricate process takes just over 1 second from start to finish and requires coordination of pharyngeal contraction and UES relaxation (Figure 9–3). The UES is only open for approximately 500 milliseconds.

Esophageal Stage

The main function of the esophagus is to transport ingested material from the mouth

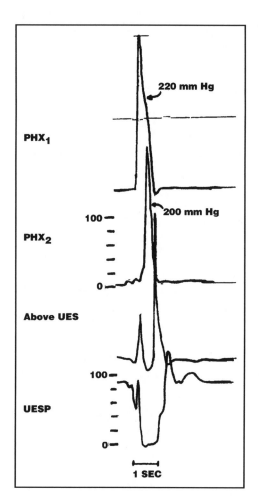

Figure 9–3. Motility tracing showing the coordinated sequence of contraction of the human pharynx and relaxation of the upper esophageal sphincter (UES). The 4 recording sites are spaced at 3-cm intervals, with the lowest in the UES high-pressure zone (UESP), the second from bottom located just proximal to the UES, and the next 2 sites at 3-cm (PHX2) and 6-cm (PHX1) distances proximally. The sequential contraction in the pharynx is noted in the 2 proximal recording sites. Movement of the UES orad followed by UES relaxation and subsequent descent of the UES during the swallow generates the "M" configuration shown at the third recording site. The apparently longer UES "relaxation" seen in the distal sensor is an artifact produced by the movement of the sphincter orad away from the transducer during swallowing. The actual time of UES relaxation is approximately 0.5 seconds as shown in the recording located second from the bottom.

to the stomach. This active process requires contraction of both the longitudinal and circular muscles of the tubular esophagus and coordinated relaxation of the sphincters. At the onset of swallowing, the longitudinal muscle contracts and shortens the esophagus to provide a structural base for the circular muscle contraction that forms the peristaltic wave. The sequential contraction of esophageal circular smooth muscle from proximal to distal generates the peristaltic clearing wave. The neuromuscular control of this activity will be described below. As opposed to other GI tract smooth muscle, the esophageal smooth muscle has a unique electrical activity pattern, showing only spiked potentials without underlying slow waves. Circular muscle contractions can be characterized into 3 distinct patterns:

1. *Primary peristalsis.* This is the usual form of a contraction wave of circular muscle that progresses down the esophagus and is initiated by the central mechanisms that follow the voluntary act of swallowing. It follows sequentially the pressure generated in the pharynx and requires approximately 8 to 10 seconds to reach the distal esophagus. The LES relaxes at the onset of the swallow and remains relaxed until it contracts as a continuation of the progressive peristaltic wave. These pressure relationships are shown in Figure 9–4.

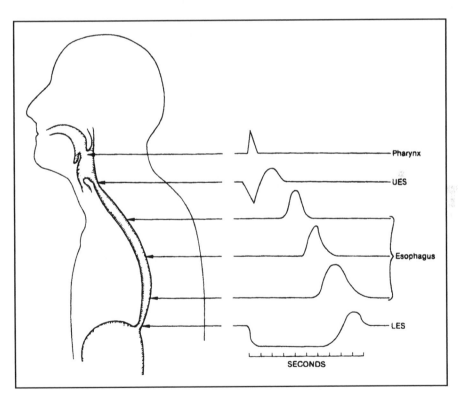

Figure 9–4. Schematic presentation of the pressure sequence of a normal primary peristaltic wave. Note the pressure complex that begins in the pharynx and progressively closes off the UES, then moves sequentially down the esophageal body and closes the LES. Also note that LES relaxation begins with the onset of the swallow and remains relaxed until the peristaltic wave reaches the distal esophagus (8–10 seconds).

2. *Secondary peristalsis.* This represents a peristaltic contraction of the circular esophageal muscle, which begins without central stimulation. That is to say, it originates in the esophagus as a result of distention and will usually continue until the esophagus is empty. Some food, particularly solid material, requires more than the single primary peristaltic wave for eventual clearance. This is accomplished by the secondary peristaltic waves. Thus, secondary peristalsis is the mechanism for clearing both ingested material and also material that is refluxed from the stomach. Experimentally, secondary peristalsis can be demonstrated by inflating a balloon in the mid-to-upper esophagus.

3. *Tertiary contractions.* This contraction pattern is identified primarily during barium x-ray studies of the esophagus.

It represents a nonperistaltic series of contractile waves that appear as localized segmented indentations in the barium column. It has no known physiologic function.

One of the interesting phenomena seen in the esophagus occurs during the process of rapid sequential swallowing (10 seconds or less between successive voluntary swallows). This process results in inhibition of peristalsis, so-called deglutitive inhibition. Peristalsis will be suspended during the continuation of a series of rapid swallows and a large "clearing wave" will occur at the completion of the swallows (Figure 9–5). This phenomenon occurs because of the inhibitory neural discharge that arises from the central swallowing center during swallowing and also because the esophageal musculature shows a refractoriness, demonstrated to persist for up to 10 seconds.[40]

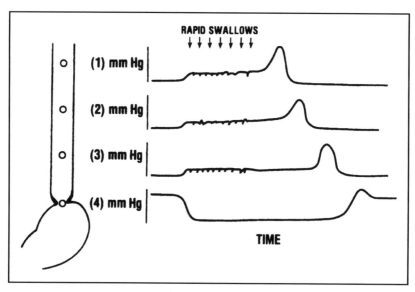

Figure 9–5. Demonstration of the phenomenon of deglutitive inhibition of the peristaltic sequence by rapid swallows separated by approximately 5-second intervals. The LES remains relaxed throughout the sequence as the esophageal body is inhibited from a peristaltic response until the termination of the swallows. At this point, the peristaltic clearing wave occurs.

Importance of the Sphincters

The esophagus is located in the thorax and has negative pressure relative to pressures in the pharynx proximally and the stomach distally. Therefore, the action of the sphincters must maintain constant closure to prevent abnormal movement of air or food into the esophagus. In the absence of a tonically contracted UES, air will flow freely into the esophagus during inspiration. In the pres-ence of a weak LES, gastric contents are not inhibited from refluxing into the distal esophagus, particularly in the recumbent position. Pressure relationships, in and around the esophagus and its sphincters, are shown in Figure 9–6.

Upper Esophageal Sphincter

The UES maintains a constant closure with its strongest forces directed in the anterior-

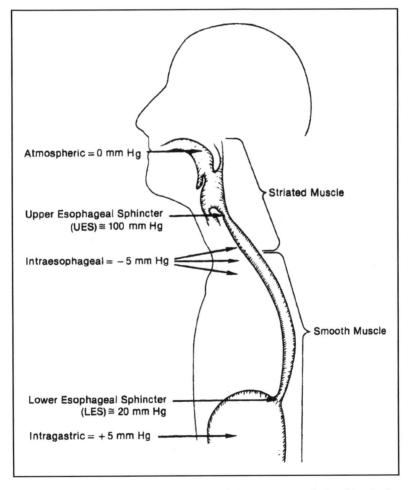

Figure 9–6. Schematic representation of the pressure relationships in the pharynx, esophagus, esophageal sphincter, and stomach. Note the negative intraesophageal pressure relative to both pharyngeal (atmospheric) pressure and intragastric pressure. Thus, the importance of the sphincters in preven-tion of abnormal movement of fluids and air is emphasized.

posterior orientation of the sling-shaped attachment of the cricopharyngeus to the cricoid cartilage. Normal pressures in the UES are approximately 100 mm Hg in the anterior-posterior direction and approximately 50 mm Hg laterally.[36]

Lower Esophageal Sphincter

The tonically contracted LES normally maintains a closing pressure 10 to 45 mm Hg greater than the intragastric pressure below. By convention, LES pressure is measured as a gradient in mm Hg higher than intragastric pressure, which is used as a zero reference (Figures 9–7 and 9–8). At the time of swallowing, the LES relaxes promptly in response to the initial neural discharge from the swallowing center in the brain and stays relaxed until the peristaltic wave reaches the end of the esophagus and produces sphincter closure. During relaxation, the pressure measured within the sphincter falls approximately to the level of gastric pressure; this is by definition "complete" relaxation. Although there has been much controversy over the years, it is now generally accepted that the LES does not have to be located within the diaphragmatic crus to maintain a constant closing pressure. Thus, the presence of a sliding hiatal hernia is not necessarily detrimental to the physiologic function of this sphincter.

The LES maintains 2 important physiologic functions; the first is its role in prevention of gastroesophageal reflux and the

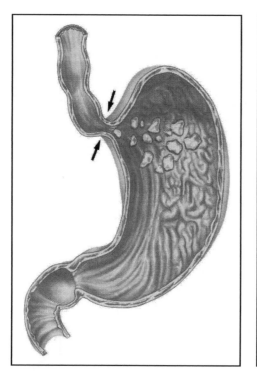

Figure 9–7. Normal lower esophageal sphincter (*arrows*) between the esophagus and the stomach. (Republished from *Quick Reference to Upper GI Motility* with the permission of Janssen Pharmaceutica.)

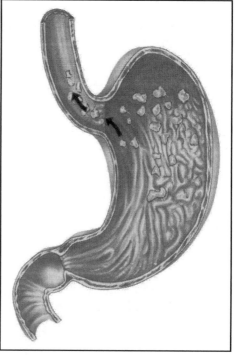

Figure 9–8. Incompetent lower esophageal sphincter. (Republished from *Quick Reference to Upper GI Motility* with the permission of Janssen Pharmaceutica.)

second is its ability to relax with swallowing to allow movement of ingested material into the stomach. The mechanism by which the circular smooth muscle of the LES maintains tonic closure has been a subject of considerable investigation over many years. At present, this is felt to be predominantly the result of intrinsic muscle activity, because investigations in animals have demonstrated that resting LES tone persists even after the destruction of all neural input by the neurotoxin tetrodotoxin.[41] In addition, truncal vagotomy does not affect resting LES pressure in humans. Calcium-channel-blocking agents, which exert their effect directly on the circular smooth muscle, will produce decreases in LES pressures in animals and humans.[42,43] There also appears to be some cholinergic tone present in many animal species and in humans, as an injection of atropine or of botulinum toxin (Botox, Allergan) has been shown to produce marked decreases in resting LES pressure.[44,45]

The mechanism of relaxation of the LES in response to a swallow has also been a subject of considerable investigation and controversy. The precise neurotransmitter responsible for this response is not definitely known. It is clear that it is not a classic cholinergic or adrenergic agent, because specific pharmacologic blockade of these mechanisms does not inhibit LES relaxation. This is a neural event. It can be reproduced in animals by stimulation of the vagus nerve, and relaxation is inhibited by tetrodotoxin.[46] Their relationships are summarized in Figure 9–9. Recent studies indicate that the neurotransmitter might be a combination of vasoactive intestinal polypeptide (VIP) and nitric oxide.[46,47]

The resting pressure of the LES is dynamic. Pressures measured over long periods of time indicate that LES pressure will vary considerably, even from minute

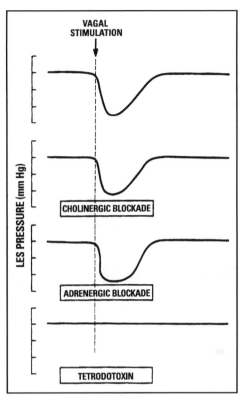

Figure 9–9. Summation of experiments in the opossum on the neural regulation of LES relaxation. Electrical stimulation of the vagus nerve produces relaxation, which is not inhibited by blocking either cholinergic or adrenergic pathways. However, the neural response is inhibited by the neurotoxin tetrodotoxin.

to minute. Much of this is due to the effect of a variety of factors that modulate pressure. These include foods ingested during meals and other events such as cigarette smoking and gastric distention. The normal LES will respond to transient increases in intra-abdominal pressure by raising its resting pressure to a greater degree than the pressure increases in the abdomen below. This normal protective mechanism guards against gastroesophageal reflux. In addition, many hormones and other peptide substances produced in the GI tract and in other areas of the body have been shown to affect LES pressure. These are summarized in Table 9–1. Many of these likely represent pharmacologic responses that have been shown to occur after intravenous injection or infusions of these substances in man or animals. Whether they represent truly physiologic actions has not been clarified in most cases. The strongest candidates for physiologic hormonal control of the LES are cholecystokinin, which helps explain the decrease in LES pressure seen after fat ingestion, and progesterone, which explains the decrease in LES pressure

that occurs during pregnancy. Finally, various neurotransmitters and pharmacologic agents have been shown to affect LES pressure. These are summarized in Table 9–2. The modulation of LES resting pressure is a complex mechanism that involves the interaction of the LES smooth muscle, neural control, and humoral factors.[48]

Controls of Esophageal Peristalsis

As noted above, esophageal peristalsis is controlled via afferent and efferent neural connections through the swallowing center in the medulla. This central mechanism regulates the involuntary sequence of muscular events that occurs during swallowing (Figures 9–10 and 9–11) and simultaneously inhibits the respiratory center in the medulla so that respiration is stopped during the pharyngeal stage of swallowing.

The direct innervation to the striated muscle of the pharynx and upper esophagus is carried via fibers from the brainstem (nucleus ambiguus) through the vagus nerve. The innervation of the smooth muscle of the distal esophagus and LES arises from the dorsal motor nucleus of the vagus

Table 9–1. Effects of Peptides and Hormones on LES Pressure

Increases LES	Decreases LES
Gastrin	Secretin
Motilin	Cholecystokinin
Substance P	Glucagon
Pancreatic polypeptide	Gastric inhibitory polypeptide (GIP)
Bombesin	Vasoactive intestinal polypeptide (VIP)
Key-enkephalin	
Pitressin	Peptide histidine isoleucine
Angiotensin	Progesterone

Table 9–2. Effects of Neurotransmitters and Pharmacologic Agents on LES Pressure

Increases LES	Decreases LES
Cholinergic (bethanechol)	Nitric oxide
(α-adrenergic)	Dopamine (β-adrenergic)
Metoclopramide	Nitrates
Cisapride	Atropine
	Calcium channel blockers
	Morphine
	Diazepam
	Theophylline

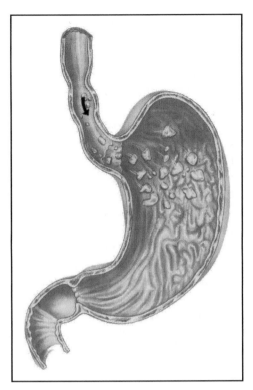

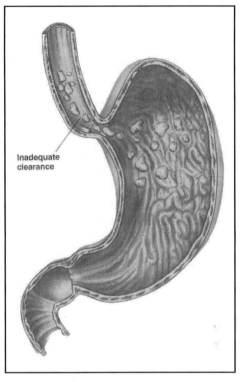

Figure 9–10. Normal esophageal peristalsis helping to move food from the esophagus to the stomach. (Republished from *Quick Reference to Upper GI Motility* with the permission of Janssen Pharmaceutica.)

Figure 9–11. Mobility disorder with dysfunctional esophageal peristalsis. (Republished from *Quick Reference to Upper GI Motility* with the permission of Janssen Pharmaceutica.)

and is carried through cholinergic visceral motor nerves to ganglia in the myenteric plexus (also known as the Auerbach plexus). Noncholinergic, nonadrenergic inhibitory nerves also course within the vagus.

The myenteric plexus in the esophageal portion of the enteric nervous system (the "brain in the gut") receives efferent impulses from the central nervous system (CNS) and sensory afferents from the esophagus. Thus, impulses travel in 2 directions through this modulating area, which interconnects and regulates signals that result in normal peristalsis in the smooth muscle of the esophagus. One manifestation of the afferent control is the regulation of peristaltic squeezing pressures, to some degree, by the size of the ingested bolus. In addition, dry swallows often fail to provide adequate stimulation for the action of the myenteric plexus as the primary regulatory mechanism of esophageal peristalsis in the smooth muscle portion, as shown by observations that bilateral cervical vagotomy in animals does not abolish peristalsis in this area.

Interesting results have been obtained from in vitro studies of esophageal smooth muscle preparations.[49] Using muscle from the opossum esophagus, it has been shown that the longitudinal smooth muscle demonstrates a sustained contraction during electrical field stimulation; this is called the "duration response." This response is neural and cholinergic, because it can be blocked with both atropine and tetrodo-toxin. The circular smooth muscle of the opossum esophagus shows a quite different response. With the onset of electrical stimulation, there is a brief, small contraction at the beginning of the stimulus, known as the "on-response." This response is quite variable and has no known physiologic role. The on-response is followed by a much larger contraction that occurs after the termination of the stimulus, known as the "off-response." This response is also neural in origin but is not cholinergic, because it is blocked only by tetrodotoxin and not atropine. Muscle strips taken from different segments of the smooth muscle portion of the esophageal body show progressively longer intervals for the off-response contraction following stimulation while moving distally in the esophagus. This phenomenon has been called the "latency gradient." These concepts are shown in Figure 9–12.

It has been proposed that these in vitro experiments from the opossum esophagus may help to explain some of the mechanisms of the development of normal peristalsis in the human smooth muscle esophagus. With the initial swallowing event, an inhibitory neural discharge is sent to the circular smooth muscle of the entire esophagus. The LES relaxes from its resting tonic state. The remainder of the esophageal smooth muscle is already relaxed and shows no measurable change. Rebound contraction occurs following the end of the brief stimulus (the off-response). The latency of the gradient for this off-response, progressing distally down the esophagus, produces the peristaltic contraction wave. Although this concept does not entirely explain all of the phenomena that have been observed in human peristaltic activity, these in vitro observations are consistent with many aspects of normal human physiology. One example is the deglutitive

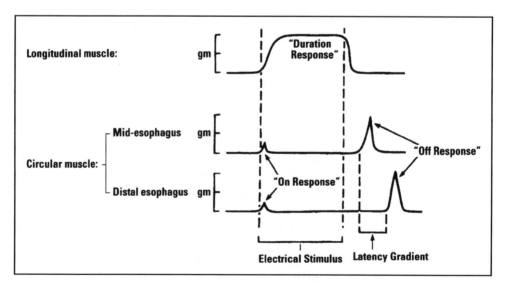

Figure 9–12. Summary of the in vitro esophageal smooth muscle responses shown in experiments in the opossum. During stimulation, the longitudinal esophageal muscle contracts throughout the stimulus; this is known as the duration response. The circular muscle shows a brief positive impulse at the beginning of stimulation; this is known as the on response. This is followed by a much greater contraction following termination of the stimulus; this is known as the off response. Delay in the latter response, progressing daily in the esophagus, produces the so-called latency gradient (gm = contraction force in grams).

inhibition referred to above. With repetitive swallowing at frequent intervals, the successive inhibitory neural impulses from the swallowing center prevent the contractions of the smooth muscle portion of the esophagus until the last swallow occurs. The off-response and the latency gradient then allow the single peristaltic clearing wave that usually follows.

Other Considerations

When gastric pressure becomes greater than LES pressure, reflux occurs. It must be remembered, however, that mechanical sphincter dysfunction is not the only cause of reflux symptoms. Gastric pathology (ie, hypersecretion and alkaline gastro-

esophageal reflux), motility disorders, and other conditions such as impaired gastric emptying (Figures 9–13 and 9–14) must be considered.

Clinical Presentation and Epidemiology of Gastroesophageal Reflux Disease: An Overview

Gastroesophageal reflux disease (GERD) is a spectrum of disease best defined as symptoms and/or signs of esophageal or adjacent organ injury secondary to the reflux of gastric contents into the esophagus or above into the oral cavity or airways. GERD is a common disorder often encountered in

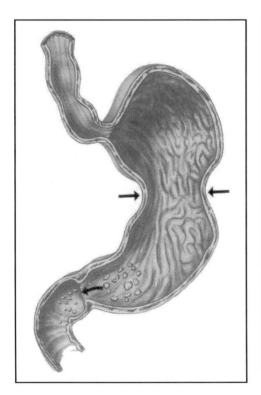

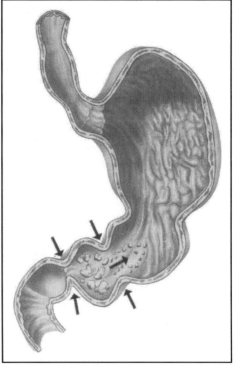

Figure 9–13. Normal gastric emptying. (Republished from *Quick Reference to Upper GI Motility* with the permission of Janssen Pharmaceutica.)

Figure 9–14. Abnormal, delayed gastric emptying. (Republished from *Quick Reference to Upper GI Motility* with the permission of Janssen Pharmaceutica.)

clinical practice and presents with a multitude of symptoms. Injury caused by GERD is defined based on symptoms or organ damage, which include esophagitis; inflammation of the larynx, pharynx, and oral cavity; or acute and/or chronic pulmonary injury. This section presents an overview of GERD, including typical, atypical, and extraesophageal presentations.

Typical Symptoms

The typical or classic symptoms of GERD are heartburn (pyrosis), defined as substernal burning occurring shortly after meals or on bending over that is relieved with antacids and regurgitation (the spontaneous return of gastric contents into the esophagus or mouth). When present together, heartburn and regurgitation establish the diagnosis with greater than 90% certainty. In clinical practice, heartburn is a daily complaint in 7% to 10% of the population in the United States and at least monthly in about 40% to 50%.[50–52] Over 20 million people in the United States have heartburn at least twice a week and use antacids or other over-the-counter (OTC) antireflux products on a regular basis. Regurgitation is experienced weekly by about 6% of the population according to one study.[51] In the same study, either heartburn or regurgitation was present weekly in 20% of patients surveyed and monthly in 59%. The prevalence of heartburn appears to decrease slightly with increasing age.

Classic heartburn is described typically by patients as a burning sensation under the breastbone with radiation upward toward the throat or mouth. Heartburn generally occurs 1 to 2 hours after meals, following heavy lifting or on bending over. Big meals, spicy foods, citrus products such as a grapefruit and orange juice, and meals high in fat are more likely to produce heartburn. Colas, coffee, teas, and even beer may have an acidic pH and cause symptoms when ingested. Heartburn may also be caused by medications (Table 9–3). Meals eaten late in the evening, close to bedtime, or taken with alcohol make patients more prone to nighttime symptoms. Patients report often that their symptoms are relieved with an over-the-counter antacid preparation, H2-receptor antagonists, or even by drinking water.

Although heartburn is often associated with the presence of regurgitation, the spontaneous experience of an acidic or bitter taste in the throat or mouth, these are not synonymous symptoms. Heartburn should not be confused with dyspepsia or a more vague epigastric distress usually localized in the upper abdominal or lower substernal area and associated with nausea, bloating, or fullness after meals. Although dyspepsia (epigastric discomfort) may be a symptom of GERD, it is neither as sensitive nor as specific a symptom as heartburn. The generic terminology of "acid indigestion" used to encompass all symptoms related to GERD is inappropriate; these symptoms must be distinguished for accurate diagnosis and therapy. Waterbrash, the sudden filling of the mouth with a clear, salty fluid, should not be confused with heartburn. This symptom reflects the increase in salivary secretion seen as a reflex response to reflux or regurgitation of gastric acid into an inflamed distal esophagus.

Heartburn is a highly specific symptom of GERD, although GERD is not the only cause. For example, a heartburnlike symptom, suspected to be due to esophageal stasis from outflow obstruction, is described often in patients with achalasia. It is felt that fermentation of undigested food in the esophagus coupled with inflammation may create a heartburnlike sensation in the absence of true GERD. Functional heart-

Table 9–3. Factors Causing Exacerbation of Heartburn

Decreases LES Pressure	*Mucosal Irritant*
Food and beverages	Food and beverages
Fats	Citrus products
Chocolate	Tomato products
Onions	Spicy foods
Carminatives	Coffee, colas, tea, beer
Coffee	
Alcohol	Medications
Smoking	Aspirin
	NSAIDs
Medications	Tetracycline
Progesterone	Quinidine
Theophylline	Potassium tablets
Anticholinergic agents	Iron salts
β-Adrenergic agonists	Alendronate
α-Adrenergic antagonists	Zidovudine
Diazepam	
Meperidine	
Nitrates	
Calcium channel blockers	

Abbreviations: LES = lower esophageal sphincter; NSAIDs = nonsteroidal anti-inflammatory drugs.

burn may also be a component of irritable bowel syndrome. However, if heartburn is the only presenting esophageal symptom, it is likely due to GERD.

Despite the sensitivity and specificity of these 2 symptoms for the diagnosis of GERD, neither the presence of heartburn and/or regurgitation nor the frequency of these symptoms is predictive of the degree of endoscopic damage to the distal esophagus. Many patients with daily heartburn will have no endoscopic abnormalities. The frequency of heartburn usually does not correlate with the severity of GERD, although nocturnal heartburn suggests the possibility of erosive esophagitis. Only 50% to 60% of patients presenting to a physician with heartburn will have erosive esophagitis

seen on a diagnostic endoscopic examination; the remainder will be diagnosed as having nonerosive GERD.[53] Severe disease, including Barrett's esophagus and peptic strictures, may present with infrequent or absent complaints of heartburn.

Most patients with esophagitis will not have progression of their disease beyond the severity of esophagitis seen at the time of initial endoscopy. In a series of 701 patients followed for up to 29 years, only 23% progressed to a more serious grade of esophagitis.[54] The patient with reflux symptoms and no evidence of esophagitis (nonerosive GERD) has even less likelihood of esophageal disease progression, with less than 15% of patients progressing to a higher grade over 6 months.[55]

Regurgitation is often associated with heartburn and GERD. When the 2 symptoms are present together, the diagnosis of GERD is highly likely. Regurgitation without heartburn should raise suspicion of Barrett's esophagus (in which acid sensitivity is reduced), achalasia, or other esophageal abnormality. Regurgitation may also be seen as a more prominent symptom in extraesophageal manifestations of GERD, particularly in patients with pulmonary symptoms of reflux, and it may be an important prognostic factor in predicting outcome of therapy.[55-57] Regurgitation is often confused by patients as vomiting. The effortless return of food or fluid in the absence of nausea is an important distinction between these 2 symptoms. Esophageal and extraesophageal symptoms associated with GERD are outlined in Table 9–4.

Extraesophageal (Atypical) Symptoms

A number of so-called atypical or extraesophageal symptoms have been associated with GERD, including unexplained substernal chest pain without evidence of coronary artery disease (noncardiac chest pain), asthma, bronchitis, chronic cough, recurrent pneumonia, hoarseness, chronic posterior laryngitis, globus sensation, otalgia, aphthous ulcers, hiccups, and erosion of dental enamel. In contrast to heartburn and regurgitation, the prevalence of these atypical or extraesophageal symptoms and their frequency in the general population have not been systematically studied until recently. In a large population-based survey of Caucasians in Olmstead County, Minnesota,[51] designed to assess the prevalence of GERD in the general population, unexplained chest pain was seen in 23% of the population yearly and in 4% at least weekly.

Table 9–4. Symptoms Associated With Gastroesophageal Reflux

Esophageal	Extraesophageal
Chest pain	Asthma or respiratory problems (ie, wheezing, shortness of breath)
Dysphagia	
Heartburn	Chronic cough
Odynophagia (rare)	Dental hypersensitivity (from loss of dental enamel)
Regurgitation	
Waterbrash	Hoarseness
	Laryngitis or laryngospasm
	Nausea
	Otalgia

The frequency of unexplained chest pain surprisingly decreased with age. Forty percent had symptoms for more than 5 years, and 5% reported severe symptoms. Asthma was reported in approximately 9%, bronchitis in approximately 20%, and chronic hoarseness in 15% of patients who had atypical GERD symptoms.

The association of these atypical symptoms with heartburn and regurgitation is controversial. In the Minnesota study,[51] patients with heartburn and regurgitation had 1 or more atypical symptoms about 80% of the time. Atypical symptoms were more common in patients with frequent GERD symptoms compared to patients with no GERD symptoms. Heartburn or regurgitation was reported in more than 80% of the patients with unexplained chest pain and in 60% with globus sensation. The only exception was asthma. Approximately 60% of patients with asthma, bronchitis, hoarseness, and pneumonia had heartburn or regurgitation. The presence of heartburn is not predictive of otolaryngologic symptoms. However, in a case control study by the Veterans Administration, patients with a discharge diagnosis of erosive esophagitis had twice the prevalence of an associated otolaryngologic symptom as compared with control patients without esophagitis.[58] Observations in patients presenting with atypical GERD show that frequent heartburn and regurgitation are uncommon complaints; however, the absence of these typical symptoms should not preclude making a diagnosis. Prospective studies using endoscopy and ambulatory pH monitoring find GERD in as many as 75% of patients with chronic hoarseness,[32] between 70% and 80% of asthmatics,[59,60] and in 20% of patients with chronic cough.[61]

Reflux is a well-recognized cause of atypical chest pain and may be responsible for many (most) of the symptoms in the 75 000 to 150 000 patients who undergo normal coronary angiography in the United States annually.[62]

Approximately 45% of these patients with unexplained chest pain can be shown to have GERD.[63] Esophagitis in this population is less common, being seen in less than 10%.[64] Endoscopically, esophagitis is seen in 30% to 40% of patients with asthma[65,66] and about 20% of patients with reflux laryngitis. Distinguishing between cardiac and noncardiac chest pain due to GERD is difficult, and they may coexist in the same patient. All of the features of cardiac angina—tight, gripping, vicelike pain radiating to the neck, shoulder, or left arm and associated with exertion—may be seen with GERD also. Long episodes of pain (greater than 1 hour), pain relieved by eating, or pain awakening from sleep are more likely esophageal symptomatology. Antacids or H2-blockers may relieve chest pain, later proven to be associated with coronary artery disease. It is therefore crucial to rule out cardiac disease before presuming GERD is the cause of chest pain. Omeprazole is an effective treatment for reflux-related, noncardiac chest pain[67]; in patients with infrequent (less than 3 times per week), noncardiac chest pain, high-dose proton pump inhibitor (PPI) therapy, such as omeprazole, may be a sensitive, specific, cost-effective strategy for diagnosing GERD.[68] However, it must be remembered that not all patients respond to PPI medications. Therefore, persistent chest pain during PPI therapy does not definitively rule out GERD as the etiology of the chest pain as the evaluation of patients with unexplained chest pain remains complex.[69] For example, the rare syndrome X is a condition involving anginal chest pain with objective signs of ischemia on exercise stress testing or myocardial scintigraphy but with normal coronary arteries on angiogram. Esophageal hypersensitivity (as opposed to gross functional abnormality) may be an associated finding in these patients, and acid suppression may improve the condition in many patients.[70] The complex relationship between reflux and chest pain remains incompletely understood. Ambulatory pH monitoring, particularly during continued PPI therapy, remains the gold standard for diagnosis of GERD in this population.

Seventy percent to 80% of patients with asthma will have associated GERD. Whether there is a cause-and-effect relationship or the coincidental presence of 2 diseases is not clear. A careful history will reveal heartburn or regurgitation in only 50%. Onset of asthma late in life, the absence of a seasonal or allergic component, and onset after a big meal, alcohol consumption, or exercise suggest GERD-related asthma. Empiric treatment with acid reflux suppression followed by pH testing in nonresponders was suggested in 1 study as the most cost-effective means of determining whether GERD is aggravating a patient's asthma.[71] This approach seems reasonable, because it has been demonstrated that PPI therapy in asthmatics with gastroesophageal reflux improves peak expiratory flow rate and quality of life.[72]

Reflux is the third most common cause of chronic cough, after postnasal drip and bronchitis, and in many cases, symptoms of postnasal drip may actually be associated with reflux. So the prevalence of reflux as an etiologic factor in chronic cough may be even higher than recognized previously. In the patient with cough, a normal chest x-ray, and no sinonasal postnasal drip, GERD should be considered as the most likely diagnosis.

Hoarseness is the most common otolaryngologic symptom of GERD. Most studies suggest that heartburn is present in only about 50% or less of otolaryngologic patients with extraesophageal manifestations (such as hoarseness) of GERD. However, some authors feel that a careful history may reveal heartburn to be present, at least occasionally, in as many as 75%.[73] Other associated symptoms of reflux laryngitis include halitosis, throat clearing, dry cough, coated tongue, globus sensation, tickle in the throat, chronic sore throat, postnasal drip, and others discussed later in this chapter. Difficulty in warming up the voice in the professional singer, voice fatigue, and intermittent laryngitis are associated symptoms. Erosion of the dental enamel may be due to GERD; however, its frequency is not known.

Complications of GERD

GERD may present with severe complications, including peptic stricture, ulceration, iron deficiency anemia, or, more important, Barrett's esophagus. Barrett's esophagus is a premalignant condition that involves a change from normal squamous epithelial lining to a metaplastic intestinal-type epithelium with typical special staining char-

acteristics. Estimates are that 2% to 10% of patients with GERD will have strictures,[74] and 10% to 15% will have Barrett's esophagus.[53,75] Dysphagia, odynophagia (painful swallowing), and upper gastrointestinal (GI) bleeding may occur with these complications of GERD. Slowly progressive dysphagia, particularly for solids, suggests peptic strictures. Liquid and solid dysphagia suggests a GERD-related motility disorder secondary to erosive esophagitis, Barrett's esophagus, or scleroderma. GERD-related motility disorders are seen with increased frequency in patients with otolaryngologic manifestations of GERD,[76] even though dysphagia is not usually a presenting symptom. Motility abnormalities pose important complications for the patient considering surgery (see Surgical Therapy for Gastroesophageal Reflux Disease). Odynophagia is uncommon in patients with reflux. Its presence suggests ulceration or inflammation, and it is seen most frequently in infectious or pill-induced esophagitis. Occasionally, esophagitis may present with occult, upper gastrointestinal bleeding or iron-deficiency anemia.[74] The frequency of these complications in patients with reflux laryngitis is not known.

Anatomy and Pathophysiology of LPR

Findings highlight the important fact that gastric acid can reflux through the esophagus to the larynx without causing esophageal injury in transit. It has been assumed that this is because distal esophageal mucosa has specialization and defense mechanisms that help it tolerate acid exposure. Esophageal protective mechanisms include peristalsis, which clears acid from the esophagus; a mucosal structure that may be specialized to tolerate intermittent acid contact; the acid-neutralizing capacity of saliva that passes through the esophagus; and bicarbonate production in the esophagus, which has been recognized since the 1980s.[77-79] Interestingly, however, if some patients stop reflux treatment after a few months, classic dyspepsia and pyrosis seem to be present commonly when symptoms recur, although this clinically observed phenomenon has not been studied formally. It should be noted that the larynx and pharynx do not have protective mechanisms, such as those found in the esophagus, to protect against mucosal injury. So, exposure to acid and pepsin that might be of no consequence in the distal esophagus may cause substantial symptoms and signs in the larynx and/or pharynx of some patients. Interestingly, preliminary data by Axford et al[80] suggest that laryngeal mucosa has different cellular defenses from those of esophageal mucosa. They also suggested that there may be specific differences in MUC gene expression and carbonic anhydrase that suggest a pattern of abnormality in patients with LPR.

In addition to prolonged vocal warm-up time, professional singers and actors may complain of vocal practice interference, manifested by frequent throat clearing and excessive phlegm, especially during the first 10 to 20 minutes of vocal exercises or singing. Hyperfunctional technique during speaking and especially singing is also associated with reflux laryngitis. This is probably due to the vocalist's unconscious tendency to guard against aspiration. Voice professionals can be helped somewhat in overcoming this secondary muscular tension dysphonia (MTD) through voice therapy with speech-language pathologists, singing voice specialists, and acting-voice specialists, but it is difficult to overcome completely until excellent reflux control has been achieved.

In addition to the paucity of typical GERD symptoms in patients with LPR, the tendency for underdiagnosis of LPR has been increased by 3 additional factors. First, the importance of various aspects of the physical examination is underappreciated. Posterior laryngitis and interarytenoid pachydermia are ignored frequently.[81] It is even more common to fail to recognize the causal relationship between reflux and edema with little or no erythema, especially if the edema is diffuse rather than most prominent on the arytenoids. Second, therapeutic medication trials may fail because patients are undermedicated (eg, a PPI only once daily) and assessed before signs of laryngopharyngeal reflux have had time to resolve (which may require a few months or more). Third, routine tests for gastroesophageal reflux disease can be falsely negative. This problem involves not only barium esophagrams, the Bernstein acid-hyperperfusion test, and radionucleotide scanning but also esophagoscopy and 24-hour pH monitor studies (depending on the norms used). Consequently, laryngologists must maintain a high index of suspicion in the presence of symptoms consistent with LPR, evaluate such patients aggressively, and interpret test results knowledgeably and with awareness of their sensitivities, specificities, limitations, and controversies.

Reflux Laryngitis and Other Otolaryngologic Manifestations of Laryngopharyngeal Reflux

Although the majority of otolaryngologists have recently acknowledged the importance of reflux in causing otolaryngologic disease, many authors have recognized the association for more than 2 decades.[1,3,4,11,12,14,16,32,82-102]

Otolaryngologists are becoming increasingly diligent about looking for erythema and edema of the mucosa overlying the arytenoid cartilages, suspecting laryngopharyngeal reflux (LPR) as the underlying problem, and treating it as the primary approach to therapy for various reflux-related conditions. However, additional information has shown that the term *laryngopharyngeal reflux* describes a complex spectrum of abnormalities, and it is important for physicians to understand the latest concepts in basic science and clinical care of LPR. Symptoms and signs related to reflux have been identified in 4% to 10% of all patients seen by otolaryngologists,[18,28,32,103] and it is probable that these estimates are low. Among patients with laryngeal and voice disorders, laryngopharyngeal reflux appears to be strongly associated with, or a significant etiologic cofactor in, about 50% of these patients. Many of the current concepts regarding reflux laryngitis and related controversies have been reviewed recently in the otolaryngologic and gastroenterologic literature.[104–106]

Other Clinical Practice Considerations

Treatment considerations in reflux patients are discussed in greater detail later in this chapter Research into appropriate treatment regimens is ongoing, and extensive additional investigation on the consequences of reflux on the larynx and all of the other mucosal surfaces above the cricopharyngeus muscle is needed.

LPR has been found in association with otitis media with effusion not only in the pediatric population but also in adults.[107] Habesoglu et al[108] studied the effects of LPR on tympanoplasty failure. They reported the results of 147 patients who underwent tympanoplasty who had laryngoscopic evidence of LPR and positive reflux finding scores. The authors suggested that these findings should be considered as a factor in the failure of tympanoplasty, and they recommended that reflux evaluation and treatment should be considered in the treatment of patients with chronic otitis media and ear disease, including eustachian tube dysfunction.[108,109] Other studies have reported that LPR and obesity are risk factors associated with lingual hypertrophy and obstructive sleep apnea.[110,111] A study by Corvo et al[112] reported significant LPR in association with patients known to have Sjögren's syndrome, confirmed by salivary analysis.

Several studies have reported the presence of pepsin and amylase in oral and tracheal secretions.[113,114] Another report[115] suggested alterations in mucin gene expression in laryngeal mucosa and/or laryngeal mucosal metaplasia due to MUC3, 4, and 5. MucSAC expression being downregulated in LPR may predispose the larynx to mucosal damage from gastric refluxate. Eckley et al[116] studied salivary epidermal growth factor in adult patients with LPR pre- and posttreatment with PPIs. Saliva samples were obtained on 20 patients with LPR before and after a 16-week course of PPI therapy and compared to a control group of 12 healthy patients. Patients with LPR had lower salivary epidermal growth factor concentrations pre- and posttreatment compared with the healthy control group. The authors suggest that this finding indicates a defective mechanism of mucosal protection. Several recent studies have shown that scintigraphic studies are useful as a screening tool for predicting aspiration in patients with LPR and GERD and in whom fundoplication surgery is being considered.[117,118] Endoscopy, olfactory function, and analysis of color and texture of laryngoscopic images also have been reported as part of the armamentarium in evaluating the presence of and/or predisposition to LPR.[119,120]

In treating LPR patients, the clinician is faced with management decisions centered on the entire aerodigestive tract. For example, the presence of pepsin in nasal lavage fluid has been documented in patients undergoing endoscopic sinus surgery.[121] LPR has been confirmed in these patients, suggesting a relationship between chronic rhinosinusitis and LPR. Nasal pepsin may prove to be an avenue of LPR screening.[121] Evidence also links LPR and chronic otitis media,[122] as discussed above, and surgical outcomes in laryngeal trauma surgery have proven better in patients with preoperative and postoperative PPI treatment.[123] Therefore, many different patient groups may benefit from reflux evaluation and treatment.

Pepsin has been found in tracheoesophageal puncture sites, as reported by Bock et al.[124] They performed tissue biopsy and collected secretions in 17 patients, 12 of whom had a history of GERD/LPR, and pepsin was detected in the majority of their patients. LPR also may play a role in the pathogenesis of dental disease and sleep disorders. Several studies have shown a relationship between LPR and dental erosion.[125,126] In an animal (rat) model study, Higo et al[127] identified microscopic dental erosion and loss of surface enamel secondary to regurgitation of acid, liquid, and gas, as well as destruction of teeth and supporting structures when they were exposed to gastric and duodenal contents. Ranjitkar et al[128] reported that casein phosphopeptide-amorphous calcium phosphate can protect teeth from erosion caused by acid and bile products.

Becker et al[129] studied the role of LPR in patients with complaints of intraoral burning sensations. They placed an oropharyngeal pH monitoring probe at the level of the uvula and found no causal relationship between LPR and intraoral burning. They suggested that PPI therapy is not indicated in this patient population.

Researchers and clinicians have examined a myriad of symptoms in patients with LPR and the relationships between LPR and voice disorders, benign and malignant lesions in the larynx, chronic cough, pulmonary disease, asthma and allergy, and obstructive sleep apnea in both adults and children. Chung et al[130] examined the relationship between LPR and benign vocal fold lesions. They reported LPR in 65% of their control group, 66% of the vocal nodules group, 75% of the vocal fold polyp group, and 95% of the patients with Reinke's edema. Saleh[131] suggested links among reflux, postnasal drip, and chronic cough. Randhawa et al[132] pointed out that it is sometimes difficult to determine the cause of dysphonia, noting that the laryngeal findings on nasopharyngolaryngoscopy may be similar in patients with LPR and in those with allergy. In their small sample population, they diagnosed allergy in 10 patients and LPR in only 3 patients, which they felt raised the question of LPR being overdiagnosed.

More recent studies suggest a relationship between LPR and obstructive sleep apnea. Eskiismir and Kezirian[133] suggested that the increased respiratory efforts used by patients with obstructive sleep apnea generate increased intrathoracic pressure, which contributes to increased reflux. Suzuki et al[134] suggested that relaxation of the LES might be the mechanism of reflux in patients with mild to moderate obstructive sleep apnea. They also found reflux-induced spontaneous arousals. Karkos and colleagues[135] reported that during sleep, UES pressures decrease significantly. However, they noted a lack of controlled trials and/or meta-analyses that address the correlation between reflux, snoring, and/or apnea. In 2010, Wang et al[136] examined the concentration of pepsin detected in oropharyngeal secretions in patients with LPR and obstructive sleep apnea. In the LPR population, they found higher levels of pepsin in sputum that correlated with a higher reflux symptom index and higher reflux finding score. In obstructive sleep apnea patients, they reported no relationship between pepsin levels and Reflux Symptom Index.

Eryuksel et al[137] examined the relationship between LPR and chronic obstructive pulmonary disease. Before and following 2 months of PPI treatment, patients underwent laryngeal examinations and pulmonary function tests and were asked to complete questionnaires for LPR and chronic obstructive pulmonary disease. The authors reported significant improvement in chronic obstructive pulmonary disease symptom index and LPR symptoms and findings on laryngeal examination. de la Hoz and colleagues[138] studied reflux and pulmonary disease in 9-11 World Trade Center first responders. Their findings suggest that patients with reflux demonstrated reduced forced vital capacity, suggestive of air trapping and lower airway disease.

Physical Examination

Physical examination of patients with throat and voice complaints must be comprehensive. A thorough head and neck examination is always included, with attention to the ears and hearing, nasal patency, signs of allergy, the oral cavity, temporomandibular joints, the larynx, and the neck. In some patients with LPR severe enough to involve the oral cavity, there is also loss of dental enamel. Hence, transparency of the lower portion of the central incisors may be seen

occasionally in reflux patients, although it may be more common in patients with bulimia and those who habitually eat lemons. At least a limited general physical examination is included to look for signs of systemic disease that may present as throat or voice complaints. More comprehensive, specialized physical examinations by medical consultants should be sought when indicated.

When the patient has complaints of vocal difficulties, laryngeal examination is mandatory. It should be performed initially using a mirror or flexible fiberoptic laryngoscope, but comprehensive laryngeal examination requires strobovideolaryngoscopy for slow-motion evaluation of the vibratory margin of the vocal folds. Formal assessment of the speaking and singing voice also should be performed, when appropriate. Objective voice analysis quantifies voice quality, pulmonary function, valvular efficiency of the vocal folds, and harmonic spectral characteristics. Neuromuscular function can be measured by laryngeal electromyography (EMG). These aspects of the physical examination and tests of voice function are discussed elsewhere in the book and will not be reviewed in this chapter.

Most commonly, laryngoscopy in patients with LPR reveals erythema and edema. Classically, reflux laryngitis involves erythema of the arytenoid cartilages and frequently interarytenoid pachydermia (a knobbled or cobblestone appearance), as well as other signs[25,96,138–145] (Figures 9–15 and 9–16). However, many additional findings may be observed, including edema of the false and true vocal folds; partial effacement or obliteration of the laryngeal ventricle; pseudosulcus (a longitudinal groove extending below the vibratory margin throughout the length of the vocal fold, including the cartilaginous portion); Reinke's edema; granulomas or ulcers (most commonly in the region

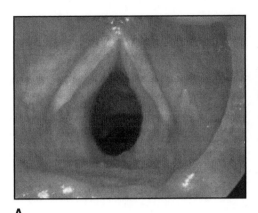
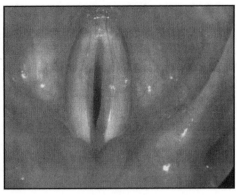

A   **B**

Figure 9–15. Open (**A**) and closed (**B**) views of the vocal folds show the bilateral inferior glottic ridges that parallel the vocal folds and prevent closure of the musculomembranous vocal folds. There is posterior laryngeal cobblestoning and arytenoid erythema and edema.

of the vocal process); nodules and other masses; an interarytenoid bar; laryngeal stenosis; and other abnormalities. Koufman et al[146] reported that edema was seen even more common than erythema, having been diagnosed in 89% of 46 patients, compared with 87% who had erythema, 19% with granuloma or granulation tissue, and 2% with ulceration.

Belafsky et al[147] developed a Reflux Finding Score (RFS) that rates signs and appears to correlate with the presence of LPR. They advocate use of this instrument in combination with the Reflux Symptom Index (RSI).[148] The reflux finding score depends on observations of subglottic edema, ventricular obliteration, erythema/hyperemia, vocal fold edema, diffuse laryngeal edema, posterior laryngeal hypertrophy, granuloma/granulation tissue, and still, thick endolaryngeal mucus. Although additional research from other centers is needed to confirm the validity and reliability of the RFS (which remains somewhat controversial), the authors found excellent inter- and intraobserver reproducibility (although all observers were practicing at the same medical center); they found the RFS to be

an accurate instrument for documenting treatment efficacy in patients with LPR, and it is used widely (including by the authors of this chapter).

In patients with severe LPR, the finding of a hyperactive gag reflex is also common; of interest, they also may have decreased laryngeal sensation. One of us (RTS) has performed functional endoscopic evaluation of sensory threshold testing on patients with LPR and found that responses were diminished prior to treatment and were improved following treatment. These findings are consistent with preliminary observations by Jonathan Aviv, MD (personal communication, 2000).

It should be noted that controversy exists regarding the significance of laryngeal findings. Credible studies of the sensitivity and specificity of laryngoscopy for diagnosis of LPR are needed, although a few initial reports exist in the literature. Carr et al[149] studied 155 children retrospectively. In a chart review of direct laryngoscopy and bronchoscopy findings, they reported a positive predictive value of 100% for the combination of posterior chronic edema with any vocal fold or ventricular abnormality.

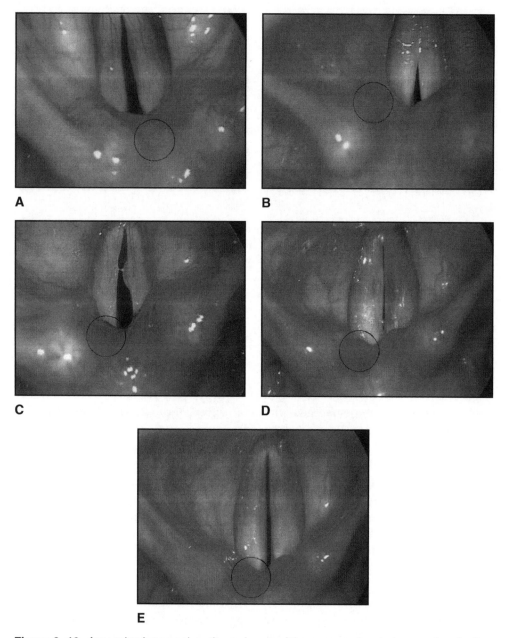

Figure 9–16. Assessing laryngeal erythema is one of the many and varied ways of evaluating laryngopharyngeal reflux (LPR). In the absence of the other irritants, acidic reflux is a major contributor to laryngeal erythema. In our center, the posterior larynx—including the medial face of the arytenoid complex, the interarytenoid area, and the posterior cricoid surface—is evaluated carefully. Erythema beyond the posterior larynx is also indicative of LPS, but our grading focuses on the posterior larynx. There are 5 categories of erythema: **A.** Normal, **B.** Mild, **C.** Moderate, **D.** Moderate-Severe, and **E.** Severe.

McMurray et al[150] evaluated 39 children prospectively with laryngoscopy, bronchoscopy, esophagoscopy, and pH monitoring prior to airway reconstruction. Full-thickness laryngeal mucosal biopsy specimens were obtained from the posterior cricoid area and the interarytenoid area, and esophageal biopsy specimens were obtained. These investigators were unable to demonstrate a correlation among pH probe data, laryngoscopic findings, and histologic findings. Hicks et al[151] studied 105 healthy, asymptomatic volunteers. On laryngoscopy, more than 80% had at least 1 "abnormal" finding, including (in order of frequency from most frequent to least) interarytenoid bar, medial arytenoid granularity, and true vocal fold erythema. This study did not perform 24-hour pH monitoring or any other tests to rule out the presence of "silent" reflux as a cause of the laryngoscopic abnormalities.

Despite many articles exploring signs and symptoms of reflux, including those cited above and other recent literature,[151–166] evidence confirming the diagnostic significance of various complaints and findings is scarce and contradictory. This is due to various problems, including the lack of a standard definition of "normal" in populations being studied. Continued interdisciplinary discourse and multicenter studies should be encouraged to answer important questions regarding the sensitivity and specificity of the many findings associated commonly with laryngopharyngeal reflux, as well as the impact of laryngopharyngeal reflux on quality of life and general health.[167]

Pathophysiology

Laryngeal abnormalities may be caused by direct injury or by a secondary mechanism. Direct injury is due to contact of acid and pepsin with laryngeal mucosa, resulting in mucosal damage.[3,95,96,168–171] Alternatively, irritation of the distal esophagus by acid may cause a reflex mediated by the vagus nerve, resulting in chronic cough and/or throat clearing, which may produce traumatic injury to the laryngeal mucosa.[83,96,172–176]

Researchers are attempting to delineate pathophysiology. To show LPR as an extra extraesophageal manifestation of GERD, Groome et al[177] hypothesized that GERD patients would have some LPR symptoms if the pathophysiology were truly common. Through a questionnaire administered to 1383 GERD patients, they determined that the prevalence of LPR increases with the severity of GERD.[177] Although based on nonstandard questionnaires, the finding suggests a relationship. A similar study sought to exclude other causes of laryngitis and found LPR in 24% of patients with reflux esophagitis. The presence of LPR was predicted best by age, hoarseness, and hiatal hernia.[178] A third study, strengthened by confirmed diagnoses of GERD and LPR with esophagogastroduodenoscopy (EGD) and 24-hour pH monitoring, respectively, similarly showed that when both GERD and non-GERD patients were treated with PPIs, laryngitis symptoms and signs improved in the GERD group only.[179] These studies seem to point toward a common pathophysiology, suggesting that laryngeal symptoms are indeed caused by acid exposure.

Bile reflux also may cause laryngeal irritation.[180,181] In addition, recent findings raise many new questions about the pathophysiology of LPR. For example, Eckley et al[182,183] report that decreased salivary epidermal growth factor may be associated with LPR and warrants further study; Altman's discovery of a proton pump in laryngeal serous cells and ducts of submucosal glands is particularly intriguing.[184] It has been established that pepsin in the larynx results in depletion of carbonic anhydrase isoenzyme III (CAI III) and squamous epithelial stress protein (Sep70), 2 laryngeal protective proteins.[185,186] Pepsin is taken up by laryngeal cells and can be reactivated by a drop in pH, as seen in LPR. Pepsin is found in the esophageal mucosa of those with LPR.[187] Interestingly, pepsin irreversibly affects CAI III at pH below 4 only in laryngeal, not esophageal, epithelium.[188] These laryngeal receptors for pepsin may be another future target for intervention. They also might explain the presence of symptoms and signs of LPR with weakly acidic reflux, as pepsin may be active to some degree at any pH between 3 and 6.5,[189] although a longer exposure time may be necessary at pH 5 or above to produce damage.[190] Possible pepsin activity at pH much above 5 remains controversial. Mucin gene (muc) expression also is downregulated in the presence of pepsin.[190,191]

Animal studies have shown that acid combined with pepsin (acid-activated enzyme) compromises the integrity of the vocal fold epithelium. In 2010, Habesoglu et al[192] reported that rats exposed to an acidic pH in the presence of pepsin developed edema of the lamina propria, submucous gland hyperplasia, and muscular atrophy. Erickson and Sivansakar[193] reported that the epithelial barrier resistance of the vocal fold is compromised when exposed to acid and pepsin. They described transepithelial resistance as a marker of epithelial barrier resistance that measures the ability to restrict movement of solute and solvents. The authors pointed out that less than 3 episodes of reflux per week could injure vocal fold mucosa, in contrast to 0 to 50 reflux events daily that are considered normal exposure in the distal esophagus.

In 2009, Johnston et al[194] reported that pepsin invades the laryngeal epithelial cells by receptor-mediated endocytosis and that pepsin activity is maximal at a pH of 2. Bulmer et al[195] in 2010 showed that the effects of acid and pepsin exposure on porcine laryngeal mucosa were similar to the effects observed in the human larynx in patients diagnosed with LPR. Samuels and Johnston[196] reported that the presence of pepsin in the airway indicates reflux. However, they reported that there are only 2 methods used to identify pepsin in the airways: immunologic and enzymatic, both of which have advantages and disadvantages. Richter[197] stated that gastric acid combined with pepsin and bile salts is known to be causally related to the development of chronic esophagitis and Barrett's esophagus. In contrast, the author reported that weak or nonacid refluxate has not been shown to cause damage to the esophageal or extraesophageal structures, including the larynx and the lungs.

Histopathologic inflammation and its association with the pathogenesis of esophageal and extraesophageal disease has been the subject of ongoing research. Some studies that have focused on histology have produced interesting findings. One found significantly increased CD8+ lymphocytes in the epithelium of patients with LPR, with proportionally more in the luminal epithelial layer. Additionally, nonclassical major histocompatibility complex (MHC) molecule expression was found to be involved in the response to refluxate, suggesting that relying upon classical markers may lead to erroneous conclusions about the response of laryngeal epithelium to reflux.[198] Wada et al[199] evaluated histopathologic inflammation of the upper esophagus in comparison with the lower esophagus. When compared with their control group, they found inflammation of the upper esophagus to be significantly greater in patients with abnormal laryngopharyngeal symptoms and significantly greater lower esophageal inflammatory histopathology in patients with classic reflux symptoms (ie, GERD).

Park et al[200] used transmission electron microscopy to examine cellular damage of the esophageal epithelium by gastric refluxate. They measured the intracellular space and quantified its dilatation. They compared 2 groups: patients who had LPR without GERD and patients who had LPR with GERD. They reported that the intracellular space of the esophageal epithelium was significantly more dilated in the LPR-with-GERD group. Amin and colleagues[201] reported that dilatation of intracellular spaces of esophageal epithelium is considered a specific marker in GERD. They studied a group of patients with LPR and sore throat in whom they found dilatation of intracellular spaces in oropharyngeal biopsy specimens. They also found dilatation of the intracellular spaces in the laryngeal mucosa in animal models exposed to pepsin.

There are important pathophysiologic differences between LPR patients and GERD patients. For example, combined upright and recumbent or nighttime reflux is typical for GI patients with GERD. Upright reflux and regurgitation also are the least common pattern in this population. However, patients with LPR are more likely to experience upright reflux commonly throughout the day,[16,28,32,202] often even in the absence of supine reflux.

We have observed some patients with LPR who experience reflux exclusively (and constantly) when they sing. Motility abnormalities have been demonstrated with higher frequency in patients with LPR, resulting in delayed acid clearance in 1 study.[203] In contrast, Postma et al[204] demonstrated that patients with GERD have significantly longer esophageal acid clearance times than those measured in patients with LPR. However, it is not unusual for LPR patients to have abnormal upper esophageal sphincter (UES)

function. In 1978, Gerhardt et al[205] showed that experimental instillation of acid in the distal esophagus in patients with esophagitis and in normal controls produces an increase in UES tone. This phenomenon does not occur normally in many patients with LPR,[103] although an increase in resting UES pressure has been demonstrated in patients with reflux laryngitis.[205] In 2010, based on their research, Szczesniak and colleagues[206] suggested upregulation of the esophago-UES relaxation as a possible mechanism in the pathophysiology of reflux laryngitis. They found that the UES relaxation reflex induced by rapid air insufflation of the esophagus is upregulated in patients with posterior laryngitis compared with healthy controls. They also found that this group of patients had a higher pharyngo-UES contractile reflex threshold, which is considered a mechanism of airway protection.

Vardouniotis et al[207] reported that a hypotensive lower esophageal sphincter (LES) is a significant pathophysiologic component of LPR, noting that complex molecular mechanisms involved in the function of the LES and genetic factors are involved in tissue protection from reflux. They reported that compared with the esophageal lining, laryngeal and pharyngeal mucosa is more susceptible to tissue damage from refluxate because the larynx is not protected by peristalsis or buffered by salivary bicarbonate. They reported that transforming growth factor–beta 1, which inhibits inflammatory response, has shown gene overexpression in postcricoid fibroblasts and that fibroblast growth factor 2 has shown decreased expression. Cheng et al[208] suggested that the microphage activation caused by gastric acid exposure should be considered also in the pathogenesis of GERD and aspiration-induced lung disease.

Chong and Jalihal[209] reported a greater percentage of LPR symptoms in patients with heterotrophic gastric mucosal patch (HGMP) of the distal esophagus. HGMP is ectopic gastric mucosa typically observed distal to the UES and thought to be congenital. Due to the fact that HGMP can produce acid, the authors suggested that this may be the etiology of LPR in some patients. In fact, in their study, patients with HGMP experienced LPR symptoms to a greater degree (73.1%) compared with their non-HGMP patients (25.9%).

Salminen and Ovaska[210] and Basseri et al[211] have reported that the endoscopic prevalence of HGMP is low, ranging from 0.1% to 10% in reported patients 16 to 75 years old. Typical symptoms in patients with HGMP include dysphagia, globus pharyngeus, cough, hoarseness, and shortness of breath. They reported that the HGMP is a source of acid production, and this has been supported by pH monitor studies showing gastric acid in this area. Parietal cells with oxyntic mucosa are the most common histologic type reported.

Laryngopharyngeal reflux can affect anyone, but it appears to be particularly common and symptomatic in professional voice users, especially singers. This is true for several reasons. First, the technique of singing involves "support" by the forceful compression of the abdominal muscles designed to push the abdominal contents superiorly and pull the sternum down. This action compresses the air in the thorax, thereby generating force for the stream of expired air, but it also compresses the stomach and works against the LES. Singing is an athletic endeavor, and the mechanism responsible for reflux in singers is similar to that associated with reflux following other athletic activities, lifting, and other conditions that alter abdominal pressure, such as pregnancy (which is also influenced by hormonal factors). It has been established clearly by Clark et al[212] that reflux is induced by exercise even in asymptomatic, young volunteers (mean age, 28 years). They demonstrated that running induced reflux more often than did exercise with less bodily agitation, such as bicycling, but both forms of aerobic exercise caused reflux, as did weightlifting in some patients. Postprandial exercise-induced reflux has a similar pattern, but with a greater amount of refluxate. It may be that the effect of exercise on reflux is even more pronounced in patients with GERD or LPR than it is in research subjects with no history of reflux symptoms, although this question has not been studied.

Second, many singers do not eat before performing because a full stomach interferes with abdominal support and promotes reflux. Performances usually take place at night. Consequently, the singer returns home hungry and eats a large meal before going to bed.

Third, performance careers are particularly stressful. Psychological stress has been associated with esophageal motility disorders (which may be associated with reflux) and with other gastroenterologic conditions, such as irritable bowel syndrome.[213] Psychological stress alone acts to increase the amplitude of esophageal contractions.[214] Stress also may affect the production of gastric acid. If psychological stress increases LPR, it may create a vicious cycle. Pharyngeal stimulation may cause transient LES relaxation directly, or it may lower the threshold for triggering gastric distention.[215]

Fourth, many singers pay little attention to good nutrition, frequently consuming caffeine, fatty foods (including fast foods), spicy foods, citrus products (especially lemons), and tomatoes (including pizza and spaghetti sauce). In addition, because of the great demands that singers place on their voices, even slight alterations caused by peptic mucositis of the larynx produce symptoms that may impair performance.

Thus, singers are more likely to seek medical care because of reflux symptoms than are individuals with fewer vocal demands. However, careful inquiry and physical examination reveal similar problems among many nonsinger patients. Most of the voice problems associated with reflux laryngitis appear to be due to direct mucosal damage from proximal reflux. The effects of distal reflux alone on laryngeal function have not been studied.

Voice abnormalities and vocal fold pathology may be due to reflux of gastric acid onto the vocal folds. Severe coughing may cause vocal fold hemorrhage or mucosal tears, sometimes leading to permanent dysphonia by causing a scar that obliterates the layers of the lamina propria and adheres the epithelium to deeper layers. Aspiration caused by reflux also makes reactive airway disease difficult to control. Even mild pulmonary obstruction impairs voice support. Consequently, afflicted patients subconsciously strain to compensate with muscles in the neck and throat, which are designed for delicate control, not for power source functions.[216,217] This behavior is typically responsible for the development of vocal fold nodules and other lesions related to voice abuse. Although it appears likely that some extraesophageal symptoms of reflux are due to stimulation of the vagus nerve rather than (or in addition) to topical irritation, the role of vagal reflexes in reflux laryngitis remains to be clarified.

Posterior Laryngitis and Related Conditions

In addition to erythema and edema, more serious vocal fold pathology may be caused by reflux laryngitis. In 1968, Cherry and Margulies[96] recognized that reflux laryngitis might be a causative factor in contact ulcers and granulomas of the posterior portion of the vocal folds, conditions that are discussed in detail below. They also observed that treatment of peptic esophagitis resulted in resolution of vocal process granulomas. Delahunty and Cherry[97] followed up on this observation by applying gastric juice to the vocal processes of 2 dogs and applying saliva to the vocal processes of a third dog who was used as a control. The control dog's vocal folds remained normal; the other dogs developed granulomas at the sites of repeated acid application. The experiment by Delahunty and Cherry is particularly interesting. The posterior portion of the left vocal fold of 2 dogs was exposed to gastric acid for a total of only 20 minutes per day, 5 days out of every 7, for a total of 29 days of exposure in a 39-day period. A total of 20 minutes out of 24 hours may not seem like an extensive exposure period; however, erythema and edema were apparent in both dogs by the fourth day of the first week. At the beginning of the second week, the larynges appeared normal after the 2-day rest period. However, visible reaction was provoked within 2 days after application was resumed, and the vocal folds never regained normal appearance. Marked inflammation, thickening, and irregularities were apparent in both dogs by the fourth week, and epithelial slough at the site of acid contact occurred on day 29 in 1 dog and day 32 in the other. Granulation tissue appeared shortly thereafter. A similar procedure was performed on a control animal by applying saliva instead of gastric juice to the vocal fold, and the vocal fold remained normal. This research suggests that even relatively short periods of acid exposure may cause substantial abnormalities in laryngeal mucosa. Since then, numerous authors have recognized the importance of reflux laryngitis as a causative factor in laryngeal ulcers and granulomas, including intubation granuloma.[12,13,77,83,96,218–221] In addition to its etiological involvement in intubation granuloma, reflux laryngitis has long been recognized as a contributing factor to posterior glottic stenosis, especially following intubation.[222] Olson[7] has suggested that it may also be a causative factor in cricoarytenoid joint arthritis through chronic inflammation and ulceration, beginning on the mucosa and involving the synovial cricoarytenoid joint. We have encountered this problem, as well. In addition to posterior glottic and supraglottic stenosis, subglottic stenosis has been reported as a complication of reflux.[104,223]

Laryngeal Granulomas

Laryngeal granulomas are a particularly vexing problem for patients and their physicians. Granulomas, like contact ulcers of the larynx, usually occur on the posterior aspect of the vocal folds, often on or above the cartilaginous portion. They may be unilateral, although it is also common to see a sizable granuloma on one side and a contact ulcer on the other. Patients with ulcers or granulomas may complain of pain (laryngeal or referred otalgia), a globus sensation, hoarseness, painful phonation, and occasionally hemoptysis. Surprisingly, even large granulomas are often asymptomatic. These benign lesions usually contain fibroblasts, collagenous fibers, proliferated capillaries, leukocysts, and sometimes ulceration. Although the term *granuloma* is universally accepted, these laryngeal lesions actually are not granulomas histopathologically, but rather chronic inflammatory lesions. However, granulomas and ulcers may mimic more serious lesions such as carcinoma, tuberculosis, and granular cell tumor. Consequently, the clinical diagnosis of laryngeal granuloma must always be made with caution and must

be considered tentative until the patient has been followed over time and a good response to treatment has been observed.

Understanding the etiology of laryngeal ulcers and granulomas is essential to clinical evaluation and treatment. Traditionally, ulcers and granulomas in the region of the vocal processes have been associated with trauma, especially intubation injury. However, they are also seen in young, apparently healthy professional voice users with no history of intubation or obvious laryngeal injury. In fact, the vast majority of granulomas and ulcerations (probably even those from intubation) are caused or aggravated by laryngopharyngeal reflux disease. In some patients, muscular tension dysphonia producing forceful vocal process contact may be contributory or causal.

Evaluation of patients with laryngeal ulcers or granulomas begins with a comprehensive history and physical examination. In addition to elucidating specific voice complaints and their importance to the individual patient's life and profession, the history is designed to reveal otolaryngologic and systemic abnormalities that may have caused dysphonia. Special attention is paid to symptoms of voice abuse and of laryngopharyngeal reflux, as listed above. It must be remembered that reflux laryngitis is commonly not accompanied by pyrosis or dyspepsia in these patients. The history also seeks specifically symptoms consistent with asthma, including voice fatigue following extensive voice use. Exercise-induced asthma can be provoked by the exercise of voice use, and even mild reactive airway disease undermines the power source of the voice and may lead to compensatory muscular tension dysphonia and consequent laryngeal granuloma or ulcer. Inquiry also investigates systematically all body systems for evidence of other diseases that present with laryngeal pathology. It is important to include a psychological assessment. Excessive stress may lead to increased acid production, abnormal esophageal function, and symptomatic reflux and to muscular tension dysphonia. In such cases, it is important to identify and treat the underlying stressor, as well as the symptomatic expressions of the stress.

Mirror examination usually reveals the presence of a granuloma or ulcer, but more sophisticated evaluation is invaluable. In the presence of suspected laryngeal granuloma or ulcer, the author (RTS) routinely performs strobovideolaryngoscopy using both flexible and rigid endoscopes. Flexible endoscopic examination reveals patterns of phonation and is extremely helpful in identifying muscular tension dysphonia and determining phonatory behaviors associated with forceful adduction. Recent observations (Steven Zeitels, MD, personal communication, 1997, and the author's [RTS] experience) suggest that some granuloma patients have a vocal fold closure pattern with initial forceful vocal process contact. This implies an adduction strategy with lateral cricoarytenoid dominance, and this observation is important in the treatment of granulomas that are refractory to therapy (medical and/or surgical) or granulomas that recur. Rigid laryngeal stroboscopic examination provides magnified, detailed information of the lesions under slow-motion light, allowing analysis of their composition (solid granulomas versus fluid-filled cysts) and their effects on phonation. This examination also permits assessment of other areas of the vocal folds to rule out separate lesions (eg, vocal fold scar) that may be the real cause of the patient's voice complaint.

Evaluation also includes at least a formal assessment by a speech-language patholo-gist (SLP) skilled in voice evaluation and care. In the author's (RTS) center, we also include objective voice analysis and a vocal stress assessment with a singing voice specialist (even with nonsingers). In addition to a laryngologist, SLP, and singing voice specialist, other members of the voice team are often used, depending on the patient's problems. Additional team members include an acting-voice specialist, psychologist, psychiatrist, otolaryngologic nurse clinician, and consulting pulmonologist, neurologist, gastroenterologist, and others. The information provided by these evaluations helps establish the degree to which voice abuse/misuse is present, and it guides the design of an individualized therapy plan.

Reflux must be suspected in virtually all cases of granuloma. It can be evaluated by 24-hour pH monitor, barium swallow with water siphonage (routine barium swallows are not satisfactory for diagnosing reflux, and the accuracy of barium swallow even with water siphonage is debatable), other tests, and/or a therapeutic trial of medical management. If there is historical evidence of prolonged reflux symptoms, endoscopic evaluation to rule out Barrett's esophagus is often advisable. It may be appropriate to biopsy the presumed granuloma at the same time. If a therapeutic trial of medications without confirmatory tests is elected, marked improvement in symptoms and signs should occur following daily use of a PPI (before breakfast and dinner) within 2 to 3 months. Treatment for laryngopharyngeal reflux should be aggressive.

The efficacy of oral corticosteroids for treatment of laryngeal granulomas and ulcers has not been proven, but they are used commonly on the basis of anecdotal evidence, especially for small- or medium-sized granulomas and ulcers that appear acutely inflamed. For these conditions, low doses of steroids for longer periods are usually given, such as triamcinolone 4 mg twice a day for 3 weeks. Steroid inhalers are not recommended. They may lead to laryngitis or laryngeal *Candida* infections, and prolonged use may cause vocal fold atrophy.

At the end of 2 months of therapy including antireflux measures, voice therapy, and possibly steroids, substantial improvement in the appearance of the larynx should be seen. Ulcers should be healed, and granulomas should be substantially smaller. Patients should be examined after 1 month to be certain that the lesions are not enlarging. If they appear worse, biopsy should be performed promptly. However, it should be noted that complete healing may take 8 months or more.[224,225] Repeated strobovideolaryngoscopic examinations allow comparison of lesion size over time. If improvements are noted, aggressive therapy and close follow-up can be continued until the mass lesion disappears or stabilizes. If the mass does not disappear, or if response to the first 2 months of aggressive therapy produces no substantial improvement, biopsy should be performed to rule out carcinoma and other diseases. If the surgeon is reasonably certain that the lesion is a granuloma, injection of an aqueous steroid preparation (such as dexamethasone) into the base of the lesion at the time of surgery may be helpful. As long as a good specimen is obtained, the laser may be used for resection of suspected granulomas because the lesions are usually not on the vibratory margin, and they often are friable. However, the author (RTS) usually uses traditional instruments to avoid the third-degree burn caused by the laser (even with a microspot) in the treatment of this chronic, irritative condition.

It is essential that causative factors, especially reflux and voice abuse, be treated preoperatively and controlled strictly following laryngeal surgery. The patient is kept on therapeutic doses of a PPI prior to surgery and for at least 6 weeks following surgery. Surgeons should not hesitate to use omeprazole (Prilosec) 20 mg as frequently as 4 times a day or the equivalent dose of another PPI under these circumstances and, if necessary, to add an H2-blocker (ranitidine, 300 mg) at bedtime. Following surgery, absolute voice rest (writing pad) is prescribed until the surgical area has remucosalized. This is usually approximately 1 week and virtually never longer than 10 to 14 days. There are no indications for more prolonged absolute voice rest, although relative voice rest (limited voice use) is recommended routinely. Voice therapy is reinstituted on the day when phonation is resumed, and frequent short therapy sessions and close monitoring are maintained throughout the healing period.

As previously stated, granulomas recur in some patients. In all such cases, aggressive reevaluation of reflux with 24-hour pH monitor studies is warranted because granulomas are seen commonly in patients with reflux laryngitis. Often endoscopy and biopsy of esophageal and postcricoid mucosa are appropriate. Twenty-four-hour pH monitor studies should be conducted not only off all medications but also when the patient is taking a PPI or H2-blocker. A few patients are resistant to PPIs and will have normal acid secretions despite even 80 mg of omeprazole daily or the equivalent dose of another PPI, and some patients may respond to PPIs initially and then develop resistance. In such patients, H2-blockers may be effective. When medical management of reflux is insufficient, laparoscopic fundoplication can be considered for patients with recurring granuloma. Voice use must also be optimized and monitored with the help of the SLP, always, and other members of the voice team when indicated. The laryngologist and voice therapists must be sure that good vocal technique is carried over outside the medical office into the patient's daily life.

Occasionally, even after excellent reflux control (including fundoplication), surgical removal including steroid injection into the base of the granulomas, and voice therapy, patients may develop multiply recurrent granulomas. Medical causes other than reflux and muscular tension dysphonia must be ruled out, particularly granulomatous diseases, including sarcoidosis and tuberculosis, and neoplasm such as granular cell tumors. Pathology slides from previous surgical procedures should be reviewed. When it has been established that the recurrent lesions are typical laryngeal granulomas occurring in the absence of laryngopharyngeal reflux, the cause is almost always phonatory trauma. When voice therapy has been insufficient to permit adequate healing, some of these uncommonly difficult patient problems can be solved by temporary paresis of selected vocal fold adductor muscles (particularly the lateral cricoarytenoid) using botulinum toxin (Botox, Allergan, Irvine, California) injection. Although this treatment approach has been effective, it is not utilized ordinarily as initial therapy and is appropriate only for selected cases.

Delayed Wound Healing

In addition to its possible carcinogenic potential, the chronic irritation of reflux laryngitis may be responsible for failure of wound healing. Reflux appears to delay the resolution not only of vocal process ulcers and granulomas but also of healing following vocal fold surgery. For this reason, otolaryngologists are becoming increasingly aggressive about diagnosing and treating reflux before subjecting patients to vocal fold surgery, even for conditions unrelated to the reflux.

Stenosis

As noted above, laryngeal stenosis has been associated with reflux.[32,84,104,105] Koufman[32] has reported laryngopharyngeal reflux in 92% of his patients with laryngeal stenosis, all of whom were documented by 24-hour pH monitoring studies. This is consistent with an earlier report by Little et al[3] in which the authors were able to produce nonhealing ulcerations and subglottic stenosis experimentally in canines by applying gastric acid and pepsin to injured subglottic mucosa. Long-term control of laryngopharyngeal reflux is essential to success in treating laryngeal stenosis.

Globus Pharyngeus

The sensation of a lump in the throat or globus pharyngeus is associated commonly with laryngopharyngeal reflux. The literature on the association of globus with reflux does not provide definitive guidance.[15,16,89,90,225-229] However, reflux has been found in 23% to 90% of patients with globus.[32,90,225-228,230,231]

Smit et al[231] studied 27 patients with globus pharyngeus alone, 20 patients with hoarseness alone (more than 3 months' duration), and 25 patients with both globus and hoarseness. Using dual-probe pH monitoring, pathologic reflux was diagnosed if patients had a pH below 4 for more than 0.1% of the total time, more than 0.2% of time in the upright position, and more than 0% of the time in the supine position in the proximal probe, or if they had more than 3 reflux episodes with pH below 4. The proximal probe was placed visually at the UES, and the distal probe was 15 cm from the proximal probe. Only 30% of patients with globus but without hoarseness had pathologic reflux. Similar findings were reported by Wilson et al[227] (23%), Curran et al[228] (38%), and Hill et al[230] (30.8%). Smit et al[231] found that only 35% of patients with hoarseness alone had pathologic reflux. However, 72% (18 of 25) of patients with globus and hoarseness had pathologic reflux. Sixty-five percent of patients with pathologic GERD had abnormal findings during esophagoscopy, including 2 patients with Barrett's mucosa. The diagnosis of laryngopharyngeal reflux should be considered in patients with globus pharyngeus, and diagnostic evaluation and therapeutic trial with PPIs are warranted.[231–233]

Laryngospasm

Laryngospasm is forceful, involuntary adduction of the vocal folds. It is associated with airway obstruction that is often severe enough to cause the patient to panic. Typically, laryngospasm occurs suddenly and without warning. It may be precipitated by laughing or exercise, or it may occur with no apparent precipitating event. Nighttime attacks that awaken the patient are common. Reflux is a well-recognized cause of laryngospasm. The mechanism may be related to chemoreceptors on the epiglottis that respond to a pH of 2.5 or below by eliciting laryngospasm.[233] Loughlin and Koufman[234] also demonstrated that this reflex is dependent on a functioning superior laryngeal nerve. In our experience, laryngopharyngeal reflux is the cause of paroxysmal laryngospasm in nearly all patients with this condition, and most respond to aggressive antireflux therapy.

Muscle Tension Dysphonia

The relationship between laryngopharyngeal reflux and muscle tension dysphonia

remains uncertain, but there is reason to consider an association possible. Koufman and coworkers[32] found a 70% incidence of laryngopharyngeal reflux in patients with structural vocal fold lesions associated commonly with muscle tension dysphonia, including nodules, Reinke's edema, hematoma, ulcers, and granuloma. Chronic reflux laryngitis causes irritation that leads not only to an inflammatory response but also to laryngeal hyperirritability. Laryngospasm is the extreme manifestation of this condition. However, hyperfunctional posturing of the laryngeal muscles in response to chronic irritation, or as a defense against unpredictably timed episodes of laryngeal aspiration of acid, conceivably could lead to hyperfunctional patterns of voice use. Alternatively, in some patients, laryngopharyngeal reflux and muscle tension dysphonia may occur coincidentally, but injury to the vocal fold mucosa by acid and pepsin may make the vocal folds more prone to injury and to the development of structural lesions associated with phonotrauma. Traditionally, otolaryngologists and speech-language pathologists have viewed muscle tension dysphonia as a primary condition in the majority of cases. In the author's (RTS) opinion, a high percentage of patients with muscle tension dysphonia have an underlying disorder such as reflux laryngitis or superior laryngeal nerve paresis that may have been responsible for the patient's hyperfunctional voice disorder. In all patients with voice abnormalities, including muscle tension dysphonia, it is essential to seek out and treat the primary etiological condition.

Paroxysmal vocal fold movement disorder is a laryngeal dystonia characterized by intermittent glottic obstruction by adduction of the vocal folds on inspiration. It is also called paradoxical vocal fold adduction, respiratory dysphonia, and other names, including paradoxical vocal fold movement disorder (PVFMD). Yelken et al[235] point out that PVFMD "mimics asthma," and patients are often diagnosed incorrectly initially. In their patients, they reported no relationship between asthma attacks and severity and PVFMD. However, they found LPR and allergy to be prevalent in their patients with PVFMD.

Cough associated with PVFMD was studied by Murry and colleagues.[236] They suggested that chronic cough associated with PVFMD might be due to laryngeal sensory deficits secondary to chronic acid exposure in the laryngopharynx, which triggers the cough reflex. They suggested also that the cough reflex could be an adaptive mechanism to clear particulate matter from the laryngopharynx.

Reinke's Edema

Prolonged acid/pepsin irritation of the laryngeal mucosa can result in significant alterations in laryngeal tissues, including carcinoma, as discussed below. Reinke's edema appears to be one such tissue alteration. Koufman[32] demonstrated abnormal 24-hour pH monitoring results in a majority of their patients with Reinke's edema, and this is consistent with our experience. In the author's (RTS) opinion, in many cases, it is unclear whether reflux is the primary cause of Reinke's edema or is a cofactor with other laryngeal mucosal irritants such as smoking, hyperfunctional voice use, or hypothyroidism. However, we evaluate all patients with Reinke's edema for reflux and treat LPR aggressively. Many patients seeking optimal restoration of voice quality require surgical treatment despite good reflux control, voice therapy, smoking cessation, and correction of any thyroid abnormalities. Good reflux control should be maintained long term, but it is especially critical in the immediate postoperative period, as discussed previously in the section on delayed wound healing.

Carcinoma

The association of gastroesophageal reflux disease with Barrett's esophagus and esophageal carcinoma has been well established. It is now thought possible that LPR is associated with laryngeal malignancy, as well.[237-241] Delahunty[78] biopsied the posterior laryngeal mucosa in a patient with reflux laryngitis and reported epithelial hyperplasia with parakeratosis and papillary down-growth. In the 1980s, Olson and others[1] reported on patients (including young, nonsmokers, nondrinkers) with posterior laryngeal carcinoma in whom he believed reflux to be a cofactor. This issue was addressed also by Morrison.[242] He reported 6 cases of vocal fold carcinoma in patients who had severe reflux but had never smoked. In 1997, Olson[243] reaffirmed that the relationship between reflux and cancer is not conclusive.

The mechanisms by which reflux may cause laryngeal cancer remains speculative. Both smoking and alcohol consumption promote reflux by lowering lower esophageal sphincter pressure, impairing esophageal motility and mucosal integrity, increasing gastric acid secretion, and delaying gastric emptying. So, a high incidence of reflux in laryngeal cancer patients who smoke and drink is not surprising. However, the association does not explain how LPR may act as a cofactor in these patients or as a primary factory in patients who do not smoke and drink. Richtsmeier et al[244] have suggested that a deficiency in T-cell mediated immunity is causally related to immunodeficiency in cancer patients. There is a subgroup of suppressor T cells with histamine-type 2 receptors. Cimetadine, a histamine-type 2 receptor antagonist, inhibits the expression of suppressor T cells and enhances immune responses. Richtsmeier et al[245] found that skin test anergy in laryngeal cancer can be reversed by cimetadine. This led El-Serag et al[246] to recommend the use of an H2-blocker not only to treat reflux in laryngeal cancer patients but also to address their underlying immune dysfunction, although this thinking is not accepted widely.

Although some questions remain regarding the relationship between LPR and laryngeal carcinoma, the studies cited above, as well as more recent evidence,[246] suggest that the 2 conditions are probably associated. At present, patients with laryngeal cancer, or those at risk to develop laryngeal cancer, should be screened for reflux; antireflux therapy should be instituted when it is present. Cancer surveillance is reasonable even in patients without known risk factors other than chronic LPR. The long-term efficacy of such treatment with regard to prevention of malignancy remains unknown, but we have seen resolution of laryngeal structural abnormalities, including suspicious leukoplakia, in patients with LPR alone, and even in patients who continue smoking and consuming alcohol. Koufman and Burke[247] have had similar experiences.

In 1988, Ward and Hanson[248] recognized reflux as a potential cofactor for the development of laryngeal cancer, particularly in nonsmokers. In 1991, Koufman[32] documented LPR in 84% of 31 consecutive patients with laryngeal carcinoma, only 58% of whom were active smokers. Freije et al[249] reviewed retrospectively 23 patients with T1 and T2 carcinomas of the larynx, and they concluded that GERD plays a role in the etiology of carcinoma of the larynx particularly in patients who lack typical risk factors (14 of their patients had quit smoking more than 15 years prior to developing laryngeal

carcinoma) and may act as a co-carcinogen in smokers and drinkers. In 1997, Koufman and Burke[247] felt that the causal relationship between LPR and laryngeal malignancy remained unproven but noted that most patients who develop laryngeal malignancy have LPR in addition to being smokers. Until more definitive data are available, we believe that long-term antireflux therapy in these patients should be considered.

Research has shown that GERD is a factor in the development of esophageal cancer.[249] Studies also have examined the potential carcinogenic role of LPR. Conflicting data exist, complicated recently by published stories that show no carcinogenic effects but that were limited by short periods of acid injury.[250,251] Although some studies have shown LPR as a risk factor in animal models, others have not, and the true relationship between LPR and laryngeal malignancy remains uncertain. However, there are enough data indicating a possible link to suggest that at present, known reflux patients should be screened for laryngeal cancer and be made aware of this risk.[252]

Given the risk of esophageal adenocarcinoma in reflux patients, the value of EGD screening has been assessed. It has been argued that LPR symptoms are better indicators of esophageal adenocarcinoma than are gastroesophageal symptoms.[253] Studies have shown esophagitis in 12% to 18% of LPR patients and in 3% to 7% Barrett's metaplasia patients.[254,255] Additionally, in patients on long-term PPIs, *Helicobacter pylori* is known to accelerate the loss of specialized gastric glands, causing atrophic gastritis and gastric cancer.[256] *H pylori*, breath, or fecal testing or biopsy may screen for this infection. Diagnosis of hiatal hernia would also potentially affect treatment and is facilitated by EGD. Some have suggested routine EGD for patients complaining of heartburn; others suggest it for all LPR patients.[254]

Until the true relationship is defined, screening with either transnasal esophagoscopy or EGD (which may be performed at the time of routine colonoscopy in appropriate patients) is advisable. Many gastroenterologists are now advising visualization of the larynx during EGD. This has led to the diagnosis of LPR in up to 4.6% of patients undergoing EGD for GERD.[257]

Recent literature reflects ongoing research on the causal effects of gastric refluxate (pepsin) and the carcinogenic effects on the larynx, pharynx, and upper airway epithelium.[258–262]

LPR has been considered a risk factor in the development of squamous cell carcinoma of the larynx, but it remains unproven.

Sudden Infant Death Syndrome and Other Pediatric Considerations

Laryngopharyngeal reflux is important in the pediatric population, although it has been studied much less extensively than has reflux in adults. Unlike adults, infants and young children are unable to complain of symptoms associated with LPR. Nevertheless, LPR has been associated with various problems in infants and children, including halitosis, dysphonia, laryngospasm, laryngomalacia, asthma, pneumonia, sleep apnea, and sudden infant death syndrome (SIDS).[6,24,263–285] The diagnosis can be established by laryngoscopy and bronchoscopy, and 24-hour pH monitor studies. Children can be treated with H2-blockers and/or PPIs, and fundoplication is appropriate in selected cases, particularly in patients with life-threatening complications of reflux.

Evidence suggests that SIDS may be causally related to acid reflux into the larynx. Hence, SIDS must join laryngeal and esophageal cancer at the top of the list of serious otolaryngologic consequences of reflux laryngitis. Wetmore[263] investigated the effects of acid on the larynges of maturing rabbits by applying solutions of acid or saline at 15-day intervals up to 60 days of age. Because the larynx is not only a site of resistance in the airway but also contains the afferent limb for reflexes that regulate respiration, he discovered that acid exposure resulted in significant obstructive, central, and mixed apnea. Gasping respirations and frequent swallowing were observed as associated symptoms. Central apnea occurred in all age groups but had a peak incidence at 45 days. Acid-induced obstructive apnea in rabbits is similar to obstructive apnea previously recognized in human infants with gastroesophageal disease. However, the demonstration of acid-induced central apnea produced by acid stimulation of the larynx is more ominous. Central apnea has been demonstrated in other animal models as a result of different forms of laryngeal stimulation. Central apnea resulting in fatal asphyxia has also been described in several animal models. Wetmore's study[263] suggests that gastroesophageal reflux alone is capable of triggering fatal central apnea. This is particularly compelling when one recognizes that the peak incidence of central apnea occurring at 45 days in the rabbit corresponds well within the peak incidence of SIDS in humans, which occurs between 2 and 4 months of age.

Otolaryngologists should be aware of the prevalence of LPR/GERD in children and infants. Studies have shown that reflux is associated commonly with regurgitation and vomiting, disturbed sleep patterns, colic, gastrointestinal pain, croup, and hoarseness in the pediatric population.[265–288]

Monitoring of pH is valuable to infants with laryngitis, including pharyngeal monitoring, which may diagnose undertreated LPR or LPR missed on esophageal monitoring.[289] LPR is a known common cause of hoarseness in children and should be in the differential diagnosis of dysphonia.[290] It may be misdiagnosed as recurrent croup when reflux triggers intermittent airway obstruction.[291] The diagnosis of LPR is still often missed in children with hoarseness or frequent respiratory disorders.

Barreto et al[292] examined the laryngeal and phonatory effects associated with untreated growth hormone deficiencies. Values for roughness, breathiness, and strain were higher, and LPR signs were also more common in this population. More research is needed. Otolaryngologists should be familiar with this association.

Ongoing research continues to examine the relationship between LPR and otitis media in children. Several studies have confirmed the presence of pepsin and pepsinogen in children with otitis media with effusion.[293,294] One study reported positive *H pylori* results in 6 of 31 children (19%) with middle ear effusion.[295] Miura et al[296] suggested that reflux disease in children with chronic otitis media with effusion appears to be factorial, but the "cause-effect" relationship is unclear. They suggested that, based on current research, "anti-reflux therapy for otitis media cannot be endorsed." Other studies have identified increased presence of reflux in children with upper respiratory infections associated with cough, runny nose, otitis media, and chronic rhinosinusitis.[297–299] Another study reported the presence of pepsin in the tears of children with LPR.[300] Andrews and Orobello[301] compared biopsies of the posterior cricoid region and nasopharyngeal pH results in diagnosing LPR in children. They reported their retrospective review of 63 patients ages 6 months to 17 years and found 80% of patients tested positive for reflux by both methodologies. Katra et al[295] investigated the relationship between *H pylori* in hyperplasia of the adenoids and reflux episodes in children

detected by impedance and pH monitoring. Their study population was small, 30 children with a mean age of 5.34 years. The children underwent adenoidectomy and pH/impedance monitoring with a proximal impedance sensor 1 cm above the UES. Their results confirmed their hypothesis that reflux episodes that reached the UES could have a significant role in *H pylori* reaching lymphoid tissue in the nasopharynx and the development of adenoid hyperplasia in children.

Diagnostic Tests for Reflux

The approach to diagnosis of laryngopharyngeal reflux (LPR) in a general or otolaryngologic practice includes careful physical examination and diagnostic testing. This section discusses the use of each of these modalities in the management of GERD in general, with specific reference to the otolaryngologic patient (Table 9–5).

Table 9–5. Diagnostic Tests for Gastroesophageal Reflux

Is reflux present?
  Barium swallow
  pH monitoring

Is there mucosal injury?
  Barium swallow (air contrast) study
  Endoscopy
  Mucosal biopsy

Are symptoms due to reflux?
  Therapeutic trial
  pH monitoring (with symptom index)

Can prognostic or preoperative information be obtained?
  Esophageal manometry
  pH monitoring

Therapeutic Trial

When a patient presents with typical heartburn and regurgitation, diagnostic studies may not be needed. Relief of symptoms after a therapeutic trial with H2-antagonists, prokinetic agents, or PPIs for 8 to 12 weeks can confirm that the symptoms are secondary to GERD. Because heartburn generally is absent in the otolaryngologic patient, the end point of the therapeutic trial is dependent on other presenting symptoms, and diagnostic tests are often necessary to confirm the diagnosis. Historical clues that otolaryngologic symptoms may be due to GERD, specifically LPR, include morning hoarseness, halitosis, excess phlegm, dry mouth, throat clearing, and others.

If a therapeutic trial is used in a patient with suspected GERD and otolaryngologic symptoms, higher doses of antireflux therapy, usually with a PPI, for longer periods of time are needed. However, neither the cost-effectiveness nor clinical efficacy of any medical regimen in patients with LPR has been tested. We currently use a PPI twice a day initially for a minimum of 8 to 12 weeks as a therapeutic trial for laryngeal symptoms suspected to be due to reflux.

It should be emphasized that patients with reflux laryngitis frequently require more intensive therapy with higher doses of H2-blockers or earlier use of PPIs than patients with dyspepsia in the absence of laryngeal symptoms and signs. In addition to monitoring symptoms and signs of reflux laryngitis, response to treatment is best judged by combined intraesophageal and intragastric pH monitoring of patients while they are receiving treatment. Such studies are worthwhile even when patients are taking PPIs, because some patients are omeprazole-resistant,[168,169] and resistance to other proton pump inhibitors may occur, as well. Our recent observations suggest that

omeprazole resistance also can develop in patients who respond well initially to the medication. Moreover, it must be recognized that a normal pH 24-hour monitor study does not indicate the absence of reflux. Rather, it demonstrates the absence of acid reflux. Regurgitation of pH-neutral liquid may still be present and may produce symptoms, especially in singers and actors. Study of this phenomenon and its optimal management is needed badly. At the present time, although there are no data to support the superiority of surgery over medical therapy for LPR patients, it appears that selected patients may benefit from surgery over medicine, especially considering the efficacy and decreased morbidity associated with laparoscopic fundoplication and the potential costs and risks associated with the use of H2-blockers or PPIs for periods of many years. If endoscopic suturing and Stretta techniques prove efficacious, one or both of these techniques may be useful, but at present, they have not been studied in LPR or compared to surgery or medical therapy.

Barium Radiographs

Barium studies are relatively inexpensive and widely available for use in the diagnosis of esophageal disease. When evaluating the esophagus, a double-contrast barium swallow is needed for optimal assessment. An upper GI (gastrointestinal) series usually results in insufficient evaluation of esophageal function, concentrates excessively on the stomach and duodenum, and does not give enough attention to potential mucosal or motility abnormalities in the esophagus. A hiatal hernia is the most common abnormality seen on barium swallow. However, up to 60% of the adult population will have a hiatal hernia,[302] making this a nonspecific finding and not diagnostic of

GERD. Free reflux is seen in up to 30% of "normal" patients and may be absent in up to 60% of patients with GERD established by pH monitoring,[303] making the barium study an insensitive and nonspecific study for GERD. It has been suggested that reflux of barium to or above the carina or to the thoracic inlet is indicative of the potential for aspiration and is useful as an aid in the diagnosis of GERD-associated laryngitis. There are no prospective or controlled studies to substantiate this clinical impression. This finding is reported usually with the patient in the supine position, making this observation of relatively little use. The so-called high reflux on a barium study has not been well correlated with proximal acid exposure on ambulatory pH monitoring. Barium swallow with water siphonage has been used to aid in the diagnosis of reflux in otolaryngology patients. Patients may show abnormalities on barium swallow with water siphonage, which may be interpreted as confirming a diagnosis of pathologic reflux, although interpretations should be made with caution as the true positive predictive value has not been confirmed. However, barium swallow with water siphonage has more value than recognized by many radiologists. The literature on this subject was reviewed in 1994 by Ott.[302] Because early reports revealed a wide discrepancy in reflux detection rates, barium esophagrams were considered insensitive, and provocative tests (ie, water siphonage) were believed to increase the sensitivity at the expense of specificity. Thompson et al[303] found that a reflux detection rate increased to 70% when using the water siphonage test, as compared with 26% for spontaneous reflux. However, this gain in sensitivity may be counterbalanced by the low specificity of this test.

In professional singers and actors especially, barium swallow with water siphonage seems to provide a good clinical approximation of daily reflux episodes. To optimize mucosal function, it is essential for singers and actors to remain well hydrated. Consequently, they drink large amounts of water, routinely carry water bottles with them, and drink substantial quantities shortly before they sing. This routine behavior is similar to the water siphon portion of the barium swallow, which raises the question of whether positive water siphonage tests may provide useful information, at least in professional voice users, even when a 24-hour pH monitor study is normal. Specific mucosal abnormalities on double-contrast barium studies, such as thickening of esophageal mucosal folds, erosions, or esophageal ulcers, are seen in a minority of patients with GERD, making this study relatively insensitive for this diagnosis. The diagnosis of Barrett's esophagus is conclusive also by a barium swallow.

The optimal use of the barium study is to evaluate patients with suspected complications of GERD, such as motility abnormalities or peptic stricture that are commonly seen in patients with solid and/ or liquid dysphagia. A barium swallow can identify rings, webs, or other obstructive lesions, including carcinoma, that are seen in patients with dysphagia, but these are unusual complications of GERD. A solid bolus such as a marshmallow or a barium cookie can be given to help localize the site of obstruction in a patient with solid dysphagia.

Although the barium swallow allows demonstration that reflux is occurring and can demonstrate mucosal injury, it is of inconsistent value in establishing a diagnosis of GERD. Its best use is in evaluation of the patient with dysphagia, and it should be performed in conjunction with endoscopy in these patients. Nevertheless, in some patients, barium esophagram provides important additional information that may be missed without radiologic imaging or esophagoscopy.[28,303,304] In a series of

128 patients, for example, barium studies showed esophagitis in 18%, a lower esophageal ring in 14%, and peptic stricture in 3% of patients.[305,306] Consequently, if endoscopy is not planned, patients with LPR should be considered for further evaluation by barium swallow.

Radionucleotide Studies

Scintigraphic studies have been suggested as valuable in diagnosis of GERD.[307] A radioisotope (Technetium 99m-sulfur colloid) marker is mixed with a measured quantity of liquid (usually H_2O), and graded abdominal compression is used to unmask reflux. Originally proposed as a sensitive test, its reliability has been questioned, and it is no longer considered a useful investigation.[308]

Endoscopy

Endoscopy is used to document mucosal disease and establish a diagnosis of erosive esophagitis or Barrett's metaplasia. When patients with frequent heartburn and regurgitation are studied prospectively, erosive esophagitis is seen in 45% to 60% of patients.[309] The others will have nonerosive disease (mucosal edema, hyperemia, or a normal-appearing esophagus). Erosive esophagitis suggests a serious form of GERD in which patients require continuous medical therapy with a PPI or antireflux surgery for effective symptom relief and healing. Barrett's esophagus is seen in 10% to 15% of reflux patients undergoing endoscopy.[94] Unfortunately, there is no classic presentation of Barrett's esophagus, but it is most common in white males over 50 years of age.[75]

Erosive esophagitis is uncommon in patients with extraesophageal symptoms.

Although 50% of patients with unexplained chest pain and normal coronary arteries have GERD, the prevalence of erosive esophagitis is 10% or less.[64] GERD-associated asthma and evidence of esophagitis on endoscopy have been reported in 30% to 40% of adult patients.[59,60] In patients with reflux laryngitis, erosive esophagitis is seen in only 20% to 30%, making this study of low diagnostic yield in GERD.[16]

There are no absolute indications for endoscopy in the patient with suspected GERD. In general, endoscopy is performed in patients who do not respond to a therapeutic trial of medical therapy, patients with symptoms for greater than 5 years to rule out Barrett's metaplasia, and patients with the "alarm" symptoms of dysphagia—odynophagia, weight loss, anemia, or gastrointestinal bleeding.[310]

Endoscopic findings may help predict the prognosis and outcome of medical therapy. Patients with erosive esophagitis will almost always require long-term PPI therapy for healing and symptom relief. Recurrence of erosive esophagitis is seen in up to 80% of patients within 3 to 6 months following the discontinuation of medications[311]; these patients usually require continuous pharmacologic therapy for effective long-term control. Because patients with nonerosive esophagitis seldom progress to more severe forms of esophagitis, they can be managed with a range of pharmacologic treatments. Endoscopy is useful for long-term treatment planning in difficult to manage cases.

Given the rarity of erosive esophagitis, we do not use endoscopy routinely as the initial study in patients with suspected GERD-related otolaryngologic disease, chest pain, asthma, or cough, preferring ambulatory dual-probe pH monitoring or a therapeutic trial of antireflux medications as the initial diagnostic test.

Esophageal Biopsy

Biopsy and cytology are of limited value in evaluation of the patient with GERD unless Barrett's esophagus or malignancy is suspected, and the author (POK) biopsies only the esophagus in these patients. The light microscopic signs of GERD—elongation of rete pegs and hyperplasia of the basal cell layer—do not distinguish between acute and chronic disease and do not help predict response to therapy. The microscopic signs of active esophagitis, polymorphonuclear leukocytes and eosinophils, are seen in a minority of adult patients, so they are insensitive diagnostic findings. Biopsy may be more useful in the pediatric population where the frequency of these findings is higher.

If Barrett's metaplasia is suspected, a systematic biopsy protocol should be followed to confirm the diagnosis and rule out dysplasia or carcinoma. Endoscopic surveillance with biopsies to rule out dysplasia every 1 to 2 years is the current standard of practice for management of patients with Barrett's metaplasia.[74]

Prolonged Ambulatory pH Monitoring

Prolonged (16–24 hour) pH monitoring is the most important study to quantify esophageal reflux and determine whether symptoms are related to GERD. The study is performed by placing an antimony catheter (2-mm diameter) transnasally into the distal esophagus with an electrode placed 5 cm above the lower esophageal sphincter, which is identified by esophageal manometry (Figure 9–17). Precise positioning is important for accuracy in the interpretation of results. The probe is connected to a small microcomputer that is worn on a belt or clipped to the waist so that the patient can be monitored in an ambulatory setting. Activity can be tailored to provoke reflux in the setting in which symptoms are typically produced. For example, a patient with chronic hoarseness who sings professionally will be reminded to sing during the study. We have found some patients who reflux constantly during singing and rarely at other times (see Figure 9–17).

Multiple electrodes can be placed on a single catheter to monitor intragastric and intraesophageal pH, distal esophageal, and proximal esophageal acid exposure, or all 3 simultaneously. Abnormal acid exposure in the proximal esophagus, just below the upper esophageal sphincter, predicts the potential for aspiration in patients with otolaryngologic symptoms. An intragastric electrode allows monitoring of the gastric acid response to antireflux therapy. Several investigators have placed probes above the upper esophageal sphincter in the hypopharynx[312,313] to document reflux above the UES, thus being more certain of aspiration as the cause of symptoms. Unfortunately, this placement creates difficulty in standardizing the distance between the proximal and distal probes and causes difficulty in placement of the distal esophageal probe 5 cm above the LES, the standard used in developing normal values. Probes in the hypopharynx can be uncomfortable, normal values are not available, and pharyngeal probe data are occasionally subject to interpretation error, including incorrect diagnosis of reflux due to probe drying and acidic food or liquid ingestion, both artifacts resulting in a drop of pH to less than 4 that is not a true reflux episode. Some investigators who believe that pharyngeal probe placement is important and that data are valid and reliable, for example, Koufman and colleagues,[312] place the proximal probe

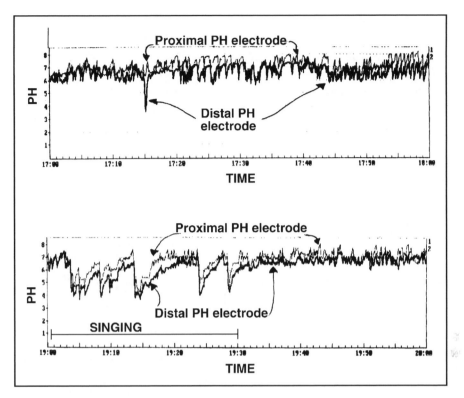

Figure 9–17. Dual-electrode pH probe monitoring while singing for a 30-minute period of the 1 hour shown. The patient experienced typical heartburn, and increased proximal and distal acid exposure was prominent during singing.

immediately above the cricopharyngeus, posterior to the larynx. This position prevents drying of the probe and reportedly produces valid data. They consider any pharyngeal acid exposure (even 1 episode) abnormal. Although placement of the proximal probe (just above the cricopharyngeus or just below it) remains controversial, the need for dual-probe pH monitoring is clear. Without a proximal probe, the sensitivity of single-probe esophageal pH monitoring has been shown to be only 62% for LPR; that is, 38% of patients had pharyngeal reflux with distal esophageal parameters that were considered within normal limits. At present, normal values for distal reflux at 5 cm above the lower esophageal sphincter

and for proximal reflux 20 cm above the sphincter are available, making this a more useful protocol.[95,313] Normal values vary slightly between laboratories and should be included with reports from the laboratory performing the procedure.

The microcomputer (data logger) has a symptom button that allows recording of up to 6 symptoms during a single study. The patient is asked to push the symptom button as well as to record symptoms on a diary card. This allows correlation of reflux events with symptoms in order to determine a symptom index,[314] which is especially valuable in patients with asthma, cough, and chest pain and allows correlation between symptoms and reflux in patients who have continued symptoms on medical therapy. Symptom correlation in the otolaryngologic patient may be more difficult on a single study, particularly when symptoms are continuous and not produced by a single reflux episode. This scenario is more likely in patients with laryngitis or chronic sore throat. Other symptoms such as throat clearing, cough, or symptoms provoked by singing may be correlated with single reflux episodes.

Prolonged pH monitoring is used in patients with heartburn to establish a diagnosis when symptoms have not responded to a trial of antireflux therapy and endoscopy is negative. In this case, a single-channel pH probe can be placed with the distal probe 5 cm above the lower esophageal sphincter. Symptoms are correlated with reflux, and reflux frequency is assessed. Patients with known GERD who have heartburn and regurgitation not responding to medical therapy can be monitored while still on therapy with a dual-channel intragastric and distal esophageal probe to assess the adequacy of gastric acid suppression, to assess esophageal reflux frequency, and to correlate symptoms with reflux events. Patients with continued esophageal acid exposure and/or symptoms may require additional therapy.

Patients with otolaryngologic symptoms, or other upper airway symptoms suggestive of GERD, are ideal candidates for prolonged ambulatory pH monitoring. We prefer performing monitoring early in the clinical course to establish a diagnosis and symptom correlation when possible. Dual-channel pH monitoring with one electrode 5 cm above the LES and a second probe 20 cm above in the proximal esophagus just below the UES (Figure 9–18) is our procedure of choice. Abnormal distal esophageal acid exposure can be documented, establishing a diagnosis of GERD. Abnormal proximal reflux can be

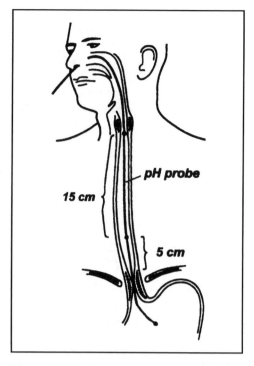

Figure 9–18. A dual-channel antimony pH probe with electrodes 15 cm apart. Distal electrode is placed 5 cm above the lower esophageal sphincter. Proximal electrode is 20 cm above the lower sphincter just below the upper esophageal sphincter.

demonstrated, suggesting the potential for aspiration and lending stronger probability that the otolaryngologic symptom is due to GERD. If symptom correlation can be demonstrated, this will establish the diagnosis. The presence of proximal reflux appears to predict the response to medical therapy in patients with pulmonary disease.[315–317] This is less clear in the otolaryngologic patient. A small percentage of patients will have normal percent time of distal esophageal acid exposure but demonstrable increased frequency of proximal reflux or reflux into the hypopharynx. This is seen in up to 30% of patients with otolaryngologic symptoms. In one study of 10 patients with reflux laryngitis, 3 of 10 (30%) demonstrated hypopharyngeal reflux with normal distal acid exposure.[318] In a larger, retrospective series of patients with pulmonary disease, 12% of patients reviewed had only abnormal proximal reflux[317]—a group that would have been diagnosed incorrectly as normal had only a single-channel study been performed. These patients should be considered abnormal and treated aggressively. Studies in our laboratory have shown that dual-electrode pH recording can document abnormal distal and proximal esophageal reflux induced by singing. A singing challenge (shown in Figure 9–17) can also unmask significant reflux in patients with otherwise normal 24-hour pH monitor studies.

Studies in adults with a variety of otolaryngologic symptoms demonstrate abnormal amounts of acid in reflux in up to 75% of patients.[16] Abnormal acid exposure has been documented in upright and supine positions, although upright reflux seems more common. Ambulatory pH monitoring is most useful in assessing response to antireflux therapy, particularly in the patient who has failed to respond to a therapeutic trial of a PPI twice daily for 8 to 12 weeks. Intragastric, distal esophageal, and proximal esophageal pH can be monitored while therapy is continued. Adequacy of intragastric acid suppression can be assessed, as can the presence of esophageal acid exposure and correlation between reflux events and symptoms. This study is particularly valuable in patients who do not respond (or are resistant) to PPIs. If acid reflux is still present, treatment can be increased or modified. If adequate acid suppression is achieved and symptoms persist, alternative diagnosis can be sought. However, the definition of "adequate acid suppression" is more complex than it might appear. For example, Shi et al[317] reviewed 771 consecutive patients who had undergone 24-hour pH monitoring studies. Statistically significant associa-

tion was found between symptoms during reflux episodes in 96 patients (12.5%) with esophageal acid exposures that were within the laboratory's normal values. In these patients, the duration of reflux episodes was shorter and the pH of reflux episodes was higher than in patients who were diagnosed with GERD. The authors hypothesized that the underlying pathological feature in these patients was hypersensitivity to acid. However, there are other possible explanations. For example, it is possible that normative values have been established at levels higher than desirable.

An area of some controversy is the evaluation of the patient with continued symptoms but no esophageal acid exposure on 24-hour pH monitoring. This is when a question of alkaline or pH-neutral reflux may be raised. Current pH monitoring technology makes it possible to detect bilirubin pigment (bile) by use of a bilitec probe in addition to standard probes used for 24-hour pH monitoring. However, current data using this technique suggest that esophageal bile reflux rarely, if ever, occurs in the absence of acid reflux, making the bilitec probe useful only in select patients (see Approach to the Patient With GERD, below). The diagnosis of alkaline reflux should not be made based solely on the rise in pH above 7; careful analysis of pH rises above 7 coupled with symptom correlation may suggest alkaline reflux, but it is rarely, if ever, diagnosed conclusively by pH testing. A new approach to detecting pH-neutral reflux utilizes measurements of electrical impedance at numerous points along an esophageal probe. This device detects the presence of liquid in the esophagus regardless of pH, and sequential measurements along the chain of sensors indicate whether the liquid is traveling from proximal to distal or is refluxing from distal to proximal. This technology is now available commercially and has proven useful. However, the decision to proceed with surgical management for the suspicion of alkaline or pH-neutral reflux is a clinical one and must be made after careful consultation among the health care team, including the patient. Current pH technology cannot confirm this diagnosis definitively.

Although prolonged pH monitoring is used extensively in the evaluation of patients with suspected LPR, controversy exists as to its overall sensitivity and specificity. This is particularly important when addressing the issue of hypopharyngeal reflux. A study by Shaker and colleagues[318] found a similar number and duration of hypopharyngeal reflux events in control subjects and patients with suspected LPR. Another study[319] revealed no major difference between hypopharyngeal acid exposure in 36 patients with LPR signs and symptoms and healthy controls. Using a newer methodology for triple-probe monitoring, Maldonado et al[320] found a 10% prevalence of abnormal pH in normal controls. These data remind us of the importance of standardization of measurement of hypopharyngeal reflux to optimally understand the causal relationship between this phenomenon and LPR.

Sato et al[321] described their experience using a tetra-probe 24-hour pH monitoring system. The proximal probe is placed in the hypopharynx; a second probe is placed in the mid-esophagus; the third probe is placed a few centimeters above the LES (but not specifically 5 cm); and the distal sensor in placed in the stomach. This system is advantageous in that it measures pH simultaneously at all 4 sites, providing information regarding the relationship of these values. However, in our opinion, there are significant disadvantages associated with failure to have a sensor 5 cm above the LES, a standard site that permits comparison

with other literature. In a separate report,[322] the authors described their results using the tetra-probe 24-hour pH monitoring system to evaluate patterns of LPR and GERD and to determine the validity of using pH 5 as an indicator of LPR. The data suggest that pH levels less than 4 and less than 5 are indicative of significant LPR events. An interesting study was reported in 2010 by Zelenik et al.[323] They performed a prospective dual-probe pH monitoring study in 46 patients with complaints of globus pharyngeus for more than 3 months. They collected data from this group using a pH less than 4 and from a second data group using pH both less than 4 and less than 5. Extraesophageal reflux was found in 23.9% of their patients using analysis of pH less than 4. When data were calculated using pH both less than 4 and less than 5, they found extraesophageal reflux in an additional 4 (8.7%) patients whose reflux had not been detected when pH less than 4 alone was used.

In addition, abnormal findings on pH monitoring do not necessarily predict patient response to therapy. Similarly, a placebo-controlled study[324] of 145 patients treated with either esomeprazole or placebo found that symptomatic or laryngeal improvement was independent of pre-therapy pH-monitoring results. The apparent dichotomy in the clinical usefulness of hypopharyngeal pH monitoring is likely due to several key factors:

1. Lack of consensus on the duration and amount of reflux that constitute abnormal pharyngeal acid exposure
2. High operator dependence and variability of probe positioning (eg, use of manometry vs direct visualization)
3. Variable sensitivity of pH monitoring in detecting reflux, which may vary from day to day[325]

All these variables have been reported to result in a diagnostic yield from 14% to 83%.[326] The yield may improve with better data evaluation parameters. Reichel and Issing[327] suggest the use of reflux area indices of 4 and 5, which would include time at pH 5. The data regarding pepsin activity at pH 5 have generated somewhat less controversy than the data on activity at higher pH. The reflux area index is calculated from the number and duration of proximal reflux events and the degree to which the pH drops below a given value.[327] Incorporating several data points and including a reflux area index of 5 may increase the sensitivity of pH monitoring.

As such, 24-hour pH monitoring cannot be used to conclusively establish or rule out reflux as the cause of suspected LPR. Until the value of other tests such as wireless esophageal pH monitoring and/or impedance monitoring (see later section) has been established, an empiric trial with an effective dose of PPI remains the most important determinant of the relationship between reflux and LPR symptoms.

Ongoing research continues to examine the value of pH impedance monitoring in the diagnosis and treatment of patients with LPR.[328–333] In 2015, Gooi et al[334] reported the findings of the American Bronchoesophageal Association (ABBA) evaluation of the changes in the management and evaluation of patients with LPR over a 10-year period between 2002 and 2012. A total of 426 ABBA members were e-mailed questionnaires to be completed online, of whom 63 (14.8%) responded. Their responses showed that dual pH probe testing remained highly regarded for sensitivity and specificity in the evaluation of LPR but was being used less often in 2012 compared to 2002 (63.8% vs 78.3%, respectively). Empirical medical management of LPR was more common in 2012 (82.6% compared to 56.3% in 2002).

Telemetry Capsule pH Monitoring

The development of telemetry capsule-based (tubeless) pH monitoring has added to laryngologists' armamentarium and ability to monitor patients with suspected reflux disease. The system is safe, well tolerated, and reliable, allowing 48-hour assessment of esophageal acid exposure. It is unobtrusive, is comfortable, and allows longer duration of acid monitoring. Its use in LPR has not been studied, and the technology is limited by current inability to place the capsule proximally due to discomfort and bulk. Further refinements in methodology, recording protocols, and diagnostic accuracy have made this an extremely useful test in typical GERD patients. One of us (POK) uses the telemetry capsule to perform off-therapy monitoring in patients prior to antireflux surgery to be certain that abnormal acid exposure is present prior to an operation. This new technology will likely become valuable in assessing patients with LPR.[335]

Role of Combined Multichannel Intraluminal Impedance pH

Combined multichannel intraluminal impedance (MII) and pH monitoring is a promising technique that identifies gas, liquid, and mixed gastroesophageal reflux and allows differentiation of them into acid (pH 7) types. The current catheter allows simultaneous monitoring of intragastric and distal esophageal pH with the ability to assess the height of refluxate from 3 to 17 cm above the LES. Early data suggest that a number of patients with so-called extraesophageal disease may have symptoms associated with weak acid or nonacid reflux, although the clear relationship of this type of reflux to LPR remains to be studied.

Wu[336] reported that combining MII and dual-channel pH monitoring increased the diagnostic yield by ~10% compared with combined MII and single-channel pH monitoring systems. Lee and colleagues[337] reported a 2-fold increase in diagnosing reflux in patients with LPR symptoms, using combined dual-channel impedance/pH-metry. Loots et al[338] reported that the addition of MII to standard pH monitoring increased the yield of symptom association in children and infants with confirmed reflux. Combined MII/pH monitoring is a useful tool in evaluating all patients with persistent symptoms of acid-suppressive therapy, particularly those with LPR.[339]

Pharyngeal Monitoring

Although the gold standard for diagnosis always has been pH testing, many physicians rely on the Reflux Finding Score (RFS) and Reflux Symptom Index (RSI) as means to diagnose laryngopharyngeal reflux (LPR) and indications to begin treatment with PPI or H2-blockers. In addition, many believe that a reduction in RSI/RSF scores reflects improvement or resolution of LPR. However, numerous studies have raised questions about the utility or validity of these indicators, and over the safety and effectiveness of empiric prescription of antireflux medications. In a 2011 prospective study of 82 participants (72 patients and 10 controls), Musser et al[340] studied the agreement between RSI, RFS, and pH probe findings at pH levels of 4 and 5. Regardless of which pH criterion was used, RSI and RFS failed to identify the LPR patients from controls and failed to correlate with severity of disease. In addition, in 2005, Park et al[341] evaluated 57 patients with globus sensation with 24-hour pH probe, RSI, and RFS scores. In this study, RFS and RSI showed low specificity, and

there was no significant difference between test and control groups. These findings suggest that both RSI and RFS should not be used as the sole diagnostic test for initiating PPI therapy.

Routine, long-term use of PPI in patients with elevated RSI/RFS, without proven LPR, may be ill-advised because of potential complications of therapy discussed elsewhere in this chapter. In addition, while PPIs are widely prescribed, resolution of LPR symptoms has been equivocal and often incomplete. Patients presenting with symptoms consistent with LPR are difficult to diagnose definitively, with most technologies providing no solid evidence on which a diagnosis or treatment can be based.[342]

Borrowing from the standards of gastroesophageal reflux disorder (GERD), the suggested definition of LPR has been a single episode of pH <4 or 1% total time below a pH of 4 on dual-lumen probe.[343–345] Although standard 24-hour monitor technique has good diagnostic utility for the presence of LPR, it often causes significant patient discomfort, both in placement and throughout the monitoring period.[346,347] Other studies have reported lack of sleep and dysphagia with a dual-lumen probe.[348] Hence, patients who alter their eating and sleeping habits may have tests that are not representative of their disease state. A new probe has been developed for monitoring the oropharyngeal pH and for the diagnosis of at least severe LPR. Multiple studies have demonstrated the ability of this device to detect reflux events compared to a traditional pH probe.

In 2009, Golub et al[348] studied 15 patients with symptoms of LPR by simultaneously placing a dual-lumen pH probe and the Restech (Houston, Texas) oropharyngeal probe. This study revealed that the correlation between the 2 probes for reflux events was 0.95 ($p < .001$). In a separate study, Wiener et al[346] compared the Restech probe to 3 traditional pH probes (2 esophageal, 1 pharyngeal) in 15 patients with symptoms of LPR. In this study, all events detected by the Restech probe were preceded by events in the distal esophagus. This study revealed the Restech probe to be a sensitive device that can detect pH events that originate in the distal esophagus and migrate toward the oropharynx.

In addition to the high correlation with traditional pH, the Restech probe offers some significant advantages. First, sensors in the conventional pH probe require a liquid environment to function properly. Traditional probes placed in the oropharynx have a tendency to dry out and lead to "false-positive" readings (pseudo-reflux). The Restech probe does not require a liquid environment to provide real-time pH readings. Second, the sensors for traditional probes are located on the side of the catheter, which leads to the possibility of masking by the mucosal wall and "false-negative" readings. The sensor on the Restech probe is located on the teardrop-shaped tip, which decreases the possibility of mucosal masking. Furthermore, the placement of a traditional probe requires manometric (radiographic in infants) confirmation of placement. The placement of the Restech probe can be confirmed visually with simple oropharyngeal examination by localizing the red LED light in the catheter tip.

Recently, multiple studies have addressed the utility of the Restech probe in a clinical setting. A study by Friedman et al[349] revealed that in a group of 163 patients with suspected LPR, there was no correlation between RSI and the oropharyngeal environment. In addition, the calculated positive and negative predictive values for RSI and severe reflux (positive Ryan score) were 44.3% and 58.7%, respectively. The authors recommend that diagnosis and treatment

decisions regarding LPR should be on the basis of symptoms (RSI), signs (RSF or oropharyngeal findings), and a confirmatory test (pH testing). In a prospective study[350] of 18 patients with symptoms of LPR, 100% of patients with positive Ryan scores (by Restech) responded to PPI therapy, while less than half of those with a negative study responded. While the specific pH profile of Ryan-negative PPI responders needs to be elucidated, these results suggest that the Restech probe may be useful in determining which patients will respond to PPI therapy. In a separate 2011 study by Friedman et al,[351] 143 patients were offered either empiric PPI treatment (70 patients) or Restech-based treatment (73 patients) for symptoms of LPR. This study revealed that patients tested with the Restech probe had significantly greater compliance with medication (68.5% vs 50%, $p = .019$) and lifestyle modification (82.2% vs 25.7%, $p < .01$) as well as significantly greater reduction in RSI (36.6% vs 24%, $p = .023$). Collectively, these studies suggest Restech has utility in the diagnosis of LPR and selection of patients who might benefit from treatment, as well as in improving patient compliance.

Based on current literature and the side effect profile of antireflux medication, questions must be considered about whether to treat all symptomatic patients empirically without first determining their oropharyngeal pH profile. More research is needed (and is in progress). If the Restech probe is really as reliable and valid as traditional dual lumen probes and offers some advantages over dual lumen probes placed below the UES or in the oropharynx, it may become a standard diagnostic tool. While often associated with GERD, LPR is a different disease state that presents its own set of problems in terms of diagnosis and treatment protocols. This becomes especially true with patients in the "gray zone" presenting with mild to moderate reflux. Currently, multiple groups are using the Restech probe to help better determine disease state/severity. This determination should lead to improved ability to predict those who will respond well to standard antireflux therapy versus those who need more aggressive management. Equally important is the elimination of empiric treatment for those who do not have LPR and faster workup to identify the true etiology of their symptoms and signs.

Esophageal Manometry

Manometry will establish abnormal LES pressure or esophageal motility and is necessary preoperatively to evaluate contraction amplitude in the esophageal body. A single measurement of LES pressure is rarely low in patients with GERD. In the author's (POK) experience, only 4% of patients with GERD have a low LES pressure.[352] Esophageal motility abnormalities are found more frequently. The most common finding appears to be ineffective esophageal motility (IEM) (amplitude of contraction in the distal esophagus less than 30 mm Hg occurring with 30% or more of water swallows). In our experience, this is the most common abnormality in patients with GERD, seen in approximately 35% of patients with esophagitis.[352] IEM appears even more common in GERD-related laryngitis, asthma, and cough.[57] Esophageal manometry is performed prior to antireflux surgery to establish the presence or absence of ineffective esophageal motility. The surgeon will usually perform a Nissen fundoplication (360° wrap) in patients with normal peristalsis and a Toupet procedure (240° wrap) in patients with significant IEM. Patients with IEM and respiratory symptoms do not appear to respond as well

to antireflux surgery if respiratory complaints are the presenting symptom.

Esophageal manometry is important also for proper placement of probes for pH monitoring. Although the proximal probe can be positioned accurately by direct vision using a flexible fiberoptic laryngoscope, mirror, or telescope, without manometry there is no way to position the distal probe precisely. However, when compared to manometry, even proximal probe placement was accurate in only 70% of cases in the study by Johnson et al.[353] Distal probe placement was accurate in just 40% of cases using estimated interprobe distance. Using fixed interprobe distances of 15 cm and 20 cm, distal probe placement was accurate in only 3% (for 15 cm) or 40% (for 20 cm) of cases. These errors are critical because the normative values for distal esophageal acid exposure were established with the distal probe positioned 5 cm above the LES.[354–357] Even slight modifications in the distance between the distal probe and the lower esophageal sphincter cause substantial changes in acid exposure data.[358–361]

Hiatal Hernia

A hiatal hernia is not predictive of reflux as a cause of the patients' symptoms.[362] Up to 60% of patients over the age of 60 will demonstrate a hiatal hernia identified on barium swallow examination. One study suggested that only 9% of patients with a radiographically demonstrated hernia have typical reflux symptoms.[77] Hernias do change the relationship of the LES and crural diaphragm. The LES is displaced above the diaphragm. The low pressure in the hernia can act as a reservoir for acid, allowing earlier reflux during LES relaxations, and may delay esophageal clearance.[363] Patients with large hernias who also have low LES pressure may be more prone to reflux[364] if changes occur in intra-abdominal pressure.

Evaluation for *Helicobacter pylori*

H pylori appears to play a role in the development of chronic type B gastritis, gastroduodenal ulcer disease, and gastric carcinoma.[365,366] Its significance in gastroesophageal reflux disease remains uncertain, and it is unclear whether it is necessary to treat *H pylori* in reflux patients, or even advisable to do so. *H pylori* can be detected through serologic determination of immunoglobin (IgG) antibodies to the organism. This blood test is performed using an enzyme-linked immunosorbent assay (ELISA)/2-step indirect sandwich assay on directly coated microtiter plates.[367] This test is believed to have a sensitivity of 94% and specificity of 85%.[367]

Researchers continue to examine the relationship between *H pylori* infection, LPR, and laryngeal diseases.[368,369] Siupsinskiene et al[370] performed a prospective case control study to examine the presence of *H pylori* through biopsy of the larynx in patients with laryngeal cancer and patients with benign laryngeal disease, including LPR and vocal fold polyps. They examined the biopsy results from 67 adult patients with benign and malignant laryngeal disease and compared them with a control group of 11 patients. They reported *H pylori* infection in greater than one-third of the patients studied, with the majority found in patients with laryngeal cancer (46.2%) and in those with chronic laryngitis (45.5%). The authors reported that these findings differed significantly from the control group (9.1%) (*p* < .05), adding that they found

no significant relationship between LPR-related symptoms and *H pylori* detected in the larynx. They stated that *H pylori* can colonize in patients with benign laryngeal disease and laryngeal cancer, but that further research is needed. Another study by Islam et al[371] also examined the presence of *H pylori* in patients with benign and malignant laryngeal disease. They performed a prospective study of 50 patients who underwent microlaryngoscopy over a 2-year period. Their patient population was diagnosed as having LPR based on a Reflux Symptom Index (RSI) greater than 12 and a Reflux Finding Score (RFS) greater than 6. The patients were diagnosed with *H pylori* based on a positive urea breath test, HP citotoxin-associated gene A(CAGA)-IgG, and HP-IGG test results. Intraoperatively, 2 surgical specimens were obtained, one from the interarytenoid area and one from the primary vocal fold lesion. The authors reported that *H pylori* was not found in any interarytenoid specimen, and they found no histologic evidence of *H pylori* in the vocal fold pathology specimens. They also reported "there was no difference between RSS-positive and RSS-negative patients in terms of HP-IGG and UBT," adding that "the presence of HP in the gastric mucosa does not have an effect on the RSS and RSI." Their study conclusions disagree with other reports in the literature and with the author's (RTS) experience.

Campbell et al[372] reviewed the role of *H pylori* in laryngopharyngeal reflux. Their objective was to determine the prevalence of *H pylori* among patients with LPR and to determine whether *H pylori* eradication would lead to greater improvement in patients with laryngopharyngeal reflux as compared to standard proton pump inhibitor therapy alone. In their study, they reported an overall prevalence of *H pylori* of 43.9% in patients with LPR. Their prevalence rate was determined by meta-analysis of 13 publications, most of which reported studies conducted in southeast Europe and western Asia. The authors felt that it remained unclear whether a rate of 43.9% justified recommended investigating and treating LPR patients for *H pylori*. Additionally, they pointed out that eradication of *H pylori* had been successful in significantly reducing some symptoms of LPR and that the relationship requires further study.

In a separate article on *H pylori* infection, Diaconu et al[373] at the University of Medicine and Pharmacy in Bucharest, Romania, provided a comprehensive review of *H pylori* diagnosis and treatment over the years. They stated that the clinical manifestations of *H pylori* range from asymptomatic gastritis to gastrointestinal malignancy. They found that mucosa-associated lymphoid tissue (MALT) lymphoma is a low-grade, B-cell, marginal zone lymphoma and that *H pylori* has been detected in more than 75% of patients with MALT lymphoma. They stated that the eradication of *H pylori* prevents the return of ulcers and ulcer complications even after appropriate medications such as PPIs are stopped. They also reported that several diseases such as idiopathic thrombocytopenic purpura (ITP), iron deficiency anemia, and vitamin B12 deficiency also have been associated with *H pylori* infection. The authors stated that the most common initial treatment includes triple therapy, including the use of a proton pump inhibitor, amoxicillin, and clarithromycin.

Choe et al[374] observed that the standard triple therapy for treatment of *H pylori* has yielded very low treatment success in Korea. According to their article, Korea is an area of high clarithromycin resistance. They conducted a study adding elemental bismuth (240 mg bid) in addition to rabeprazole 20 mg, metronidazole 750 mg, and amoxicillin 1 g daily (PAM-B therapy) for 14 days. The study compared PAM-B therapy with the standard triple treatment for *H pylori* infection in 270 randomized patients. They reported high success in both groups, 88.1% and 83.0%, respectively. Six weeks after treatment, the *H pylori* was eradicated. They recommend PAM-B therapy as an alternative to standard triple therapy for first-line eradication of *H pylori* in Korea.

Approach to the Patient With GERD-Related Otolaryngologic Abnormalities

In patients with GERD-related otolaryngologic complaints, a thorough history, physical examination, and laryngoscopy should be performed (Figure 9–19). If dysphagia is present, a functional endoscopic evaluation of swallowing (FEES) or videoendoscopic swallowing evaluation should be considered, and a barium swallow should be obtained to rule out stricture or motility abnormalities. The clinician's dilemma revolves around the choice of early diagnostic testing with prolonged pH monitoring or institution of a therapeutic trial of medication. The "best" approach is not clear. Although diagnostic testing with ambulatory pH monitoring would be ideal, there are several limitations: (1) pH monitoring is not always available, (2) the sensitivity and specificity are clearly not 100%, (3) patients do not reflux with the same frequency every day, and (4) variability in both distal and proximal esophageal acid exposure time in patients with extraesophageal GERD is common, increasing the possibility of a false-negative pH study if physiologic acid exposure is seen on a single study.

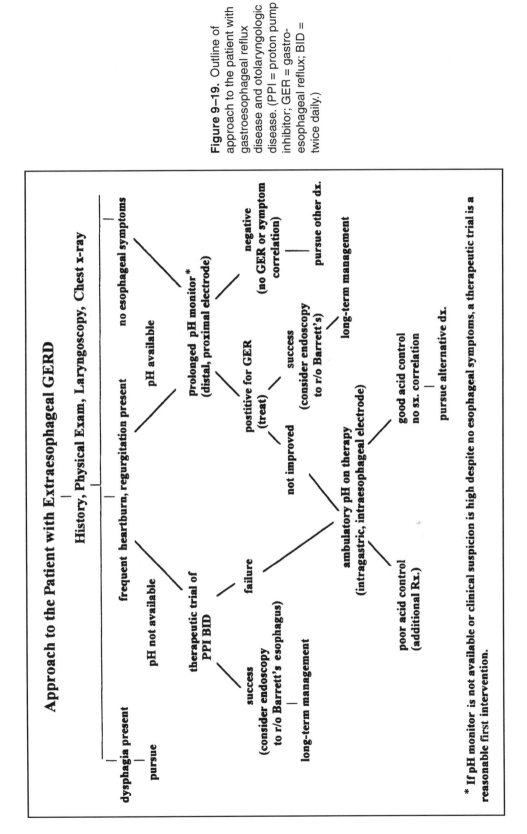

Figure 9–19. Outline of approach to the patient with gastroesophageal reflux disease and otolaryngologic disease. (PPI = proton pump inhibitor; GER = gastro-esophageal reflux; BID = twice daily.)

237

If the history and laryngoscopic examination raise a high clinical suspicion of GERD or LPR, if prolonged monitoring is not available, if frequent heartburn and regurgitation are present, or if there is endoscopic documentation of GERD or LPR, a therapeutic trial of antireflux therapy is a reasonable initial choice. An early study with empiric omeprazole, 40 mg at bedtime, in patients with suspected reflux laryngitis found a 67% response in patients with laryngeal symptoms suggestive of GERD.[375] Another study found 70% success with empiric omeprazole 20 mg BID for a similar time period.[376] We use a trial of a PPI twice daily in combination with dietary and behavior modification initially for 8 to 12 weeks. If the patient does not respond, pH monitoring should be performed while PPI therapy is continued. A dual-channel probe with intragastric and distal esophageal electrodes should be placed to ascertain adequate gastric acid suppression and to assess the presence of esophageal acid exposure. If distal esophageal acid exposure is seen more than 1.2% of the time, this is definitely abnormal and additional medical therapy is indicated.[377] "Normal" esophageal acid exposure, particularly when any proximal esophageal acid exposure is documented, may not always be a negative study. A positive symptom index may be seen even in patients with "normal" distal acid exposure, and this, too, is abnormal and warrants additional therapy. The absence of any esophageal acid exposure and presence of adequate gastric acid suppression (pH >4, 50% of total time) suggests adequate medical therapy in most patients, and an alternative diagnosis should be considered. If GERD-associated otolaryngologic disease is documented, endoscopy is indicated in many cases to rule out Barrett's esophagus prior to initiating long-term medical therapy or surgery.

Outcomes Measures

In addition to using instruments discussed elsewhere such as the Voice Handicap Index (VHI)[378] that were designed to measures outcomes of voice disorders, Belafsky, Postma, and Koufman[379] have introduced "The Reflux Finding Score (RFS)." The RFS depends on observations of subglottic edema, ventricular obliteration, erythema/hyperemia, vocal fold edema, diffuse laryngeal edema, posterior laryngeal hypertrophy, granuloma/granulation tissue, and thick endolaryngeal mucus. Although additional research from other centers is needed to confirm the validity and reliability of the RFS, the authors found excellent inter- and intraobserver reproducibility (although all observers were practicing at the same medical center); they found the RFS to be an accurate instrument for documenting treatment efficacy in patients with LPR. Other quality-of-life evaluations have highlighted the impact of GERD and LPR on patient function.[380,381] The Pharyngeal Reflux Symptom Questionnaire was developed by Andersson et al.[382] It is a self-administered questionnaire specific for LPR patients. They compared this tool with the LPR-Health Related Quality of Life and the reflux symptom index and reported strong correlation. The authors also reported that the questionnaire discriminated between patients without and with LPR. Several reports[383,384] have suggested that anxiety, depression, and depression symptoms can impact subjective responses to quality-of-life tools and symptom indices and thus diminish the predictive value of symptom assessment, which raises concern about the usefulness of these tools. Researchers in China[385] reported significantly higher Voice Handicap Index scores and higher depression scores in their patients with LPR.

Nishimura et al.[386] evaluated postoperative LPR in patients who had undergone surgery for esophageal cancer. They proposed a classification system for grading findings on endoscopy to facilitate more accurate diagnosis of LPR in this patient population.

Behavioral and Medical Management of Gastroesophageal Reflux Disease

Treatment of the patient with GERD requires careful consideration of the primary symptom presentation, degree of mucosal injury, and the presence or absence of complications. Treatment focuses on 4 goals: elimination of symptoms, healing of mucosal injury if present, management of complications, and maintenance of symptomatic remission. Treatment should combine lifestyle modifications, pharmacologic therapy, and appropriate use of antireflux surgery. GERD is a chronic condition that may recur quickly if therapy is stopped or medication dosage is decreased; therefore, long-term therapy is the key to effective management and often requires continuous full prescription doses of appropriate medications. Symptom relief and mucosal healing in GERD are directly related to control of intragastric acid secretion (the time during which gastric pH is less than 4) and reduction of esophageal acid exposure.[387] Clinical trials in patients with symptomatic erosive esophagitis suggest that a careful and systematic stepwise approach to medical therapy will result in satisfactory symptom relief in over 90% of patients.[388]

In contrast, there have been relatively few clinical trials of treatment involving patients with asthma, cough, laryngopharyngeal reflux (LPR), and other extraesoph-ageal manifestations of GERD. Most trials have been uncontrolled, and maintenance trials are lacking. Treatment is based on the principles for treating patients with heartburn and erosive esophagitis and observations from available clinical trials and clinical experience. As a general rule, patients with LPR and the other extraesophageal manifestations of GERD require higher doses of pharmacologic therapy, usually with PPIs twice daily, with longer periods of treatment needed to achieve complete relief of symptoms compared to patients with heartburn and erosive esophagitis. Although relief of symptoms, healing of mucosal injury, and maintenance of remission are still the primary goals, assessing these end points is somewhat more difficult as the "gold standard" for diagnosis is not always clear. The principles of the medical treatment of GERD with specific emphasis on LPR and other extraesophageal manifestations of GERD are discussed below.

Lifestyle Modification and Patient Education

Simple and effective changes in lifestyle are crucial in controlling symptoms of GERD. Educating patients about the recurring nature and chronicity of GERD and LPR is crucial to compliance with long-term medical management. Studies with overnight pH monitoring have shown a significant decrease in total esophageal acid exposure after elevation of the head of the bed 6 inches compared to sleeping flat.[388] Recent studies continue to support the critical importance of head of bed elevation in the management of LPR.[389,390] A similar effect can be produced by placing a foam rubber wedge under the patient's mattress. A long (full length) wedge is preferable to tilt the whole mattress rather than bending it at the waist level. The use of pillows in lieu of a wedge or head-of-the-bed elevation cannot be recommended, because bending of the waist and change in body position may paradoxically increase intra-abdominal pressure and increase reflux. In addition, if patients roll over on their stomachs while sleeping on pillows, bending backward may result in lower back pain, which may lead them to stop complying with instructions to elevate their torsos. An effective alternative approach is to instruct patients to preferentially sleep lying on their left side. This will place the esophagogastric junction in an advantageous position above the gastric contents and has been shown to significantly decrease recumbent reflux.[391]

Elimination or decreasing of gastric irritants from the diet will reduce symptoms. These agents include citrus juices, tomato products, coffee (both caffeinated and decaffeinated), and alcohol. Colas, tea, and other acidic fluids are often overlooked as potential gastric and esophageal irritants.[392] A meal high in fat will increase postprandial reflux episodes in patients with GERD,[393] so a low-fat diet is recommended. Chocolate and other carminatives will decrease lower esophageal pressure (LES) and increase reflux frequency,[394] as will onions, and should be eliminated from the diet (Table 9–6). Koufman[395] evaluated the clinical impact of a low-acid diet on therapeutic outcome in patients treated for LPR. She studied a group of 20 patients with persistent signs and symptoms of LPR despite twice-daily use of a PPI and a histamine-2 (H2) blocker at bedtime. The low-acid diet described by Koufman eliminated all foods and beverages with a pH less than 5. The patients were placed on this diet for a minimum of 2 weeks, and both the Reflux Symptom Index and the Reflux Finding Score were determined before and after the diet. Koufman's findings show that both the clin-

Table 9–6. Lifestyle Modifications for Treatment of Gastroesophageal Reflux

Elevation of head of bed (6 inches)—avoid waterbed

Dietary modifications
1. Lower fat, higher protein
2. Avoid specific irritants
   a. Citrus juices
   b. Tomato products
   c. Coffee, tea
   d. Alcohol
   e. Colas
   f. Onions
3. No eating prior to sleeping (allow at least 2 hours)
4. Avoid chocolate, carminatives (lower LES pressure)

Decrease or stop smoking

Avoid potentially harmful medications
1. Affect LES pressure
   a. Anticholinergics
   b. Sedatives/tranquilizers
   c. Theophylline
   d. Prostaglandins
   e. Calcium-channel blockers
2. Potentially cause esophageal injury
   a. Potassium tablets
   b. Ferrous sulfate
   c. Antibiotics (gelatin capsules), eg, tetracycline
   d. NSAIDs, aspirin
   e. Alendronate

Abbreviation: LES = Lower esophageal sphincter.

ical signs and symptoms in these patients who had had persistent symptoms despite PPI treatment improved following an acid-free diet. Gastric distention provides the major stimulus for transient lower esophageal sphincter relaxation (TLESR), the most common abnormality responsible for individual reflux episodes. Eating large, high-fat meals increases gastric distention and slows gastric emptying, probably increasing TLESRs. Going to sleep on a full stomach or lying down after a meal also creates a stimulus for TLESR and is likely to increase reflux. It is therefore critical to remind patients to avoid eating within 2 to 3 hours of sleep and to avoid recumbency after a meal, especially if reflux occurs when they are supine (which is not always the case with LPR).[394] An interesting study by Hamdan et al[396] studied the effects of fasting vs nonfasting (12 hours) on LPR findings in 22 males and reported no significant effects on LPR symptoms in this population (RSI scores), or in RFSs of laryngeal examinations. Smoking may decrease LES pressure and delay esophageal clearance, increasing reflux frequency and potentially mucosal injury. This is likely due to the effects of nicotine.

Smoking may decrease the effectiveness of H2-receptor antagonists, especially at night (when reflux injury is more severe due to delayed esophageal clearance of refluxate); however, the effect of smoking on the action of PPIs is not known. Clearly, smoking can be detrimental to overall health—exacerbation of GERD is no exception. One study examined the effects of lifestyle modifications, including raising the head of the bed 6 inches, eliminating meals before bedtime, and using antacids in the treatment of patients with respiratory symptoms and GERD. Outcomes were compared to patients not using antireflux measures for 2-month periods. In this study, both esophageal and respiratory symptoms were reported to improve with lifestyle modifications compared to no antireflux therapy. However, no objective changes were noted in pulmonary function and endoscopy was not performed.[389] This suggests that the addition of the conservative measures outlined in Table 9–6 is useful in treatment of extraesophageal GERD. No studies have specifically examined lifestyle modifica-

tions in patients with LPR. However, we routinely recommend the use of these conservative measures as patients often reflux during the postprandial period, even when they are upright.

The importance of including lifestyle modifications as part of a treatment program at a time when very efficacious drug therapy, such as PPIs, is available has been debated. All clinical trials have included these lifestyle changes as part of treatment, so the effect of eliminating them is not known. These lifestyle modifications are easy to explain and implement and are of low economic cost. Based on symptom severity and control, patients can decide for themselves how diligent they should be. Some patients with mild, infrequent symptoms may avoid regular prescription medications by following these modifications as recommended. They appear somewhat less likely to be sufficient in many voice professionals, especially in singers who experience upright reflux when they sing due to increased intra-abdominal pressure that occurs with proper voice support. However, if 24-hour pH monitor studies show that these patients do not experience supine and/or nocturnal reflux, it may be unnecessary for them to elevate the head of the bed. Head of bed elevation can be a substantial inconvenience for performers who may spend 200 nights per year or more in hotel rooms. Therapies for such patients should be rational and individualized on the basis of symptoms, signs, and test results.[82]

The diagnoses represented within the gluten sensitivity spectrum are as diverse and nebulous as are its presenting symptoms, as we have discussed elsewhere[397] and are reviewing here. One of the best categorizations found in the recent literature subdivides gluten sensitivity into allergic, autoimmune, and nonallergic/nonautoimmune, or simply immune.[398] The allergy category includes wheat allergy (WA) or food allergy, wheat-dependent exercise-induced anaphylaxis (WDEIA), occupational or Baker's asthma, and contact urticaria. The autoimmune category includes celiac disease (CD), dermatitis herpetiformis, and gluten ataxia. Nonceliac gluten sensitivity (NCGS) belongs to the third category, which is the newest and least studied but also the most intriguing. The scientific community is just beginning to recognize the existence of NCGS as a disease with distinct pathophysiologic and epidemiologic characteristics. While the prevalence of CD in the United States is between 0.5% and 1%,[399] epidemiologic studies place NCGS prevalence in the United States slightly higher, with best estimates ranging from 0.55% to 6%.[400,401]

Gluten sensitivity, including CD and NCGS, presents with gastrointestinal and extraintestinal symptoms. The most common GI complaints include irritable bowel syndrome (IBS)–like symptoms (eg, bloating, abdominal pain, bowel habit abnormalities such as diarrhea and/or constipation) and even symptoms of GERD (heartburn and regurgitation).[402] For example, between 2004 and 2010, 5896 patients were seen at the Center for Celiac Research, University of Maryland.[403] The criteria for gluten sensitivity were fulfilled by 347 (6%) of the patients seen. Their symptoms included abdominal pain (68%); eczema and/or rash (40%); headache (35%); "foggy mind" (34%); fatigue (33%); diarrhea (33%); depression (22%); anemia (20%); numbness in the legs, arms, or fingers (20%); and joint pain (11%). Other studies have confirmed these symptoms in this population.[404,405] Gluten sensitivity, particularly CD, also has been associated with an increased risk of other autoimmune disorders such as autoimmune thyroiditis, type I diabetes mellitus, Addison disease, Crohn's and ulcerative colitis, myasthenia gravis, and psoriasis.[403] It is

equally important to recognize that some of these patients have minimal or no symptoms, making it even more difficult to select those who would benefit from a diagnostic workup. Fasano et al[404] found that 41% of patients with positive serology for CD were asymptomatic. This problem is compounded further by the nonspecific nature of extraintestinal symptoms, the variable effect of gluten on an individual's immune system, the observation that many patients are already on a gluten-free diet (GFD) or a low fermentable oligo-di-monosaccharides and polyols (FODMAP) diet at the time of presentation, and the possibility that other extraintestinal symptoms may be linked but not yet identified. It is conceivable, given the current evidence linking gluten sensitivity with GERD, that the signs and symptoms attributed to LPR also might be linked to gluten sensitivity in this population, but this possibility has not been studied.

At the present time, there are insufficient data linking CD and NCGS with LPR. Conversely, studies have identified that the esophagus is not spared in patients with gluten sensitivity. Consistent data are now available on the presence of disturbed motility of the esophagus, along with the stomach, small intestine, gallbladder, and colon of untreated patients with CD.[406–413] Using esophageal manometry, Usai et al[411] studied the presence of specific esophageal motor disorders in this population. They reported motor abnormalities in 67% of 18 patients with CD. They consisted of nutcracker esophagus (50%), low pressure in LES associated with simultaneous contractions (11%), and frequent repetitive contractions (22%). No subjects in the control group (34 patients) and the ulcerative colitis group (9 patients) had these manometric abnormalities. Additional interesting findings in the study group were the presence of dysphagia in 50% (vs 9% of controls) and odynophagia in 14% (vs 0% of controls) of 36 patients with CD.

There have been studies exploring GERD in the gluten-sensitive population, primarily those with CD. The findings show that GERD symptoms are more common in patients with CD than in the general population. In a study by Nachman et al,[412] 30% of patients complained of moderate-to-severe GERD symptoms at the time of CD diagnosis (defined as score >3 in the Gastrointestinal Symptoms Rating Scale), a rate 6-fold higher than the rate seen in healthy controls (5.7%). A GFD has been shown to improve symptoms of GERD in patients with CD, irrespective of PPI therapy.[411–414] Because GERD-like symptoms can be a presentation of active celiac disease and non-celiac gluten sensitivity, some studies have concluded that celiac disease should be considered, and investigated, by means of serology or with duodenal biopsies during EGD, in patients with refractory GERD, especially if these patients exhibit other signs or symptoms suggestive of CD.[415]Although Collin et al[416] argued against screening for CD in patients with reflux esophagitis, concluding that GERD is not a major manifestation of CD, they also commented that a GFD may result in symptomatic relief of reflux symptoms in patients with CD. The study also did not explore this question in patients with NCGS.

A study by Lamanda et al[413] documented esophageal erosive lesions in 23% of 65 adult patients diagnosed with CD over a year, a prevalence far above that which was established for the general population. Cuomo et al[417] monitored esophageal pH in 15 out of the 39 celiac patients included in their case series; 14 out of 15 showed pathologic pH levels. Furthermore, lower esophageal sphincter (LES) pressure values trended lower than those observed in healthy controls, although the differences did not reach

statistical significance. There is interesting literature illustrating the relationship that exists between GERD and GFD in patients with CD. A GFD alone reduces severity of both heartburn and regurgitation significantly in adults with CD.[418,419] In patients with CD treated with PPI, a GFD also reduced the risk of recurrence of GERD-related symptoms after discontinuation of antisecretory treatment. Nachman et al[412] found that after 3 months from the start of the GFD, GERD-related symptom scores had decreased significantly in their series of adult patients with CD, reaching values similar to those of healthy controls. Lamanda et al[413] showed that GERD symptoms had remitted in 91% of adult patients with CD after 4 weeks of treatment with PPI at standard doses, with no relapse in any case after 12 months of follow-up on GFD. A GFD also has been shown to prevent recurrence of GERD-related symptoms in patients with CD who have both erosive and nonerosive esophatitis.[405,406] Long-term benefits of a GFD on GERD symptoms still persist in the event of partial compliance.[415]

The potential association between LPR and gluten sensitivity was not investigated until our (RTS) preliminary study. In our practice, this connection has become more apparent after a growing number of patients have reported improvement in symptoms usually associated with LPR while following a GFD.

Numerous mechanisms have been proposed to explain the association of gluten sensitivity and GERD. In summary, they have included nutrient malabsorption affecting gastroesophageal motility, GI hormonal derangements causing decreased LES pressures and dysmotility, and the inflammatory reaction to gluten resulting in increased mucosal permeability.[396,397] Wex et al[418] report that zonulin, a protein involved in the regulation of interepithelial permeability in the intestines of CD patients, may be implicated because it was found to be expressed in esophageal epithelial cells, as well. In addition to these potential mechanisms, Iovino[405] has proposed the possible involvement of neurotransmitters and the direct toxic effect of gluten on muscular tissues. In a similar manner, one or more of these potential mechanisms could contribute to the presence of LPR in these patients.

Tursi[415] reported on 3 patients with GERD refractory to antisecretory treatment who were diagnosed with CD after duodenal biopsies and who had rapid and long-lasting remission of symptoms after starting a GFD. In one example, a 24-year-old woman had persistent GERD symptoms despite esomeprazole 80 mg/day. Twenty days after starting PPI therapy, celiac disease was diagnosed based on histologic evaluation, and the patient was started immediately on a GFD. Symptoms improved within 7 days and disappeared completely within 2 weeks of GFD despite cessation of PPI therapy, and she remained symptom free 6 months later.

Lucendo[406] acknowledged this observation by stating that the lack of response to PPI therapy to improve GERD symptoms, even after increasing the doses, could be the key for suspecting and actively excluding CD. Regardless of the pathophysiology of GERD symptoms in patients with CD, the question arises whether GFD should be added to antisecretory treatment, because it appears that symptom improvement may be more related in these patients to gluten suppression than to medication. In his editorial, Tursi[415] proposed avoiding antisecretory medications altogether and instead using antacids such as sodium alginate to treat nonerosive GERD in patients with CD until gluten elimination reversed clinical symptoms.

The current literature has shown that GERD is more prevalent in patients with CD and that it responds favorably to GFD. Pending future studies, a similar observation is likely to be established between GERD and NCGS. The impact of gluten sensitivity on LPR, however, represents a new frontier of untapped research potential. From our clinical observations and identifications of current gaps in existing knowledge, it can be concluded that further research investigating this potential relationship is warranted. We have incorporated consideration for possible gluten sensitivity into our routine assessment of patients with suspected LPR (Figure 9–20). At a minimum, the knowledge presented here should prove useful for laboratory screening and referring patients to our gastroenterology colleagues if suspicion for gluten sensitivity arises. Following the most recent literature and national guidelines on CD and NCGS including the American College of Gastroenterology (ACG),[420,421] our practice has initiated laboratory testing for patients with LPR, particularly when refractory to antisecretory reflux therapy or when indicated by the patient's history. This laboratory panel includes the following:

- Tissue transglutanimase (TTG) IgA, IgG
- Deamidated gliadin peptide (DGP) IgA, IgG
- Antigliadin antibody (AGA) IgA, IgG
- Total IgA
- Wheat-specific IgE
- HLA-DQ genotyping

Some laboratories have incorporated reflex testing into their celiac disease panels to look for tissue transglutaminase IgG if total IgA is low, for example, because 2% to 3% of patients with celiac disease also have IgA deficiency. HLA DQ2 or DQ8 is present in nearly 100% of patients with celiac disease, while it is present in 50% of patients

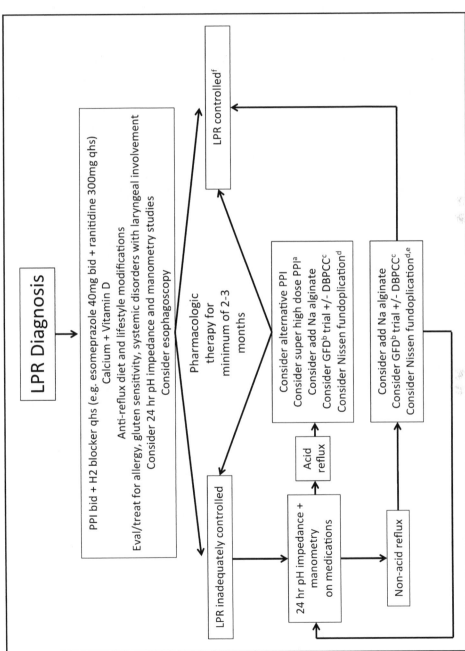

Figure 9–20. Laryngopharyngeal reflux algorithm incorporating gluten sensitivity evaluation and management. [a]Portnoy JE, Gregory ND, Cerull CE, et al. Efficacy of super high dose proton pump inhibitor administration in refractory laryngopharyngeal reflux: a pilot study. *J Voice.* 2014;28(3):369–377. [b]Gluten-free diet may be considered at any step in the pathway with serologic testing recommended prior to initiation. [c]DBPCC = double-blind placebo controlled (gluten) challenge. [d]Repeat 24-hour pH impedance with manometry off antisecretory medications is recommended 3 months post-Nissen fundoplication. [e]Nissen fundoplication is likely to be therapeutic for non–acid reflux laryngitis, especially if a positive symptom index during 24-hour pH impedance testing. [f]Nissen fundoplication should be considered for patients who do not want to use antisecretory medications long term.

Diagram content:

LPR Diagnosis

PPI bid + H2 blocker qhs (e.g. esomeprazole 40mg bid + ranitidine 300mg qhs)
Calcium + Vitamin D
Anti-reflux diet and lifestyle modifications
Eval/treat for allergy, gluten sensitivity, systemic disorders with laryngeal involvement
Consider 24 hr pH impedance and manometry studies
Consider esophagoscopy

Pharmacologic therapy for minimum of 2–3 months

LPR controlled[f]

LPR inadequately controlled

24 hr pH impedance + manometry on medications

Acid reflux

Non-acid reflux

Consider alternative PPI
Consider super high dose PPI[a]
Consider add Na alginate
Consider GFD[b] trial +/- DBPCC[c]
Consider Nissen fundoplication[d]

Consider add Na alginate
Consider GFD[b] trial +/- DBPCC[c]
Consider Nissen fundoplication[d,e]

with NCGS and 30% to 40% of the general population. This test, along with AGA IgG (positive in 56% of patients with NCGS), presently are the only 2 commercially available laboratory tests that have been shown to be positive more often in NCGS patients than in the general population. Algorithms have been developed to help guide evaluation and workup,[422-424] and our approach is summarized in Table 9–7. If CD is diagnosed or if NCGS is suspected, a GFD trial may be recommended, along with referrals to a gastroenterologist and a nutritionist.

Medications that decrease esophageal pressures and promote reflux include anticholinergics, sedatives or tranquilizers, tricyclic antidepressants, theophylline, nitrates, and calcium-channel blocking agents. Many other drugs are known to cause direct esophageal injury (pill-induced esophagitis).[425] The most common are KCl (potassium chloride) tablets, iron sulfate, gelatin capsule antibiotics, nonsteroidal anti-inflammatory drugs (NSAIDs), and alendronate (Fosamax).[426] These should be used with caution in patients with GERD. Although there is no direct evidence that these agents cause GERD, they can cause esophageal injury and may make mucosal injury from reflux more severe (see

Table 9–7. Laboratory Evaluation of Gluten Sensitivity

Lab Test	Can Test on Gluten-Free Diet?	Indication	Sensitivity	Specificity
Tissue transglutaminase (TTG)				
TTG IgA	No	Celiac disease	98%	98%
TTG IgG	No	Celiac disease	70%	95%
Deamidated gliadin peptide (DGP)				
DGP IgA	No	Celiac disease	88%	95%
DGP IgG	No	Celiac disease	80%	98%
Anti-gliadin antibody (AGA)				
AGA IgA	No	Celiac disease	85%	90%
AGA IgG	No	Celiac disease/ **NCGS**	85% (CD)	80% (CD)
Endomysial Antibody IgA	No	Celiac disease	95%	99%
Wheat specific IgE	No	Wheat allergy (IgE)	83%	43%
HLA DQ2 and DQ8	Yes	Celiac disease/ **NCGS**	~100% (CD)	Low; varies depending on population

Abbreviations: CD = celiac disease; NCGS = nonceliac gluten sensitivity.

Table 9–6). The effects of these agents vary from patient to patient. Experience suggests that none of these drugs greatly exacerbates GERD, so discontinuing a needed agent is usually not necessary, especially with concomitant use of PPIs.

Over-the-Counter Agents

Numerous antacids and over-the-counter H2-receptor antagonists are available to treat patients with symptomatic reflux. These agents should be used exclusively to treat symptoms such as heartburn that is intermittent and as adjuncts to prescription therapy for breakthrough symptoms. Symptom relief is similar with equipotent antacids and all of the H2-antagonists available over the counter. Because patients with LPR often require long-term (or lifetime) therapy with high doses of PPIs or H2-blockers in full prescription doses, management with over-the-counter (low-dose) H2-blockers is rarely adequate.

The use of antacids remains controversial. Experts agree that they should be superfluous if *sufficient* doses of acid suppression medication therapy are used. However, there are differences of opinion regarding the level of control achieved in most patients on the customary doses of PPIs (omeprazole 40 mg daily, or the equivalent) and on the importance of occasional episodes of breakthrough reflux. It is well known that reflux may still occur on daily 40-mg doses of omeprazole or 60 mg of lansoprazole. This has been confirmed by pH monitor studies often in clinical settings, and some patients require higher doses for complete acid suppression. The occasional reflux episodes experienced by many patients on 40 mg of omeprazole per day may be "normal" and not significant; however, in patients with LPR, especially voice professionals, any laryngeal acid exposure is detrimental. Rather than doing 24-hour pH studies on medication for every patient with LPR or prescribing even higher doses of PPIs routinely, some physicians use antacids, H2-blockers, and/or lifestyle modifications in addition to PPIs. The antacids are used at bedtime and before strenuous exercise (such as singing). This regimen may be useful for singers whose laryngeal appearance improves, but incompletely, on PPIs.

More recently, in treating patients with laryngopharyngeal reflux, PPIs have been combined with an H2-blocker at bedtime, for reasons discussed below. Clearly, research into optimal treatment regimens is needed.

Vardar et al[427] reported on the effect of alginate in patients with GERD and hiatal hernia. They pointed out that alginate-based formulations often are used in combination with proton pump inhibitor therapy to control the symptoms of heartburn and regurgitation. They stated that alginate decreased acid reflux most effectively within the first hour after eating a meal.

However, they noted that there are limited data regarding the mechanisms and the effects of this dual therapy. They found no definitive effect of alginate on the height of proximal migration of reflux events in the patients with or without hiatal hernia.

In 2018, Takeuchi et al[428] discussed the efficacy of treating gastroesophageal reflux disease and functional dyspepsia (FD). They evaluated the efficacy of acotiamide in combination with a standard dose of rabeprazole for treatment of GERD. Acotiamide is a new prokinetic agent that is an acetylcholinesterase inhibitor. It is approved for use in Japan; approval of its use is pending in the United States. They pointed out that patients with GERD and FD often experience heartburn and epigastric fullness after standard dose proton pump inhibitor use for more than

8 weeks. They concluded that acotiamide 300 mg per day in combination with rabeprazole 10 mg per day or 20 mg a day relieved symptoms in patients with overlap of GERD and FD, heartburn, and epigastric fullness after standard dose PPI administration for more than 8 weeks. They suggested that the combination therapy might be an alternative option for persistent symptoms in these patients.

Foocharoen et al[429] examined the efficacy of omeprazole and domperidone versus combining alginic acid and proton pump inhibitor therapy in reducing symptoms of gastroesophageal reflux disease in patients who had shown only partial response to PPIs alone. They concluded that domperidone and algycon were equally effective treatments in combination with omeprazole. However, they found that approximately 17% (of 148) of their patients showed no significant response. They recommend further study of combination therapy combining algycon and domperidone with a PPI.

Baclofen

Baclofen relaxes skeletal muscle and is used primarily to treat spasticity. It is a GABA receptor agonist that has been used effectively to treat reflux.[430] In 2012, Cossentino et al[431] published the results of a randomized clinical trial that showed that baclofen was associated with a significant decrease in upright reflux. Upright reflux is common in patients with LPR. Abbasinazari et al[432] compared omeprazole with a combination of omeprazole and sustained-release baclofen (SR baclofen) and demonstrated that the combination therapy works better than omeprazole alone for treatment of regurgitation and heartburn (although they used only 20 mg per day of omeprazole in both arms of the study). Scarpellini

et al[433] showed that baclofen does not alter the intragastric acid pocket but limits its extension into the esophagus by an increase in postprandial LES pressure. In 2014, a meta-analysis found that there was good evidence to suggest that baclofen is useful for treatment of reflux, but the authors recommended a large, well-designed study.[434] Baclofen has been shown to be effective in the treatment of children with refractory reflux.[435] It may also be helpful for treatment of chronic cough,[436,437] rumination, and supragastric belching/aerophagia,[438] and reflux-induced sleep disturbances.[439] Baclofen comes as 10-mg and 20-mg pills. It is given in divided doses (3 times daily or 4 times daily), and daily total doses range from 20 to 80 mg per day. It can be started at 5 mg 3 times daily and increased by 15 mg per day every 3 days. When discontinued, the dose should be tapered gradually, not stopped abruptly.

H2-Receptor Antagonists

Since their introduction in the late 1970s, H2-receptor antagonists have been the mainstay of the treatment of GERD. The only mechanism of action of these drugs is to inhibit gastric acid secretion; they have no effect on LES pressure or esophageal clearance. The 4 H2-blockers (cimetidine, ranitidine, famotidine, and nizatidine) are equal in efficacy when used in equivalent doses. These agents are extremely well tolerated in all age groups and have been shown to relieve heartburn completely in 60% of patients treated.[440] Healing of mucosal abnormalities in the esophagus is less frequent and often overestimated, being seen in 0% to 82% (mean = 48%) of patients.[441] The best results are seen in patients with nonerosive esophagitis where success rates are as high as 75%.[442,443] Higher doses of

H2-antagonists, up to 4 times daily, are usually needed to treat erosive esophagitis[443]; however, the cost of this double-dose therapy is greater and therapy is not as clinically effective as using a single daily dose of PPIs. Maintenance of heartburn relief and healing of esophageal mucosal injury is seen in only 25% to 50% of patients treated with continuous therapy of traditional doses of H2-antagonists (eg, ranitidine 150 mg twice daily) for 1 year.[443]

H2-receptor antagonists are remarkably safe agents. Side effects are rarely seen with greater frequency than placebo in clinical trials. Rare cases of hepatitis, qualitative platelet defects, and mental confusion with intravenous administration have been reported. Drug interactions are extremely rare, although they seem to be slightly more prevalent with cimetidine. Caution should be exercised in patients on Dilantin, warfarin, and theophylline, although clinically problems are rare.[441]

Cimetidine has also been associated with male infertility. Although the cause-and-effect relationship has not been proven, impotence and gynecomastia have also been reported as possible complications. An uncontrolled study by Van Thiel et al[444] reported that the concentration of sperm in 7 males was reduced during treatment with cimetidine (Tagamet) 300 mg qid for 9 weeks. In only 1 patient did the count fall below the lower limit of normal of 50 000 000/mL (ie, 45 000 000/mL). After the treatment period, the concentrations returned to pretreatment levels. In contrast, a controlled double-blind study by Enzmann et al[445] on spermatogenesis in 30 normal males who received cimetidine (300 mg qid or 400 mg hs) or placebo for 6 months did not demonstrate any effects of cimetidine on spermatogenesis, sperm count, sperm motility and morphology, or fertilizing capacity in vitro, and the blood levels of androgen and gonadotropin were unchanged in this study population.

Carlson et al[446] studied the endocrine effects of cimetidine after acute and chronic administration in both men and women. These investigators noted the rise in prolactin levels after the acute intravenous administration of cimetidine (Tagamet). However, no acute change in the prolactin levels was noted after oral administration (300 mg cimetidine) or intravenous injection (50 mg cimetidine). The patients taking cimetidine on a chronic oral basis experienced no significant changes in serum prolactin, testosterone, free testosterone, estradiol, LH (luteinizing hormone), or FSH (follicle-stimulating hormone). The authors concluded that it is likely that the impotence and breast changes occasionally seen during cimetidine therapy are due to peripheral antagonism of androgen action rather than to alterations in circulating hormone levels.

Winters et al[447] analyzed the effects of cimetidine on androgen binding to the human prostate, testes, and semen. They found that cimetidine competed for dihydrotestosterone (DHT) binding sites in the human prostate and no apparent binding to the testes or semen. In agreement with Carlson et al, these authors postulate that androgen antagonism may be the mechanism of the endocrine side effects of cimetidine in men.

Jensen and coworkers[448] studied the use of cimetidine to determine the long-term efficacy of medical management in 22 patients with gastric hypersecretory states (20 patients had Zollinger-Ellison syndrome and 2 had idiopathic hypersecretions). Of the 22 patients followed, 11 reported impotence, breast tenderness, gynecomastia, or some combination of these symptoms. The remaining 11 patients were asymptomatic. The mean dose of cimetidine in the patients with impotence or breast changes tended to be higher than those in patients without these side effects (5.3 ± 3.5 vs 3 ± 1.3 g per day). This dosage is more than 4 times that used in the therapy of uncomplicated gastric or duodenal ulcers where impotence and gynecomastia have been reported extremely rarely.

Malagelada et al[449] also studied the long-term use of cimetidine in 18 patients with Zollinger-Ellison syndrome. The patients received an average cimetidine dose of 2 g/day and were followed for an average of 28.9 months (range: 7–59 months). Unlike Jensen's findings, none of these patients presented with major side effects. There were no reports of impotence among this group; however, 1 patient developed tender gynecomastia.

These problems have not been reported prominently with other H2-antagonists (which have not been studied as extensively), but complications can occur with all of the medications in this class, and physicians should be familiar with them. It is also helpful to warn patients that H2-receptor antagonists may result in increased blood alcohol levels and functional impairments after consumption of amounts of alcohol that would be considered safe in the absence of H2-receptor antagonist therapy. This problem is particularly prominent with cimetidine.[450]

There are few trials in which H2-receptor antagonists have been evaluated systematically in the treatment of extraesophageal GERD, and all of the reported trials have been in patients with either asthma or chronic cough. The largest study by Larrain et al[65] randomized patients to placebo, cimetidine 300 mg 4 times a day, or antireflux surgery in a 6-month treatment trial. Most of the patients had mild GERD. Before treatment, heartburn was seen less than once a week in all patients, and 66% had no evidence of esophagitis by endoscopic examination. All patients had abnormal esophageal acid exposure during prolonged pH monitoring. Both pulmonary and esophageal symptoms were improved in the cimetidine and surgery groups compared to placebo. However, the response to surgical therapy was statistically superior to medical therapy. Response was slower in patients with extraesophageal reflux than in typical patients with heartburn, with many patients achieving optimal response only after 4 to 6 months of treatment.[66]

Another study comparing ranitidine, 150 mg 3 times daily, with antireflux surgery showed a statistical advantage for antireflux surgery.[449] These studies reinforce that the superior control of esophageal acid exposure seen after antireflux surgery compared to that of H2-blockers may be needed for optimal relief of pulmonary (and other extraesophageal) symptoms. Several other short-term studies using H2-receptor antagonists in doses from 150 mg ranitidine at bedtime up to 150 mg 3 times a day for periods of 1 to 8 weeks have consistently demonstrated improvement in heartburn. However, they demonstrate limited improvement in objective changes of pulmonary function and symptoms at the end of these 8-week trials.[451–454] Improvements in respiratory symptoms, if they occurred, lagged weeks behind esophageal symptoms. Clinical experience confirms these findings.

Cimetidine has been used successfully in unblinded and uncontrolled trials of patients with chronic cough associated with GERD. Improvement of cough has been reported in 70% to 100%.[455–458] Time to symptom improvement was quite prolonged, usually about 161 to 179 days. Patients with heartburn as the primary GERD symptom usually improved in 1 to 3 weeks. Despite reports of clinical improvement, no correlation was seen between clinical response and reduction in esophageal acid exposure by prolonged pH monitoring, which was performed at the end of the study. Although they were used extensively before the introduction of PPIs, there are no definitive studies in which H2-receptor antagonists have been used to treat LPR. Currently, we use them in patients who are unable to tolerate PPIs and in those who have symptoms from nocturnal acid secretion despite the use of PPIs. If they are to be used, high-dose therapy is required, using as a minimum the equivalent dose of ranitidine, 150 mg 4 times a day (Table 9–8).

Prokinetic Agents

Drugs that increase LES pressure and accelerate esophageal clearance and gastric emptying are ideal agents to "correct" one of the pathogenic problems underlying GERD. Unfortunately, the results seen with the 2 most commonly prescribed prokinetic agents, metoclopramide and cisapride, have been somewhat disappointing in treating GERD. Equal efficacy is seen with either agent. Heartburn relief can be achieved with cisapride in close to 60% of patients when 10 mg is given 4 times a day and is equal in

Table 9–8. Standard Medical Therapy for Gastroesophageal Reflux

Agents	Dosage
Promotility agents	
Metoclopramide	5–10 mg 4 times a day
Cisapride	10 mg 4 times a day (available only for "Compassionate use"
Acid suppressive agents	
H₂-receptor antagonists[a]	
Cimetidine	400 mg 2 times a day (nonerosive symptomatic disease)
	800 mg 2 times a day (erosive esophagitis)
Ranitidine	150 mg 4 times a day (nonerosive symptomatic disease)
	150 mg 4 times a day (erosive esophagitis)
Famotidine	20 mg 2 times a day (nonerosive symptomatic disease)
	40 mg 2 times a day (erosive esophagitis)
Nizatidine	150 mg 2 times a day (all forms of reflux disease)
Proton pump inhibitors[b]	
Omeprazole	20 mg a day (AM) acute maintenance therapy
Lansoprazole	30 mg a day (acute)
	15 mg a day (maintenance)
Pantoprazole	40 mg a day (acute and maintenance)
Esomeprazole	20–40 mg once a day (healing)
Rabeprazole	20 mg a day (acute and maintenance)

[a]Also available over-the-counter in reduced dose for medication as needed.
[b]Higher doses are required for treatment of extraesophageal disease. See text.

efficacy compared with H2-receptor antagonists.[459] Studies suggest that comparable heartburn relief can be achieved with 20 mg twice a day, a dose that will increase compliance.[460] Cisapride has been withdrawn from the US market because of concerns over cardiac side effects. Limited access through the manufacturer is still possible but difficult.

The central nervous system side effects of metoclopramide (drowsiness, irritability, extrapyramidal effects) make its use problematic, particularly in the elderly and in voice professionals. Because cisapride does not cross the blood-brain barrier, these side effects are not seen, so it has largely replaced metoclopramide as the prokinetic agent of choice. The major side effects of cisapride are diarrhea (about 10%) and nausea. Prolongation of the QT interval and development of ventricular arrhythmias may be seen in patients on cisapride who are treated concomitantly with macrolide antibiotics (eg, erythromycin) or antifungal agents.[461] Use of these drugs in combination should be avoided. Metoclopramide is available in the United States for routine use.

Cisapride's major use was in patients with mild or nonerosive esophagitis who have nocturnal heartburn. Superior symptom relief and healing in combination with H2-receptor antagonists are seen when compared to either drug alone. However, cost and compliance issues with this combination offer no advantage over PPIs.

Prokinetic agents have been used alone or in combination therapy with H2-antagonists for treatment of cough, predominantly in children, but they have not been extensively studied in the treatment of cough-related asthma and/or LPR. Improvement in cough was seen in 64.5% to 100% of patients in 2 uncontrolled studies.[462–465] Cisapride was studied in 22 infants aged 4 to 26 weeks with abnormal sleep patterns characterized by apneic episodes and associated GERD by pH monitoring,[462] as well as in a group of 19 children aged 3 months to 10 years (mean: 7 years) with either nocturnal cough, wheezing, or bronchitis, all of whom also had GERD by pH monitoring.[462] Apnea, night cough, and asthma symptoms were improved in 70% to 90%. Objectively, GERD was decreased by pH monitoring after treatment. A third study evaluating the use of cisapride in 27 children (mean age 6 years) with refractory asthma and GERD confirmed by pH monitoring reported partial or complete improvement in respiratory symptoms in 80% after 3 months of treatment.[466]

A preliminary study by Khoury et al,[467] a double-blind controlled trial in 16 adult patients with pulmonary symptoms and GERD documented by ambulatory pH monitoring, compared cisapride, 10 mg 4 times a day, with placebo and showed significant improvement in FEV1 and FVC in patients on cisapride compared to placebo. No improvement in objective assessment of esophageal acid exposure by ambulatory pH monitoring or in esophageal symptoms could be documented. Prokinetic agents have not been studied for efficacy in patients with LPR.[468]

Proton Pump Inhibitors Are the Most Effective Nonsurgical Treatment for GERD

Treatment of GERD with extraesophageal manifestations, including LPR, remains a topic of much debate. However, otolaryngologists and laryngologists prescribe PPI therapy, often in combination with an H2-antagonist (typically before bedtime), but the daily dosages of PPIs prescribed vary among treating physicians.[469,470]

Proton pump inhibitors (omeprazole, lansoprazole, rabeprazole, pantoprazole, and esomeprazole) inhibit the H+K+ATPase enzyme that catalyzes the terminal step of acid secretion in the parietal cells. Profound acid inhibition is possible with these agents, resulting in improved symptom relief and healing of erosive disease. Several studies have shown increasing evidence that PPI treatment is effective in controlling the symptoms of LPR such as dysphonia and hoarseness.[471–479] A single daily dose of either omeprazole or rabeprazole will produce a 67% to 95% (mean 83%) rate of symptom relief and healing of erosive esophagitis.[469] A large trial comparing omeprazole 20 mg daily to lansoprazole 30 mg daily showed comparable healing rates of over 85% after 8 weeks of therapy.[471] Successful, complete symptom relief and healing of erosive esophagitis is seen in 85% of patients when continuous therapy is given over 1 year.[471] Continuous therapy is significantly superior to alternative day or weekend therapy and to H2-receptor antagonists in the long-term treatment of GERD. Continuous therapy with omeprazole 20 to 60 mg a day has been shown to maintain complete symptom relief and healing for up to 5 years even in patients refractory to H2-antagonists.[473] This study illustrates several key points: long-term remission is possible in up to 100% of patients if adequate doses of PPIs are used, up to 30% of patients refractory to H2-antagonists will require either twice-daily or more frequent dosing of PPIs, and most patients respond to stable doses of omeprazole long term without the development of tolerance. A preliminary report of continued follow-up of the same patient group shows continued success of omeprazole for 11 years. Relapse occurred in 1 patient per 9 years of treatment, with minimal side effects.[474]

Combination therapy with PPIs and prokinetics is used commonly in patients whose reflux is difficult to manage. Unfortunately, no studies have shown a statistical advantage for combination therapy compared to increasing the dose of PPIs. Proton pump inhibitors appear to have their best effect when given before a meal; if more than a single dose is required, they should be given in divided doses twice daily before breakfast and dinner[477] or more frequently. Omission of breakfast will reduce the efficacy of the PPIs.[476] If PPIs are used in combination with antacids, the medications should be separated by about an hour with the antacids being taken about one-half hour after meals. If an H2-antagonist is added, it should be given at bedtime. Data suggest that combining a PPI twice daily with an H2-antagonist at bedtime may be particularly helpful. Peghini et al[477] demonstrated nocturnal gastric acid breakthrough between 2 AM and 5 AM in a majority of patients and normal volunteers taking PPI twice daily. In a follow-up study, Peghini et al[478] suggested that this nocturnal acid breakthrough is histamine related, and they demonstrated that an H2-blocker (ranitidine 300 mg) at bedtime is more effective than bedtime omeprazole for controlling residual nocturnal acid secretion.

There are clinical situations in which difficulty swallowing mandates alternative methods of administrating proton pump inhibitors. Multiple studies with omeprazole and 2 studies with lansoprazole have shown that these proton pump inhibitors can be given to patients who are unable to ingest intact capsules by opening the capsule and mixing the intact granules with water, preparing a bicarbonate-based suspension, administering the capsules in apple or orange juice, or sprinkling the granules on applesauce or yogurt. The capsules should not be crushed.[479] Adequate control of intragastric pH has been demonstrated when omeprazole suspension is given via percutaneous gastrostomy, jejunostomy, or nasogastric tube. This is particularly useful in postoperative patients prone to aspiration, patients at risk for stress ulceration, or the patient on chronic enteral feeding via gastrostomy tube.

Since omeprazole and lansoprazole were introduced, additional PPIs have become available. Rabeprazole, pantoprazole, and esomeprazole have slightly different pharmacokinetic profiles, and they have been studied less extensively than omeprazole and lansoprazole, but all 5 PPIs appear effective for GERD and probably for LPR. Omeprazole has been studied for treatment of posterior laryngitis and was found to improve symptoms and signs of LPR.[480] It is important to recognize that symptoms improve before signs in most cases. A recent study by Belafsky et al[481] supports this common clinical observation. They noted that symptoms improved maximally during the first 2 months of therapy, but laryngeal findings improved slightly during the first 2 months and continued improving for at least the first 6 months of therapy.

Proton pump inhibitors have an excellent safety profile with no side effects greater than placebo seen in clinical trials. The major side effects, headache and diarrhea, are quite rare. There has been concern about long-term safety of PPIs because of their profound acid suppression. Current evidence suggests this fear is unjustified, as ample gastric acid is produced in a 24-hour period to allow for normal protein digestion, iron and calcium absorption, and to prevent bacterial overgrowth and maintain B12 absorption. The most important concern with long-term use of PPIs is hyperplasia of enterochromaffin-like (ECL) cells and development of gastric carcinoid tumors because of hypersecretion of gastrin. As of this writing, there have been no reports of gastric carcinoid or any gastric malignancy with up to 11 years of omeprazole.[474] Hyper-

plasia of ECL cells is seen in 4% or less of patients on PPIs. A recent study suggested that patients on long-term omeprazole who were infected with *H pylori* developed atrophic gastritis (a proposed precursor of gastric adenocarcinoma) at a more rapid rate than patients who were not infected, prompting these authors to recommend screening and treatment of *H pylori* in patients on long-term proton pump inhibitors.[482] A US Food and Drug Administration (FDA) panel determined that these data are insufficient to support this recommendation.[483] No specific laboratory monitoring—in particular, serum gastrin—is required for patients on long-term PPIs.

Several clinical trials have been conducted using PPIs in patients with extra-esophageal symptoms, principally asthma and LPR. All of the trials were conducted with omeprazole. Two short-term studies, one with omeprazole 20 mg once a day for 4 weeks[484] and the other with 20 mg twice daily for 6 weeks, showed an improvement in pulmonary function tests on omeprazole compared to placebo. However, little change in bronchodilator use or asthma scores could be demonstrated. A longer trial by Boeree et al,[485] a randomized double-blind controlled trial in 36 patients comparing omeprazole 40 mg twice daily to placebo for 3 months, showed a reduction in nocturnal cough during treatment with omeprazole compared to placebo. However, objective changes in FEV1 and other pulmonary function tests were not seen. The study by Meier et al[486] using omeprazole 20 mg twice daily found that 6 of 11 patients who failed to improve on omeprazole also did not heal their esophagitis. This suggests that acid suppression was inadequate in these patients. The patients who did have control of their asthma also had healed their esophagitis, reinforcing the fact that adequate acid control can relieve pulmonary symptoms.

Important insights into the treatment of patients with extraesophageal GERD come from a well-designed study by Harding et al[57] in which 30 patients with documented asthma and proven GERD by prolonged pH monitoring were treated with increasing doses of omeprazole beginning with 20 mg a day, increasing by 20 mg daily after every 8 weeks of treatment for 3 months or until esophageal acid exposure was reduced to "normal." Normalization of esophageal acid exposure resulted in improvement in pulmonary symptoms in 70% of patients. There are several important observations from this trial: 8 of 30 patients (28%) required more than 20 mg of omeprazole daily to normalize esophageal acid exposure; many patients required the entire 3-month period of treatment to achieve optimal symptom relief with improvement progressing continuously over the 3-month period; a favorable response to omeprazole was seen in patients who presented with frequent regurgitation (more often than once a week) and/or abnormal proximal acid exposure demonstrated by ambulatory pH monitoring (see Reflux Laryngitis and Other Otolaryngologic Manifestations of Laryngopharyngeal Reflux). The study emphasizes the importance of adequate esophageal acid control to achieve improvement in patients with extraesophageal symptoms. Complete elimination of esophageal acid exposure is often necessary in patients with extraesophageal disease (including LPR) to effectively relieve symptoms. The author (DOC) requires that esophageal pH be greater than 4 for 99% of the time during prolonged pH monitoring while on proton pump inhibitor therapy before accepting that acid suppression is optimal. In selected cases, even that is not adequate in patients with LPR if the 1% period of reflux includes proximal acid exposure with persistent laryngeal symptoms and signs.

Hanson et al[487] evaluated 16 patients with posterior laryngitis (LPR) who had failed to respond to initial treatment with conservative, lifestyle measures for a 6-week period, with omeprazole 40 mg daily for at least 6 weeks. Laryngeal and esophageal symptom scores improved significantly at the end of 6 weeks compared to preomeprazole scores. Objective improvement compared to pretreatment values was also seen when the larynx was evaluated by a blinded investigator using videolaryngoscopy. Six patients had improvement in their laryngoscopic scores but not in laryngeal symptom scores. Symptoms relapsed within 6 weeks in all patients after therapy was stopped. Poorer response was seen in patients with abnormal proximal esophageal acid exposure on ambulatory pH monitoring. It is reasonable to speculate that 40 mg a day of omeprazole was inadequate therapy for these patients and that they might have responded to higher doses or to a regimen combining other medications.

The same authors studied 182 patients with posterior laryngitis and at least one of the following symptoms: postnasal drip, persistent or recurrent sore throat, cough, or hoarseness.[487] Patients were treated sequentially with conservative lifestyle modifications for an initial period of 6 to 12 weeks followed by famotidine 20 mg at bedtime for 6 weeks. Omeprazole 20 mg at bedtime was given to nonresponders. Omeprazole was then increased in 20-mg increments every 6 weeks until 80 mg a day was reached. Laryngitis was characterized as mild if posterior laryngeal erythema was seen; moderate if marked erythema, secretions, and mucosal granularity were present; and severe if ulceration, granulation tissue, or hyperkeratosis was seen. Patients with mild symptoms and minimal laryngeal changes responded to conservative doses of famotidine, whereas patients with severe laryngitis required PPIs.[487] These studies emphasize variability in response of patients with LPR, the need to treat for longer periods before seeing a response when disease is severe, the need for higher doses of PPIs, and the rapid relapse of symptoms when therapy is discontinued, emphasizing that long-term treatment is often needed in patients with LPR.

Wo et al[488] studied 22 patients with posterior laryngitis felt to be secondary to GERD and diagnosed by indirect laryngoscopy, using an 8-week trial of omeprazole 40 mg at bedtime. Laryngeal symptoms improved in 67% of these patients. Increasing omeprazole to 40 mg twice a day in nonresponders did not improve response. Relapse was seen in 40% when omeprazole was stopped. There were no predictors of response, although nocturnal symptoms were more common in nonresponders. Perhaps this group had nocturnal acid breakthrough and continued to reflux despite high-dose PPI therapy. It is likely that results would have been improved if omeprazole were given twice daily (before breakfast and dinner), a treatment regimen that produces superior acid suppression to other modes of administration of this drug. The response rate to omeprazole in this trial does, however, support empiric therapy for LPR.

Metz and colleagues[489] studied 10 patients with laryngitis documented by endoscopy who also had GERD diagnosed by abnormal ambulatory pH monitoring. They used 40 mg omeprazole as a single daily dose and found improvement in 7 of 10 (70%) patients at the end of 8 weeks. Jaspersen and colleagues[490] studied 34 patients with laryngeal symptoms, laryngoscopic changes of LPR, and erosive esophagitis treated with omeprazole 20 mg a day for 4 weeks, reporting improvement in esophagitis and laryngeal symptoms in 32 of 34 patients (92%). No comment was made

about laryngeal examinations. These studies were uncontrolled but showed excellent results with omeprazole. Although lansoprazole has not been studied in this patient population, comparable healing rates for omeprazole 20 mg and lansoprazole 30 mg a day, respectively, are seen in erosive esophagitis,[490] suggesting that this PPI should be equally effective in patients with LPR and other extraesophageal disease.

El-Serag and colleagues[491] performed a randomized controlled trial in 20 patients with LPR comparing lansoprazole 30 mg bid to placebo. After 16 weeks, 50% of the treated patients had complete relief of LPR symptoms compared to 10% with placebo. Laryngeal findings were not highlighted.

Clinicians must be cognizant of the fact that PPI therapy is not universally effective. Failure rates are high in patients receiving a PPI only once daily.[492] In addition, a morning dose of omeprazole has been shown to last an average of only 13.8 hours.[493] The problem of nocturnal acid breakthrough has been discussed above and may be viewed as effectively limiting the duration of the evening dose of PPI to a period of 7½ hours.[494] In addition, a few patients produce substantial (or normal) acid levels even when receiving high doses of PPIs. Amin et al[492] studied LPR patients receiving PPIs up to 4 times a day and reported a medical treatment failure rate of 10%. At the author's (RTS) voice center,[494] we evaluated the use of super high-dose PPI administration in a group of patients that appeared refractory to standard twice-daily PPI dosing in controlling their LPR. A retrospective review of 35 medical records of patients (ages 20–76 years) who were treated with high-dose PPI therapy was conducted. Three blinded raters compared RSS scores and 24-hour pH impedance scores on standard and super high-dose PPI therapy. RSS scores revealed some improvement in reports of laryngeal symptom pathology, with the most significant changes noted on standard high-dose therapy. The authors concluded that neither RSS nor 24-hour impedance scores appeared to be sufficient enough to detect improvement in LPR with these results, given a relatively small sample population. Lee et al[495] examined the effects of PPI therapy for LPR related to age. They conducted a prospective study at 3 medical centers of 264 patients diagnosed with LPR between 2010 and 2012. Thirty-five patients were lost to follow-up, so results are reported on 135 males and 94 females. The patients were grouped according to age. There were 111 patients in the oldest group (ages 60–79), 83 patients aged 40 to 59 years, and 35 patients aged 18 to 39 years. All patients received lansoprazole 15 mg twice daily for 3 months. RSI, RSS, and LPR-HRQLL (health-related quality of life) data were recorded pretreatment, at 1 month on treatment, and at 3 months post-PPI treatment. Based on the scores at all 3 intervals, the older patients' results reflected less response to PPI therapy in regard to their symptoms and quality of life as compared to the younger patients.

A prospective, placebo-controlled study of PPI therapy for patients with LPR was published by El-Serag and Sonnenberg[496] in which 22 patients from a Veterans Administration hospital population were treated with lansoprazole 30 mg twice daily or placebo for 3 months. Subjects underwent esophagoscopy, 24-hour pH monitor studies, and indirect laryngoscopy using a laryngeal telescope. The lower sensor was 5 cm above the LES, and the sensors were separated by 15 cm. Their primary outcome criterion was complete resolution of laryngeal symptoms. Of the 20 patients (out of 22) who finished the study and had all information available, 11 received lansoprazole and 9 received placebo. Seven patients were complete responders, 6 of whom received

lansoprazole and 1 of whom received placebo. The difference was statistically significant. At the end of this study, 58% of the patients treated with lansoprazole had complete ($n = 2$) or partial ($n = 5$) resolution of laryngeal signs of reflux (posterior laryngitis), and 30% of the placebo-treated group had partial resolution of laryngeal signs (none had complete resolution). The authors concluded that lansoprazole is effective in the treatment of LPR. The study was well designed, but the population was fairly small, and a VA hospital population is not necessarily comparable with the general population (21/22 subjects were male; mean age was 59 years in the lansoprazole group and 65 years in the placebo group).

In 2001, Noordzij et al[497] reported on 53 patients with reflux laryngitis. Of these, 30 subjects were enrolled, who had more than 4 episodes of proximal reflux during their 24-hour monitor study. Fifteen received omeprazole 40 mg twice daily, and the other 15 received placebo. The study lasted for 2 months. They assessed symptoms and laryngeal signs of LPR. During 24-hour pH monitor studies, the upper sensor was placed under flexible laryngoscopic guidance 1 cm above the UES, and the distal sensor was 18 cm from the proximal sensor. The patients were instructed to avoid behavioral activities known to have an effect on gastroesophageal reflux. The mean age (years) in the treatment group was 51.7 and in the placebo group, 45.3. Subjects were fairly evenly divided by gender. There were large differences in initial symptom severity between the omeprazole and placebo groups for some symptoms. The authors reported that most symptom scores improved for both groups, although mild hoarseness and throat clearing may be treated effectively by omeprazole, but they also concluded that there was a placebo effect. It is interesting that laryngoscopic findings showed no improvement in either group. Although complete resolution of laryngeal signs commonly takes many months, improvement in erythema usually is seen in less than 2 months, and improvements in edema often are seen during this time, as well. Their results may have been due to the fact that abnormalities in laryngeal signs were very mild in the entire study population (in blind subjective assessments, the 5 laryngeal signs were all rated in the 0–1 range). Hence, very little change in laryngeal findings could be expected. Findings might be different in a population with more severe disease.

In 2003, Eherer et al[498] reported a placebo-controlled, double-blind crossover study of the effects of pantoprazole on LPR. They assessed 62 patients. Twenty-four showed reflux on 24-hour pH monitoring, and 21 were entered into the study. The proximal sensor was located 1 to 3 cm above the UES, and the distal sensor was placed 15, 18, or 21 cm below the upper sensor. Studies monitoring pH were performed for each subject prior to entry into the study and between its 3-month arms. The requirement for 2 pH monitoring studies and the duration of the study (>6 months) may be responsible for the fact that only 14 patients completed all portions of the research protocol. All subjects were nonsmokers. However, the methodology makes no mention of preventing patients from adopting behavioral changes that might have contributed to improvements in both groups. The authors reported that both pantoprazole and placebo were associated with "marked improvement" in laryngitis scores and that there was no significant difference between the 2 groups after 3 months. After a 2-week washout period, a second pH monitoring study confirmed persistence of reflux in most subjects. Switching the placebo group to pantoprazole resulted in further improvement of laryngitis scores. In the pantopra-

zole group switched to placebo, a minority of patients had recurrence of symptoms and signs. Changes in symptom scores were not significantly different between the 2 groups. After reversal of treatments, there was also no significant change in symptoms, although 1 patient who switched from pantoprazole to placebo had a severe recurrence of symptoms. Like the study by Noordzij et al,[497] these results are somewhat difficult to interpret because of the fairly mild severity of LPR in both groups. For example, the maximum possible score for esophageal symptoms was 48 (the higher, the worse). The esophageal score prior to treatment was 11 in the placebo/pantoprazole group and 3.3 in the pantoprazole/placebo group.

Similarly, the maximum laryngeal symptom score was 72. The pretreatment placebo/pantoprazole score was 17.4, and the pantoprazole/placebo score was 14.6. Hence, there was not much room for improvement, and these patients had mild disease, in which spontaneous fluctuations in severity are common. This problem, combined with the small number of subjects, raises questions about the conclusions of this otherwise well-designed study from which the authors deduced that pantoprazole may be helpful in relieving acute symptoms but that the advantage of long-term treatment has been overestimated. Substantially larger numbers and inclusion of patients with long-term, moderate-to-severe symptoms and signs will be needed to assess these concerns definitively.

Other recent studies of LPR also have failed to provide incontestable answers to questions about diagnostic accuracy and treatment efficiency.[499,500]

Bruley des Varannes et al[501] reported that the superiority of PPIs over other drugs has been well established for both short- and long-term treatment of GERD. Patients with erosive esophagitis are more responsive to PPIs than patients with nonerosive reflux disease. PPIs also have become widely used and have been proven to be safe and effective in the management of GERD in children, although to date, only omeprazole, lansoprazole, and esomeprazole are approved for use in children.[502,503]

A randomized placebo-controlled study revealed improved LPR symptoms compared with placebo after 12 weeks of treatment with rabeprazole 20 mg twice daily.[504] The authors reported a relapse of symptoms 6 weeks after stopping PPI therapy, suggesting that LPR requires longer duration of treatment. Many clinicians still advocate the use of empiric therapy with twice-daily PPI dosing for 6 to 12 weeks (on average) as a diagnostic tool in patients with suspected LPR.[505,506] However, we believe that this is not an adequate approach, particularly for nonresponders, as some patients may produce acid even when taking 2 or more PPIs daily. Monitoring of pH while on medications is invaluable in detecting these patients, and for many patients, PPI treatment must be continued indefinitely.

Dadabhai and Friedenberg[507] reported that rabeprazole has a faster onset of action in comparison with other PPIs. They cited rabeprazole's high pKa of 5, which facilitates activation at a higher pH, as a possible reason for its faster onset. They described rabeprazole's pathway of metabolism as nonenzymatic, thus making it less affected by the genetic polymorphisms of the CYP2C19 on which the other PPIs depend.

In 2010, Fass et al[508] reported the results of a randomized, placebo-controlled study that evaluated the effectiveness of esomeprazole twice daily in their patients with LPR, all of whom had undergone endoscopy and pH monitor testing. Following the 3-month trial, the results revealed no significant difference in videostroboscopic reflux finding score and no significant difference

in acoustic measures after treatment, comparing the esomeprazole group and the placebo group. The patients completed a voice use and quality diary and a symptom diary pretreatment and at the end of the study, and no significant differences were found in these between the 2 groups.

Recognizing that PPI therapy is not universally effective, caution must be exercised in interpretation of available literature. An insightful analysis by Johnston et al[509] revealed that in a recent meta-analysis, all but 2 studies fell within a funnel plot. The only 2 that did not show PPI effect were flawed by publication bias. Meta-analyses commonly magnify inherent flaws in the included studies, and more rigorous studies need to be performed. A randomized, double-blind, placebo-controlled study[510] revealed improvement in reflux finding score and reflux symptom index after treatment with esomeprazole in both placebo and PPI groups for 6 weeks. However, diffuse laryngeal edema showed significantly greater improvement in the PPI group, and ventricular obliteration and laryngeal erythema trended toward greater improvement in the PPI group. Posterior laryngeal hypertrophy improved significantly in the PPI group only. Lifestyle modifications were not instituted, so improvement was probably from medical intervention. Whereas a placebo effect has been shown repeatedly, including in this study, improvements were greater in the PPI group in several parameters.

Belafsky et al[511] describe the presence of esophagopharyngeal reflux—as distinct from LPR—which should also be considered as a possible cause for treatment failures. This disorder is characterized by regurgitation of proximal esophageal contents into the laryngopharynx secondary to inadequate volume clearance and dysmotility, rather than acid and peptic injury.

Further studies are needed to elucidate this process, as treatment with antireflux medications, prokinetics, dilatation, and diet modification ameliorates symptoms in 50% of affected individuals.[511] We also have noted substantial problems associated with intraesophageal (or esophagopharyngeal) reflux in some patients after fundoplication, as well as in other patients who have not undergone surgery.

Side Effects of PPIs

Clinical experience suggests that most patients with LPR have chronic gastroesophageal reflux and require long-term medical therapy or antireflux surgery, or both. Of note, it is common for laryngeal reflux findings and symptoms to take longer to resolve than esophageal symptoms. Also, symptoms often improve before clinical findings, which may take 6 months or longer to reverse.[512] Reichel et al[513] noted control of LPR symptoms on daily PPI after an average of 4 weeks when combined with lifestyle modifications. Resistant cases could be treated with twice-daily medication at higher doses. Improvement can be seen not only in symptoms and signs but also in objective assessments, such as acoustic parameters. Jin et al[514] reported that jitter, shimmer, and harmonic-to-noise ratio improved significantly after 1 to 2 months of treatment. The dose of PPIs and other medications and the decision to perform antireflux surgery should be individualized to maintain symptom relief and mucosal healing. The evidence suggests that long-term medical therapy is safe and that tolerance or tachyphylaxis is extremely rare.

A review article[515] and editorial[516] (from which the following 9 paragraphs are adapted) highlight many of the potential problems encountered in patients who receive PPI treatment for many months or years. PPIs are fairly safe, especially compared with many other prescription drugs, but adverse effects occur and should be known to physicians who prescribe PPIs. In 2008, Davies et al[517] studied almost 12 000 patients treated with esomeprazole over an 8-month period, with an average treatment duration of 26 weeks. Only 119 events were reported as possibly related to the medication. The few serious adverse effects were hypersensitivity reactions, including 3 cases of angioedema and 2 cases of anaphylaxis that were possibly related to the medication. This study did not examine long-term effects of PPI treatment.

PPIs are designed to cause hypochlorhydria. Therefore, they may interfere with calcium absorption. Numerous studies have confirmed that PPIs impair calcium absorption, and perhaps the best-known study showed an association between PPI use and hip fracture. Interestingly, Yang et al's study[518] showed that with long-term PPI use, risk for hip fracture was greater in men than in women. It has been speculated that this was due to the fact that many women use calcium replacement after menopause, and most men do not. At present, many of us are counseling our patients on long-term PPIs to take calcium and vitamin D supplementation while more is being learned about this problem. Since then, there have been more than 30 studies investigating the effects of PPIs on bone density, and it is now uncertain that the risk exists. For example, data from the study of women's health across the nation (SWAN) were analyzed.[519] This was a multiethnic, multicenter, community-based cohort report related to menopause. The association of bone mineral density changes associated with PPI and H2-antagonist users was examined. The subjects included 207 new users of PPIs, 185 new users of H2-antagonists, and 1676 nonusers. Subjects were followed for a period of approximately 10 years, and their median age was 50. The results of the study showed no difference in annual measurements of bone mineral density changes in any of the 3 groups.

Calcium absorption is not the only potential nutritional problem associated with long-term PPI use. It is also possible that vitamin B12 and iron levels may be affected in some patients taking PPIs for long periods of time.[520]

Diarrhea caused by *Clostridium difficile* has been associated with virtually all antibiotics. In 2008, Aseeri et al[521] suggested that the use of PPIs may increase the risk for diarrhea under some circumstances. They felt that the inhibition of gastric acidity impaired the body's defenses against ingested bacteria. However, this study was performed in hospitalized patients, and the implications for the general healthy population remain uncertain. This is a problem that has not been encountered widely in outpatient clinical practice.

Similarly, there has been a suggestion that PPIs may be associated with an increased risk of community-acquired pneumonia. However, there are shortcomings in the papers that have studied this issue, and the conclusions of some of the studies suggesting an association remain controversial.

One of the most striking adverse effects described recently is the interaction between at least some PPIs and clopidogrel. Well-executed studies have pointed out that some PPIs reduce the biological action of clopidogrel, decreasing its effect and increasing the risk for serious cardiovascular problems, including myocardial infarction.[522,523] Clearly there is a problem with concomitant use of omeprazole and clopidogrel. This is of particular concern, not only because omeprazole is readily available over the counter, but also because

many insurance companies require patients to use omeprazole (because it is inexpensive) before permitting use of a later-generation PPI. Interactions between other PPIs and clopidogrel remain under study.

Other potential adverse effects may be associated with long-term PPI use, including atrophic gastritis, possibly progressing to metaplasia and adenocarcinoma,[524] hypergastrinemia (an increase in circulating gastrin hormone that has been associated with the development of carcinoid tumors of the gastric mucosa in rats),[525] and other problems.

Potential side effects associated with PPI therapy include headache, diarrhea, and dyspepsia in less than 2% of users. Switching to another PPI can be considered if this occurs. Chapman et al[515] reviewed complications of PPI treatment. New discussions have been raised regarding associations with vitamin and mineral deficiencies, new data on infections including community-acquired pneumonia and *C difficile*, associations of PPI use with long bone fractures, and cardiovascular events in patients receiving concomitant therapy with clopidogrel (Plavix). Clopidogrel is a platelet activation inhibitor used as a "blood thinner" in many patients with cardiovascular disorders, often in association with aspirin. The FDA issued warnings regarding the potential for adverse cardiovascular events among clopidogrel users taking PPI therapy in 2009 and regarding the potential for wrist, hip, and spine fractures among PPI users in 2010. In late 2012, the FDA issued a class warning for *C difficile* infections.

In an editorial published in *ENT Journal*, the authors provided a summary review of adverse side effects associated with PPI use, widely prescribed in the United States.[516] They and others have cited the research of several reporters and their discussions. Further studies reported that chronic PPI use was associated with chronic and acute kidney disease and with interstitial nephritis.[526,527] The author reported that in 2011, the FDA issued a warning that prolonged use of PPIs may not be beneficial.[528] Cheungpasitporn et al[529] reported that meta-analysis of multiple observational studies revealed a 40% increased risk of low magnesium levels in patients using PPIs compared to participants not using PPIs. They also cited an increased incidence of C difficile infections, increased risk of bone fractures secondary to decreased calcium absorption and subsequent decrease in bone density, increased rates of pneumonia, and an increase in myocardial events in patients taking PPIs and clopidogrel has been reported.[530-536]

In 2014, Shin et al[537] stated that recent reports have suggested that PPI therapy may worsen vitiligo, but the effects on the melanocytes are yet to be determined. They performed an in vivo study of the effects of PPIs on the melanogenesis. They examined zebrafish embryos to investigate the effects of PPIs on pigmentation. They measured TIR (tirosinate) activity and tirosinase-related protein-1 (PRP-1) by Western blot technique. The results suggested that functional inhibition of melanization may cause or aggravate vitiligo in predisposed patients on PPI therapy.

Two recent studies examined the association between PPI usage and the risk of myocardial infarction.[537,538] Both studies' results showed that the data support an association of PPI use with the increased risk of myocardial infarction. Shah et al[538] reported, however, that they did not find an associated risk of cardiovascular events with the use of H2-blockers. Shih et al[539] pointed out that despite the increased risk of myocardial infarction, the benefits of PPIs "may outweigh the risk of adverse cardiovascular effects, with the number needed to detect harm of 400 per 1357" in their study.

Their study utilized the propensity score-matching analysis and a second using case-crossover analysis that included 126 367 PPI users and 126 367 propensity score matches for PPI nonusers.

Two recent reviews demonstrated evidence that PPI therapy reduces the absorption of protein-bound vitamin B12 but did not generate enough clinical evidence to document B12 deficiency in chronic PPI users or the need to check B12 levels. Recent studies have suggested that in elderly, institutionalized, long-term PPI users, B12 deficiency is more likely to develop and should be considered.[519] Researchers at Kaiser Permanente in Oakland, California, performed a case-control study over a period of 14 years to see if there is an association between vitamin D deficiency and use of acid-suppressing drugs and reported that both PPIs and H2-receptor antagonists may lead to malabsorption of vitamin B12 due to suppression of gastric acid.[520]

Semb et al,[540] researchers from the Department of Gastroenterology at Zealand University Hospital in Denmark, published a case report on persistent, severe hypomagnesemia believed to be caused by a proton pump inhibitor that resolved after laparoscopic fundoplication. Their patient had been on long-term PPI use and had had persistent hypomagnesemia with severe symptoms at presentation. The patient was unable to stop the proton pump inhibitor therapy because of severe reflux symptoms and was dependent on weekly intravenous infusions of magnesium until magnesium levels finally normalized. He underwent laparoscopic fundoplication and had an uneventful perioperative and postoperative course. Following the surgery, he no longer needed PPI therapy, and his magnesium levels remained normal.

Gastric acid is needed to allow absorption of nonheme iron and enhance iron salt dissociation from ingested food. Iron deficiency anemia has been reported in patients with atrophic gastritis, gastric resection, or vagotomy. To date, no data are available demonstrating the development of iron deficiency anemia in normal subjects on PPI therapy.

By their effects in increasing gastric pH levels, PPIs may encourage growth of gut microflora and increase susceptibility to organisms such as *Salmonella, Campylobacter jejuni, Escherichia coli, C difficile, Vibrio cholera*, and *Listeria*. An increased susceptibility in PPI users for *Salmonella, Campylobacter,* and *C difficile* infections was found in a systematic review.[530,531] Current recommendations are to carefully evaluate the need for PPI therapy in hospitalized patients who need intravenous antibiotics to reduce risk for *C difficile*.

Tergast et al[541] reviewed the dose-dependent impact of PPIs on spontaneous bacterial peritonitis in 2018. They investigated potential relevance and effect of the PPI dose on the incidence and clinical course of spontaneous bacterial peritonitis. Their study included 613 consecutive patients who had advanced cirrhosis. Their proton pump inhibitor dosage was considered, and the patients were followed for the development of spontaneous bacterial peritonitis as well as the incidence of the reported complications, including acute kidney injury, hepatic encephalopathy, and mortality. The authors reported that the incidence of spontaneous bacterial peritonitis did not differ between the proton pump inhibitor group and the non–proton pump inhibitor group, or between patients taking high-dose (>40 mg/day) proton pump inhibitors and those taking a dose between 10 and 40 mg per day. However, they noted that proton pump inhibitor use had a negative effect on the course of spontaneous bacterial peritonitis. Between the 2 study populations, they found

a higher incidence of acute kidney injury (71% vs 43%) and severe hepatic encephalopathy (15% vs 0%) in the PPI group. They reported an increased mortality (24% vs 0%) in the PPI group within 28 days after the onset of spontaneous peritonitis diagnosis. Additionally, they found no effect of proton pump inhibitors on acute kidney injury, hepatic encephalopathy, and mortality in patients who did not have spontaneous bacterial peritonitis. They recommended that high-dose proton pump inhibitors be used carefully in these patients.

Otani and Banerji[542] discussed the evaluation and management of immediate and delayed hypersensitivity reactions to proton pump inhibitors. They pointed out that proton pump inhibitors are the most commonly prescribed medications in the United States and are generally tolerated well. However, rarely both immediate and delayed immune-mediated hypersensitivity reactions have been reported. They noted that a desensitization protocol can be used when PPI use cannot be avoided in an allergic patient.

Li et al[543] examined the effect of proton pump inhibitors and their association with the accelerated development of cirrhosis, hepatic decompensation, and hepatocellular carcinoma in noncirrhotic patients with chronic hepatitis C infection. They concluded that in veterans with chronic hepatitis C virus infection, increased proton pump inhibitor use was associated with a dose-dependent risk of the progression of chronic liver disease to cirrhosis and additionally an increased risk of hepatocellular carcinoma and hepatic decompensation. However, the effect of PPIs on noncirrhotic patients with chronic liver disease is uncertain, and evidence of damage has not been established.

Dado et al[544] reported a case of severe iron deficiency anemia associated with long-term proton pump inhibitor use. The authors noted that proton pump inhibitors had been used in clinical practice for more than 25 years and have generally replaced H2-blockers as the first line of therapy. They stated that proton pump inhibitors cause few side effects during short-term use. However, long-term use has come under greater scrutiny due to inappropriateness in some cases, interactions with other drugs, potential for adverse side effects including hip fractures, *C difficile* infection, pneumonia, vitamin and mineral deficiencies, and cardiac events. They presented the case of a 50-year-old male with severe iron deficiency anemia due to malabsorption suspected to be caused by long-term PPI use. An extensive medical workup failed to reveal any definitive source of bleeding. The patient had been started on omeprazole in 2005 and remained on proton pump inhibitors through 2015. He was noted to be anemic first in February 2012 and iron studies had shown a ferratin level of 5 in September 2013. He had been treated with iron supplementation with good compliance but never had significant improvement in his iron studies or his anemia. They suggested that long-term PPI administration might have contributed to the patient's observed iron deficiency and anemia, but no causal relationship was established by evidence.

In 2017, in the *Journal of Gastroenterology and Hepatology*, Jung et al[545] discussed standard and double-dose intravenous proton pump inhibitor therapy for prevention of bleeding after endoscopic resection of gastric neoplasms. The effective dosing or scheduling of proton pump inhibitors for the prevention of delayed bleeding following that endoscopic procedure remains unclear. Their study included 166 patients with gastric adenoma or early gastric cancer. Following the endoscopic procedure, each subject was randomly selected to receive either pantoprazole 40 mg intravenously every 24 hours or 40 mg every 12 hours. The patients underwent a second-look endoscopic procedure 2 days after their original resection to evaluate for signs of rebleeding in these 2 groups. Their findings showed that intravenous pantoprazole 40 mg every 24 hours and every 12 hours for 2 days were equally effective following endoscopic resection.

Takeda et al[546] reported a case of fundic gland polyps associated with long-term proton pump inhibitor therapy. Their 44-year-old male patient had tarry stool and presented to the hospital with a hemoglobin of 8. He was found to have upper GI bleeding from polyps formed like fundic gland during long-term PPI administration. He was treated with endoscopic resection of the polyps. The authors suggested that this case presentation demonstrates the rarity of bleeding from such polyps and that long-term administration of PPIs might have been causally related. They recommended further study.

Yu et al[547] assessed a previous meta-analyses that had reported that proton pump inhibitor therapy was associated with increased incidence of spontaneous bacterial peritonitis in cirrhotic patients. They stated that the conclusion was based on case-control studies, but the association between PPI use and the mortality from spontaneous bacterial peritonitis had not been confirmed. The authors concluded after reviewing literature that included 10 case-control and 6 cohort studies (8145 patients were analyzed) that it was not possible to determine that PPI therapy increased the risk of spontaneous bacterial peritonitis. They recommended future prospective study to clarify this association.

An increased risk for community-acquired pneumonia is difficult to demonstrate in association with PPI therapy.

A meta-analysis showed that the overall risk for pneumonia was higher among users of PPIs. If only randomized controlled trial data are analyzed, H2-receptor antagonists rather than PPIs have been associated with an elevated risk for hospital-acquired pneumonia.[533] A more recent meta-analysis did find an increased risk for pneumonia associated with PPI use, but the results were confounded by methodologic issues. Paradoxically, short duration of use was associated with increased odds of community-acquired pneumonia but chronic use was not.[534] No definite recommendation can be given in this complex area.

Arai et al[548] examined whether acid-suppressive drugs and PPI therapy increased the risk of pneumonia in acute stroke patients. The authors performed a retrospective study to investigate the relationship between acid-suppressive drugs and pneumonia in acute stroke. They restricted the subjects to those who were susceptible to pneumonia. Their study found 3875 patients who were admitted with acute stroke to the hospital from January 2006 through January 2016. They stated that 555 patients met inclusion criteria for this study. They excluded patients who had been receiving acid-suppressive medications before admission ($n = 23$), presented with pneumonia on admission ($n = 5$), underwent surgery and/or mechanical ventilation during the first 2 weeks of hospitalization ($n = 167$), received antibiotics during the entire 2 weeks after admission ($n = 14$), and those whose data were missing ($n = 11$). However, after those exclusions, 335 patients were included in this study. They evaluated patients with acute stroke who were outside critical care and susceptible to pneumonia and found that PPI use was significantly associated with an increase of pneumonia while H2-blockers were not. The authors pointed out several limitations of their study, but they concluded that the use of PPI was associated with pneumonia in acute stroke patients susceptible to pneumonia, while the use of H2-blockers was not. They recommend that prophylactic PPI therapy in acute stroke patients may have to be avoided in those at high risk for pneumonia.

Several other interesting studies[547,549–554] have been reported regarding the association of proton pump inhibitors versus H2-receptor antagonists and the risk of pneumonia in patients with stroke,[549] the association of pump inhibitor use with the development of progression of albuminuria among Japanese patients with diabetes,[550] risk factors for poor outcome in community-onset *C difficile* infection,[551] a randomized clinical trial looking at the impact of gastrointestinal risk factor screening and prophylactic proton pump inhibitor therapy in patients receiving dual antiplatelet therapy,[552–554] and the relationship between chronic rhinosinusitis and gastroesophageal reflux in adults.[555] In addition, Sella et al[555] evaluated meta-analyses to determine the association between PPI use with infectious and inflammatory diseases. They concluded that PPI use may be a risk factor for development of infections caused by *Clostridium difficile* and other infectious diseases. It should be remembered that those conclusions are limited by the quality of the papers included in the meta-analyses. The authors also examined gut microbiota during PPI use and found increased presence of Streptococcaceae and Enterococcaceae (risk factors for *C difficile* infection) and decreased *Faecalibacterium* (an anti-inflammatory microorganism) using high-throughput, microbial 165 RNA gene sequencing.

Clinical studies in patients taking PPI therapy have shown mixed results regarding fracture. The study with the longest clinical follow-up matched cases with abnormal bone mineral density (osteoporosis) at the hip or lumbar vertebrae (T-score ≤−2.5) to controls with normal bone mineral density (T-score ≥1). PPI use was not associated with having osteoporosis in either the hip or the lumbar spine for PPI use more than 1500 doses over the previous 5 years. In the longitudinal study, no significant decrease was observed in bone mineral density at either site attributable to PPI use. This suggests that the association between PPI use and hip fracture was probably related to factors independent of osteoporosis.[556]

In a recent meta-analysis, the pooled odds ratio (OR) for fracture was 1.29 (95% confidence interval [CI], 1.18–1.41) with PPIs and 1.10 (95% CI, 0.99–1.23) with H2-receptor antagonist use compared with nonuse. Another study showed that the hip fracture risk among PPI users was seen only in persons with at least one other fracture-risk factor.[557] A meta-analysis covering 1 521 062 patients showed significant risk for spine fractures (OR, 1.50; 95% CI, 1.32–1.72; $p < .001$). For hip fractures, there was an increased risk for fractures with PPIs (OR, 1.23; 95% CI, 1.11–1.36; $p < .001$). Overall, an OR of 1.2 is seen for PPIs, and an OR of 1.08 is seen for H2-receptor antagonists (95% CI, 1–1.18; $p = .06$). Again, short duration of PPI use may be associated with increased risk for developing hip fracture (OR, 1.24; 95% CI, 1.19–1.28), but not in long-term PPI users (OR, 1.3; 95% CI, 0.98–1.7).[558] No change in bone mineral density was seen in patients using PPIs continuously for 5 to 10 years in a Canadian study[559] despite the finding of a lower baseline bone mineral density in those same patients.

Soen[560] pointed out that many observational studies have suggested an association between PPI use and the increased risk of hip and vertebral fractures. He stated that there is no evidence of duration effect found by meta-analysis. He stated that a mechanism through which PPI use might increase the risk of fracture has not been proven and that "overall, PPI use dos not interfere with calcium absorption in most instances and, therefore, it is unlikely that PPI influence fracture risk through interfering with absorption of dietary calcium." Moreover, he stated that he does not recommend discontinuing PPI use in patients with a history of fracture or in those patients with increased risk of fracture. He stated that further controlled, randomized studies are needed.

Although association between PPI use and hip fracture (or osteoporosis) remains controversial, a 2018 systematic review and meta-analysis reported a statistically significant increased risk of hip fracture (26% increase) in PPI users compared with nonusers.[561]

In 2009, the FDA issued a warning regarding the potential for increased adverse cardiovascular events in concomitant users of PPIs and clopidogrel, particularly users of omeprazole, lansoprazole, and esomeprazole. In vitro, the antiplatelet activity of clopidogrel requires activation by cytochrome (CY) P2C19, which is the same pathway through which PPIs are metabolized. Although overall studies have been conflicting, the newest data suggest that dexlansoprazole does not inhibit platelets in vitro to the same degree as do the 3 former PPIs. Pantoprazole appears to have less inhibition as well. A meta-analysis (23 studies) focused on primary myocardial infarction, stroke, stent occlusion, death, and secondary outcomes (rehospitalization for cardiac symptoms or revascularization procedures).[562] Outcomes from the 2 randomized controlled trials did not show an increased risk for adverse outcomes. Meta-analysis of primary and secondary outcomes showed an increased risk difference for all studies. Essentially, the risk for adverse cardiac outcomes was 0% based on data from well-controlled randomized trials.[563] Data from retrospective studies and the addition of probable vascular events slightly but significantly increased the risk estimates, likely due to lack of adjustment for potential confounders. Recent consensus is that PPIs can be used with clopidogrel if they are clinically indicated.

Würtz and Grove[564] discussed the use of proton pump inhibitors in cardiovascular disease and drug interactions with antiplatelet drugs. They pointed out that aspirin is used widely in the treatment of cardiovascular disease. Upper GI complications, including ulcers and bleeding, are relatively common during antiplatelet treatment, and thus proton pump inhibitors are prescribed often. Pharmacodynamic studies have suggested an interaction between proton pump inhibitors and clopidogrel, and clinical studies have been conducted to evaluate the impact of this action. They stated it had been reported that PPIs may attenuate the antiplatelet effect of aspirin, but they stated that more research is needed to confirm or refute that finding.

Xie et al[565] published a study that allegedly showed an increased risk of death in patients taking PPIs compared with H2-blockers. Unfortunately, the study was fundamentally flawed.[566] An association was reported, but there was no basis to establish causation. This retrospective study did not indicate why PPIs were used versus H2-blockers in any individual patient. It is possible that H2-blockers were prescribed for people with few or no symptoms, and PPIs were used for patients who were symptomatic and sicker, but such details are not reported in the paper. About two-thirds of their patients had no reported indication for needing either a PPI or an H2-blocker. There were no data about patient compliance, and specifically there was no indication that the patients were actually taking the medications as prescribed. Moreover, the study looked at people who died in as few as 91 days following initiation of PPI therapy. The study period was only about 5 years. It is important to understand the shortcomings of such work. Publications of this nature can easily be misunderstood (ie, believed) and lead to patients who need PPIs avoiding them because of invalid "research." It is important for all physicians to read published studies carefully not only for content but more importantly for validity.

Ohmure et al[567] evaluated proton pump inhibitor use for sleep bruxism in a randomized clinical trial. Their study population was small (12 patients). These patients underwent polysomnography to diagnose sleep bruxism and assessment of GI symptoms using symptom index and esophagogastroduodenoscopy (EGD). All patients also underwent electromyography of masticatory muscle activity. In total, 41.7% of the patients were diagnosed clinically with gastroesophageal reflux, and mild reflux was confirmed by EGD in 6 patients. They performed EMG of the left masseter muscle and audio-video recording on days 4 and 5 of administrated 10 mg of rabeprazole or placebo. They found that PPI administration yielded a significant reduction in frequency of EMG bursts and grinding noise. The authors did not recommend the clinical initiation of proton pump inhibitor therapy for treatment on the basis of their small study population, but they did assert that this trial suggested potential value of treatment of gastroesophageal reflux in patients with sleep bruxism. They recommended larger studies.

A comprehensive paper investigating the possible association of PPI use with the risk of dementia appeared is a large study that includes a comprehensive review of references on the subject. While the study does not provide definitive answers and contains weaknesses (many of which are acknowledged by the authors), Gomm et al[568] provide data that raise serious questions about the possible association of PPI use and dementia, and the study warrants increased consideration of this possible risk, as well as additional research. The study reviewed insurance data from 73 679 participants in the German health system. They were 75 years of age or older and free of dementia at the beginning of the study according to the records. The study revealed a significantly increased risk of incident dementia in patients receiving PPI medication, in comparison with those not receiving PPIs (hazard ratio of 1.44; $p < .001$). The risk was slightly higher in males than in females. Potential confounding factors were controlled as well as possible in a study of this design, and this included analysis of depression (the condition with the highest risk associated with incident dementia), age (also associated), diabetes, polypharmacy, and others. Use of anticholinergic medications (a known risk factor for dementia) also was considered. The 3 most common PPIs used were omeprazole, pantoprazole, and esomeprazole. The risk was slightly greater with esomeprazole than with the other 2 more common medications. Patients on rabprazole were included in the study, as well. The association between PPI use and dementia was clear, although causation could not be established in this study. The authors offered several speculations regarding mechanism. Lansoprazole and omeprazole cross the blood-brain barrier and have the potential to affect the brain directly. PPI use appears to increase beta-amyloid levels in the brain in mice, a substance associated with Alzheimer's disease, and it is possible that PPIs may alter degradation of brain substances, some of which is pH dependent. Unfortunately, the authors did not have information on vitamin B12

levels in their cohort. Vitamin B12 deficiency has been associated with PPI use and can cause dementia. If this is the primary mechanism, then it is possible that the dementia risk can be mitigated or eliminated by maintaining B12 levels. However, substantial further research will be required to determine causation. The authors also mentioned that antihypertensive drugs such as calcium channel blockers and renin-angiotensin system blockers may prevent dementia, but there are no data on whether simultaneous use of these medications with PPIs would alter the dementia risk. Interestingly, Gomm et al also found that the risk of incident dementia associated with PPIs decreased gradually with age, with the highest risk occurring between 75 and 79 years of age. This is also true of potential confounding factors associated with dementia such as depression and stroke. Despite numerous strengths, the study was limited by the inability to completely rule out effects of confounding factors (eg, educational level and ApoE4 allele status were unknown). The authors also were unable to differentiate between different causes of dementia, such as vascular dementia vs Alzheimer's disease. In addition, although not mentioned in their article, it is possible (unlikely) that there is an association between reflux and dementia (as opposed to between reflux treatment with PPIs and dementia). This could be studied by comparing a group of treated reflux patients with a group of untreated reflux patients, but such data were not available in Gomm et al's study and were also not available in any other research, so far. The statistical association between PPI use and the risk of dementia warrants further research and careful consideration of the risks of treatment with PPIs vs nontreatment in each individual patient. If it is shown eventually that there is a causal relationship between

PPIs and dementia, then clearly alternative treatment approaches will need to be considered, possibly including increased referral for antireflux surgery to minimize or avoid use of all antireflux medication.

In 2017, Vaezi and colleagues[569] discussed the possible complications of proton pump inhibitor therapy, as well as recent media reports citing safety issues regarding the use of proton pump inhibitors that had caused concern and fear among the general population. They pointed out that many patients have self-discontinued their PPI therapy due to safety concerns. The authors point out that prescribers need to evaluate the evidence objectively when considering any reported association of complications that might be related to PPI therapy. The authors stated that "evidence is inadequate to establish causal relationships between PPI therapy and many of the proposed associations. Residual confounding related to study design and the overextrapolation of quantitatively small estimates of effect size have probably led to much of the current controversy about PPI safety." They suggested that increasing PPI dosage and continued chronic therapy in those who do not respond to initial empiric therapy should be discouraged. The authors pointed out that there has been a large increase in the number of published studies on PPI-related adverse effects in recent years. The authors stated that "virtually the entire evidence base regarding PPI-related safety concerns consists of observational studies. We need to have a clear understanding of the meaning of a 'statistically significant' but modest association from such studies." They point out that like all drugs, proton pump inhibitors should be used at the most effective dose for the shortest period of time and that current evidence linking PPI use to serious long-term adverse consequences has been weak and insubstantial.

In a study at the University of Bologna, Eusebi and colleagues[570] reviewed the risks of long-term proton pump inhibitor use. Their findings were similar to those reported by Vaezi et al.[569] These authors pointed out that proton pump inhibitors are among the most commonly prescribed class of drugs and that there has been increasing concern regarding the safety of long-term usage. They stated that the clinical evidence of adverse effects was often weak. The authors noted that long-term side effects have been studied, including the interaction with other drugs, reduced intestinal absorption of vitamins and minerals, kidney damage, and dementia. They reviewed the most recent literature pertaining to these adverse effects and their associations to proton pump inhibitor use. The potential adverse effects of long-term PPI treatment they reviewed included risk of fracture, hypomagnesemia, vitamin B12 deficiency, dementia, cardiovascular risk, renal disease, *C difficile* infection, pneumonia, fundic gland polyps, gastric cancer, and colon cancer. The authors found that underlying biological mechanisms were possible; however, the clinical evidence of adverse effects is often weak and cannot be associated definitively with PPI use. They recommend further randomized controlled trials for evaluation of these proposed associations. They stated "in most cases when based on available evidence, PPI benefits seem to outweigh potential adverse effects."

Other Treatment Options

A novel approach to the treatment of pharyngolaryngeal reflux was introduced by Smoak and Koufman.[571] They studied the effects of chewing regular sugarless gum or sugarless gum containing bicarbonate on pharyngeal and esophageal pH. They demonstrated significant increases in mean pharyngeal and esophageal pH for both types of gum, but the improvements were more pronounced with sugarless gum containing bicarbonate. The beneficial effects of chewing bicarbonate gum lasted twice as long as the actual gum-chewing periods (25 minutes vs 49 minutes), and the beneficial effects of gum chewing were significantly greater than the buffering effect in control subjects obtained by eating a meal. In some patients, gum chewing completely abolished reflux episodes on 24-hour pH monitor study. Additional study is needed, but it appears as if gum chewing may be useful adjunctive antireflux therapy.

Durkes and Sivansakar[572] examined bicarbonate effects on vocal fold mucosal epithelium exposed to acid in 32 viable porcine vocal folds. Their findings suggest that bicarbonate has potential therapeutic effects in reducing acidic pH abnormalities associated with laryngeal pathology, including reflux, inflammation, and carcinogenesis.

Koufman and Johnston[573] have shown the potential value of using alkaline water. Our experience suggests that this has value for some patients. She also has suggested using atomized alkaline water (pH 11) through a handheld sprayer as an inhalant (personal communication, 2015). Koufman has found that inhaling a topical spray of alkaline water resolves arytenoid erythema and improves symptoms of LPR, although formal confirmation by Koufman and others is pending.

Helicobacter pylori

If a decision is made to treat *H pylori* after its presence has been proven, a combination of agents is used. Triple therapy with clarithromycin, metronidazole, and a PPI has been reported as efficacious, and there are few side effects.[574] At present, our therapy consists of a PPI twice daily, clarithromycin 500 mg twice daily, and amoxicillin 1 g twice daily for 1 week.

Surgical Therapy for Gastroesophageal Reflux Disease

Although comparison studies are inconclusive, it is likely that long-term medical therapy with PPIs and antireflux surgery are equal options for most patients with regard to acid injury, and the choice can be left to the patients in consultation with their treating physicians. Acid suppression does not always provide adequate control of symptoms in patients who note symptoms from suspected pH-neutral or alkaline reflux, especially singers; although this has not been demonstrated by clinical trials, such patients may be considered for surgical therapy.[575–577]

The history of surgical therapy for the treatment of gastroesophageal reflux began with Phillip Allison,[578] who was the first to correlate the symptoms of hiatal hernia with gastroesophageal reflux. His repair, described in 1951, emphasized the need to place the gastroesophageal junction intra-abdominally to improve its function. This maneuver alone, however, was found to be associated with a high rate of symptom recurrence. More sophisticated attempts at securing the gastroesophageal junction below the diaphragm culminated with the posterior gastropexy described by Hill in 1967.[579] This operation is still in use, although it has largely been replaced by fundoplication.

Rudolph Nissen[580] described his gastric fundic wrap in 1956. His innovations were followed by a flurry of interest in surgical management for this disease. However, over the past 2 decades, surgical treatment for reflux has become much less commonly utilized, owing to the introduction of more effective medical therapy, specifically H2-blockers and PPIs.

In 1991, the first reports of laparoscopic antireflux surgery (Nissen fundoplication) were published.[581] Minimally invasive approaches to this disease made operations more acceptable to gastroenterologists and patients, leading to a resurgence in interest for surgical correction of gastroesophageal reflux disease (GERD). Since the initial clinical reports in 1991, numerous studies have been published on the laparoscopic approach to antireflux surgery.[582–585]

Medical therapy is effective in controlling acid reflux in the majority of patients with GERD. However, while usually effective in controlling symptoms, medical therapy does not correct the mechanical abnormality that causes reflux. Patients often require long-term or indefinite courses of medications, as discontinuation frequently leads to recurrence of symptoms. In a series of 196 patients with severe esophagitis responsive to omeprazole, 82% developed recurrent erosions within 6 months after cessation of therapy.[185] Moreover, the consequences of long-term acid suppression are unknown.

In 1992, Spechler[586] compared the outcome of medical vs surgical therapy for complicated GERD. Surgery was significantly more effective, resulting in greater patient satisfaction, higher lower esophageal sphincter (LES) pressures, lower grades of esophagitis, and lower levels of esophageal acid exposure. This study had an average 2-year follow-up but was done without the use of PPIs.

However, in the follow-up study in 2001, Spechler et al[587] found no significant long-term differences between the groups in terms of grade of esophagitis, frequency of treatment of esophageal stricture and subsequent antireflux operations, SF-36 standardized physical and mental component scale scores, and overall satisfaction with antireflux therapy. They suggested that antireflux surgery should not be advised with the expectation that patients with GERD will no longer need to take antisecretory medications or that the procedure will prevent esophageal cancer among those with GERD and Barrett's esophagus. So et al[588] compared laparoscopic fundoplication results in patients complaining of atypical symptoms with results in patients who had typical GERD symptoms (heartburn and regurgitation). They found that postoperative relief of atypical symptoms was less satisfactory and more difficult to predict than relief of heartburn and regurgitation. The only predictors of relief of atypical symptoms were preoperative response to pharmacologic acid suppression and dual-probe pH testing (only in patients with laryngeal symptoms). Preoperative relief of atypical symptoms with use of a PPI or H2-blocker was associated significantly with successful surgical outcome. Findings of other authors who have assessed the effects of antireflux surgery on atypical symptoms have been variable.[589–602] For example, Larrain et al[65] found that antireflux surgery produced symptomatic improvement in GERD-related asthma and reduced the need for bronchodilators. However, Pitcher et al[603] found that antireflux surgery did not correct reflux-related asthma reliably. In 1996, Hunter et al[604] reported atypical symptom improvement rates of 80% to 91% in patients undergoing laparoscopic fundoplication, with particularly good results in the subset of patients with laryngopharyngeal symptoms. Although the role of antireflux surgery remains controversial, in our experience, it has proven valuable in appropriately selected voice patients.

Proton pump inhibitors continue to be the primary treatment for symptoms of LPR by most otolaryngologists. However, some patients' symptoms appear refractory to medical management with PPIs (twice or more daily dosing), and another subset of symptomatic patients is not willing to take daily medications for an extended period of time. At our voice center (RTS et al),[605] we performed a retrospective review of the patients' medical records to examine the effectiveness of antireflux surgery on LPR symptoms refractive to medical treatment in 25 professional voice users ranging in age from 14 to 75 years, most of whom did not meet traditional surgical criteria. Twenty-four-hour pH impedance studies were performed pre- and postoperatively. Reflux finding scores were graded (blind raters) pre- and postoperatively; these scores revealed no significant differences pre- and postoperatively with good inter- and intra-rater reliability. This was not a great surprise, since most patients were on 2, 3, or 4 doses of PPI at the time of the preoperative study. Postoperative 24-hour pH impedance studies postlaprascopic Nissen fundoplication revealed a significant decrease in reflux episode. Approximately 60% of patients were on no medication postoperatively, and 76% of patients who had been on BID PPI dosing and 86% who had been on super-high-dose PPI (3 or 4) administration reported satisfaction with the results of Nissen fundoplication in managing their symptoms. DeMeester scores also were normal before and after surgery and not helpful for outcomes assessments. Our findings also suggest the Reflux Finding Score may lack sensitivity as a tool for monitoring the severity of LPR symptoms.

A study by Trad et al[606] examined the long-term outcomes of patient satisfaction and symptom resolution in a group of patients who underwent transoral incisionless fundoplication (TIF) for GERD and/or LPR symptoms. Thirty-four patients had a confirmed diagnosis of GERD that was not controlled medically with antisecretory drugs (PPIs) and reported unwillingness to continue taking medications. All 34 patients underwent TIF surgery using the esophX. Follow-up data were obtained on 28 of 34 patients: 50% of the study population was female, 50% male, with a mean age of 57 years. The authors reported that "standard TIF-2 protocol was used and resulted in reduction of hiatal hernia and restored GE junction anatomy (heal grade 1)." They reported no postoperative complication in any patient. Follow-up at 14 months found 82% (23 of 28) patients were off daily PPIs and 68% (19 of 28) reported improvement in their symptoms compared to preoperatively. They utilized the RSI to evaluate LPR symptoms, including throat clearing, cough, and hoarseness, and reported that these symptoms were eliminated in 63% (17 of 28) patients.

Fahin et al[607] also examined the effect of laparoscopic antireflux surgery on laryngeal symptoms, physical findings, and voice analysis. They performed a prospective analysis on 2 groups of patients preoperatively and 2 years after laparoscopic antireflux surgery (LARS). Group 1 included 41 patients (24 men) with GERD and LPR symptoms. Group 2 included 26 patients (16 men) with GERD and no LPR symptoms. All patients underwent EGD, 24-hour pH monitoring, or M11-pH monitoring. Patients completed RSI and VHI-10 questionnaires. Laryngeal findings were evaluated by blinded otolaryngologists utilizing the RFS and the GRBS scale. The Multi-Dimensional Voice Program (MDVP) was used for objective voice measurements. Follow-up for both groups was at approximately 25 months following surgery. The authors reported that group 1 had significantly lower RSI and RF scores following surgery. They stated further that "LARS substantially improved RFS, RSI, and VH1 in carefully selected patients with GERD, especially the signs and symptoms related to the larynx and voice." The authors pointed out that "indications for LARS are limited in patients with LPR" but suggested that their findings support consideration of the procedure in the management of patients' LPR.

Hoppo et al[608] studied the role of hypopharyngeal multichannel intraluminal impedance (HM11) testing in patients undergoing antireflux surgery for reflux disease associated with chronic cough. The authors defined cough as lasting greater than or equal to 8 weeks and of undetermined etiology. They performed HM11 testing on 314 symptomatic patients, looking for high esophageal reflux (2 cm distal to the upper esophageal sphincter). Forty-nine patients were identified as having chronic cough, and 36 of the 49 patients (73%) were found to have abnormal proximal exposure. Sixteen of the 36 patients underwent antireflux surgery, and 81% (13 patients) reported resolution of cough. The authors suggest that HM11 aids in the diagnosis of LPR and potentially in identifying those patients who might benefit from antireflux surgery.

Another study by Mazzoleni et al[609] suggests that 24-hour pH impedance (pH-M11) is not reliable for the diagnosis of LPR and that oropharyngeal (OP) pH monitoring with the Dx-pH probe is a better diagnostic tool. They studied 36 patients with both tests concomitantly and reported weak correlations between results of both tests. They suggest that the etiology of pH alteration is uncertain, thus making determination of the best test for diagnosing LPR problematic.

Toomey et al[610] compared the results of patients with GERD who underwent transoral incision-less fundoplication (TIF) with those patients who underwent Toupet or

Nissen fundoplication between 2010 and 2013. They performed a case-controlled study of 20 patients in the 3 cohorts: those undergoing TIF, those undergoing laprascopic Nissen fundoplication, and those undergoing Toupet fundoplication. Their case-control data included age, preoperative DeMeester scores, and body mass index. They found that the patients undergoing TIF procedures had shorter operative times and shorter hospitalization time. In all 3 procedures, patients reported "dramatic and similar reduction in symptom frequency and severity." Patients reported experiencing symptoms less than once a month included 83% following TIF, 80% after Nissen fundoplication, and 92% after Toupet fundoplication. They concluded that TIF is safe and effective as compared to Nissen and Toupet procedures and recommended they continue use.

Du et al[611] reviewed laparoscopic Nissen fundoplication versus anterior 180-degree fundoplication for the treatment of gastroesophageal reflux disease. They searched the literature and found 6 randomized controlled trials (RCTs) that compared laparoscopic Nissen fundoplication (LNF) (360 degrees) with laparoscopic anterior fundoplication (LAF) (180 degrees). They studied the data comparing the benefits and adverse results of both techniques and compared the findings utilizing meta-analysis. The authors found that the procedures were equally effective in controlling GERD symptoms, and patients reported a comparable degree of satisfaction postoperatively. They stated that LNF was associated with higher incidence of postoperative dysphagia compared to the 180-degree LAF. However, the 180-degree LAF required more reoperations for recurrent reflux symptoms.

Oor et al[612] evaluated 17-year outcomes comparing laparoscopic versus conventional (open) Nissen fundoplication. In total, 111 patients were included in their study, 60 patients underwent laparoscopic Nissen fundoplication, and 51 underwent open Nissen fundoplication. Seventeen years after the procedures, most patients reported symptomatic relief and no differences in GERD symptoms or dysphagia. The authors reported that 17 years following Nissen fundoplication, 60% of the patients they studied remained off of PPI therapy, and 16% had required reoperation for recurrent GERD and/or dysphagia.

Zhang et al[613] compared Nissen fundoplication versus proton pump inhibitor therapy for the treatment of laryngopharyngeal reflux. The study focused on the results of pH-monitoring and symptomatic assessment scale for inclusion in this study. Seventy patients were diagnosed with LPR and type I hiatal hernia between 2014 and 2015. In their study population, over 30 patients had undergone laparoscopic Nissen fundoplication, and 39 patients had been treated with PPI therapy alone. Fifty-three patients in the LNF group completed reviews and follow-up for 2 years. The authors reported that there was significant improvement in the RSI and LPR symptom index scores after 2-year follow-up in both groups, and they recommended that the clinical diagnosis of LPR should be assessed with pH-monitoring, manometry, and a symptom index. They stated that laparoscopic Nissen fundoplication achieved better improvement than proton pump inhibitors in the treatment of LPR in patients who had type I hiatal hernia.

Martin Del Campo et al[614] examined the effectiveness of laparoscopic Nissen fundoplication in improving reflux symptoms and quality of life in patients with class I and class II obesity. They noted that patients with class I obesity and refractory gastroesophageal reflux disease often do not qualify for bariatric surgery and that

laparoscopic Nissen fundoplication for these patients remains controversial. The authors performed a prospective study of patients undergoing laparoscopic Nissen fundoplication between 2009 and 2014. Their study cohorts were defined based on body mass index (BMI) at the time of surgery. They defined nonobese patients as having a body mass index of less than 30 kg/m^2, class I obese patients with a body mass index between 30 and 34.9 kg/m^2, and class II obese patients as having a body mass index of 35 to 39.9 kg/m^2. In total, 167 patients underwent LNF during this study; 76 were nonobese, 53 were class I obese, and 47 had class II obesity. The authors studied outcomes using the gastroesophageal reflux symptom score and the gastroesophageal reflux disease health-related quality-of-life questionnaires. After 18 months, all patients reported improvement: 86% in the nonobese group, 83% in the class I obesity group, and 79% in the class II obesity patient group remained free of proton pump inhibitor medications postoperatively. The authors suggested that laparoscopic Nissen fundoplication helps quality of life 18 months postoperatively in nonobese and in class I and class II obese patients.

Although Nissen fundoplication has remained the gold standard for surgical treatment of gastroesophageal disease, 2 recent studies[615,616] have compared the use of magnetic sphincter augmentation (MSA) Nissen fundoplication as a newer treatment for gastroesophageal reflux disease. Both studies recommended MSA as an alternative treatment for GERD based on short-term studies with results showing significantly reduced reflux symptoms, increased quality of life, and reportedly gas-bloating due to shorter operative times. Both studies suggest that this procedure is an excellent alternative to fundoplication for the treatment of GERD, but it has not been studied for LPR.

Indications for Surgical Therapy

Indications for surgery include persistent symptomatology despite reasonable medical management and patient intolerance to medications. Surgery may also be an option for patients who are concerned about the costs and consequences of long-term medical therapy. In patients whose symptom control requires continuous medical therapy, surgery is an important option. Patients with complicated gastroesophageal reflux disease, manifesting in Barrett's metaplasia, stricture, or ulceration, and those who require long-term therapy should also be considered for surgery.

In the past, surgery for GERD was recommended infrequently due to the risks associated with abdominal surgery under general anesthesia, significant postoperative discomfort, and the recognition of substantial long-term complications such as dysphagia, "gas bloat," and others. Since the initial description of the operation by Rudolph Nissen in 1956, the operation has undergone significant modifications that have lessened the incidence of postoperative complications.[580] In addition, the introduction of the laparoscopic approach to antireflux surgery has minimized the postoperative discomfort and many of the risks. It has also shortened postoperative recuperation from 6 to 8 weeks to 2 to 3 weeks, allowing patients to return to normal activities in an acceptable period of time.

Preoperative Evaluation

Thorough preoperative evaluation is essential to successful surgical management of GERD. Although the typical patient with this disorder has well-recognized gastrointestinal symptoms, GERD may underlie certain cases of asthma and other respiratory diseases, laryngitis, chronic cough, and chest pain. In addition, other upper gastrointestinal conditions may present with symptoms similar to those seen with GERD. Thus, it is critical to firmly establish the diagnosis and to exclude other conditions.

Further goals of preoperative evaluation are to assess the anatomy and physiology of the swallowing mechanism and stomach. Adequacy of esophageal motility and gastric emptying are important preoperative considerations, because disorders in either of these areas will affect the choice of a surgical procedure. It is also important to document complications of reflux, specifically the presence or absence of Barrett's metaplasia, ulceration, or stricture.

The preoperative evaluation should include the following:

1. A complete history and physical examination is especially important both to determine symptoms related to reflux and to exclude other conditions. Evaluation of the general medical status is also crucial.

2. Upper gastrointestinal endoscopy is important to exclude other lesions and to assess for the presence or absence of Barrett's metaplasia. Stricture and ulceration may also be seen. The presence or absence of *H pylori* may be determined.

3. Roentgenographic barium contrast study of the upper gastrointestinal tract defines the anatomy of the esophagus and stomach, as well as the relationship of the gastroesophageal junction of the hiatus. The length of the esophagus is easily assessed. A foreshortened esophagus would alter surgical management significantly, as discussed below. The presence of a sliding or paraesophageal

hernia can be assessed. In addition, other anatomic abnormalities of the esophagus and stomach can be identified, such as strictures, webs, masses, or diverticula. Furthermore, this is a dynamic study allowing the radiologist to assess the motility of the esophagus and the emptying function of the stomach. Although reflux of barium is not always identified, the absence of this finding does not rule out the presence of reflux; demonstration of significant reflux of barium during this radiographic procedure is almost always considered abnormal. An assessment of gastric emptying also can be performed. This information can be obtained from the upper GI series or from a gastric emptying study. It is important to document the status of gastric emptying prior to surgical intervention that occurs in the area of the vagal trunks, as there have been occasional reports of postoperative gastroparesis.

4. Twenty-four-hour pH monitoring is considered the most accurate test for documenting the presence of abnormal acid reflux. This is particularly useful in patients who present with atypical symptoms such as asthma, chronic cough, hoarseness, chest pain, and others. This study quantifies the amount of abnormal reflux, its relationship to symptomatology, its presence in upright or supine positions, and the relationship of reflux episodes to time of day and specific activities. Although it is not strictly obligatory to obtain this study in patients with typical symptoms of reflux and evidence of reflux by other means (eg, endoscopic evidence of ulcerative esophagitis or Barrett's metaplasia), having this study is a useful baseline to help objectively assess postoperative results.

5. Esophageal manometry is obligatory in the preoperative evaluation of the patient with GERD. This essential study provides information regarding lower esophageal sphincter (LES) pressure, length, and relaxation. It also provides vital information regarding esophageal motility. Major motility abnormalities of the esophagus alter the choice of surgical procedure.

6. Other studies and evaluations include pulmonary function testing and comprehensive voice evaluations in selected patients. These are particularly valuable in patients presenting with atypical symptoms.

Although definitive information on the incidence, true causal relationship, and importance (relative to the risk of untreated LPR) of many of these adverse effects remains unknown, it is important for otolaryngologists to be aware of the potential problems associated with all of the medications we prescribe frequently.

Review of these potential problems is not intended to suggest that PPI therapy is overprescribed or should not be prescribed. The consequences of untreated LPR can be substantial and potentially life threatening. However, much of the research on adverse events of PPIs is known widely by otolaryngologists. Otolaryngologists need to make an extra effort to remain current on new findings so that we can counsel and treat our patients optimally. Caution should be exercised particularly when using PPIs in patients with acute coronary syndromes, and cardiology consultation should be considered when PPIs are necessary in patients taking clopidogrel.

Refractory cases may be particularly challenging. Inadequate medication dosage, resistance to medication, reactivity to non-acid reflux in adequately controlled patients, and misdiagnosis are all potential factors. Medication dosages can be increased as discussed above, as can the frequency of administration, although such modifications are "off label." Promotility agents and histamine receptor antagonists can be added. Monitoring of pH during medication use can be useful in determining the cause of persistent signs and symptoms in patients receiving treatment for LPR.

Reimer et al[617] described symptom-producing rebound acid hypersecretion following withdrawal of PPI therapy after 2 months. Acid-related symptoms occurred in a group of healthy volunteers after treatment was stopped, which the authors interpreted as suggesting that rebound acid hypersecretion may result in PPI dependency. We believe that it is also possible because of healing of sensors that were not functional due to long-term acid exposure but recover on PPIs. Hence, it is not uncommon for LPR patients who have never had heartburn to develop heartburn during treatments with PPIs (especially at low doses) or after PPIs are stopped. Patients who choose long-term medical therapy can be reasonably expected to avoid acid-induced mucosal injury, without risk for serious complications. Although comparison studies are inconclusive, it is likely that in most patients, long-term medical therapy with PPIs and antireflux surgery are equivalent options for minimizing acid injury, and the choice can be left to the patient in consultation with the treating physician. Acid suppression does not always provide adequate control of symptoms in patients who note symptoms from suspected pH-neutral or alkaline reflux, especially singers; although this has not been demonstrated by clinical trials, such patients may be considered for surgical therapy.

Current Operations for Correction of Gastroesophageal Reflux Disease

Antireflux procedures can be classified into 2 groups: those that involve some form of fundoplication and those that do not. They can also be classified by surgical approach, specifically whether performed through the abdomen or through the chest. Additionally, all of these operations can be done open or with minimally invasive techniques (laparoscopic and thoracoscopic approaches).

In selecting an antireflux operation, all preoperative information needs to be considered. Esophageal function and motility affect the choice of operation. When motility is normal, the Nissen fundoplication with a full 360° wrap is the operation of choice. Conversely, with major motility abnormalities, a partial fundoplication is usually preferable.

Second, the length of the esophagus is important. Esophageal shortening should be treated with the addition of a gastroplasty. Third, the presence or absence of hypersecretions of gastric acid may play a role in choice of surgical procedure. An acid-reducing procedure such as a selective vagotomy may be considered in addition to the antireflux procedure. Fourth, the finding of a significant gastroparesis preoperatively may prompt consideration of an additional gastric procedure such as a pyloroplasty at the time of antireflux repair.

Surgical Repairs Involving Fundoplication

Nissen Fundoplication. In 1956, Rudolph Nissen[580] described his 360° gastric fundic wrap. Since that time, modifications regarding the length and looseness of the wrap have been made, allowing the most effective antireflux procedure with minimal morbidity. Currently, this is the most popular antireflux procedure. The steps in performing fundoplication, which are similar whether the approach is open or laparoscopic, include:

1. Incision of the gastrohepatic omentum at the gastroesophageal junction to expose the esophagus and the diaphragmatic crura (Figures 9–21 and 9–22)
2. Identification and preservation of the anterior and posterior vagus nerves (Figure 9–23)
3. Circumferential dissection of the esophagus (Figure 9–24)

4. Assessment of mobility of the fundus
   a. Mobilization of the fundus by division of the short gastric vessels if the fundus is not sufficiently floppy (Figure 9–25)
   b. With a sufficiently floppy fundus, mobilization of the short gastric vessels can occasionally be omitted, creating a Rossetti modification of the Nissen fundoplication
5. Closure of the crura (Figure 9–26)
6. Construction of a loose fundoplication around the distal esophagus just proximal to the gastroesophageal junction. This is performed over a large (54–56 Fr) dilator and is created 2 cm in length (Figure 9–27).

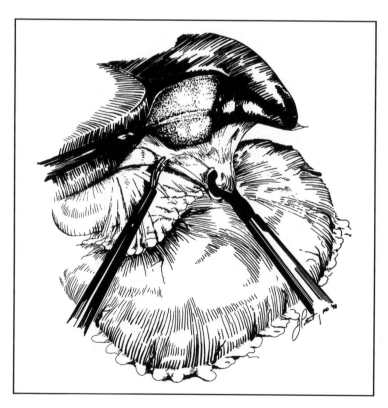

Figure 9–21. Incision of gastrohepatic omentum.

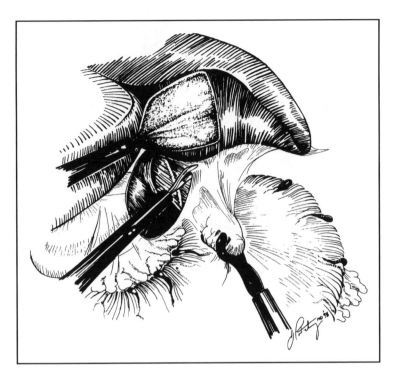

Figure 9–22. Exposure of esophagus and diaphragmatic crura.

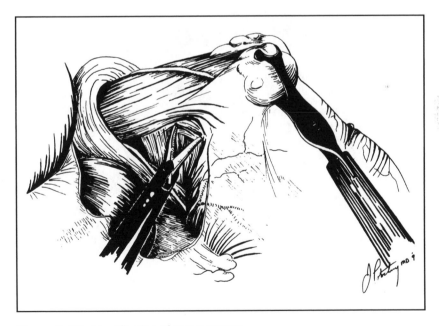

Figure 9–23. Identification of vagus nerves.

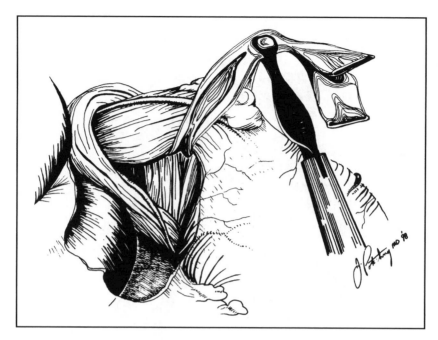

Figure 9–24. Circumferential dissection of the esophagus.

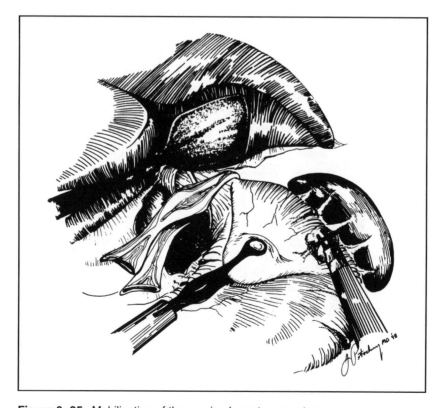

Figure 9–25. Mobilization of the proximal greater curvature.

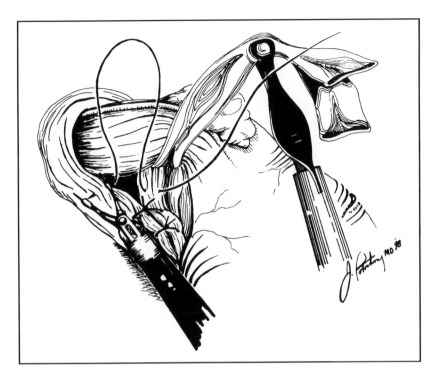

Figure 9–26. Closure of the crura.

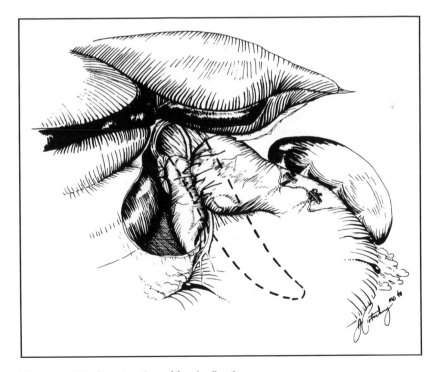

Figure 9–27. Construction of fundoplication.

The Laparoscopic Approach. In the 1990s, the first reports of laparoscopic antireflux surgery were published.[581] They described a minimally invasive surgical approach to treatment of this disease with low mortality and morbidity. The laparoscopic approach can be used in most patients undergoing antireflux surgery and has become the approach of choice. Contraindications to a laparoscopic antireflux operation include major coagulopathy, severe obstructive pulmonary disease, and possibly pregnancy. Prior abdominal surgery is not a contraindication. Reoperative antireflux surgery usually cannot be performed laparoscopically. Occasionally, a laparoscopic approach may be attempted but generally, conversion to an open procedure is necessary. This is usually due to severe central obesity or a large left lobe of the liver, both of which preclude adequate visualization of the relevant anatomy.

The patient is placed on the operating table in lithotomy and reverse Trendelenburg positions. This allows the surgeon to be positioned between the patient's legs, which facilitates 2-handed dissection essential to satisfactory performance of this procedure. However, the 2-handed technique also can be used effectively with the patient in the supine position, having the surgeon on the left side of the table and modifying port placement somewhat (Figure 9–28).

A 12-mm port is positioned to the right of the xiphoid for the liver retractor. Right upper quadrant and left upper quadrant 10-mm ports are positioned, functioning as dissecting ports. An additional 10-mm port is placed in the midline for placement of the camera, and a 10-mm port is placed in the left mid-abdomen for retraction of the stomach. The left lobe of the liver is retracted upward, exposing the gastroesophageal junction. A laparoscopic Babcock clamp is utilized to pull down the fundus, exposing the hiatus.

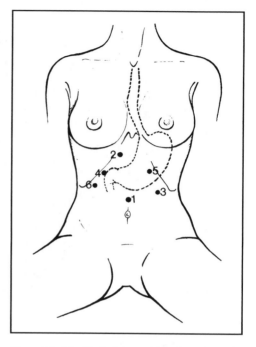

Figure 9–28. Port placement for laparoscopic fundoplication: (1) 30° laparoscope; (2) liver retractor; (3) stomach retractor; (4) dissecting port; (5) dissecting port; (6) optional dissecting port.

The gastrohepatic omentum overlying the gastroesophageal junction is incised, and the right crus is identified. The right crus is then dissected away from the right lateral wall of the esophagus. The left crus is then identified and dissected away from the left side of the esophagus. The esophagus is then retracted upward, and the posterior aspect of the esophagus is dissected under direct vision. To avoid perforation, it is important to perform the esophageal dissection under direct vision at all times. Furthermore, dissection should not stray from the esophagus, because dissection in the pleural space can occur, causing pneumothorax. Once the esophagus is circumferentially dissected, a Penrose drain is placed around it, and the Babcock clamp previously used to retract the fundus is repositioned on the Penrose drain. The anterior (left) and posterior (right) vagus nerves are identified. The posterior nerve is excluded from the Penrose drain.

The fundus is then inspected to assess its mobility. In most cases, it is advisable to divide the short gastric vessels to allow for a loose, tension-free wrap. This can be accomplished using the harmonic scalpel or using clips. The proximal third of the greater curvature is mobilized in this manner.

The diaphragmatic opening is made appropriately snug. This is performed with a 54- to 56-Fr dilator within the esophagus to avoid making the closure too tight. Once the diaphragmatic closure is completed, the dilator is retracted into the mid-esophagus by the anesthesiologist or an assistant. The fundus is then drawn around the posterior surface of the esophagus. The wrap is accomplished over the 54- to 56-Fr dilator by placing three 2-0 silk sutures. These sutures are placed from the fundus to the esophagus to the other side of the fundus in each instance. The abdomen is then irrigated and hemostasis is ensured. All trocars are removed under direct vision, and port sites are closed.

The Transthoracic Approach. Indications for performing an antireflux procedure via the thorax are:

1. Reoperative antireflux surgery
2. Patients who require concomitant procedures on the intrathoracic esophagus
3. Patients with coexistent left pulmonary pathology that requires surgery
4. Patients with a foreshortened esophagus
5. Obese patients in whom an abdominal approach may afford poor visualization
6. Surgeon preference

Partial Fundoplication. In the presence of esophageal dysmotility, partial fundoplication is the operation of choice. This can be performed through a thoracic approach such as a Belsey Mark IV partial fundoplication, which creates a 240° anterior partial fundoplication. Alternatively, the Toupet partial fundoplication can be performed transabdominally as an open or laparoscopic procedure. The technical aspects of this procedure are similar to those for a Nissen fundoplication with the exception of the wrap. After mobilization of the fundus and pulling it around posterior to the esophagus, the fundus is sutured to the right crus using three 2-0 silk sutures.

The anterior aspect of the fundus is then sutured to the esophagus. The fundus is similarly sutured to the left crus and anteriorly along the left side of the esophagus. This wrap necessitates placement of 12 sutures in the 4 rows (Figure 9–29).

Collis Gastroplasty

In patients with a foreshortened esophagus, a Collis gastroplasty is utilized to lengthen the esophagus. This is followed by a partial or complete fundoplication around the gastric tube with placement of the repair intraabdominally (Figure 9–30).

Nonfundoplication Repairs (Gastropexy)

In 1967, Lucius Hill[579] described his experience with posterior gastropexy. After his initial series, approximately 20% of his patients had recurrence of reflux symptoms with long-term follow-up. This led to modifications of the technique to include calibration of the lower esophageal sphincter pressure intraoperatively. The physiologic basis of the current Hill operation is that the lower esophageal sphincter segment is restored to the high-pressure environment of the abdomen and secured in that position by anchoring the gastroesophageal junction to the median actuate ligament posteriorly. The hiatal hernia defect is corrected, and

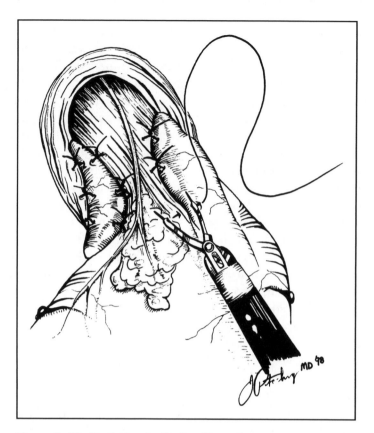

Figure 9–29. Partial fundoplication (Toupet).

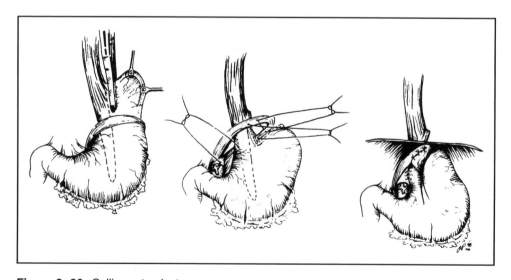

Figure 9–30. Collis gastroplasty.

284

the lower esophageal sphincter pressure is restored using intraoperative manometry (Figure 9–31).

The Hill repair has been described utilizing an open or laparoscopic technique.[579] The following steps are common to both:

1. The crura are dissected.
2. The anterior and posterior vagus nerves are identified and preserved.
3. The esophagus is dissected circumferentially.
4. The medial aspect of the gastric fundus is mobilized from its adhesions to the diaphragm, which occasionally also includes division of several short gastric vessels.

5. The preaortic fascia is dissected down to the area of the median actuate ligament.
6. The esophageal hiatus is loosely closed around the esophagus.
7. Sutures are placed in the anterior and posterior phreno-esophageal bundles, avoiding the esophagus. Three such sutures are placed.
8. Intraoperative manometry is performed. Sutures are placed through the imbricated bundles and carried through the preaortic fascia.
9. Additional sutures are placed from the fundus through the diaphragm to further reinforce the reconstructed gastroesophageal sphincter.

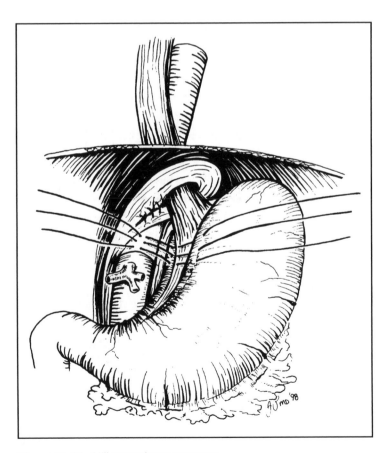

Figure 9–31. Hill posterior gastropexy.

Postoperative Care

Patients are admitted to the hospital pre-operatively. A nasogastric tube is not used routinely. Antireflux medications are not restarted. On the first postoperative day, patients undergo an upper gastrointestinal contrast study using water-soluble contrast to rule out the presence of a leak. If no leak is identified, the patient is asked to swallow a small amount of barium to better delineate the postoperative anatomy and to assess emptying function of the esophagus and stomach. Clear liquids are started on the first postoperative day, and diet is advanced as tolerated. With laparoscopic surgery, patients are generally discharged on the second postoperative day. Some degree of minor transient dysphagia is common, but in nearly all cases, this resolves within 8 to 12 weeks.

Patients are seen in follow-up at 2 weeks. At 3 and 12 months, patients are asked to undergo repeat 24-hour pH monitoring and esophageal manometry.

Operative Complications

In general, antireflux surgery, whether performed open or closed, is safe. In several large series, mortality rates are essentially zero.[578-597] Wound complications such as infection and herniation are seen slightly more often with the open technique. In addition, splenic injury is reported as occurring in 1% to 2% of open fundoplications, but it is very rarely, if ever, seen with the laparoscopic approach.

Complications following laparoscopic antireflux surgery include those common to all operations, those specific to laparoscopy, and those related to the specific surgical procedure. Operative complications common to all procedures include bleeding and infection. Bleeding complications are rarely, if ever, seen with laparoscopic antireflux surgery. It is virtually never necessary to transfuse patients. Wound infection is also extremely uncommon. Another complication common to many operations performed under general anesthesia is pulmonary emboli. In our series of 70 laparoscopic antireflux procedures, this complication occurred in 2.8% of patients. In no instance was it fatal.[587]

Complications specific to laparoscopy include trocar injuries, hypercapnea requiring ventilation, pneumothorax, and pneumomediastinum. Trocar injures are rare. We utilize an open technique for inserting the initial trocar and have not had any injuries. Many patients have pneumothorax. As part of the author's (DMS) original protocol, all patients underwent routine chest x-ray in the recovery room, and this finding was incidentally noted commonly. In all instances, patients were asymptomatic, and the pneumothorax resolved on follow-up chest x-ray the next day. In addition, pneumomediastinum with air occasionally tracking into the subcutaneous tissues of the neck and chest was also seen. In all instances, these findings resolved within 24 hours.

Complications specific to the operation include persistent dysphagia, defined as dysphagia still present more than 3 months after surgery. In the literature, patients have required reoperation for this complication, although we have not had that experience in our series to date.

Occasionally, persistent dysphagia can be corrected with endoscopic dilatation. Postoperative gastroparesis is occasionally seen and thought to be due to edema around the vagus nerves secondary to the operative dissection. This complication is rare and is effectively treated with prokinetic agents such as cisapride or metoclopramide. This phenomenon is generally transient, and these medications can be discontinued several weeks after surgery.

Esophageal or gastric perforation occurring intraoperatively has also been described. Should these complications be recognized intraoperatively, they can be repaired laparoscopically. However, this requires an experienced surgeon well versed in advanced laparoscopic techniques. Failure to recognize these complications may lead to septic complications, which frequently requires a return to the operating room. Fortunately, these are also rare.

Results

Many studies report the efficacy of antireflux surgery with 90% of patients demonstrating symptom control. The laparoscopic approach achieves similar outcomes to open antireflux surgery, although follow-up is shorter.

Professional voice users often will demonstrate reflux during singing. This reflux may be acidic or pH neutral. This subgroup of patients does well following surgery with improved vocal quality and strength, although some of these patients will still require antireflux medication, at least occasionally.

Endoscopic Antireflux Therapy

Although medical and surgical therapies for GERD are extremely successful, well-studied, and effective alternatives for patients with need for long-term therapy, many patients would prefer a nonsurgical, nonpharmacologic option for treatment of their symptoms. This has led to extensive research and development of endoscopic procedures designed to treat GERD. Four of

these procedures are approved by the FDA for treatment of GERD: radiofrequency energy delivery to the gastroesophageal junction (Stretta, Curon Medical, Fremont, California); transoral flexible endoscopic suturing (EndoCinch, Bard, Murray Hill, New Jersey); injection of a biocompatible, nonbiodegradable copolymer to reinforce the muscular layer of the LES (Enteryx, Boston Scientific, Natick, Massachusetts); and an endoscopic, full-thickness plicator device (NDO plicator). All attempt to reduce reflux by mechanically altering the LES. The exact mechanism for their efficacy is unknown.

Several key generalizations can be made. To date, a relatively small number of patients have been studied, follow-up time is relatively short (≤3 years), and a few major side effects have been reported. Studies have been performed in patients with heartburn and regurgitation.

All patients treated have had good response to PPIs. Only patients with mild erosive esophagitis (grade 2 or less) and small hiatal hernias have been evaluated. Therefore, patients with severe erosive esophagitis, Barrett's esophagus, and other manifestations of GERD (cough, asthma, LPR) have not been studied. Although long-term side effects are few, chest pain, dysphagia, and fever are seen immediately after the procedure in most patients. Unfortunately, several deaths have been associated with the procedures (Stretta and Enteryx); other rare major complications such as pleural effusion, esophageal perforation, and aspiration have also been reported.

Stretta

Six months after therapy, patients in an open-label study in the United States who were treated with radiofrequency energy showed an improvement in heartburn score, regurgitation, quality of life, and patient satisfaction compared with baseline without any changes in esophageal motility.[618]

The initial study reported no major complications. At 6 months, 70% were not on any antisecretory therapy and 87% were able to discontinue PPIs. At 1-year follow-up, more than 60% continued to be off antisecretory therapy and had sustained improvement in heartburn. Unfortunately, serious side effects have been reported to the FDA, including aspiration, pleural effusion, atrial fibrillation, and deaths in the first 1000 procedures performed.

Stretta has been studied in a prospective, sham-controlled study.[619] Sixty-four patients were randomly assigned to radiofrequency energy delivery to the gastroesophageal junction (35 patients) or to a sham procedure (29 patients). Radiofrequency energy delivery significantly improved GERD symptoms and quality of life compared with the sham procedure (61% of patients in the treatment group compared with 33% of patients who received a sham procedure ceased to have daily heartburn symptoms), but it did not decrease esophageal acid exposure or medication use at 6 months. Symptom improvement persisted 12 months after treatment, and no perforations or deaths were reported.

Yan et al[620] compared the effect of the Stretta procedure with results of Toupet fundoplication for the treatment of gastroesophageal and extraesophageal symptoms. The authors evaluated 98 patients diagnosed with GERD-related extraesophageal symptoms between 2011 and 2012. All patients underwent the Stretta procedure or laparoscopic toupet fundoplication (LTF). The patients were followed for 3 years. Forty-seven patients underwent the Stretta procedure and 51 patients underwent the LTF procedure. Ninety patients were avail-able for the 3-year follow-up. The authors found that the patients in the LTF group were more satisfied with quality of life than those with the Stretta procedure. However, they pointed out that 2 patients in the LTF group had severe dysphagia 2 weeks following the procedure and required dilation postoperatively. The authors stated that both procedures are safe and effective for the control of GERD-related and extra-esophageal symptoms of reflux and in the reduction of proton pump inhibitor therapy.

EndoCinch

The second approved procedure, endoluminal gastroplication (EndoCinch), was reported initially in a multicenter trial of 64 patients with heartburn more often than 3 times a week, dependence on antisecretory medication, mild erosive esophagitis, and abnormal 24-hour pH monitoring. They were treated with EndoCinch, an endoscopic suturing system designed to create an "internal placation" of the stomach.[621]

In this uncontrolled trial, improvement in the number of reflux episodes was seen. No change in upright, recumbent, or total esophageal acid exposure was seen at 3 and 6 months. Sixty-two percent of patients were able to decrease drugs to less than 4 doses of antisecretory medications per month. Improvement was seen in patient satisfaction, heartburn severity, and heartburn score compared with the initial measurements. With the exception of a "stitch" perforation that required short-term hospitalization, no major complications were reported. To date, no sham trial has been reported in full manuscript form using this method.

More recently, a 2-year follow-up study in 33 patients originally treated with this endoscopic device was reported.[622] After a mean follow-up of 25 months, heartburn severity and score and frequency of regurgitation showed continued improvement compared with baseline measurements. However, only 8 patients (25%) initially on PPIs were completely off antisecretory medications, with 9% taking half or less of their initial dose. Forty percent required full-dose medications, and 6% had undergone a laparoscopic Nissen fundoplication because of the therapeutic failure.

In an open-label, multicenter US trial,[623] 85 patients with GERD were treated with endoluminal gastroplication. At 12 and 24 months postoperatively, 59% and 52%, respectively, showed heartburn symptom resolution, and 73% and 69% decreased their PPI use by at least 50%. Eleven patients had adverse events, only 2 of which were serious: 1 patient had severe dysphagia necessitating removal of the plications, and 1 had severe bronchospasm requiring intubation to allow completion of the procedure. These data are disappointing and suggest that long-term efficacy of this procedure as designed originally will not be forthcoming.

Enteryx

The Enteryx procedure was granted approval by the FDA in April 2003. The procedure is performed by injecting a biopolymer (ethylene vinyl alcohol, EVA) into the muscular layer of the LES under fluoroscopic guidance. The proposed mechanism of action is based on enhancing the gastroesophageal barrier against reflux via a space-occupying effect, inducing fibrosis in the area of injection, and altering the compliance of the sphincter during gastric distention.[623,624]

In the expanded, multicenter, open-label, international clinical trial of Enteryx implantation for GERD,[625] promising results at 12 and 24 months were reported: 78% and 72%, respectively, of patients were able to reduce their previous PPI dose by at least 50%, and 78% and 80% reported significant improvements of their heartburn-related quality-of-life symptoms during the same time periods. None of the patients had what was considered a potentially life-threatening adverse event. The most common adverse event was transient retrosternal chest pain in 85% of patients, which resolved with prescription pain medications in 84% of affected patients. One of the 144 enrolled patients developed a paraesophageal fluid collection diagnosed at 6 weeks after the procedure, which resolved completely with intravenous antibiotics.

In a randomized, single-blind, prospective, multicenter clinical trial in Europe,[626] 64 patients with classic heartburn symptoms controlled on PPI therapy were randomized into 2 groups of equal sizes to receive either the Enteryx procedure or a sham procedure consisting of a standard upper endoscopy and were followed before allowing for crossover for 3 months. Eighty-one percent of patients in the Enteryx group achieved ≥50% reduction of their PPI use compared with 53% of those in the sham group, and 68% of patients in the Enteryx group vs 41% of patients in the sham group ceased PPIs completely. More Enteryx-treated (81%) than sham-treated (19%) patients did not undergo retreatment. Pain, odynophagia/dysphagia, and fever were the most common adverse events in the Enteryx group. An esophageal ulcer with extrusion of the copolymer was noted in 1 patient. Preliminary results of the US multicenter trial were recently reported with results similar to the European trial. Overall, although pH studies have shown statistical improvement from baseline, normalization is seen in less than one-third of patients.

Although few major side effects have been reported in the organized clinical trials, at least 1 procedure-related death has been reported, as well as case reports of mediastinitis and pleural effusion.

Endoscopic Full-Thickness Plicator

This system creates a transmural plication 1 cm distal to the esophageal-gastric junction, reinforcing the competency of the gastroesophageal barrier. It was granted premarket approval by the FDA in April 2003.

Data on the intermediate-term safety and efficacy of this device were published recently in a multicenter North American trial[627]; 64 patients requiring maintenance antisecretory therapy for chronic heartburn received a single endoscopic full-thickness plication in the gastric cardia 1 cm distal to the gastroesophageal junction. Of the 57 patients who completed the 12-month follow-up, 70% were off PPI therapy. Median heartburn-related quality-of-life scores improved significantly compared with baseline both while not taking PPIs and while taking such medication. Normal pH scores were observed in 30% of patients. Common procedure-related adverse events included sore throat (41%) and abdominal pain (20%), resolving spontaneously after several days. The same group had reported 6 serious adverse events during the initial follow-up at 6 months[626]: 2 patients experienced severe dyspnea, 1 developed pneumothorax, 1 pneumoperitonum, 1 gastric perforation, and 1 fundic mucosal abrasion. None resulted in long-term patient injury.

In 2010, Velanovich[628] reported his experience using Esophyx, a device for endoscopic fundoplication. Esophyx was used in 24 patients; 20 had symptoms and signs of GERD and 4 had been diagnosed with LPR. Four of the 24 patients had recurrent symptoms following Nissen procedures. He suggested that much research is still needed and that endoscopic fundoplication is most effective in patients with mild-to-moderate symptoms of GERD and those with small hiatal hernias. Its value for patients with LPR has not been established.

Transoral Incisionless Fundoplication

Testoni et al[629] reported on the use of transoral incisionless fundoplication for gastroesophageal reflux disease. The authors stated that over the past few years, transoral incisionless fundoplication (TIF) has proven to be an effective therapeutic option as an alternative to other medical and surgical therapy. Their review described the steps of the transoral incisionless fundoplication using both the EsophyX device and the MUSE system. The authors pointed out that there have only been prospective observational studies for TIF using the EsophyX device and that there are only limited data available for TIF with the MUSE system. Both procedures involve endoscopic stapling. The authors pointed out that as with all new surgical interventions, despite encouraging short- and medium-term outcomes, the long-term efficacy of TIF needs further assessment and controlled trials, especially the MUSE technique.

Summary and Role in LPR

The concept of endoscopic therapy is excellent, and its potential is exciting. Nonetheless, we are early in our evaluation of these evolving techniques. No organized clinical trials have been done or are in process in LPR. Therefore, efficacy in these difficult-to-treat patients cannot be predicted. Based on the current outcomes in patients with heartburn, the best that one might expect is the opportunity to reduce PPI dosage. More data on efficacy and safety are needed before we can recommend these techniques widely. Patients should be reminded that medical therapy is safe and surgery a reasonable alternative when performed by an experienced surgeon. Francis et al[630] examined the role of antireflux surgery in patients with signs and symptoms of LPR refractory to medical management with PPIs. They pointed out the controversy regarding the role of fundoplication in patients with PPI-refractory symptoms and abnormal nonacid reflux by pH impedance monitoring. In their patients, 59% reported symptom improvement postsurgery. They defined preoperative refractory symptoms as <50% improvement following at least 12 weeks of twice-daily PPI therapy. Their patients underwent esophagogastroduodenoscopy, wireless 48-hour pH monitoring, and esophageal motility testing off acid suppression to determine their baseline acid exposure. The patients also underwent 24-hour impedance pH monitoring while on twice-daily PPI therapy. The authors could not confirm that the impedance of pH parameter measured while on therapy was a predictor of symptom response following fundoplication.

If endoscopic antireflux therapy is considered, patients should have it only after careful consideration of the alternatives and with clear understanding of the absence of long-term data and the small but real risk for major complications. At present, these procedures should not be considered as indicated for those who have failed medical therapy.

Conclusion

Antireflux surgery is a safe, effective therapeutic alternative in the management of gastroesophageal reflux disease. In expert hands, laparoscopic antireflux surgery is safe, is effective, and corrects the underlying cause of reflux with minimal morbidity and high patient satisfaction. It eliminates the problems of pH-neutral reflux and the need for prolonged use of acid-suppressing medications. Surgery should be considered as an appropriate option in the treatment of reflux disease. Newer endoscopic approaches to improve the function of the LES require further refinement and study. They have potential to be less invasive and less morbid than even laparoscopic surgery. If they prove to be safe and effective, if they do not affect adversely the results of subsequent laparoscopic fundoplication for patients in whom they fail, and if they are not associated with an excessive number of serious complications, then they may become desirable therapeutic options for patients with LPR, especially professional voice users. However, at present, preliminary data do not justify their routine use for patients with LPR.

References

1. Olson NR. The problem of gastroesophageal reflux. *Otolaryngol Clin North Am.* 1986;19:119–133.
2. Menon AP, Schefft GL, Thach BT. Apnea associated with regurgitation in infants. *J Pediatr.* 1985;106:625–629.
3. Little FB, Koufman JA, Kohut RI, Marshall RB. Effect of gastric acid on the pathogenesis of subglottic stenosis. *Ann Otol Rhinol Laryngol.* 1985;94:516–519.

4. Kambic V, Radsel Z. Acid posterior laryngitis. Aetiology, histology, diagnosis and treatment. *J Laryngol Otol.* 1984;98:1237–1240.

5. Feder RJ, Michell MJ. Hyperfunctional, hyperacidic, and intubation granulomas. *Arch Otolaryngol.* 1984;110:582–584.

6. Belmont JR, Grundfast K. Congenital laryngeal stridor (laryngomalacia): etiologic factors and associated disorders. *Ann Otol Rhinol Laryngol.* 1984;39:430–437.

7. Olson NR. Effects of stomach acid on the larynx. *Proc Am Laryngol Assoc.* 1983;104:108–112.

8. Ohman L, Olofsson J, Tibbling L, Ericsson G. Esophageal dysfunction in patients with contact ulcer of the larynx. *Ann Otol Rhinol Laryngol.* 1983;92:228–230.

9. Bain WM, Harrington JW, Thomas LE, Schaefer SD. Head and neck manifestations of gastroesophageal reflux. *Laryngoscope.* 1983;93:175–179.

10. Orenstein SR, Orenstein DM, Whitington PF. Gastroesophageal reflux causing stridor. *Chest.* 1983;84:301–302.

11. Ward PH, Berci G. Observations on the pathogenesis of chronic non-specific pharyngitis and laryngitis. *Laryngoscope.* 1982;92:1377–1382.

12. Ward PH, Zwitman D, Hanson D, Berci G. Contact ulcers and granulomas of the larynx: new insights into their etiology as a basis for more rational treatment. *Otolaryngol Head Neck Surg.* 1980;88:262–269.

13. Goldberg M, Noyek AM, Pritzker KP. Laryngeal granuloma secondary to gastroesophageal reflux. *J Otolaryngol.* 1978;7:196–202.

14. Chodosh PL. Gastro-esophago-pharyngeal reflux. *Laryngoscope.* 1977;87:1418–1427.

15. Toohill RJ, Kuhn JC. Role of refluxed acid in pathogenesis of laryngeal disorders. *Am J Med.* 1997;103(5A):100S–106S.

16. Wiener GJ, Koufman JA, Wu WC, et al. Chronic hoarseness secondary to gastroesophageal reflux disease: documentation with 24-hr ambulatory pH monitoring. *Am J Gastroenterol.* 1989;84:1503–1508.

17. Sataloff RT, Spiegel JR, Hawkshaw MJ. Strobovideolaryngoscopy: results and clinical value. *Ann Otol Rhinol Laryngol.* 1991;100(9):725–727.

18. Koufman JA, Wiener GJ, Wu WC, Castell DO. Reflux laryngitis and its sequelae: the diagnostic role of ambulatory 24-hour pH monitoring. *J Voice.* 1988;2(1):78–89.

19. Toohill RJ, Ulualp SO, Shaker R. Evaluation of gastroesophageal reflux in patients with laryngotracheal stenosis. *Ann Otol Rhinol Laryngol.* 1998;107:1010–1014.

20. Ross JA, Noordzji JP, Woo P. Voice disorders in patients with suspected laryngopharyngeal reflux disease. *J Voice.* 1998;12:84–88.

21. Rothstein SG. Reflux and vocal disorders in singers with bulimia. *J Voice.* 1988;12:89–90.

22. Kuhn J, Toohill RJ, Ulualp SO, et al. Pharyngeal acid reflux events in patients with vocal cord nodules. *Laryngoscope.* 1998;108:1146–1149.

23. Gumpert L, Kalach N, Dupont C, Contencin P. Hoarseness and gastroesopahgeal reflux in children. *J Laryngol Otol.* 1998;112:49–54.

24. Halstead LA. Role of gastroesophageal reflux in pediatric upper airway disorders. *Otolaryngol Head Neck Surg.* 1999;120:208–214.

25. Al Sabbagh G, Wo JM. Supraesophageal manifestations of gastroesophageal reflux disease. *Semin Gastrointest Dis.* 1999;10:113–119.

26. Hanson DG, Jiang JJ. Diagnosis and management of chronic laryngitis associated with reflux. *Am J Med.* 2000;108(suppl 4a):112S–119S.

27. Grontved AM, West F. pH monitoring in patients with benign voice disorders. *Acta Otolaryngol Suppl.* 2000;543:229–231.

28. Koufman JA, Amin MR, Panetti M. Prevalence of reflux in 113 consecutive patients with laryngeal and voice disorders. *Otolaryngol Head Neck Surg.* 2000;123:385–388.

29. Poelmans J, Tack J, Feenstra L. Chronic middle ear disease and gastroesophageal

reflux disease: a causal relation? *Otol Neurotol.* 2001;22:447–450.

30. Tasker A, Dettmar PW, Panetti M, et al. Reflux of gastric juice and glue ear in children. *Lancet.* 2002;359(9305):493.

31. Loehrl TA, Smith TL, Darling RJ, et al. Autonomic dysfunction, vasomotor rhinitis, and extraesophageal manifestations of gastroesophageal reflux. *Otolaryngol Head Neck Surg.* 2002;126:382–387.

32. Koufman JA. The otolaryngologic manifestations of gastroesophageal reflux disease (GERD): a clinical investigation of 225 patients using ambulatory 24-hour pH monitoring and an experimental investigation of the role of acid and pepsin in the development of laryngeal injury. *Laryngoscope.* 1991;101(4, pt 2)(suppl 53):1–78.

33. Sataloff RT. *Professional Voice: The Science and Art of Clinical Care.* 3rd ed. San Diego, CA: Singular Publishing Group; 2005.

34. Rosen DC, Sataloff RT. *The Psychology of Voice Disorders.* San Diego, CA: Singular Publishing Group; 1997:1–284.

35. Li Q, Castell JA, Castell DO. Manometric determination of esophageal length. *Am J Gastroenterol.* 1994;89:722–725.

36. Gerhardt DC, Shuck TL, Bordeaux RA, Winship DH. Human upper esophageal sphincter. *Gastroenterology.* 1978;75:268–274.

37. Winans CS. Manometric asymmetry of the lower esophageal high-pressure zone. *Am J Dig Dis.* 1977;22:348–354.

38. Meyer GW, Austin RM, Brady CE, et al. Muscle anatomy of the human esophagus. *J Clin Gastroenterol.* 1986;8:131–134.

39. Weisbrodt NW. Neuromuscular organization of esophageal and pharyngeal motility. *Arch Intern Med.* 1976;136:524–531.

40. Meyer GW, Gerhardt DC, Castell DO. Human esophageal response to rapid swallowing: muscle refractory period of neural inhibition? *Am J Physiol.* 1981;241:G129–G136.

41. Goyal RK, Rattan S. Genesis of basal sphincter pressure: effect of tetrodotoxin on the lower esophageal sphincter in oposum in vivo. *Gastroenterology.* 1976;71:62–67.

42. Richter JE, Sinar DR, Cordova CM, Castell DO. Verapamil—a potent inhibitor of esophageal contractions in the baboon. *Gastroenterology.* 1982;82:882–886.

43. Richter JE, Spurling TJ, Cordova CM, Castell DO. Effects of oral calcium blocker, diltiazem, on esophageal contractions. *Dig Dis Sci.* 1984;29:649–656.

44. Dodds WJ, Dent J, Hogan WJ, Arndorfer RC. Effect of atropine on esophageal motor function in humans. *Am J Physiol.* 1981;240:G290–G296.

45. Pasricha PJ, Ravich WJ, Kalloo AN. Effects of intragastric botulinum toxin on the lower esophageal sphincter in piglets. *Gastroenterology.* 1993;105:1045–1049.

46. Goyal RK, Rattan S, Said SI. VIP as a possible neurotransmitter of non-cholinergic non-adrenergic inhibitory neurones. *Nature.* 1980;288:378–380.

47. Sanders KM, Ward SM. Nitric oxide as a mediator of nonadrenergic non-cholinergic neurotransmission. *Am J Physiol.* 1992;262(3, pt 1):C379–C392.

48. Castell DO. The lower esophageal sphincter. Physiologic and clinical aspects. *Ann Intern Med.* 1975;83:390–401.

49. Christensen J, Lund GF. Esophageal responses to distention and electrical stimulation. *J Clin Invest.* 1969;48:408–419.

50. *A Gallop Survey on Heartburn Across America.* New York, NY: The Gallop Organization Inc; 1968.

51. Locke GR III, Talley NJ, Fett SL, et al. Prevalence and clinical spectrum of gastroesophageal reflux: a population-based study in Olmstead County, Minnesota. *Gastroenterology.* 1997;112:448–456.

52. Nebel OT, Fornes MF, Castell DO. Symptomatic gastroesophageal reflux: incidence and precipitating factors. *Am J Dig Dis.* 1976;21:953–956.

53. Winters C Jr, Spurling TJ, Chobanian SJ, et al. Barrett's esophagus: a prevalent, occult complication of gastroesophageal reflux disease. *Gastroenterology.* 1987;92:118–123.

54. Ollyo JB, Monnier P, Fontollier C, et al. The natural history, prevalence and incidence of reflux esophagitis. *Gullet.* 1993;3 (suppl):3–10.

55. Pace F, Santalucia F, Bianchi Porro G. Natural history of gastro-oesophageal reflux disease without esophagitis. *Gut.* 1991;32: 845–848.

56. Schnatz PF, Castell JA, Castell DO. Pulmonary symptoms associated with gastroesophageal reflux: use of ambulatory pH monitoring to diagnose and to direct therapy. *Am J Gastroenterol.* 1996;91:1715–1718.

57. Harding SM, Richter JE, Guzzo MR, et al. Asthma and gastroesophageal reflux: acid suppressive therapy improves asthma outcome. *Am J Med.* 1996;100:395-405.

58. el-Serag HB, Sonnenberg A. Comorbid occurrence of laryngeal or pulmonary disease with esophagitis in United States military veterans. *Gastroenterology.* 1997;113: 755–760.

59. Harding SM, Guzzo MR, Richter JE. Prevalence of GERD in asthmatics without reflux symptoms. *Gastroenterology.* 1997;4:A141.

60. Sontag SJ, O'Connell S, Khandelwal S, et al. Most asthmatics have gastroesophageal reflux with or without bronchodilator therapy. *Gastroenterology.* 1990;99:613–618.

61. Irwin RS, French CL, Curley FJ, et al. Chronic cough due to gastroesophageal reflux: clinical, diagnostic, and pathogenic aspects. *Chest.* 1993;194:1511–1517.

62. Katz PO, Castell DO. Approach to the patient with unexplained chest pain. *Am J Gastroenterol.* 2000;7:95(8)(suppl):S4–S8.

63. Hewson EG, Sinclair JW, Dalton CB, Ritcher JE. Twenty-four-hour esophageal pH monitoring: the most useful test for evaluating noncardiac chest pain. *Am J Med.* 1991;90:576–583.

64. Cherian P, Smith LF, Bardham KD, et al. Esophageal tests in the evaluation of non-cardiac chest pain. *Dis Esophagus.* 1995;8: 129–133.

65. Larrain A, Carrasco E, Galleguillos F, et al. Medical and surgical treatment of non-allergic asthma associated with gastroesophageal reflux. *Chest.* 1991;99:1330–1335.

66. Sontag SJ, Schnell TG, Miller TQ, et al. Prevalence of oesophagitis in asthmatics. *Gut.* 1992;33:872–876.

67. Achem SR, Kolts BE, MacMath T, et al. Effects of omeprazole versus placebo in treatment of noncardiac chest pain and gastroesophageal reflux. *Dig Dis Sci.* 1997; 42(10):2138–2145.

68. Fass R, Fennerty B, Ofman JJ, et al. The clinical and economic value of a short course of omeprazole in patients with non-cardiac chest pain. *Gastroenterology.* 1998; 115:42–49.

69. Achem SR, DeVault KR. Unexplained chest pain at the turn of the century. *Am J Gastroenterol.* 1999;94(1):5–8.

70. Börjesson M, Albertsson P, Dellborg M, et al. Esophageal dysfunction syndrome X. *Am J Cardiol.* 1998;82:1187–1191.

71. O'Connor JF, Singer ME, Richter JE. The cost-effectiveness of strategies to assess gastroesophageal reflux as an exacerbating factor in asthma. *Am J Gastroenterol.* 1999; 94(6):1472–1480.

72. Levin TR, Sperling RM, McQuaid KR. Omeprazole improves peak expiratory flow rate and quality of life in asthmatics with gastroesophageal reflux. *Am J Gastroenterol.* 1998;93(7):1060–1063.

73. Govil Y, Khoury R, Katz PO, et al. Antireflux therapy improves symptoms in patients with reflux laryngitis [Abstract]. *Gastroenterology.* 1998;114:562.

74. Spechler SJ. Complications of gastroesophageal reflux disease. In: Castell DO, ed. *The Esophagus.* Boston, MA: Little, Brown and Company; 1992:543–556.

75. Lieberman DA, Oehlke M, Helfand M. Risk factors for Barrett's esophagus in community based practice. *Am J Gastroenterol.* 1997;92:1293–1297.

76. Fouad YM, Koury R, Hattlebakk JG, Katz PO, Castell DO. Ineffective esophageal motility: the most common motility disorder in patients with GERD-associated respiratory symptoms. *Am J Gastroenterol.* 1999;94:1464–1467.

77. Johnson LF. New concepts and methods in the study and treatment of gastroesopha-

geal reflux disease. *Med Clin North Am.* 1981;65:1195–1222.

78. Delahunty JE. Acid laryngitis. *J Laryngol Otol.* 1972;86(4):335–342.

79. Sataloff RT. The human voice. *Sci Am.* 1993;267:108–115.

80. Axford SE, Sharp N, Ross PE, et al. Cell biology of laryngeal epithelial defenses in health and disease: preliminary studies. *Ann Otol Rhinol Laryngol.* 2001;110(12): 1099–1108.

81. Kamel PL, Hanson D, Kahrilas PJ. Omeprazole for the treatment of posterior laryngitis. *Am J Med.* 1994;96:321.

82. Sataloff RT. Professional singers: the science and art of clinical care. *Am J Otolaryngol.* 1981;8:251–266.

83. Spiegel JR, Sataloff RT, Cohn JR, et al. Respiratory function in singers: medical assessment, diagnoses and treatments. *J Voice.* 1988;2(1):40–50.

84. Hallewell JD, Cole TB. Isolated head and neck symptoms due to hiatus hernia. *Arch Otolaryngol.* 1970;92:499–501.

85. Ossakow SJ, Elta G, Colturi T, et al. Esophageal reflux and dysmotility as the basis for persistent cervical symptoms. *Ann Otol Rhinol Laryngol.* 1987;96:387–392.

86. Kuriloff DB, Chodosh P, Goldfarb R, Ongseng F. Detection of gastroesophageal reflux in the head and neck: the role of scintigraphy. *Ann Otol Rhinol Laryngol.* 1989;98:74–80.

87. Lumpkin SM, Bishop SG, Katz PO. Chronic dysphonia secondary to gastroesophageal reflux disease (GERD): diagnosis using simultaneous dual-probe prolonged pH monitoring. *J Voice.* 1989;3:351–355.

88. McNally PR, Maydonovitch CL, Prosek RA, et al. Evaluation of gastroesophageal reflux as a cause of idiopathic hoarseness. *Dig Dis Sci.* 1989;34:1900–1904.

89. Katz PO. Ambulatory esophageal and hypopharyngeal pH monitoring in patients with hoarseness. *Am J Gastroenterol.* 1990; 85:38–40.

90. Freeland AP, Adran GM, Emrys-Roberts E. Globus hystericus and reflux oesophagitis. *J Laryngol Otol.* 1974;88:1025–1031.

91. Pesce G, Caligaris F. Le laringiti posteriori nella pathologia dell'apparato digerente. *Arch Ital Laringol.* 1966;74:77–92.

92. Vaughan CW, Strong MS. Medical management of organic laryngeal disorders. *Otolaryngol Clin North Am.* 1984;17:705–712.

93. Barkin RL, Stein ZL. GE reflux and vocal pitch. *Hosp Pract.* 1989;24(10A):20.

94. Jacob P, Kahrilas PJ, Herzon G. Proximal esophageal pH-metry in patients with "reflux laryngitis." *Gastroenterology.* 1991; 100:305–310.

95. Wilson JA, White A, von Haacke NP, et al. Gastroesophageal reflux and posterior laryngitis. *Ann Otol Rhinol Laryngol.* 1989; 98:405–410.

96. Cherry J, Margulies S. Contact ulcer of the larynx. *Laryngoscope.* 1968;78:1937–1940.

97. Delahunty JE, Cherry J. Experimentally produced vocal cord granulomas. *Laryngoscope.* 1968;78:1941–1947.

98. Gaynor EB. Gastroesophageal reflux as an etiologic factor in laryngeal complications of intubation. *Laryngoscope.* 1988;98:972–979.

99. Lillemoe KD, Johnson LF, Harmon JW. Role of the components of the gastroduodenal contents in experimental acid esophagitis. *Surgery.* 1982;92:276–284.

100. Johnson LF, Harmon JW. Experimental esophagitis in a rabbit model: clinical relevance. *J Clin Gastroenterol.* 1986;8(suppl 1): 26–44.

101. Cherry J, Seigel CI, Margulies SI, Donner M. Pharyngeal localization of symptoms of gastroesophageal reflux. *Ann Otol Rhinol Laryngol.* 1970;79:912–914.

102. von Leden H, Moore P. Contact ulcer of the larynx. Experimental observations. *Arch Otolaryngol.* 1960;72:746–752.

103. Toohill RJ, Mushtag E, Lehman RH. Otolaryngologic manifestations of gastroesophageal reflux. In: Sacristan T, Alvarez-Vincent JJ, Bartual J, et al, eds. *Proceedings of XIV World Congress of Otolaryngology—Head and Neck Surgery.* Amsterdam, The Netherlands: Kugler & Ghedini Publications; 1990:3005–3009.

104. Koufman JA, Amin M. Laryngopharyngeal reflux and voice disorders. In: Rubin

JS, Sataloff RT, Korovin GS, eds. *Diagnosis and Treatment of Voice Disorders*. 2nd ed. Clifton Park, NY: Delmar Thomson Learning; 2003:381–392.

105. Ormseth EJ, Wong RK. Reflux laryngitis: pathophysiology, diagnosis and management. *Am J Gastroenterol.* 1999;94(10):2812–2817.

106. Richter JE, Hicks DM. Unresolved issues in gastroesophageal reflux-related ear, nose and throat problems. *Am J Gastroenterol.* 1997;92(12):2143–2144.

107. Sone M, Katayama N, Kato T, et al. Prevalence of laryngopharyngeal reflux symptoms: comparison between health checkup examinees and patients with otitis media. *Otolaryngol Head Neck Surg.* 2012;146(4): 562–566.

108. Habesoglu TE, Habesoglu M, Kalaycik C, et al. Gastroesophageal reflux disease and tympanoplasty surgical outcome: is there a relationship? *J Laryngol Otol.* 2012;126(6): 580–585.

109. Brunworth JD, Mahboubi H, Garg R, et al. Nasopharyngeal acid reflux and eustachian tube dysfunction in adults. *Ann Otol Rhinol Laryngol.* 2014;123(6):415–419.

110. Rodrigues MM, Dibbern RS, Santos VJ, Passeri LA. Influence of obesity on the correlation between laryngopharyngeal reflux and obstructive sleep apnea. *Braz J Otorhinolaryngol.* 2014;80(1):5–10.

111. Sung MW, Lee WH, Wee JH, et al. Factors associated with hypertrophy of the lingual tonsils in adults with sleep-disordered breathing. *JAMA Otolaryngol Head Neck Surg.* 2013;139(6):598–603.

112. Corvo MA, Eckley CA, Liquidato BM, Castilho GL, Arruda CN. pH salivary analysis of subjects suffering from Sjogren's syndrome and laryngopharyngeal reflux. *Braz J Otorhinolaryngol.* 2012;78(1):81.

113. Sole ML, Conrad J, Bennett M, et al. Pepsin and amylase in oral and tracheal secretions: a pilot study. *Am J Crit Care.* 2014; 23(4):334–338.

114. Garland JS, Alex CP, Johnston N, Yan JC, Werlin SL. Association between tracheal pepsin, a reliable marker of gastric aspiration, and head of bed elevation among ventilated neonates. *J Neonatal Perinatal Med.* 2014;7(3):185–192.

115. Ali Mel-S, Bulmer DM, Dettmar PW, Pearson JP. Mucin gene expression in reflux laryngeal mucosa: histological and in situ hybridization observations. *Int J Otolaryngol.* 2014;2014:264075.

116. Eckley CA, Sardinha LR, Rizzo LV. Salivary concentration of epidermal growth factor in adults with reflux laryngitis before and after treatment. *Ann Otol Rhinol Laryngol.* 2013;122(7):440–444.

117. Falk GL, Beattie J, Ing A, et al. Scintigraphy in laryngopharyngeal and gastroesophageal reflux disease: a definitive diagnostic test? *World J Gastroenterol.* 2015;21(12): 3619–3627.

118. Falk M, Van der Wall H, Falk GL. Differences between scintigraphic reflux studies in gastrointestinal reflux disease and laryngopharyngeal reflux disease and correlation with symptoms. *Nucl Med Commun.* 2015;36(6):625–630.

119. Günbey E, Gören I, Ünal R, Yilmaz M. An evaluation of olfactory function in adults with gastro-esophageal reflux disease [published online October 19, 2015]. *Acta Otolaryngol.* 2016;136(2):214–218.

120. Krawczyk M, Scierski W, Ryzkiel I, et al. Endoscopic evidence of reflux disease in the larynx. *Acta Otolaryngol.* 2014;134(8): 831–837.

121. Ozmen S, Yücel OT, Sinici I, et al. Nasal pepsin assay and pH monitoring in chronic rhinosinusitis. *Laryngoscope.* 2008;118(5): 890–894.

122. Bercin S, Kutluhan A, Yurttas V, et al. Evaluation of laryngopharyngeal reflux in patients with suspected laryngopharyngeal reflux, chronic otitis media and laryngeal disorders. *Eur Arch Otorhinolaryngol.* 2008;265:1539–1543.

123. Kantas I, Balatsouras DG, Kamargianis N, et al. The influence of laryngopharyngeal reflux in the healing of laryngeal trauma. *Eur Arch Otorhinolaryngol.* 2009;266:253–259.

124. Bock JM, Brawley MK, Johnston N, et al. Analysis of pepsin in tracheoesophageal

puncture sites. *Ann Otol Rhinol Laryngol.* 2010;119:799–805.

125. Cengiz S, Cengiz MI, Sarac YS. Dental erosion caused by gastroesophageal reflux disease: a case report. *Cases J.* 2009;2:8018.

126. Roth DF, Ferguson BJ. Vocal allergy: recent advances in understanding the role of allergy in dysphonia. *Curr Opin Otolaryngol Head Neck Surg.* 2010;18:176–181.

127. Higo T, Mukaisho K, Ling ZG, et al. An animal model of intrinsic dental erosion caused by gastro-oesophageal reflux disease. *Oral Dis.* 2009;15:360–365.

128. Ranjitkar S, Kaidonis JA, Richards LC, Townsend GC. The effect of CPP-ACP on enamel wear under severe erosive conditions. *Arch Oral Biol.* 2009;54:527–532.

129. Becker S, Schmidt C, Berghaus A, Tschiesner U, Olzowy B, Reichel O. Does laryngopharyngeal reflux cause intraoral burning sensations? A preliminary study. *Eur Arch Otolaryngol.* 2011;268:1375–1381.

130. Chung JH, Tae K, Lee YS, et al. The significance of laryngopharyngeal reflux in benign vocal mucosal lesions. *Otolaryngol HNS.* 2009;141:369–373.

131. Saleh H. Rhinosinusitis, laryngopharyngeal reflux and cough: an ENT viewpoint. *Pulm Pharmacol Ther.* 2009;22:127–129.

132. Randhawa PS, Mansuri S, Rubin JS. Is dysphonia due to allergic laryngitis being misdiagnosed as laryngopharyngeal reflux? *Logoped Phoniatr Vocol.* 2010;35:1–5.

133. Eskiizmir G, Kezirian E. Is there a vicious cycle between obstructive sleep apnea and laryngopharyngeal reflux disease? *Med Hypotheses.* 2009;73:706–708.

134. Suzuki M, Saigusa H, Kurogi R, et al. Arousal in obstructive sleep apnea patients with laryngopharyngeal and gastroesophageal reflux. *Sleep Med.* 2010;11:356–374.

135. Karkos PD, Leong SC, Benton J, Sastry A, Assimakopoulos DA, Issing WJ. Reflux and sleeping disorders: a systematic review. *J Laryngol Otol.* 2009;123:372–374.

136. Wang L, Liu X, Liu YL, et al. Correlation of pepsin measured laryngopharyngeal reflux disease with symptoms and signs. *Otolaryngol HNS.* 2010;143:765–771.

137. Eryuksel E, Dogan M, Olgun S, Kocak I, Celikel T. Incidence and treatment results of laryngopharyngeal reflux in chronic obstructive pulmonary disease. *Eur Arch Otorhinolaryngol.* 2009;266:1267–1271.

138. de la Hoz RE, Christie J, Teamer JA, et al. Reflux symptoms and disorders and pulmonary disease in former World Trade Center rescue and recovery workers and volunteers. *J Occup Environ Med.* 2008;50:1351–1354.

139. Ward PH, Berci G. Observations on the pathogenesis of chronic non-specific pharyngitis and laryngitis. *Laryngoscope.* 1982; 92:1377–1382.

140. Von Leden H, Moore P. Contact ulcer of the larynx. Experimental observations. *Arch Otolaryngol.* 1960;72:746–752.

141. Kjellen G, Brudin L. Gastroesophageal reflux disease and laryngeal symptoms. Is there really a causal relationship? *ORL J Otorhinolaryngol Relat Spec.* 1994;56:287–290.

142. Groome M, Cotton JP, Borland M, et al. Prevalence of laryngopharyngeal reflux in a population with gastroesophageal reflux. *Laryngoscope.* 2007;117:1424–1428.

143. Lai YC, Wang PC, Lin JC. Laryngopharyngeal reflux in patients with reflux esophagitis. *World J Gastroenterol.* 2008;14: 4523–4528.

144. Qua CS, Wong CH, Gopala K, Goh KL. Gastro-oesophageal reflux disease in chronic laryngitis: prevalence and response to acid-suppressive therapy. *Aliment Pharmacol Ther.* 2007;25:287–295.

145. Galli J, Calo L, Agostino S, et al. Bile reflux as possible risk factor in laryngopharyngeal inflammatory and neoplastic lesions. *Acta Otorhinolaryngol Ital.* 2003;23:377–382.

146. Koufman JA, Wiener GJ, Wu WC, Castell DO. Reflux laryngitis and its sequelae: the diagnostic role of ambulatory 24-hour pH monitoring. *J Voice.* 1988;2(1):78–89.

147. Belafsky PC, Postma GN, Koufman JA. The validity and reliability of the Reflux Finding Score (RFS). *Laryngoscope.* 2001;111: 1313–1317.

148. Belafsky PC, Postma GN, Koufman JA. The validity and Reliability of the Reflux Symptom Index (RSI). *J Voice.* 2002;16:274–277.

149. Carr MM, Nguyen A, Poje C, et al. Correlation of findings on direct laryngoscopy and bronchoscopy with presence of extraesophageal reflux disease. *Laryngoscope.* 2000;110:1560–1562.

150. McMurray JS, Gerber M, Stern Y, et al. Role of laryngoscopy, dual pH probe monitoring, and laryngeal mucosal biopsy in the diagnosis of pharyngoesophageal reflux. *Ann Otol Rhinol Laryngol.* 2001;110:299–304.

151. Hicks DM, Ours TM, Abelson T, et al. The prevalence of hypopharynx findings associated with gastroesophageal reflux in normal volunteers. *J Voice.* 2002;16:564–579.

152. Close LG. Laryngopharyngeal manifestations of reflux: diagnosis and therapy. *Eur J Gastroenterol Hepatol.* 2002;14(suppl 1): S23–S27.

153. Tauber S, Gross M, Issing WJ. Association of laryngopharyngeal symptoms with gastroesophageal reflux disease. *Laryngoscope.* 2002;112:879–886.

154. Vaezi MF. Ear, nose, and throat manifestations of gastroesophageal reflux disease. *Clin Perspect Gastroenterol.* 2002;5:324–328.

155. Book DT, Rhee JS, Toohill RJ, Smith TL. Perspectives in laryngopharyngeal reflux: an international survey. *Laryngoscope.* 2002;112(8, pt 1):1399–1406.

156. Branski RC, Bhattacharyya N, Shapiro J. The reliability of the assessment of endoscopic laryngeal findings associated with laryngopharyngeal reflux disease. *Laryngoscope.* 2002;112:1019–1024.

157. Noordzij JP, Khidr A, Desper E, et al. Correlation of pH probe–measured laryngopharyngeal reflux with symptoms and signs of reflux laryngitis. *Laryngoscope.* 2002;112:2192–2195.

158. Marambaia O, Andrade NA, Varela DG, et al. Laryngopharyngeal reflux: prospective study that compares early laryngoscopic findings and 2-channel 24-hour pH monitoring. *Rev Brasil Otorrinolaryngol.* 2002; 68:527–531.

159. Siupsinskiene N, Adamonis K. Diagnostic test with omeprazole in patients with posterior laryngitis. *Medicina (Kaunas, Lithuania).* 2003;39:47–55.

160. Vaezi MF. Sensitivity and specificity of reflux-attributed laryngeal lesions: experimental and clinical evidence. *Am J Med.* 2003;115(suppl 3A):105S–108S.

161. Issing WJ. Gastroesophageal reflux—a common illness? [in German]. *Laryngorhinootologie.* 2003;82:118–122.

162. Maronian N, Haggitt R, Oelschlager BK, et al. Histologic features of reflux-attributed laryngeal lesions. *Am J Med.* 2003;115 (suppl 3A):105S–108S.

163. Burati DO, Duprat ADC, Eckley CA, et al. Gastroesophageal reflux disease: analysis of 157 patients. *Rev Brasil Otorrinolaringol.* 2003;69:458–462.

164. Wang JH, Lou JY, Dong L, et al. Epidemiology of gastroesophageal reflux disease: a general population-based study in Xi-an of Northwest China. *World J Gastroenterol.* 2004;10:1647–1651.

165. Ahmad I, Batch AJ. Acid reflux management: ENT perspective. *J Laryngol Otol.* 2004;118:25–30.

166. Grillo C, Maiolino L, Caminiti D, et al. Gastroesophageal reflux and otolaryngologic diseases. *Acta Medica Mediterrancea.* 2004;20:155–158.

167. Lenderking WR, Hillson E, Crawley JA, et al. The clinical characteristics and impact of laryngopharyngeal reflux disease on health-related quality of life. *Value Health.* 2003;6:560–565.

168. Gaynor EB. Gastroesophageal reflux as an etiologic factor in laryngeal complications of intubation. *Laryngoscope.* 1988;98: 972–979.

169. Lillemoe KD, Johnson LF, Harmon JW. Role of the components of the gastroduodenal contents in experimental acid esophagitis. *Surgery.* 1982;92:276–284.

170. Johnson LF, Harmon JW. Experimental esophagitis in a rabbit model. Clinical relevance. *J Clin Gastroenterol.* 1986;8(suppl 1): 26–44.

171. Cherry J, Siegel CI, Margulies SI, Donner M. Pharyngeal localization of symptoms of

gastroesophageal reflux. *Ann Otol Rhinol Laryngol.* 1970;79:912–914.

172. Chen MY, Ott DJ, Casolo BJ, et al. Correlation of laryngeal and pharyngeal carcinomas and 24-hr pH monitoring of the esophagus and pharynx. *Otolaryngol Head Neck Surg.* 1998;119:460–462.

173. Ludemann JP, Manoukian J, Shaw K, et al. Effects of simulated gastroesophageal reflux on the untraumatized rabbit larynx. *J Otolaryngol.* 1998;27:127–131.

174. Ward PH, Berci G. Observations on the pathogenesis of chronic non-specific pharyngitis and laryngitis. *Laryngoscope.* 1982; 92:1377–1382.

175. Von Leden H, Moore P. Contact ulcer of the larynx. Experimental observations. *Arch Otolaryngol.* 1960;72:746–752.

176. Kjellen G, Brudin L. Gastroesophageal reflux disease and laryngeal symptoms. Is there really a causal relationship? *ORL J Otorhinolaryngol Relat Spec.* 1994;56: 287–290.

177. Groome M, Cotton JP, Borland M, et al. Prevalence of laryngopharyngeal reflux in a population with gastroesophageal reflux. *Laryngoscope.* 2007;117:1424–1428.

178. Lai YC, Wang PC, Lin JC. Laryngopharyngeal reflux in patients with reflux esophagitis. *World J Gastroenterol.* 2008;14: 4523–4528.

179. Qua CS, Wong CH, Gopala K, Goh KL. Gastro-oesophageal reflux disease in chronic laryngitis: prevalence and response to acid-suppressive therapy. *Aliment Pharmacol Ther.* 2007;25:287–295.

180. Galli J, Calo L, Agostino S, et al. Bile reflux as possible risk factor in laryngopharyngeal inflammatory and neoplastic lesions. *Acta Otorhinolaryngol Ital.* 2003;23:377–382.

181. Adhami T, Goldblum JR, Richter JE, et al. The role of gastric and duodenal agents in laryngeal injury: an experimental canine model. *Ann J Gastroenterol.* 2004;99:2098–2106.

182. Eckley CA, Michelsohn N, Rizzo LV, et al. Salivary epidermal growth factor concentration in adults with reflux laryngitis.

Otolaryngol Head Neck Surg. 2004;131: 401–406.

183. Eckley CA, Costa HO. Salivary EGF concentration in adults with chronic laryngitis caused by laryngopharyngeal reflux. *Rev Brasil Otorrinolaringol.* 2003;69:590–597.

184. Altman KW, Haines GK III, Hammer ND, Radosevich JA. The H+/K+-ATPase (proton) pump is expressed in human laryngeal submucosal glands. *Laryngoscope.* 2003; 113:1927–1930.

185. Johnston N, Dettmar PW, Lively MO, et al. Effect of pepsin on laryngeal stress protein (Sep70, Sep53, and Hsp70) response: role in laryngopharyngeal reflux disease. *Ann Otol Rhino Pharyngol.* 2006;115:47–58.

186. Johnson N, Knight J, Dettmar PW, et al. Pepsin and carbonic anhydrase isoenzyme III as diagnostic markers for laryngopharyngeal reflux disease. *Laryngoscope.* 2004; 114:2129–2134.

187. Johnston N, Wells CW, Blumin JH, et al. Receptormediated uptake of pepsin by laryngeal epithelial cells. *Ann Otol Rhinol Laryngol.* 2007;116:934–938.

188. Johnston N, Bulmer D, Gill GA, et al. Cell biology of laryngeal epithelial defenses in health and disease: further studies. *Ann Otol Rhinol Laryngol.* 2003;112:481–491.

189. Johnston N, Dettmar PW, Bishworkarma B, et al. Activity/stability of human pepsin: implications for reflux attributed to laryngeal disease. *Laryngoscope.* 2007;117:1036–1039.

190. Ylitalo R, Thibeault SL. Relationship between time of exposure of laryngopharyngeal reflux and gene expression in laryngeal fibroblasts. *Ann Otol Rhinol Laryngol.* 2006;115:775–783.

191. Samuels TL, Handler E, Syring ML, et al. Mucin gene expression in human laryngeal epithelia: effect of laryngopharyngeal reflux. *Ann Otol Rhinol Laryngol.* 2008;117: 688–695.

192. Habesoglu TE, Habesoglu M, Surmeli M, et al. Histological changes of rat soft palate with exposure to experimental laryngopharyngeal reflux. *Auris Nasus Larynx.* 2010;37:730–736.

193. Erickson E, Sivansakar M. Simulated reflux decreases vocal fold epithelial barrier resistance. *Laryngoscope*. 2010;120:1569–1575.

194. Johnston N, Wells CW, Samuels TL, Blumin JH. Pepsin in non-acidic refluxate can damage hypopharyngeal epithelial cells. *Ann Otol Rhinol Laryngol*. 2009;118:677–685.

195. Bulmer DM, Ali MS, Brownlee IA, Dettmar PW, Pearson JP. Laryngeal mucosa: its susceptibility to damage by acid and pepsin. *Laryngoscope*. 2010;120:777–782.

196. Samuels TL, Johnston N. Pepsin as a marker of extraesophageal reflux. *Ann Otol Rhinol Laryngol*. 2010;119:203–208.

197. Richter JE. Role of gastric refluxate in gastroesophageal reflux disease: acid, weak acid and bile. *Am J Med Sci*. 2009;338:89–95.

198. Rees LEN, Pazmany L, Gutowska-Owsiad D, et al. The mucosal immune response to laryngopharyngeal reflux. *Am J Respir Crit Care Med*. 2008;177:1187–1193.

199. Wada T, Sasaki M, Kataoka H, et al. Gastroesophageal and laryngopharyngeal reflux symptoms correlate with histopathologic inflammation of the upper and lower esophagus. *J Clin Gastroenterol*. 2009;43:249–252.

200. Park S, Chun HJ, Keum B, et al. An electron microscope study—correlation of gastroesophageal reflux disease and laryngopharyngeal reflux. *Laryngoscope*. 2010;120:1303–1308.

201. Amin SM, Abdel Maged KH, Naser AY, Aly BH. Laryngopharyngeal reflux with sore throat: an ultrastructural study of oropharyngeal epithelium. *Ann Otol Rhinol Laryngol*. 2009;118:362–367.

202. Ossakow SJ, Elta G, Colturi T, et al. Esophageal reflux and dysmotility as the basis for persistent cervical symptoms. *Ann Otol Rhinol Laryngol*. 1987;96:387–392.

203. Fouad YM, Khoury RM, Hatlebakk JG, Katz PO, Castell DO. Ineffective esophageal motility (IEM) is more prevalent in reflux patients with respiratory symptoms. *Gastroenterology*. 1998;114(suppl 1):A123. Abstract 6506.

204. Postma GN, Tomek MS, Belafsky PC, Koufman JA. Esophageal acid clearance in otolaryngology patients with laryngopharyngeal reflux. *Ann Otol Rhinol Laryngol*. 2001;110:1114–1116.

205. Gerhardt DC, Shuck TJ, Bordeaux RA, Winship DH. Human upper esophageal sphincter. Response to volume, osmotic and acid stimuli. *Gastroenterology*. 1978;75:268–274.

206. Szczesniak MM, Williams RB, Brake HM, Maclean JC, Cole IE, Cook IJ. Upregulation of the esophago-UES relaxation response: a possible pathophysiological mechanism in suspected reflux laryngitis. *Neurogastroenterol Motil*. 2010;22:381–386.

207. Vardouniotis AS, Karatzanis AD, Tzortzaki E, et al. Molecular pathways and genetic factors in the pathogenesis of laryngopharyngeal reflux. *Eur Arch Otorhinolaryngol*. 2009;266:795–801.

208. Cheng CM, Hsieh CC, Lin CS, et al. Macrophage activation by gastric fluid suggests MMP involvement in aspiration-induced lung disease. *Immunobiology*. 2010;215:173–181.

209. Chong VH, Jalihal A. Heterotopic gastric mucosal patch of the esophagus is associated with higher prevalence of laryngopharyngeal reflux symptoms. *Eur Arch Otorhinolaryngol*. 2010;267:1793–1799.

210. Salminen P, Ovaska J. Heterotopic gastric mucosal patch in patients with reflux laryngitis: an entity of clinical interest? *Surg Laparosc Endosc Percutan Tech*. 2009;19:361–363.

211. Basseri B, Conklin JL, Mertens RB, Lo SK, Bellack GS, Shaye OA. Heterotopic gastric mucosa (inlet patch) in a patient with laryngopharyngeal reflux (LPR) and laryngeal carcinoma: a case report and review of literature. *Dis Esophagus*. 2009;22:E1–E5.

212. Clark CS, Kraus BB, Sinclair J, Castell DO. Gastroesophageal reflux induced by exercise in healthy volunteers. *JAMA*. 1989;261:3599–3601.

213. Spechler SJ, Castell DO. Non-achalasia esophageal motility abnormalities. In: Castell DO, Richter JE, eds. *The Esophagus*.

4th ed. Philadelphia, PA: Lippincott; 2004: 262-274.

214. Tack J, Janssens J. The esophagus and non-cardiac chest pain. In: Castell DO, Richter JE, eds. *The Esophagus*. 4th ed. Philadelphia, PA: Lippincott; 2004:635-647.

215. Mittal RK. Pathophysiology of gastroesophageal reflux disease: motility factors. In: Castell DO, Richter JE, eds. *The Esophagus*. 4th ed. Philadelphia, PA: Lippincott; 2004:412-413.

216. Sataloff RT. The human voice. *Sci Am*. 1993;267:108-115.

217. Spiegel JR, Sataloff RT, Cohn JR, Hawkshaw M, Epstein J. Respiratory function in singers: medical assessment, diagnoses and treatments. *J Voice*. 1988;2:40-50.

218. Koufmna JA, Wiener GJ, Wu WC, Castell DO. Reflux laryngitis and its sequelae: the diagnostic role of ambulatory 24-hour pH monitoring. *J Voice*. 1988;2(1):78-89.

219. Gould WJ, Sataloff RT, Spiegel JR. *Voice Surgery*. St. Louis, MO: CV Mosby; 1993.

220. Teisanu E, Heciota D, Dimitriu T, et al. Tulburari Faringolaringiene la Bolnavii cu reflux gastroesofagian. *Rev Chir Oncol Radio ORL Oftalmol Stomatol Otorinolaringol*. 1978;23:279-286.

221. Miko TL. Peptic (contact ulcer) granuloma of the larynx. *J Clin Pathol*. 1989;42:800-804.

222. Bogdassarian RS, Olson NR. Posterior glottic laryngeal stenosis. *Otolaryngol Head Neck Surg*. 1980;88:765-772.

223. Fligny I, Francois M, Aigrain Y, et al. [Subglottic stenosis and gastroesophageal reflux]. *Ann Otolaryngol Chir Cervicofac*. 1989;106:193-196.

224. Havas TE, Priestley J, Lowinger DS. A management strategy for vocal process granulomas. *Laryngoscope*. 1999;109:301-306.

225. Koufman JA. Contact ulcer and granuloma of the larynx. In: Gates G, ed. *Current Therapy in Otolaryngology–Head and Neck Surgery*. 5th ed. St. Louis, MO: Mosby; 1994: 456-459.

226. Delahunty JE, Ardran GM. Globus hystericus: a manifestation of reflux oesophagitis? *J Laryngol Otol*. 1970;84:1049-1054.

227. Wilson JA, Pryde A, Piris J, et al. Pharyngoesophageal dysmotility in globus sensation. *Arch Otolaryngol Head Neck Surg*. 1989; 115:1086-1090.

228. Curran AJ, Barry MK, Callanan V, Gormley PK. A prospective study of acid reflux and globus pharyngeus using a modified symptom index. *Clin Otolaryngol Allied Sci*. 1995;20(6):552-554.

229. Shaker R, Milbrath M, Ren J, et al. Esophagopharyngeal distribution of refluxed gastric acid in patients with reflux laryngitis. *Gastroenterology*. 1995;109:1575-1582.

230. Hill J, Stuart RC, Fung HK, et al. Gastroesophageal reflux, motility disorders and psychological profiles in the etiology of globus pharyngis. *Laryngoscope*. 1997;107: 1373-1377.

231. Smit CF, van Leeuwen AMJ, Mathus-Vliegen LMH, et al. Gastropharyngeal and gastroesophageal reflux in globus and hoarseness. *Arch Otolaryngol Head Neck Surg*. 2000;126:827-830.

232. Malcomson KG. Radiological findings in globus hystericus. *Br J Radiol*. 1966;39:583-586.

233. Koufman JA, Blalock PD. Functional voice disorders. *Otolaryngol Clin North Am*. 1991;24:1059-1073.

234. Loughlin CJ, Koufman JA. Paroxysmal laryngospasm secondary to gastroesophageal reflux. *Laryngoscope*. 1996;106:1502-1505.

235. Yelken K, Yilmaz A, Guven M, Eyibilen A, Aladag I. Paradoxical vocal fold motion dysfunction in asthma patients. *Respiratory*. 2009;14:729-733.

236. Murry T, Branski RC, Yu K, Cukier-Blaj S, Duflo S, Aviv JE. Laryngeal sensory deficits in patients with chronic cough and paradoxical vocal fold movement disorder. *Laryngoscope*. 2010;120:1576-1581.

237. Spechler SJ, Goyal RK. Barrett's esophagus. *N Engl J Med*. 1986;315:362-371.

238. MacDonald WC, MacDonald JB. Adenocarcinoma of the esophagus and/or gastric cardia. *Cancer*. 1987;60:1094-1098.

239. Garewal HS, Sampliner R. Barrett's esophagus: a model premalignant lesion for adenocarcinoma. *Prev Med*. 1989;18:749-756.

240. Reid BJ. Barrett's esophagus and esophageal adenocarcinoma. *Gastroenterol Clin North Am.* 1991;20:817–834.

241. Chow WH, Finkle WD, McLaughlin JK, et al. The relation of gastroesophageal reflux disease and its treatment to adenocarcinomas of the esophagus and gastric cardia. *JAMA.* 1995;274(6):474–477.

242. Morrison M. Is chronic gastroesophageal reflux a causative factor in glottic carcinoma? *Otolaryngol Head Neck Surg.* 1988; 99:370–373.

243. Olson NR. Aerodigestive malignancy and gastroesophageal reflux disease. *Am J Med.* 1997;103(5A):975–995.

244. Richtsmeier WJ, Eisele D. In vivo anergy reversal with cimetadine in patients with cancer. *Arch Otolaryngol Head Neck Surg.* 1986;112:1074–1077.

245. Richtsmeier WJ, Styczynski P, Johns ME. Selective, histamine-mediated, immunosuppression in laryngeal cancer. *Ann Otol Rhinol Laryngol.* 1987;96:569–572.

246. El-Serag HB, Hepworth EJ, Lee P, Sonnenberg A. Gastroesophageal reflux disease is a risk factor for laryngeal and pharyngeal cancer. *Am J Gastroenterol.* 2001;96: 2013–2018.

247. Koufman JA, Burke AJ. The etiology and pathogenesis of laryngeal carcinoma. *Otolaryngol Clin North Am.* 1997;30:1–19.

248. Ward PH, Hanson DG. Reflux as an etiological factor of carcinoma of the laryngopharynx. *Laryngoscope.* 1988;98:1195–1199.

249. Freije JE, Beatty TW, Campbell BH, et al. Carcinoma of the larynx in patients with gastroesophageal reflux. *Am J Otolaryngol.* 1996;17(6):386–390.

250. Ling ZQ, Mukaisho K, Hidaka M, et al. Duodenal contents reflux-induced laryngitis in rats: possible mechanism of enhancement of the causative factors in laryngeal carcinogenesis. *Ann Otol Rhinol Laryngol.* 2007;116:471–478.

251. Del Negro A, Araujo MR, Tincani AJ, et al. Experimental carcinogenesis on the oropharyngeal mucosa of rats with hydrochloric acid, sodium nitrate, and pepsin. *Acta Cir Bras.* 2008;23:337–342.

252. Qadeer MA, Colabianchi N, Strome M, et al. Gastroesophageal reflux and laryngeal cancer: causation or association? *Am J Otolaryngol.* 2006;27:119–128.

253. Reavis KM, Morris CD, Gopal DV, et al. Laryngopharyngeal reflux symptoms better predict the presence of esophageal adenocarcinoma than typical gastroesophageal reflux symptoms. *Ann Surg.* 2004;239: 849–858.

254. Reichel O, Issing WJ. Should patients with pH-documented laryngopharyngeal reflux routinely undergo oesophagogastroduodenoscopy? A retrospective analysis. *J Laryngol Otol.* 2007;121:1165–1169.

255. Perry KA, Enestyedt CK, Lorenzo CS, et al. The integrity of esophagogastric junction anatomy in patients with isolated laryngopharyngeal reflux symptoms. *J Gastrointest Surg.* 2008;12:1880–1887.

256. Kuipers EJ. Helicobacter pylori and the risk and management of associated diseases: gastritis, ulcer disease, atrophic gastritis and gastric cancer. *Aliment Pharmacol Ther.* 1997;11(suppl 1):71–88.

257. Katsinelos P, Kountouras J, Chatzimavroudis G, et al. Should inspection of the laryngopharyngeal area be part of routine upper gastrointestinal endoscopy? A prospective study. *Dig Liver Dis.* 2009;41:283–288.

258. Sandner A, Illert J, Koitzsh S, Unverzagt S, Schon I. Reflux induces DNA strand breaks and expression changes of MMP1+9+14 in a human miniorgan culture model. *Exp Cell Res.* 2013;319(19):2905–2915.

259. Kelly EA, Samuels TL, Johnston N. Chronic pepsin exposure promotes anchorage-independent growth and migration of a hypopharyngeal squamous cell line. *Otolaryngol Head Neck Surg.* 2014;150(4):618–624.

260. LeBlanc B, Lewis E, Caldito G, Nathan CA. Increased pharyngeal reflux in patients treated for laryngeal cancer: a pilot study. *Otolaryngol Head Neck Surg.* 2015;153(5): 791–794.

261. Samuels TL, Pearson AC, Wells CW, Stoner GD, Johnston N. Curcumin and anthocyanin inhibit pepsin-mediated cell damage

and carcinogenic changes in airway epithelial cells. *Ann Otol Rhinol Laryngol.* 2013; 122(10):632–641.

262. Little PJ, Matthews BL, Glock MS, et al. Extraesophageal pediatric reflux: 24-hour double-probe pH monitoring of 222 children. *Ann Otol Rhinol Laryngol Suppl.* 1997;169:1–16.

263. Wetmore RF. Effects of acid on the larynx of the maturing rabbit and their possible significance to the sudden infant death syndrome. *Laryngoscope.* 1993;103:1242–1254.

264. Landler U. Hollwarth ME, Uray E, et al. Esophageal function of infants with sudden infant death—risk [in German]. *Klin Padiatr.* 1990;202(1):37–42.

265. Kurza R, Schenkeli R, Hollwarth M, et al. Sleep apnea in infants and the risk of SIDS [in German]. *Monatsschr Kinderheilkd.* 1986;134(10):17–20.

266. Benhamou PH, Dupont C. Relationship between gastroesophageal reflux and severe malaise in infants [in French]. *Presse Med.* 1992;21(35):1673–1676.

267. Spitzer AR, Boyle JT, Tuchman DN, et al. Awake apnea associated with gastroesophageal reflux: a specific clinical syndrome. *J Pediatr.* 1984;104:200–205.

268. McCulloch K, Vidyasagar D, Infantile apnea. *Am Fam Physician.* 1986;34(3): 105–114.

269. Jeffery HE, Rahilly P, Read DJ. Multiple causes of asphyxia in infants at high risk for sudden infant death. *Arch Dis Child.* 1983;58(2):92–100.

270. Camfield P, Camfield C, Bagnell P, Rees E. Infant apnea syndrome. A prospective evaluation of etiologies. *Clin Pediatr.* 1982; 21(11):684–687.

271. Mark JD, Brooks JG. Sleep-associated airway problems in children. *Pediatr Clin North Am.* 1984;31(4):907–918.

272. Rosen CL, Frost JD Jr, Harrison GM. Infant apnea: polygraphic studies and follow-up monitoring. *Pediatrics.* 1983;71(5): 731–736.

273. Haney PJ. Infant apnea: findings on the barium esophagram. *Radiology.* 1983;148(2): 425–427.

274. Kahn A, Rebuffat E, Sottiaux M, et al. Sleep apneas and acid esophageal reflux in control infants and in infants with an apparent life-threatening event. *Biol Neonate.* 1990; 57(3–4):144–149.

275. Ramet J. Cardiac and respiratory reactivity to gastroesophageal reflux: experimental data in infants. *Biol Neonate.* 1994;6: 240–246.

276. Paton JY, Macfadyen U, Williams A, Simpson H. Gastro-oesophageal reflux and apnoeic pauses during sleep in infancy—no direct relation. *Eur J Pediatr.* 1990;149(10): 680–686.

277. Paton JY, Nanayakkara CS, Simpson H. Observations on gastro-oesophageal reflux, central apnoea and heart rate in infants. *Eur J Pediatr.* 1990;149(9):608–612.

278. Buts JP, Barudi C, Moulin D, et al. Prevalence and treatment of silent gastro-oesophageal reflux in children with recurrent respiratory disorders. *Eur J Pediatr.* 1986;145(5):396–400.

279. Rahilly PM. The pneumographic and medical investigation of infants suffering apparent life threatening episodes. *J Paediatr Child Health.* 1991;27(60):349–353.

280. Sacre L, Vandenplas Y. Gastroesophageal reflux associated with respiratory abnormalities during sleep. *J Pediatr Gastroenterol Nutr.* 1989;9(1):28–33.

281. Vandenplas Y, Deneyer M, Verlinden M, et al. Gastroesophageal reflux incidence and respiratory dysfunction during sleep in infants: treatment with cisapride. *J Pediatr Gastroenterol Nutr.* 1989;8(1):31–36.

282. Halpern LM, Jolley SG, Tunell WP, et al. The mean duration of gastroesophageal reflux during sleep as an indicator of respiratory symptoms from gastroesophageal reflux in children. *J Pediatr Surg.* 1991; 26(6):686–690.

283. Graff MA, Kashlan F, Carter M, et al. Nap studies underestimate the incidence of gastroesophageal reflux. *Pediatr Pulmonol.* 1994;18(40):258–260.

284. Gomes H, Lallemand P. Infant apnea and gastroesophageal reflux. *Pediatr Radiol.* 1992;22(1):8–11.

285. Kurz R, Hollwarth M, Fasching M, et al. Combined disturbance of respiratory regulation and esophageal function in early infancy. *Prog Pediatr Surg.* 1985;18:52–61.

286. Singareddy R, Moole S, Calhoun S, Vocalan P, Tsaoussoglou M. Medical complaints are more common in young school-aged children with parent reported insomnia symptoms. *J Clin Sleep Med.* 2009;5:549–553.

287. Indrio F, Riezzo G, Raimondi F, Cavallo L, Francavilla R. Regurgitation in healthy and non-healthy infants. *Ital J Pediatr.* 2009; 35:39.

288. Van Houtte E, Van Lierde K, Claeys S. Pathophysiology and treatment of muscle tension dysphonia: a review of the current knowledge. *J Voice.* 2011;25:202–207.

289. Ulualp SO, Rodriguez S, Cunningham S, et al. Pharyngeal pH monitoring in infants with laryngitis. *Otolaryngol Head Neck Surg.* 2007;137:776–779.

290. Block BB, Brodsky L. Hoarseness in children: the role of laryngopharyngeal reflux. *Int J Ped Otorhinolaryngol.* 2007;71: 1361–1369.

291. Hoa M, Kingsley EL, Coticchia JM. Correlating the clinical course of recurrent croup with endoscopic findings: a retrospective observational study. *Ann Otol Rhinol Laryngol.* 2008;117:464–469.

292. Barreto VM, D'Avila JS, Sales NJ, et al. Laryngeal and vocal evaluation in untreated growth hormone deficient adults (IGHD). *Otolaryngol HNS.* 2009;140:37–42.

293. Dogru M, Kuran G, Haytoglu S, Dengiz R, Arikan OK. Role of laryngopharyngeal reflux in the pathogenesis of otitis media with effusion. *J Int Adv Otol.* 2015; 11(1):66–71.

294. Abdel-Aziz MM, El-Fattah AM, Abdalla AF. Clinical evaluation of pepsin for laryngopharyngeal reflux in children with otitis media with effusion. *Int J Pediatr Otorhinolaryngol.* 2013;77(10):1765–1770.

295. Katra R, Kabelka Z, Jurovcik M, et al. Pilot study: association between *Helicobacter pylori* in adenoid hyperplasia and reflux episodes detected by multiple intraluminal

impedance in children. *Int J Pediatr Otorhinolaryngol.* 2014;78(8):1243–1249.

296. Miura MS, Mascaro M, Rosenfeld RM. Association between otitis media and gastroesophageal reflux: a systematic review. *Otolaryngol Head Neck Surg.* 2012;146(3):345–352.

297. Martines F, Salvago P, Ferrara S, et al. Factors influencing the development of otitis media among Sicilian children affected by upper respiratory tract infections. *Braz J Otorhinolaryngol.* 2016;82(2):215–222.

298. Nation J, Kaufman M, Allen M, Sheyn A, Coticchia J. Incidence of gastroesophageal reflux disease and positive maxillary antral cultures in children with symptoms of chronic rhinosinusitis. *Int J Pediatr Otorhinolaryngol.* 2014;78(2):218–222.

299. Luo HN, Yang QM, Sheng Y, et al. Role of pepsin and pepsinogen: linking laryngopharyngeal reflux with otitis media with effusion in children. *Laryngoscope.* 2014; 124(7):E294–E300.

300. Iannella G, Di Nardo G, Plateroti R, et al. Investigation of pepsin in tears of children with laryngopharyngeal reflux disease. *Int J Pediatr Otorhinolaryngol.* 2015;79(12): 2312–2315.

301. Andrews TM, Orobello N. Histologic versus pH probe results in pediatric laryngopharyngeal reflux. *Int J Pediatr Otorhinolaryngol.* 2013;77(5):813–816.

302. Ott DJ. Gastroesophageal reflux: what is the role of barium studies? *Am J Roentgenol.* 1994;162:627–629.

303. Thompson JK, Koehler RE, Richter JE. Detection of gastroesophageal reflux: value of barium studies compared with 24-hour pH monitoring. *Am J Roentgenol.* 1994; 162:621–626.

304. Ott DJ, Wu WC, Gelfand DW. Reflux esophagitis revisited: prospective analysis of radiologic accuracy. *Gastrointest Radiol.* 1981;6:1–7.

305. Richter JE, Castell DO. Gastroesophageal reflux. Pathogenesis, diagnosis, and therapy. *Ann Intern Med.* 1982;97:93–103.

306. Sellar RJ, DeCaestecker JS, Heading RC. Barium radiology: a sensitive test for gastro-

oesophageal reflux. *Clin Radiol.* 1987;38: 303–307.

307. Malmud LS, Fisher RS. Radionuclide studies of esophageal transit and gastroesophageal reflux. *Semin Nucl Med.* 1982;12(2): 104–115.

308. Jenkins AF, Cowan RJ, Richter JE. Gastroesophageal scintigraphy: is it a sensitive test for gastroesophageal reflux disease? *J Clin Gastroenterol.* 1985;7:127.

309. Ismail-Beigi F, Horton PF, Pope CE Jr. Histological consequences of gastroesophageal reflux in man. *Gastroenterology.* 1970;58: 163–174.

310. DeVault KR, Castell DO. Guidelines for the diagnosis and treatment of gastroesophageal reflux disease. *Arch Intern Med.* 1995; 155:2165–2173.

311. Hetzel DJ, Dent J, Reed WD, et al. Healing and relapse of severe peptic esophagitis after treatment with omeprazole. *Gastroenterology.* 1988;95:903–912.

312. Koufman JA. Personal communication. June 2004.

313. Johnson LF. DeMeester TR. Twenty-four hour pH monitoring of the distal esophagus. *Am J Gastroenterol.* 1974;62:325–332.

314. Wiener GJ, Richter JE, Copper PA, et al. The symptom index: a clinically important parameter of ambulatory 24-hour esophageal pH monitoring. *Am J Gastroenterol.* 1988;83(4):358–361.

315. Dobhan R, Castell DO. Normal and abnormal proximal esophageal acid exposure: results of ambulatory dual probe pH monitoring. *Am J Gastroenterol.* 1993;88:25–29.

316. Schnatz PE, Castell JA, Castell DO. Pulmonary symptoms associated with gastroesophageal reflux: use of ambulatory pH monitoring to diagnose and to direct therapy. *Am J Gastroenterol.* 1996;91:1715–1718.

317. Shi G, des Varannes SB, Scarpignato C, Le Rhun M Galmiche J-P. Reflux related symptoms in patients with normal oesophageal exposure to acid. *Gut.* 1995;37:457–464.

318. Shaker R, Bardan E, Gu C, et al. Intrapharyngeal distribution of gastric acid refluxate. *Laryngoscope.* 2003;113:1182–1191.

319. Bilgen C, Ogut F, Kesimli-Dinc H, et al. The comparison of an empiric proton pump inhibitor trial vs. 24-hour double-probe pH monitoring in laryngopharyngeal reflux. *J Laryngol Otol.* 2003;117:386–390.

320. Maldonado A, Diederich L, Castell D, et al. Laryngopharyngeal reflux identified using a new catheter design: defining normal values and excluding artifacts. *Laryngoscope.* 2003;113:349–355.

321. Sato K, Umeno H, Chitose S, Nakashima T. Tetraprobe, 24-hour pH monitoring for laryngopharyngeal reflux: a technique for simultaneous study of hypopharynx, esophagus and stomach. *J Laryngol Otol.* 2009;123(suppl 31):117–122.

322. Sato K, Umeno H, Chitose S, Nakashima T. Patterns of laryngopharyngeal and gastroesophageal reflux. *J Laryngol Otol.* 2009; 123(suppl 31):42–47.

323. Zelenik K, Matousek P, Urban O, Schwarz P, Starek I, Kominek P. Globus pharyngeus and extraesophageal reflux: simultaneous pH <4.0 and pH <5.0 analysis. *Laryngoscope.* 2010;120:2160–2164.

324. Vaezi MF, Richter J, Stasney CR, et al. A randomized double-blind placebo controlled study of acid suppression for the treatment of suspected laryngopharyngeal reflux. *Gastroenterology.* 2004;126:A40.

325. Ulualp SO, Toohill RJ, Shaker R, et al. Outcomes of acid suppressive therapy in patients with posterior laryngitis. *Otolaryngol Head Neck Surg.* 2001;124:16–22.

326. El-Sayed Ali M. Laryngopharyngal reflux: diagnosis and treatment of a controversial disease. *Curr Opin Allergy Clin Immunol.* 2008;8:28–33.

327. Reichel O, Issing WJ. Impact of different pH thresholds for 24-hour dual probe pH monitoring in patients with suspected laryngopharyngeal reflux. *J Laryngol Otol.* 2008;122(5):485–489.

328. Friedman M, Hamilton C, Samuelson CG, et al. The value of routine pH monitoring in the diagnosis and treatment of laryngopharyngeal reflux. *Otolaryngol Head Neck Surg.* 2012;146(6):952–958.

329. Carroll TL, Fedore LW, Aldahlawi MM. pH impedance and high-resolution manometry in laryngopharyngeal reflux disease high-dose proton pump inhibitor failures. *Laryngoscope*. 2012;122(11):2473–2481.

330. Komatsu Y, Hoppo T, Jobe BA. Proximal reflux as a cause of adult-onset asthma: the case for hypopharyngeal impedance testing to improve the sensitivity of diagnosis. *JAMA Surg*. 2013;148(1):50–58.

331. Vailati C, Mazzoleni G, Bondi S, et al. Oropharyngeal pH monitoring for laryngopharyngeal reflux: is it a reliable test before therapy? *J Voice*. 2013;27(1):84–89.

332. Jette ME, Gaumnitz EA, Birchall MA, Welham NV, Thibeault SL. Correlation between reflux and multichannel intraluminal impedance pH monitoring in untreated volunteers. *Laryngoscope*. 2014; 124(10):2345–2351.

333. Becker V, Graf S, Schlag C, et al. First agreement analysis and day-to-day comparison of pharyngeal pH monitoring with pH/impedance monitoring in patients with suspected laryngopharyngeal reflux. *J Gastrointest Surg*. 2012;16(6):1096–1101.

334. Gooi Z, Ishman SL, Bock JM, Blumin JH, Akst LM. Changing patterns in reflux care: 10-year comparison of ABEA members. *Ann Otol Rhinol Laryngol*. 2015;124(12): 940–946.

335. Pandolfino JE, Kahrilas PJ. Prolonged pH monitoring: Bravo capsule. *GI Clin North Am*. 2005;15:307–318.

336. Wu JCY. Combined multichannel intraluminal impedance and pH monitoring for patients with suspected laryngopharyngeal reflux: is it ready to use? *J Neurogastroenterol Motil*. 2010;16:108–109.

337. Lee BE, Kim GH, Ryu DY, et al. Combined dual channel impedance/pH-metry in patients with suspected laryngopharyngeal reflux. *J Neurogastroenterol Motil*. 2010; 16:157–165.

338. Loots CM, Benninga MA, Davidson GP, Omari TI. Addition of pH-impedance monitoring (pH-MII) to standard pH monitoring increases the yield of symptom

339. Tutuian R, Castell DO. Reflux monitoring: role of combined multi-channel intraluminal impedance and pH. *GI Clin North Am*. 2005;15:361–371.

340. Musser J, Kelchner L, Nelis-Strunjas J, Montorse M. A comparision of rating scales used in the diagnosis of estraesophagel reflux. *J Voice*. 2011;25:293–300.

341. Park K, Choi S, Kwon S, Yon S, Kim S. Diagnosis of laryngopharyngeal reflux among globus patients. *Otolaryngol Head Neck Surg*. 2006;134:81–85.

342. Barry D, Vaezi M. Laryngoparyngeal reflux: more questions than answers. *Cleveland Clin J Med*. 2010;77(5):327–334.

343. Qadeer MA, Phillips CO, Lopez AR, et al. Proton pump inhibitor therapy for suspected GERD-related chronic laryngitis: a meta-analysis of randomized controlled trials. *Am J Gastroenterol*. 2006;101(11): 2646–2654.

344. Ford CN. Evaluation and management of laryngopharyngeal reflux. *JAMA*. 2005; 294(12):1534–1540.

345. Belafsky PC, Postma GN, Koufman JA. Validity and reliability of the Reflux Symptom Index (RSI). *J Voice*. 2002;16(2): 274–277.

346. Wiener GJ, Tsukashima R, Kelly C, et al. Oropharyngeal pH monitoring for the detection of liquid and aerosolized supraesophagel gastric reflux. *J Voice*. 2009; 23(4):498–504.

347. Koufman JA. The otolaryngologic manifestations of gastroesophageal reflux disease (GERD): a clinical investigation of 225 patients using ambulatory 24-hour pH monitoring and an experimental investigation of the role of acid and pepsin in the development of laryngeal injury. *Laryngoscope*. 1991;101(4, pt 2)(suppl 53):1–78.

348. Golub JS, Johns MM 3rd, Lim JH, DelGaudio JM, Klein AM. Comparison of an oropharyngeal pH probe and a standard dual pH probe for the diagnosis of laryngopha-

ryngeal reflux. *Ann Otol Rhinol Laryngol.* 2009;118(1):1–5.

349. Friedman M, Hamiliton C, Samielson CG, et al. The value of routine pH monitoring in the diagnosis and treatment of laryngopharyngeal reflux. *Otolaryngol Head Neck Surg.* 2012;146(6):952–958.

350. Vailati C, Mazzoleni G, Bondi S, Passaretti S, Bussi M, Testoni P. Oropharyngeal pH-monitoring with the Restech probe for laryngo-pharyngeal reflux: a new reliable test before PPI therapy? *Gastroenterology.* 2012;142(5 suppl 1):S-424.

351. Friedman M, Maley A, Kelley K, et al. Impact of pH monitoring on laryngopharyngeal reflux treatment: improved compliance and symptom resolution. *Otolaryngol Head Neck Surg.* 2011;144(4):558–562.

352. Barrett J, Peghini P, Katz P, et al. Ineffective esophageal motility (IEM): the most common manometric abnormality in GERD (Abstract 66.) *Gastroenterology.* 1997;112:4.

353. Johnson PE, Koufman JA, Nowak LJ, et al. Ambulatory 24-hour double-probe pH monitoring: the importance of manometry. *Laryngoscope.* 2001;111:1970–1975.

354. Johnson LF, DeMeester TR. Twenty-four hour pH monitoring of the distal esophagus. *Am J Gastroenterol.* 1974;62:325–332.

355. Rosen SN, Pope CE Jr. Extended esophageal pH monitoring. An analysis of the literature and assessment of its role in the diagnosis and management of gastroesophageal reflux. *J Clin Gastroenterol.* 1989;11:260–270.

356. Mattox H III, Richter JE. Prolonged ambulatory esophageal pH monitoring in the evaluation of gastroesophageal reflux disease. *Am J Med.* 1990;89:345–356.

357. Richter JE, Bradley LA, DeMeester TR, Wu WC. Normal 24-hour ambulatory esophageal pH values: influence of study center, pH electrode, age and gender. *Dig Dis Sci.* 1992;37:849–856.

358. Johansson KE, Tibbling L. Gastric secretion and reflux pattern in reflux oesophagitis before and during ranitidine treatment. *Scand J Gastroenterol.* 1986;21(4):487–492.

359. Haase GM, Ross MN, Gance-Cleveland B, Kolack KE. Extended four-channel esophageal pH monitoring: the importance of acid reflux patterns at the middle and proximal levels. *J Pediatr Surg.* 1988;23(1, pt 2):32–37.

360. Lehamn G, Rogers D, Cravens E, Flueckiger J. Prolonged pH probe testing less than 5 cm above the lower esophageal sphincter (LES): establishing normal control values. *Gastroenterology.* 1990;98:77.

361. Weusten BL, Akkermans LM, vanBerge-Henegouwen GP, Smout AJ. Spatiotemporal characteristics of physiological gastroesophageal reflux. *Am J Physiol.* 1994;266 (3, pt 1):G357–G362.

362. Sloan S, Rademaker AW, Kahrilas PJ. Determinants of gastroesophageal junction incompetence: hiatal hernia, lower esophageal sphincter, or both? *Ann Intern Med.* 1992;117:977–982.

363. Palmer ED. The hiatus hernia-esophagitis-esophageal stricture complex. Twenty-year prospective study. *Am J Med.* 1968;44: 566–579.

364. Sloan S. Kakrilas PJ. Impairment of esophageal emptying with hiatal hernia. *Gastroenterology.* 1991;100:596–605.

365. NIH. Consensus Conference. *Helicobacter pylori* in peptic ulcer disease. NIH Consensus Development Panel on *Helicobacter pylori* in peptic ulcer disease. *JAMA.* 1994; 272:65–69.

366. World Health Organization. Schistosomes, liver flukes and *Helicobacter pylori. IARC Monograph on the Evaluation of Carcinogen Risks to Humans.* 1994;61:177–220.

367. Nilius M, Malfertheiner P. Diagnostische Verfahren bei *Helicobacter-pylori* Infektion. In: Malfertheiner P, Hrsg. *Helicobacter pylori: Von der Grundlage zur Therapie.* Stuttgart, Germany: George Thieme Verlag; 1996:139–147.

368. Yilmaz T, Bajin MD, Gunaydin RO, Ozer S, Sozen T. Laryngopharyngeal reflux and *Helicobacter pylori. World J Gastroenterol.* 2014;20(27):8964–8970.

369. Cekin E, Ozyurt M, Erkul E, et al. The association between *Helicobacter pylori*

and laryngopharyngeal reflux in laryngeal pathologies. *Ear Nose Throat J.* 2012;91(3): E6–E9.

370. Siupsinskiene N, Jurgutaviciute V, Katutiene I, et al. *Helicobacter pylori* infection in laryngeal diseases. *Eur Arch Otorhinolaryngol.* 2013;270(8):2283–2288.

371. Islam A, Oguz H, Yucel M, et al. Does *Helicobacter pylori* exist in vocal fold pathologies and in the interarytenoid region? *Dysphagia.* 2013;28(3):382–387.

372. Campbell R, Kitty SJ, Hutton B, Bonaparte JP. The role of *Helicobacter pylori* in laryngopharyngeal reflux: a systematic review and meta-analysis. *Otolaryngol Head Neck Surg.* 2017;156(2):255–262.

373. Diaconu S, Predescu A, Moldoveanu A, et al. *Helicobacter pylori* infection: old and new. *J Med Life.* 2017;10(2):112–117.

374. Choe JW, Jung Sw, Kim SY, et al. Comparative study of *Helicobacter pylori* eradication rates of concomitant therapy vs modified quadruple therapy compromising proton-pump inhibitor, bismuth, amoxicillin, and metronidazole in Korea. *Helicobacter.* 2018;23(2):e12466.

375. Wo JM, Grist WJ, Gussack G, et al. Empiric trial of high-dose omeprazole in patients with posterior laryngitis: a prospective study. *Am J Gastroenterol.* 1997;92:2160–2165.

376. Metz DC, Childs ML, Ruiz C, Weinstein GS. Pilot study of the oral omeprazole test for reflux laryngitis. *Otolaryngol Head Neck Surg.* 1997;16:41–46.

377. Kuo B, Castell DO. Optimal dosing of omeprazole 40 mg daily: effects on gastric and esophageal pH and serum gastrin in healthy controls. *Am J Gastroenterol.* 1996; 91:1532–1538.

378. Jacobson BH, Johnson A, Grywalski C, et al. The Voice Handicap Index (VHI): development and validation. *J Speech Lang Pathol.* 1997;6:66–70.

379. Belafsky PC, Postma GN, Koufman JA. The validity and reliability of the Reflux Finding Score. *Laryngoscope.* 2001;111:1313–1317.

380. Rivicki DA, Wood M, Maton PN, et al. The impact of gastroesophageal reflux disease on health-related quality of life. *Am J Med.* 1998;104:252–258.

381. Lenderking WR, Hillson E, Rawler C, et al. The clinical characteristics and impact of laryngopharyngeal reflux disease on health-related quality of life. *Value Health.* 2003;6:560–565.

382. Andersson O, Rydén A, Ruth M, Moller RY, Finizia C. Development and validation of a laryngopharyngeal reflux questionnaire, the Pharyngeal Reflux Symptoms Questionnaire. *Scand J Gastroenterol.* 2010;45: 147–159.

383. Oyer SL, Anderson LC, Halum SL. Influence of anxiety and depression on the predictive value of the Reflux Symptom Index. *Ann Otol Rhinol Laryngol.* 2009;118:687–692.

384. Elam JC, Ishman SL, Dunbar KB, Clarke JO, Gourin CG. The relationship between depressive symptoms and Voice Handicap Index scores in laryngopharyngeal reflux. *Laryngoscope.* 2010;120:1900–1903.

385. Cheung TK, Lam PK, Wei WI, et al. Quality of life in patients with laryngopharyngeal reflux. *Digestion.* 2009;79:52–57.

386. Nishimura K, Fujita H, Tanaka Y, et al. Endoscopic classification for reflux pharyngolaryngitis. *Dis Esophagus.* 2010;23: 20–26.

387. Bell NJ, Burget DL, Howden CW, et al. Appropriate acid suppression for the management of gastro-esophageal reflux disease. *Digestion.* 1992;51(suppl 1):59–67.

388. Johnson LF, DeMeester TR. Elevation of the head of the bed, bethanecol and antacid form tablets on gastroesophageal reflux. *Dig Dis Sci.* 1981;26:673.

389. Scott DR, Simon RA. Supraesophageal reflux: correlation of position and occurrence of acid reflux-effect of head-of-bed elevation on supine reflux. *J Allergy Clin Immunol Pract.* 2015;3(3):356–361.

390. Schallom M, Dykeman B, Metheny N, Kirby J, Pierce J. Head-of-bed elevation and early outcomes of gastric reflux, aspiration and pressure ulcers: a feasibility study. *Am J Crit Care.* 2015;24(1):57–66.

391. Richter JE, Castell DO. Drugs, foods, and other substances in the cause and treat-

ment of reflux esophagitis. *Med Clin North Am.* 1981;65:1223–1234.

392. Becker DJ, Sinclair J, Castell DO, Wu WC. A comparison of high and low fat meals on postprandial esophageal acid exposure. *Am J Gastroenterol.* 1989;84:782–786.

393. Wright LE, Castell DO. The adverse effect of chocolate on lower esophageal sphincter pressure. *Am J Dig Dis.* 1975;20:703–707.

394. Dent J, Dodds WJ, Friedman RH, et al. Mechanism of gastroesophageal reflux in recumbent asymptomatic human subjects. *J Clin Invest.* 1980;65:256–267.

395. Koufman JA. Low-acid diet for recalcitrant laryngopharyngeal reflux: therapeutic benefits and their implications. *Ann Otol Rhinol Laryngol.* 2011;120:281–287.

396. Hamdan AL, Nassar J, Dowli A, Al Zaghal Z, Sabri A. Effect of fasting on laryngopharyngeal reflux disease in male subjects. *Eur Arch Otorhinolaryngol.* 2012;269(11): 2361–2366.

397. Jaworek A, Krane N, Lyons K, Sataloff RT. *Laryngopharyngeal reflux and gluten sensitivity.* Presented at: The Voice Foundation's 44th Annual Symposium on Care of the Professional Voice & International Association of Phonosurgery; Philadelphia, Pennsylvania; May 31, 2015.

398. Sapone A, Bai JC, Ciacci C, et al. Spectrum of gluten-related disorders: consensus on new nomenclature and classification. *BMC Med.* 2012;10:13.

399. Fasano A, Berti I, Gerarduzzi T, et al. Prevalence of celiac disease in at-risk and not-at-risk groups in the United States: a large multicenter study. *Arch Intern Med.* 2003; 163(3):286–292.

400. Mansueto P, Seidita A, D'Alcamo A, Carrocio A. Nonceliac gluten sensitivity: literature review. *J Am Coll Nutr.* 2014;33(1): 39–54.

401. Leonard M, Vasagar B. US perspective on glutenrelated diseases. *Clin Exp Gastroenterol.* 2014;7:25–37.

402. Volta U, Tovoli F, Cicola R, et al. Serological tests in gluten sensitivity (nonceliac gluten intolerance). *J Clin Gastroenterol.* 2012;46: 680–685.

403. Gujral N, Freeman H, Thomson ABR. Celiac disease: prevalence, diagnosis, pathogenesis, and treatment. *World J Gastroenterol.* 2012;46:680–685.

404. Fasano A, Berti I, Gerarduzzi T, et al. Prevalence of celiac disease in at-risk and not-at-risk groups in the United States, a large multicenter study. *Arch Intern Med.* 2003;163:286–292.

405. Iovino P, Ciacci C, Sabbatini F, et al. Esophageal impairment in adult celiac disease with steatorrhea. *Am J Gastroenterol.* 1998; 93:1243–1249.

406. Lucendo AJ. Esophageal manifestations of celiac disease. *Dis Esophagus.* 2011;24: 470–475.

407. Giorgetti GM, Tursi A, Brandimarte G, et al. Dysmotility-like dyspeptic symptoms in celiac patients: role of gluten and *Helicobacter pylori* infection. *Dig Liver Dis.* 2000; 32:73–74.

408. Chiarioni G, Bassotti G, Germani U, et al. Gluten-free diet normalizes mouth-to-cecum transit of a caloric meal in adult patients with celiac disease. *Dig Dis Sci.* 1997;42:2100–2105.

409. Fraquelli M, Bardella MT, Peracchi M, et al. Gallbladder emptying and somatostatin and cholecystokinin plasma levels in celiac disease. *Am J Gastroenterol.* 1999; 94:1866–1870.

410. Bai JC, Maurino E, Martinez C, et al. Abnormal colonic transit time in untreated celiacsprue. *Acta Gastroenterol Latinoam.* 1995;25:277–284.

411. Usai P, Manca R, Cuomo R, et al. Effect of gluten-free diet on preventing recurrence of gastroenterol reflux disease-related symptoms in adult celiac patients with nonerosive reflux disease. *J Gastroenterol Hepatol.* 2008;23:1368–1372.

412. Nachman F, Vazquez H, Gonzalez A, et al. Gastroesophageal reflux symptoms in patients with celiac disease and the effect of a gluten-free diet. *Clin Gastroenterol Hepatol.* 2011;9:214–219.

413. Lamanda R, Panarese A, De Stefano S. Coeliac disease and gastroesophageal non-erosive reflux: prevalence and effect

of gluten-free diet. *Dig Liver Dis.* 2009;41 (suppl 1):S90.

414. Revicki DA, Wood M, Wiklund I, Crawley J. Reliability and validity of the gastrointestinal symptom rating scale in patients with gastroesophageal reflux disease. *Qual Life Res.* 1998;7:75–83.

415. Tursi A. The treatment of gastro-esophageal reflux disease in adult celiac disease. *J Clin Gastroenterol.* 2004;38(8):724–725.

416. Collin P, Mustalahti K, Kyronpalo S, et al. Should we screen reflux oesophagitis patients for celiac disease? *Eur J Gastroenterol Hepatol.* 2004;16:917–920.

417. Cuomo A, Romano M, Rocco A, et al. Reflux oesophagitis in adult celiac disease: beneficial effect of a gluten free diet. *Gut.* 2003;52:514–517.

418. Wex T, Monkemuller K, Kuester D. Zonulin is not increased in the cardiac and esophageal mucosa of patients with gastroesophageal reflux disease. *Peptides.* 2009; 30:1082–1087.

419. Rubio-Tapia A, Hill ID, Kelly CP, et al. American College of Gastroenterology clinical guideline: diagnosis and management of celiac disease. *Am J Gastroenterol.* 2013;108(5):656–677.

420. Volta U, Tovoli F, Cicola R, et al. Serological tests in gluten sensitivity (nonceliac gluten intolerance). *J Clin Gastroenterol.* 2012;46: 680–685.

421. Leffler DA, Schuppan D. Update on serologic testing in celiac disease. *Am J Gastroenterol.* 2010;105:2520–2524.

422. Kabbani TA, Vanga RR, Leffler DA, et al. Celiac disease or non-celiac gluten sensitivity? An approach to clinical differential diagnosis. *Am J Gastroenterol.* 2014;109: 741–746.

423. Castillo NE, Thimmaiah GT, Leffler DA. The present and future in the diagnosis and management of celiac disease. *Gastroenterol Rep.* 2015;3(1):3–11.

424. Lundin KEA, Alaedini A. Non-celiac gluten sensitivity. *Gastrointest Endoscopy Clin N Am.* 2012;22:723–734.

425. Kikendall JW, Friedman AC, Oyewole MA, et al. Pill-induced esophageal injury: case reports and review of the medical literature. *Dig Dis Sci.* 1983;28:174–182.

426. de Groen PC, Lubbe DF, Hirsch LJ, et al. Esophagitis associated with the use of alendronate. *N Engl J Med.* 1996;335(14): 1016–1021.

427. Vardar R, Keskin M, Valitova E, et al. Effect of alginate in patients with GERD hiatal hernia matters. *Dis Esophagus.* 2017; 30(10):1–7.

428. Takeuchi T, Takahashi Y, Kawaguchi S, et al. Therapy of gastroesophageal reflux disease and functional dyspepsia overlaps with symptoms after usual-dose proton pump inhibitor: Acotiamide plus usual-dose proton pump inhibitor versus double-dose proton pump inhibitor. *J Gastroenterol Hepatol.* 2018;33(3):623-630.

429. Foocharoen C, Chunlertrith K, Mairiang P, et al. Effectiveness of add-on therapy with domperidone vs alginic acid in proton pump inhibitor partial response gastro-oesophageal reflux disease in systemic sclerosis: randomized placebo-controlled trial. *Rheumatology (Oxford).* 2017;56(2): 214–222.

430. Curcic J, Schwizer A, Kaufman E, et al. Effects of baclofen on the functional anatomy of the oesophagogastric junction and proximal stomach in healthy volunteers and patients with GERD assessed by magnetic resonance imaging and high-resolution manometry: a randomized controlled double-blind study. *Aliment Pharmacol Ther.* 2014;40(10):1230–1240.

431. Cossentino MJ, Mann K, Armbruster SP, Lake JM, Maydonovitch C, Wong RK. Randomised clinical trial: the effect of baclofen in patients with gastro-oesophageal reflux—a randomized prospective study. *Aliment Pharmacol Ther.* 2012;35(9): 1036–1044.

432. Abbasinazari M, Panahi Y, Mortazavi SA, et al. Effect of a combination of omeprazole plus sustained release baclofen versus omeprazole alone on symptoms of patients with gastroesophageal reflux disease (GERD). *Iran J Pharm Res.* 2014;13(4): 1221–1226.

433. Scarpellini E, Boecxstaens V, Farre R, et al. Effect on baclofen on the acid pocket at the gastroesophageal junction. *Dis Esophagus.* 2015;28(5):488–495.

434. Li S, Shi S, Chen F, Lin J. The effects of baclofen for the treatment of gastroesophageal reflux disease: a metaanalysis of randomized controlled trials. *Gastroenterol Res Pract.* 2014;2014:307805.

435. Vadlamudi NB, Hitch MC, Dimmitt RA, Thame KA. Baclofen for the treatment of pediatric GERD. *J Pediatr Gastroenterol Nutr.* 2013;57(6):808–812.

436. Xu X, Chen Q, Luang S, Lu H, Qiu Z. Successful resolution of refractory chronic cough induced by gastroesophageal reflux with treatment of baclofen. *Cough.* 2012; 8(1):8.

437. Xu XH, Yang ZM, Chen Q, et al. Therapeutic efficacy of baclofen in refractory gastroesophageal reflux-induced chronic cough. *World J Gastroenterol.* 2013;19(27): 4386–4392.

438. Blondeau K, Boecxstaens V, Rommel N, et al. Baclofen improves symptoms and reduces postprandial flow events in patients with rumination and supragastric bleching. *Clin Gastroenterol Hepatol.* 2012; 10(4):379–384.

439. Orr WC, Goodrich S, Wright S, Shepherd K, Mellow M. The effect of baclofen on nocturnal gastroesophageal reflux and measures of sleep quality: a randomized, crossover trial. *Neurogastroenterol Motil.* 2012;24(6):553–559.

440. Sontag S, Robinson M, McCallum RW, et al. Ranitidine therapy for gastroesophageal reflux disease. Results of a large double blind trial. *Arch Intern Med.* 1987;147:1485–1491.

441. Euler AR, Murdocck RH Jr, Wilson TH, et al. Ranitidine is effective therapy for erosive esophagitis. *Am J Gastroenterol.* 1993; 88:520–524.

442. Vigneri S, Termini R, Leandro G, et al. A comparison of five maintenance therapies for reflux esophagitis. *N Engl J Med.* 1995; 333:1106–1110.

443. Feldman M, Burton ME. Histamine 2-receptor antagonists: standard therapy for acid-peptic diseases. *N Engl J Med.* 1990;323:1672–1680.

444. Van Thiel DH, Gavaler JS, Smith WI Jr, Paul G. Hypothalamic-pituitary-gonadal dysfunction in men using cimetidine. *N Engl J Med.* 1979;300:1012–1015.

445. Enzmann GD, Leonard JM, Paulsen CA. Effects of cimetidine on reproductive function in men [Abstract]. *Clin Res.* 1981: 29(1):26A.

446. Carlson HE, Ippoliti AF, Swerdloff RS. Endocrine effects of acute and chronic cimetidine administration. *Dig Dis Sci.* 1981;26(5):428–432.

447. Winters SJ, Lee J, Teoen P. Competition of the histamine H2-antagonist cimetidine for androgen binding sites in man. *J Androl.* 1980;1(30):111–114.

448. Jensen RT, Collen MJ, Pandol SJ, et al. Cimetidine-induced impotence and breast changes with gastric hypersecretory states. *N Engl J Med.* 1989;308(15):383–387.

449. Malagelada JR, Edis AJ, Adson MA, et al. Medical and surgical options in the management of patients with gastrinoma. *Gastroenterology.* 1983;85:1524–1532.

450. DiPadova C, Roine R, Frezza M, et al. Effects of ranitidine on blood alcohol levels after ethanol ingestion. *JAMA.* 1992;267(1):83–86.

451. Sontag S, O'Connell SA, Greenlee HB, et al. Is gastroesophageal reflux a factor in some asthmatics? *Am J Gastroenterol.* 1987;82: 119–126.

452. Harper PC, Bergner A, Kaye MD. Antireflux treatment for asthma: improvement in patients with associated gastroesophageal reflux. *Arch Intern Med.* 1987;147:56–60.

453. Ekstrom T, Lindgren BR, Tibbling L. Effects of ranitidine treatment on patients with asthma and a history of gastro-oesophageal reflux: a double blind crossover study. *Thorax.* 1989;44:19–23.

454. Gustafsson PM, Kjellman NI, Tibbling L. A trial of ranitidine in asthmatic children and adolescents with or without pathologic gastroesophageal reflux. *Eur Respir J.* 1992;5:201–206.

455. Irwin RS, Curley FJ, French CL. Chronic cough. The spectrum and frequency of

causes, key components of the diagnostic evaluation, and outcome of specific therapy. *Am Rev Respir Dis.* 1990;141:640–647.

456. Irwin RS, Zwacki JK, Curley FJ, et al. Chronic cough as the sole presenting manifestation of gastroesophageal reflux. *Am Rev Respir Dis.* 1989;140:1294–1300.

457. Fitzgerald JM, Allen CJ, Craven MA, Newhouse MT. Chronic cough and gastroesophageal reflux. *Can Med Assoc J.* 1989; 140:520–524.

458. Waring JP, Lacayo L, Hunter J, et al. Chronic cough and hoarseness in patients with severe gastroesophageal reflux disease. Diagnosis and response to therapy. *Dig Dis Sci.* 1995;40:1093–1097.

459. Blum AL, Adami B, Bouzo MH, et al. Effect of cisapride on relapse of esophagitis. *Dig Dis Sci.* 1993;38:551–560.

460. Castell DO, Sigmund C, Patterson D, et al. Cisapride 20 mg bid provides symptomatic relief of heartburn and related symptoms in patients with symptoms of chronic mild to moderate gastroesophageal reflux disease. *Am J Gastroenterol.* 1998;93:547–552.

461. Wiseman LR, Faulds D. Cisapride. An updated review of its pharmacology and therapeutic efficacy as a prokinetic agent in gastrointestinal motility disorders. *Drugs.* 1994;47:116–152.

462. Dordal MT, Baltazar MA, Roca I, et al. Nocturnal spasmodic cough in the infant. Evolution after antireflux treatment. *Allerg Immunol (Paris).* 1994;26:53–58.

463. Dupont C, Molkhou P, Petrovic N, Freitag B. Treatment using motility of gastroesophageal reflux associated with respiratory manifestations in children [in French]. *Ann Pediatr (Paris).* 1989;36:148–150.

464. Ekstrom T, Tibbling T. Esophageal acid perfusion, airway function, and symptoms in asthmatic patients with marked bronchial hyperactivity. *Chest.* 1989;96:995–998.

465. Smyrnios NA, Irwin RS, Curley FJ. Chronic cough with a history of excessive sputum production. *Chest.* 1995;108:991–997.

466. Ing AJ, Ngu MC, Breslin AB. Chronic persistent cough and gastroesophageal reflux. *Thorax.* 1994;46:479–483.

467. Khoury R, Paoletti V, Cohn J, et al. Cisapride improves pulmonary function tests in patients with gastroesophageal (GE) reflux and chronic respiratory symptoms. *Gastroenterology.* 1998;114:712.

468. Glicksman JT, Mick PT, Fung K, Carroll TL. Prokinetic agents and laryngopharyngeal reflux disease: a systematic review. *Laryngoscope.* 2014;124(10):2375–2379.

469. Guo H, Ma H, Wang J. Proton pump inhibitor therapy for the treatment of laryngopharyngeal reflux: a meta-analysis of randomized controlled trials. *J Clin Gastroenterol.* 2016;50(4):295–300.

470. Luo H, Ma S, Gao Y, et al. The therapeutic effect of proton pump inhibitor on alleviation of hoarseness symptoms in patients with laryngopharyngeal reflux. *Lin Chung Er Bi Yan Hou Tou Jing Wai Ke Za Zhi.* 2015;29(11):997–1001.

471. Sandmark S, Carlsson R, Fausa O, Lundell L. Omeprazole or ranitidine in the treatment of reflux esophagitis. *Scand J Gastroenterol.* 1988;23:625–632.

472. Castell DO, Richter JE, Robinson M, et al. Efficacy and safety of lansoprazole in the treatment of erosive esophagitis. *Am J Gastroenterol.* 1996;91:1749–1757.

473. Klinkenberg-Knol E, Festen HP, Jansen JB, et al. Long-term treatment with omeprazole for refractory esophagitis. *Ann Intern Med.* 1994;121:161–167.

474. Klinkenberg-Knol EC. Eleven years' experience of continuous maintenance treatment with omeprazole in GERD patients [abstract 180]. *Gastroenterology.* 1991;98: 114.

475. Hatlebakk JG, Katz PO, Kuo B, Castell DO. Nocturnal gastric acidity and acid breakthrough on different regimes of omeprazole 40 mg daily. *Aliment Pharmacol Ther.* 1998;12:1235–1240.

476. Hatlebakk JG, Katz PO, Camacho-Lobato L, Castell DO. Proton pump inhibitors: better acid suppression when taken before a meal than without a meal. *Aliment Pharmacol Ther.* 2000;14:1267–1272.

477. Peghini PL, Katz PO, Bracy NA, Castell DO. Nocturnal recovery of gastric acid

secretion with twice-daily dosing of proton pump inhibitors. *Am J Gastroenterol.* 1998; 93:763–767.

478. Peghini PL, Katz PO, Castell DO. Ranitidine controls nocturnal gastric acid breakthrough on omeprazole: a controlled study in normal subjects. *Gastroenterology.* 1998; 115:1335–1339.

479. Zimmerman A, Walters JK, Katona B, Souney P. Alternative methods of proton pump inhibitor administration. *Consultant Pharmacist.* 1886;19:990–998.

480. Kamel PL, Hanson D, Kahrilas PJ. Omeprazole for the treatment of posterior laryngitis. *Am J Med.* 1994;96:321–325.

481. Belafsky PC, Postma GN, Koufman JA. Laryngopharyngeal reflux symptoms improve before changes in physical findings. *Laryngoscope.* 2001;111:979–981.

482. Kuipers EJ, Lundell L, Klinkenberg-Knol EC, et al. Atrophic gastritis and *Helicobacter pylori* infection in patients with reflux esophagitis treated with omeprazole or fundoplication. *N Engl J Med.* 1996;334: 1018–1022.

483. Proton pump inhibitor relabeling for cancer risk not warranted. *FDA Report.* 1996; 58:T&G-1–2.

484. Ford GA, Oliver PS, Prior JS, et al. Omeprazole in the treatment of asthmatics with nocturnal symptoms and gastro-oesophageal reflux: a placebo-controlled crossover study. *Postgrad Med J.* 1994:70:350–354.

485. Boeree MJ, Peters FT, Postma DS, Kleibbeuker JH. No effects of high dose omeprazole in patients with severe airway hyperresponsiveness and a symptomatic gastro-oesophageal reflux and pulmonary function in patients with obstructive lung disease. *Eur Respir J.* 1998;11(5):1070–1074.

486. Meier JH, McNally PR, Punja M, et al. Does omeprazole (Prilosec) improve respiratory function in asthmatics with gastroesophageal reflux? *Dig Dis Sci.* 1994;39: 2127–2133.

487. Hanson DG, Kamel PL, Kahrilas PJ. Outcomes of antireflux therapy for the treatment of chronic laryngitis. *Ann Otol Rhinol Laryngol.* 1995;104:550–555.

488. Wo JM, Grist WJ, Gussack G, et al. Empiric trial of high dose omeprazole in patients with posterior laryngitis: a prospective study. *Am J Gastroenterol.* 1997;92:2160–2165.

489. Metz DC, Child ML, Ruiz C, Weinstein GS. Pilot study of the oral omeprazole test for reflux laryngitis. *Otolaryngol Head Neck Surg.* 1997;116:41–46.

490. Jaspersen D, Draf W, Weber R, Hammar C-H. Effect of omeprazole on the course of treatment of reflux associated esophagitis and laryngitis. *Gastroenterology.* 1996;31: 765–767.

491. El-Serag HB, Lee P, Buchner A, et al. Lansoprazole treatment of patients with chronic idiopathic laryngitis; a placebo-controlled trial. *Am J Gastroenterol.* 2001; 96(4):979–983.

492. Amin MR, Postma GN, Johnson P, et al. Proton pump inhibitor resistance in the treatment of laryngopharyngeal reflux. *Otolaryngol Head Neck Surg.* 2001;125:374–378.

493. Chiverton SG, Howden CW, Burget DW, Hunt RH. Omeprazole (20 mg) daily given in the morning or evening: a comparison of effects on gastric acidity, and plasma gastrin and omeprazole concentration. *Aliment Pharmacol Ther.* 1992;6:103–111.

494. Portnoy JE, Gregory ND, Cerulli CE, et al. Efficacy of super high dose proton pump inhibitor administration in refractory laryngopharyngeal reflux: a pilot study. *J Voice.* 2014;28(3):369–377.

495. Lee YC, Lee JS, Kim SW, et al. Influence of age on treatment with proton pump inhibitors in patients with laryngopharyngeal reflux disease: a prospective multicenter study. *JAMA Otolaryngol Head Neck Surg.* 2013;139(12):1291–1295.

496. El-Serag HB, Sonnenberg A. Comorbid occurrence of laryngeal or pulmonary disease with esophagitis in United States military veterans. *Gastroenterology.* 1997;113:755–760.

497. Noordzij J, Khidir A, Evans BA, et al. Evaluation of omeprazole in the treatment of reflux laryngitis: a prospective, placebo-controlled, randomized, double-blind study. *Laryngoscope.* 2001;111:2147–2151.

498. Eherer AJ, Habermann W, Hammer HF, et al. Effect of pantoprazole on the course of reflux-associated laryngitis: a placebo-controlled double-blind crossover study. *Scand J Gastroenterol.* 2003;38:462–467.

499. Issing WJ, Tauber S, Folwaczny C, et al. Impact of 24-hour intraesophageal pH monitoring with 2 channels in the diagnosis of reflux-induced otolaryngologic disorders [in German]. *Laryngorhinootology.* 2003;82:347–352.

500. Bilgen C, Ogut F, Kesimli-Dinc H, et al. The comparison of an empiric proton pump inhibitor vs. 24-hour double-probe pH monitoring in laryngopharyngeal reflux. *J Laryngol Otol.* 2003;117:386–390.

501. Bruley des Varannes S, Coron E, Galmiche JP. Short and long-term PPI treatment for GERD. Do we need more-potent antisecretory drugs? *Best Pract Res Clin Gastroenterol.* 2010;24:905–921.

502. Tighe MP, Afzal NA, Bevan A, Beattie RM. Current pharmacological management of gastro-esophageal reflux in children: an evidence-based systematic review. *Paediatr Drugs.* 2009;11:185–202.

503. Romano C, Chiaro A, Comito D, Loddo I, Ferrau V. Proton pump inhibitors in pediatrics: evaluation of efficacy in GERD therapy. *Curr Clin Pharmacol.* 2011;6:41–47.

504. Lam PK, Ng ML, Cheung TK, et al. Rabeprazole is effective in treating laryngopharyngeal reflux in a randomized placebo-controlled trial. *Clin Gastroenterol Hepatol.* 2010;8:770–776.

505. Masaany M, Marina MB, Ezat WP, Sani A. Empirical treatment with pantoprazole as a diagnostic tool for symptomatic adult laryngopharyngeal reflux. *J Laryngol Otol.* 2011;125:502–508.

506. Abou-Ismail A, Vaezi MF. Evaluation of patients with suspected laryngopharyngeal reflux: a practical approach. *Curr Gastroenterol Rep.* 2011;13:213–218.

507. Dadabhai A, Friedenberg FK. Raberprazole: a pharmacologic and clinical review for acid-related disorders. *Expert Opin Drug Saf.* 2009;8:119–126.

508. Fass R, Noelck N, Willis MR, et al. The effect of esomeprazole 20 mg twice daily on acoustic and perception parameters of the voice in laryngopharyngeal reflux. *Neurogastroenterol Motil.* 2010;22:134–141, e44–e45.

509. Johnston N, Bulmer D, Gill GA, et al. Cell biology of laryngeal epithelial defenses in health and disease: further studies. *Ann Otol Rhinol Laryngol.* 2003;112:481–491.

510. Reichel O, Dressel H, Wiederanders K, et al. Double-blind, placebo-controlled trial with esomeprazole for symptoms and signs associated with laryngopharyngeal reflux. *Otolaryngol Head Neck Surg.* 2008;139: 414–420.

511. Belafsky PC, Rees CJ, Rodriguez K, et al. Esophagopharyngeal reflux. *Otolaryngol Head Neck Surg.* 2008;138:57–61.

512. Belafsky PC, Postma GN, Koufman JA. Laryngopharyngeal reflux symptoms improve before changes in physical findings. *Laryngoscope.* 2001;111:979–981.

513. Reichel O, Keller J, Rasp G, et al. Efficacy of once-daily esomeprazole treatment in patients with laryngopharyngeal reflux evaluated by 24-hour pH monitoring. *Otolaryngol Head Neck Surg.* 2007;136:205–210.

514. Jin BJ, Lee YS, Jeong SW, et al. Change of acoustic parameters before and after treatment in laryngopharyngeal reflux patients. *Laryngoscope.* 2008;118:938–941.

515. Chapman DB, Rees CJ, Lippert D, Sataloff RT, Wright SC Jr. Adverse effects of long-term proton pump inhibitor use: a review for otolaryngologists. *J Voice.* 2011; 25:236–240.

516. Sataloff RT. Proton pump inhibitor: adverse effects. *ENT J.* 2010;89(12):574–576.

517. Davies M, Wilton LV, Shakir SA. Safety profile of esomeprazole: results of a prescription-event monitoring study of 11,595 patients in England. *Drug Saf.* 2008;31: 313–323.

518. Yang YX, Lewis JD, Epstein S, Metz DC. Long-term proton pump inhibitor therapy and risk of hip fracture. *JAMA.* 2006;296: 2947–2953.

519. Solomon DH, Diem SJ, Ruppert K, et al. Bone mineral density changes among women initiating proton pump inhibitors or H2 receptor antagonists: a SWAN cohort study. *J Bone Miner Res.* 2015;30(2): 232–239.

520. Lam JR, Schneider JL, Zhao W, Corley DA. Proton pump inhibitor and histamine 2 receptor antagonist use and vitamin B12 deficiency. *JAMA.* 2013;310(22): 2435–2442.

521. Aseeri M, Schroeder T, Kramer J, Zackula R. Gastric acid suppression by proton pump inhibitors as a risk factor for *Clostridium difficile*–associated diarrhea in hospitalized patients. *Am J Gastroenterol.* 2008;103(9):2308–2313.

522. Gilard M, Arnaud B, Cornily C, et al. Influence of omeprazole on the antiplatelet action of clopidogrel associated with aspirin: the randomized, double-blind OCLA (Omeprazole Clopidogrel Aspirin) study. *J Am Coll Cardiol.* 2008;51:256–260.

523. Pezalla E, Day D, Pulliadath I. Initial assessment of clinical impact of a drug interaction between clopidogrel and proton pump inhibitors. *J Am Coll Cardiol.* 2008;52:1038–1039.

524. Eslami L, Kalantarian S, Nasseri-Moghaddam S, Majdzadeh R. Long-term proton pump inhibitor (PPI) use and the incidence of gastric (pre)malignant lesions. *Cochrane Database Syst Rev.* 2008;10.1002/14651858. CD007098.

525. Freston JW. Omeprazole, hypergastrinemia, and gastric carcinoid tumors. *Ann Intern Med.* 1994;121:232–233.

526. Lazarus B, Yuan C, Wilson FP, et al. Proton pump inhibitor use and the risk of chronic kidney disease. *JAMA Intern Med.* 2016;176(2):238–246.

527. Antoniou T, Macdonald EM, Hollands S, et al. Proton pump inhibitors and the risk of acute kidney injury in older patients: a population-based cohort study. *CMAJ Open.* 2015;3(2):E166–E171.

528. FDA Drug Safety Communication: Low magnesium levels can be associated with long-term use of Proton Pump Inhibitor drugs (PPIs) 2011. Rockville, MD: MedWatch.

529. Cheungpasitporn W, Thongprayoon C, Kittanamongkolchai W, et al. Proton pump inhibitors linked to hypomagnesemia: a systematic review and metaanalysis of observational studies. *Ren Fail.* 2015;37(7): 1237–1241.

530. Kwok CS, Arthur AK, Anibueze CI, et al. Risk of *Clostridium difficile* infection with acid suppressing drugs and antibiotics: meta-analysis. *Am J Gastroenterol.* 2012; 107(7):1011–1019.

531. Bavishi C, Dupont HL. Systematic review: the use of proton pump inhibitors and increased susceptibility to enteric infection. *Aliment Pharmacol Ther.* 2011;34: 1269–1281.

532. Zhou B, Huang Y, Li H, Sun W, Liu J. Proton-pump inhibitors and risk of fractures: an update meta-analysis. *Osteoporos Int.* 2016;27(1):339–347.

533. Eom CS, Jeon CY, Lim JW, et al. Use of acid-suppressive drugs and risk of pneumonia: a systematic review and meta-analysis. *CMAJ.* 2011;183(3):310–319.

534. Fillion KB, Chateau D, Targownik LE, et al; CNODES Investigators. Proton pump inhibitors and the risk of hospitalization for community-acquired pneumonia: replicated cohort studies with meta-analysis. *Gut.* 2014;63(4):552–558.

535. Focks JJ, Brouwer MA, von Oijen MG, et al. Concomitant use of clopidogrel and proton pump inhibitors: impact on platelet function and clinical outcome: a systematic review. *Heart.* 2013;99(8):520–527.

536. Melloni C, Washam JB, Jones WS, et al. Conflicting results between randomized trials and observational studies on the impact of proton pump inhibitors on cardiovascular events with coadministered with dual antiplatelet therapy: systematic review. *Circ Cardiovasc Qual Outcomes.* 2015;8(1):47–55.

537. Shin JM, Lee JY, Lee DY, et al. Proton pump inhibitors as a possible cause of vitiligo: an

in vivo and in vitro study. *J Eur Acad Dermatol Venereol.* 2014;28(11):1475–1479.

538. Shah NH, LePendu P, Bauer-Mehren A. Proton pump inhibitor usage and the risk of myocardial infarction in the general population. *PLoS One.* 2015;10(6):e0124653.

539. Shih CJ, Chen YT, Ou SM, Li SY, Chen TJ, Wang SJ. Proton pump inhibitor use represents an independent risk factor for myocardial infarction. *Int J Cardiol.* 2014;177: 292–297.

540. Semb S, Helgstrand F, Hjørne F, Bytzer P. Persistent severe hypomagnesemia caused by proton pump inhibitor resolved after laparoscopic fundoplication. *World J Gastroenterol.* 2017;23(37):6907–6910.

541. Tergast TL, Wranke A, Laser H, et al. Dose-dependent impact of proton pump inhibitors on the clinical course of spontaneous bacterial peritonitis. *Liver Int.* 2018;38(9): 1602-1613.

542. Otani IM, Banerji A. Immediate and delayed hypersensitivity reactions to proton pump inhibitors: evaluation and management. *Curr Allergy Asthma Rep.* 2016; 16(3):17.

543. Li DK, Yan P, Abou-Samra AB, et al. Proton pump inhibitors are associated with accelerated development of cirrhosis, hepatic decompensation and hepatocellular carcinoma in noncirrhotic patients with chronic hepatitis C infection: results from ERCHIVES. *Aliment Pharmacol Ther.* 2018;47(2):246–258.

544. Dado D, Loesch E, Jaganathan S. A case of severe iron deficiency anemia associated with long-term proton pump inhibitor use. *Curr Ther Res Clin Exp.* 2017;84:1–3.

545. Jung SW, Kim SY, Choe JW, et al. Standard and double-dose intravenous proton pump inhibitor injections for prevention of bleeding after endoscopic resection. *J Gastroenterol Hepatol.* 2017;32(4):778–781.

546. Takeda T, Asaoka D, Tajima Y, et al. Hemorrhagic polyps formed like fundic gland polyps during long-term proton pump inhibitor administration. *Clin J Gastroenterol.* 2017;10(5):478–484.

547. Yu T, Tang Y, Jiang L, et al. Proton pump inhibitor therapy and its association with spontaneous bacterial peritonitis incidence and mortality: a meta-analysis. *Dig Liver Dis.* 2016;48(4):353–359.

548. Arai N, Nakamizo T, Ihara H, et al. Histamine H2-blocker and proton pump inhibitor use and the risk of pneumonia in acute stroke: a retrospective analysis on susceptible patients. *PLoS One.* 2017;12(1): e 0169300.

549. Momosaki R, Yasunaga H, Matsui H, et al. Proton pump inhibitors versus histamine-2 receptor antagonists and risk of pneumonia in patients with acute stroke. *J Stroke Cerebrovasc Dis.* 2016;25(5):1035–1040.

550. Hayashino Y, Okamura S, Mashitani T, et al. Association of proton pump inhibitor use with the risk of the development or progression of albuminuria among Japanese patients with diabetes: A prospective cohort study [Diabetes Distress and Care Registry at Tenri (DDCRT 16)]. *Diabetes Res Clin Pract.* 2018;138:1–7.

551. Lee E, Song KH, Bae JY, et al. Risk factors for poor outcome in community-onset *Clostridium difficile* infection. *Antimicrob Resist Infect Control.* 2018;7:75.

552. Jensen BES, Hansen JM, Larsen KS, et al. Randomized clinical trial: the impact of gastrointestinal risk factor screening and prophylactic proton pump inhibitor therapy in patients receiving dual antiplatelet therapy. *Eur J Gastroenterol Hepatol.* 2017; 29(10):1118–1125.

553. Weisz G, Smilowitz NR, Kirtane AJ, et al. Proton pump inhibitors, platelet reactivity, and cardiovascular outcomes after drug-eluting stents in clopidogrel-treated patients: the ADAPT-DES Study. *Circ Cardiovasc Interv.* 2015;8(10). pii: e001952.

554. Vaduganathan M, Bhatt DL. Revisiting the clopidogrel-proton pump inhibitor interaction: from bench to bedside. *Circ Cardiovasc Interv.* 2015;8(10). pii: e003208.

555. Sella GCP, Tamashiro E, Anselmo-Lima WT, Valera FCP. Relation between chronic rhinosinusitis and gastroesophageal reflux

in adults: systematic review. *Braz J Otorhinolaryngol.* 2017;83(3):356–363.

556. Targownik LE, Lix LM, Leung S, et al. Proton-pump inhibitor use is not associated with osteoporosis or accelerated bone mineral density loss. *Gastroenterology.* 2010;138:8896–8904.

557. Corley DA, Kubo A, Zhao W, et al. Proton pump inhibitors and histamine-2 receptor antagonists are associated with hip fractures among at-risk patients. *Gastroenterology.* 2010;139:93–101.

558. Ngamreungphong S, Leonatiadis GI, Radhi S, et al. Proton pump inhibitors and risk of fracture: a systematic review and meta-analysis of observational studies. *Am J Gastroenterol.* 2011;106:1209–1218; quiz 1219.

559. Targownik LE, Leslie WD, Davison KS, et al. The relationship between proton pump inhibitor use and longitudinal change in bone mineral density: a population-based study from the Canadian Multicentre Osteoporosis Study (CaMos). *Am J Gastroenterol.* 2012;107:1361–1369.

560. Soen S. Proton pump inhibitor and bone complications. *Clin Calcium.* 2015;25(11):1667–1674.

561. Hussain S, Siddiqui AN, Habib A, et al. Proton pump inhibitors' use and risk of hip fracture: a systematic review and meta-analysis. *Rheumatol Int.* 2018;38(11):1999–2014.

562. Kwok CS, Jeevanantham V, Dawn B, Loke YK. No consistent evidence of differential cardiovascular risk amongst proton-pump inhibitors when used with clopidogrel: meta-analysis. *Int J Cardiol.* 2013;167(3):965–974.

563. Ford GA, Oliver PS, Prior JS, et al. Omeprazole in the treatment of asthmatics with nocturnal symptoms and gastro-oesophageal reflux: a placebo-controlled cross-over study. *Postgrad Med J.* 1994;70:350–354.

564. Würtz M, Grove EL. Proton pump inhibitors in cardiovascular disease: drug interactions with antiplatelet drugs. *Adv Exp Med Biol.* 2017;906:325–350.

565. Xie Y, Bowe B, Li T, et al. Risk of death among users of proton pump inhibitors: a longitudinal observational cohort of study of United States veterans. *BMJ Open.* 2017; 7:e015735.

566. McKinnon BJ, Hawkshaw MJ, Sataloff RT. Proton pump inhibitor-related mortality: let us not be dead wrong. *J Voice.* 2017; 31(5):519.

567. Ohmure H, Kanematsu-Hashimoto K, Nagayama K, et al. Evaluation of a proton pump inhibitor for sleep bruxism: a randomized clinical trial. *J Dent Res.* 2016; 95(13):1479–1486.

568. Gomm W, von Holt K, Thome F, et al. Association of proton pump inhibitors with risk of dementia: a pharmacoepidemiological claims data analysis. *JAMA.* 2016;73(4):410–416.

569. Vaezi MF, Yang YX, Howden CW. Complications of proton pump inhibitor therapy. *Gastroenterology.* 2017;153(1):35–48.

570. Eusebi LH, Rabitti S, Artesiani ML, et al. Proton pump inhibitors: risks of long-term use. *J Gastroenterol Hepatol.* 2017;32(7):1295–1302.

571. Smoak BR, Koufman JA. Effects of gum chewing on pharyngeal and esophageal pH. *Ann Otol Rhinol Laryngol.* 2001;110:1117–1119.

572. Durkes A, Sivansakar MP. Bicarbonate availability for vocal fold epithelial defense to acidic challenge. *Ann Otol Rhinol Laryngol.* 2014;123(1):71–76.

573. Koufman JA, Johnston N. Potential benefits of pH 8.8 drinking water as an adjunct in the treatment of reflux disease. *Ann Otol Rhinol Laryngol.* 121(7):431–434.

574. Goddard A, Logan R. One-week low-dose triple therapy: new standards for *Helicobacter pylori* treatment. *Eur J Gastroenterol Hepatol.* 1995;7:1–3.

575. Katz PO, Anderson C, Khoury R, Castell DO. Gastrooesophageal reflux associated with nocturnal gastric acid breakthrough on proton pump inhibitor. *Aliment Pharmacol Ther.* 1998;12:1231–1234.

576. Katzka DA, Paoletti V, Leite L, Castell DO. Prolonged ambulatory pH monitoring in patients with persistent gastroesophageal

symptoms reflux disease: testing while on therapy identifies need for more aggressive antireflux therapy. *Am J Gastroenterol.* 1996;91:2110–2113.

577. Peghini P, Katz P, Castell D. Bedtime ranitidine decreases gastric acid secretion and eliminates acid exposure overnight in a patient with Barrett's esophagus taking omeprazole, 20 mg BID. *Am J Gastroenterol.* 1997;92:1723.

578. Allison PR. Reflux esophagitis, sliding hiatal hernia, and the anatomy of repair. *Surg Gynecol Obstet.* 1951;92:419–431.

579. Hill LD. An effective operation for hiatal hernia: an eight-year appraisal. *Ann Surg.* 1967;166:681–692.

580. Nissen R. Eine einfache Operation zur Beeinflussung der Refluxoesophagitis. *Schweiz Med Wochenschr.* 1956;86:590.

581. Geagea T. Laparoscopic Nissen's fundoplication: preliminary report on ten cases. *Surg Endosc.* 1991;5:170–173.

582. Bittner HB, Meyers WC, Brazer SR, Pappas JN. Laparoscopic Nissen fundoplication: operative results and short-term follow-up. *Am J Surg.* 1994;167:193–200.

583. Collet D, Cadiere GB. Conversions and complications of laparoscopic treatment of gastroesophageal reflux disease. *Am J Surg.* 1995;169:622–626.

584. Cuschieri A, Hunter J, Wolfe B, et al. Multicenter prospective evaluation of laparoscopic antireflux surgery. *Surg Endosc.* 1993;7:505–510.

585. Fontaumard E, Espalieu P, Boulez J. Laparoscopic Nissen-Rossetti fundoplication. *Surg Endosc.* 1995;9:869–873.

586. Spechler SJ. Comparison of medical and surgical therapy for complicated gastroesophageal reflux disease in veterans. *N Engl J Med.* 1992;326:786–792.

587. Spechler SJ, Lee E, Ahnen D, et al. Long-term outcome of medical and surgical therapies for gastroesophageal reflux disease. *JAMA.* 2001;285(18):2331–2338.

588. So JB, Zeitels SM, Rattner DW. Outcomes of atypical symptoms attributed to gastroesophageal reflux treated by laparoscopic fundoplication. *Surgery.* 1998;124(1):28–32.

589. Geagea T. Laparoscopic Nissen-Rossetti fundoplication. *Surg Endosc.* 1994;8:1080–1084.

590. Hinder RA, Filipi CJ, Wetscher G, et al. Laparoscopic Nissen fundoplication is an effective treatment for gastroesophageal reflux disease. *Ann Surg.* 1994;220:472–483.

591. Jamieson GG, Watson DI, Britten-Jones R, et al. Laparoscopic Nissen fundoplication. *Ann Surg.* 1994;220:137–145.

592. McKernan JB, Laws HL. Laparoscopic Nissen fundoplication for the treatment of gastroesophageal reflux disease. *Am Surg.* 1994;60:87–93.

593. McKernan JB, Champion JK. Laparoscopic anti-reflux surgery. *Am Surg.* 1995;6:1530–1536.

594. Peters JH, Heimbucher J, Kauer WK, et al. Clinical and physiological comparison of laparoscopic and open Nissen fundoplication. *J Am Coll Surg.* 1995;180:385–393.

595. Rattner DW, Brooks DC. Patient satisfaction following laparoscopic and open antireflux surgery. *Arch Surg.* 1995;130:289–294.

596. Sataloff DM, Pursnani K, Hoyo S, et al. An objective assessment of laparoscopic anti-reflux surgery. *Am J Surg.* 1997;174:63–67.

597. Snow LL, Weinstein LS, Hannon JK. Laparoscopic reconstruction of gastroesophageal anatomy for the treatment of reflux disease. *Surg Endosc.* 1995;9:774–780.

598. Weerts JM, Dallemagne B, Hamoir E, et al. Laparoscopic Nissen fundoplication detailed analysis of 132 patients. *Surg Laparosc Endosc.* 1993;3:359–364.

599. Johnson WE, Hagen JA, DeMeester TR, et al. Outcome of respiratory symptoms after antireflux surgery on patients with gastroesophageal reflux disease. *Arch Surg.* 1996;131:489–492.

600. DeMeester TR, O'Sullivan GC, Bermudez G, Midell AI, Cimochowski GE, O'Drobinak J. Esophageal function in patients with angina-type chest pain and normal coronary angiograms. *Ann Surg.* 1982;196:488–498.

601. Perrin-Fayolle M, Gormand F, Braillon G, et al. Long-term results of surgical treat-

ment for gastroesophageal reflux in asthmatic patients. *Chest.* 1989;96:40–45.

602. Deveney CW, Benner K, Cohen J. Gastroesophageal reflux and laryngeal disease. *Arch Surg.* 1993;128:1021–1027.

603. Pitcher DE, Pitcher WD, Martin DT, Curet MJ. Antireflux surgery does not reliably correct reflux-related asthma. *Gastrointest Endosc.* 1996;43:433.

604. Hunter JG, Trus TL, Branum GD, et al. A physiological approach to laparoscopic fundoplication for gastroesophageal reflux disease. *Ann Surg.* 1996;223:673–687.

605. Weber B, Portnoy JE, Castellanos A, et al. Efficacy of anti-reflux surgery on refractory laryngopharyngeal reflux disease in professional voice users: a pilot study. *J Voice.* 2014;28(4):492–500.

606. Trad KS, Turgeon DG, Deljkich E. Long-term outcomes after transoral incisionless fundoplication in patients with GERD and LPR symptoms. *Surg Endosc.* 2012;26(3): 650–660.

607. Fahin M, Vardar R, Ersin S, et al. The effect of antireflux surgery on laryngeal symptoms, findings and voice parameters. *Eur Arch Otorhinolaryngol.* 2015;272(11):3375–3383.

608. Hoppo T, Sanz AF, Nason KS, et al. How much pharyngeal exposure is "normal"? Normative data for laryngopharyngeal reflux events using hypopharyngeal multichannel intraluminal impedance (HMII). *J Gastrointest Surg.* 2012;16(1):16–24.

609. Mazzoleni G, Vailati C, Lisma DG, Testoni PA, Passaretti S. Correlation between oropharyngeal pH-monitoring and esophageal pH-impedance monitoring in patients with suspected GERD-related extraesophageal symptoms. *Neurogastroenterol Motil.* 2014;26(11):1557–1564.

610. Toomey P, Teta A, Patel K, et al. Transoral incisionless fundoplication: is it as safe and efficacious as a Nissen or Toupet fundoplication? *Am Surg.* 2014;80(9):860–867.

611. Du X, Wu JM, Hu ZW, et al. Laparoscopic Nissen (total) versus anterior 180° fundoplication for gastro-esophageal reflux disease: a meta-analysis and systematic review. *Medicine (Baltimore).* 2017;96(37):e8085.

612. Oor JE, Roks DJ, Broeders JA, et al. Seventeen-year outcome of a randomized clinical trial comparing laparoscopic and conventional Nissen fundoplication: a plea for patient counseling and clarification. *Ann Surg.* 2017;266(1):23–28.

613. Zhang C, Hu ZW, Yan C, et al. Nissen fundoplication vs proton pump inhibitors for laryngopharyngeal reflux based on pH-monitoring and symptom-scale. *World J Gastroenterol.* 2017;23(19):3546–3555.

614. Martin Del Campo SE, Chaudhry UI, Kanji A, et al. Laparoscopic Nissen fundoplication controls reflux symptoms and improves disease-specific quality of life in patients with class I and II obesity. *Surgery.* 2017;162(5):1048–1054.

615. Chen MY, Huang DY, Wu A, et al. Efficacy of magnetic sphincter augmentation versus nissen fundoplication for gastroesophageal reflux disease in short term: a meta-analysis. *Can J Gastroenterol Hepatol.* 2017;2017:9596342.

616. Schwamels K, Nikolic M, Morales Castellano DG, et al. Results of magnetic sphincter augmentation for gastroesophageal reflux disease. *World J Surg.* 2018;42(10): 3263–3269.

617. Reimer C, Sendergaard B, Hilsted L, Bytzer P. Proton-pump inhibitor therapy induces acid-related symptoms in healthy volunteers after withdrawal of therapy. *Gastroenterology.* 2009;137:80–87.

618. Triadafilopoulos G, DiBaise JK, Nostrant TT, et al. The Stretta procedure for the treatment of GERD: 6 and 12 month follow-up of the US open label trial. *Gastrointest Endosc.* 2002;55:149–156.

619. Corley DA, Katz P, Wo JM, et al. Improvement of gastroesophageal reflux symptoms after radiofrequency energy: a randomized, sham-controlled trial. *Gastroenterology.* 2003;125:668–676.

620. Yan C, Liang WT, Wang ZG, et al. Comparison of Stretta procedure and toupet fundoplication for gastroesophageal reflux disease-related extra-esophageal symptoms. *World J Gastroenterol.* 2015;21(45): 12882–12887.

621. Filipi CJ, Lehman GA, Rothstein RI, et al. Transoral, flexible endoscopic suturing for treatment of GERD: a multicenter trial. *Gastrointest Endosc.* 2001;53:416–422.

622. Rothstein RI, Pohl H, Grove M, et al. Endoscopic gastric plication for the treatment of GERD: two-year follow-up results. *Am J Gastroenterol.* 2001;96:S35. Abstract 107.

623. Chen YK, Raijman I, Ben-Menachem T, et al. Long-term outcomes of endoluminal gastroplication: a US multicenter trial. *Gastrointest Endosc.* 2005;61:659–667.

624. Mason RJ, Hughes M, Lehman GA, et al. Endoscopic augmentation of the cardia with a biocompatible injectable polymer (Enteryx) in a porcine model. *Surg Endosc.* 2002;16:386–391.

625. Cohen LB, Johnson DA, Ganz RA, et al. Enteryx implantation for GERD: expanded multicenter trial results and interim post-approval follow-up to 24 months. *Gastrointest Endosc.* 2005;61:650–658.

626. Deviere J, Costamagna G, Neuhaus H, et al. Nonresorbable copolymer implantation for gastroesophageal reflux disease: a randomized sham-controlled multicenter trial. *Gastroenterology.* 2005;128:532–540.

627. Pleskow D, Rothstein R, Lo S, et al. Endoscopic full-thickness plication for the treatment of GERD: 12-month follow-up for the North American open-label trial. *Gastrointest Endosc.* 2005;61:643–649.

628. Velanovich V. Endoscopic, endoluminal fundoplication for gastroesophageal reflux disease: initial experience and lessons learned. *Surgery.* 2010;148:646–651.

629. Testoni PA, Mazzoleni G, Testoni SG. Transoral incisionless fundoplication for gastro-esophageal reflux disease: techniques and outcomes. *World J Gastrointest Pharmacol Ther.* 2016;7(2):179–189.

630. Francis DO, Goutte M, Slaughter JC, et al. Traditional reflux parameters and not impedance monitoring predict outcome after fundoplication in extraesophageal reflux. *Laryngoscope.* 2011;121:1902–1909.

10

The Adverse Role of Obesity in Gastroesophageal and Laryngopharyngeal Reflux Disease

Abdul-Latif Hamdan, Robert Thayer Sataloff, and Mary J. Hawkshaw

This chapter provides an overview of gastroesophageal (GERD) and laryngopharyngeal (LPRD) reflux diseases in the context of obesity as a confounding entity. The adverse role of obesity in exacerbating the frequency and severity of reflux is discussed in four sections. The first section is a review of the association between GERD and obesity. The second section summarizes the association between laryngopharyngeal reflux disease and obesity, the third section is a summary of the mechanisms by which obesity may affect GERD, and the last section reviews how reflux disease can affect voice. A detailed review of the clinical presentation, pathogenesis, diagnosis, and treatment of laryngopharyngeal reflux disease is found in Chapter 59 "Reflux and Other Gastroenterology Conditions That May Affect Voice" of the fourth edition of *Professional Voice*[1] and updated in Chapter 9 of this book.

Obesity and Gastroesophageal Reflux Disease

Gastroesophageal reflux disease is defined as retrograde movement of gastric content into the esophagus. The most common pathophysiology is dysfunction in the lower esophageal sphincter (LES) pressure and transient relaxation time.[2,3] Excessive exposure of the esophageal lining to the refluxate results in injury with typical symptoms of heartburn, epigastric discomfort (dyspepsia), and regurgitation. Commonly associated esophageal pathologies include esophageal strictures and rings, hiatal hernia, Zenker's diverticulum, and Barrett's esophagus.[2,4] The alarming increase in GERD's prevalence and comorbidities spurred numerous studies on predisposing factors. Among these, dietary changes and increase in weight are considered as particularly important. Based on a cross-sectional study by Locke et al[5] on 1524 subjects, a body mass index (BMI) above 30 kg/m^2 is associated independently with weekly reflux symptoms with an odds ratio of 2.8. Ruhl and Everhart,[6] in their follow-up on the first "National Health and Nutrition Examination Survey," reported an association between high BMI and reflux disease-related hospitalization, with a hazard ratio of 1.22. Similarly, Langergren et al[7] used personal interview on 820 subjects and reported a 0.99 odds ratio of having reflux symptoms in those with a history of obesity during adulthood in comparison with those who had no history of obesity. However, there was no association between the extent and duration of gastroesophageal reflux and BMI.

Despite the consensus on the high prevalence of reflux symptoms in obese patients, the correlation between obesity and abnormal pH-metry remains controversial. Fisher et al[8] studied the correlation between GERD and BMI in a group of 30 morbidly obese patients using pH-metry and manometry. Patients with longer esophageal exposure time (more than 5%) of a pH less than 4 had a higher body mass index than those who had an exposure time of less than 5% (56.5 vs 48.3 kg/m^2). Moreover, reflux symptom scores were higher in patients with higher BMI. El-Serag et al[9] in their cross-sectional study of 206 patients undergoing 24-hour pH-metry reported that patients with BMI greater than or equal to 30 kg/m^2 had longer and more frequent episodes of esophageal acid exposure in comparison with those with BMI lower than 25 kg/m^2. Waist circumference was among the anthropometric measures linked most strongly to obesity. In 2007, Merrouche et al[10] reported a significant association between BMI and DeMeester score, which is a composite pH score. The study was conducted on 100 morbidly obese patients who underwent bariatric surgery. Similar association was described by Ayazi et al[11] in 2009 in a group of 1659 patients. Thirteen percent of the disparities in esophageal acid exposure were associated with differences in BMI. Contrary to those reports, other investigators failed to show a significant association between weight, BMI, and abnormalities in pH-metry readings.[12–14] O'Brien[12] reported reflux using pH electrodes in only 4 out of 21 morbidly obese patients undergoing gastric bypass surgery. A decrease in pH by more than 1.5 below the intraesophageal pH was diagnostic of GERD. Similarly, Lundell et al[14] reported no significant correlation between BMI, weight, and reflux variables, namely daytime reflux and total acid exposure. The study was conducted on 50 morbidly obese patients with a mean BMI of 42.5 kg/m^2 using 24-hour ambulatory pH-metry and endoscopy.

Notwithstanding the debatable link between BMI and esophageal acid exposure, numerous studies have confirmed an association between GERD comorbidities and obesity.[15–18] In 1999, Wilson et al[15] in their retrospective case control study of 1389 patients demonstrated that excessive weight is independently and strongly associated with esophagitis with an odds ratio (OR) of 1.8. These results corroborated those of Stene-Larsen et al[16] in their study of 1224 patients undergoing esophageal endoscopic evaluation. The authors reported higher prevalence of overweight expressed as elevated weight-for-height index, in patients with grade 1 and grade 2 esophagitis and in patients with hiatal hernia. Patients with hiatal hernia and esophagitis had excessive weight of 5% whereas patients with no esophagitis and no hernia had normal weight.[16] Similarly, Labenz et al,[17] in 2004, in their analysis of risk factors for

GERD-related erosive esophagitis, identified overweight in addition to other factors such as smoking and regular intake of alcohol as independent predictors. Interestingly, a meta-analysis that included cross-sectional, cohort, and case-control studies looking at the association between obesity and GERD revealed a significant association between BMI and various esophageal pathologies. In this report by Hampel et al,[18] which included 9 studies, the authors reported a significant association between BMI, erosive esophagitis, and esophageal adenocarcinoma in 6 studies and a significant association between BMI and gastric cardiac adenocarcinoma in 4 studies. The odds ratios for GERD symptoms increased with an increase in BMI reaching 1.94 for patients with BMI greater than 30 kg/m^2.

In summary, obesity is associated significantly with gastroesophageal reflux disease. It is considered a predictor of numerous morbidities associated with GERD, including esophagitis and esophageal carcinoma.

Obesity and Laryngopharyngeal Reflux Disease

Association Between Obesity and LPRD

The term *laryngopharyngeal reflux disease* was introduced by Koufman[19] and defined as backflow of gastric contents into the laryngopharynx. When the refluxate reaches the laryngopharyngeal complex, atypical symptoms of reflux such as globus pharyngeus, throat clearing, cough, and change in voice quality may occur. These symptoms affect at least one-tenth of patients presenting to otolaryngologists.[20,21] Unlike the typical symptoms of GERD, LPRD and

its symptoms occur primarily during daytime and mostly when the patient is in the upright position.[22–24] These symptoms, as well as suboptimal response to conventional antireflux therapy used for GERD, led to numerous investigations of the underlying pathophysiology. Today, it is well established that one of the main dysfunctions is a decrease in the myogenic activity of the upper esophageal sphincter with subsequent impairment in laryngeal protection.[1,24] The absence of peristalsis and lack of salivary buffering increase the vulnerability of the laryngeal mucosa further.[25,26] Exposure of the laryngeal lining to refluxed gastric juice and aerosol usually results in inflammatory changes that lead to a myriad of symptoms and signs.[27] Despite the ubiquity of studies on the correlation between LPRD and various laryngeal and extralaryngeal diseases thoroughly reviewed in Chapter 59, "Reflux and Other Gastroenterologic Conditions That May Affect Voice" of the fourth edition of *Professional Voice*[1] and updated in Chapter 9 of this book, the link between LPRD (or extraesophageal manifestations of GERD) and obesity has scarcely been investigated. Halum et al[28] examined the correlation between abnormal pharyngeal reflux patterns and BMI in 285 patients who had a history of reflux, had positive laryngeal findings, and had undergone 24-hour pH-metry. A patient was considered to have pharyngeal reflux disease if he or she had one or more event of pH less than 4. By evaluating the BMI in those with abnormal pharyngeal acid exposure vs those with normal results, the authors found no significant correlation between BMI and number of pharyngeal reflux events. However, there was a significant correlation between BMI and esophageal reflux events (p = value of .002 with an r of 0.18). Moreover, patients with both LPRD and GERD had higher BMI in comparison to patients with normal pH-metry.[28] Given the well-known relation between GERD and LPRD clearly shown in their study, the authors recommended weight loss in obese patients with symptoms of LPRD similar to recommendations for obese patients with GERD.[28] The results of their investigation were in partial accordance with the study by Jaspersen et al on the prevalence of extraesophageal manifestations (EED) in a cohort of 6215 patients with GERD. The authors reported the presence of chronic cough in 13% and laryngeal disorders, defined as "chronic hoarseness, sore throat and persistent cough,"[29(p1516)] in 10.4%. Obesity, among other factors such as age and duration of GERD for more than 1 year, was related significantly to the prevalence of laryngeal disorders. Moreover, the prevalence of extraesophageal manifestations in patients with erosive esophagitis was significantly higher in comparison with those with nonerosive laryngitis (34.9% vs 30.5%, respectively).[29]

In parallel with the aforementioned studies on the association between LPRD and obesity, several authors investigated the interplay between LPRD, obesity, and obstructive sleep apnea (OSA).[30–32] The coexistence of OSA and LPRD in obese patients made it hard to elucidate the cause-effect relationship between obesity and LPRD. Obstructive sleep apnea also is associated with chronic inflammatory changes in the upper airway similar to those observed in patients with LPRD.[23,31] The collapse and friction of the upper airway soft tissues in patients with reduced airway may lead to mucosal inflammation with impairment in sensation.[31–35] In the study by Nguyen et al[34] on 39 patients with OSA, the authors reported significant impairment in laryngeal and pharyngeal sensory detection threshold in comparison to controls (11 mm Hg vs 8 mm Hg, respectively). Hence, upper airway inflammatory changes seen in obese patients with OSA may be due either to OSA or to LPRD, or to both. The studies on the association between LPRD and obesity in the context of OSA remain controversial. In 2013, Xavier et al[35] examined the prevalence of laryngopharyngeal reflux in a group of 74 patients who had tested positive for OSA based on the Berlin questionnaire. Using both Reflux Symptom Index (RSI) and Reflux Finding Score (RFS), the authors reported an 89% prevalence of symptoms and signs of LPRD in the total group of OSA patients. A significantly higher prevalence of laryngeal symptoms suggestive of LPRD was found in obese patients with OSA (BMI greater than 30) in comparison to nonobese patients (68% vs 58%, respectively).[35] However, it is worth noting that there was no statistically significant difference in the mean RSI score between the obese group and nonobese group (21 vs 17, respectively). A year later, Rodrigues et al[36] investigated the impact of obesity on the correlation between obstructive sleep apnea and laryngopharyngeal reflux. In their retrospective analysis of 105 patients stratified as 66 nonobese and 39 obese, the authors showed an association between the RSI score and the severity of OSA only in the obese group. The RSI almost doubled in obese patients with moderate-to-severe OSA in comparison to those with mild OSA (mean RSI of 11.3 vs 6.7, respectively). This was not observed in the nonobese group in which the RSI score was comparable in patients with mild and moderate OSA. Interestingly, the RFS did not correlate with the severity of OSA, and normal RFS means were found in all subgroups.[36] A year later, Gilani et al reported an association between GERD and OSA using a cross-sectional analysis of the "National Ambulatory Medical Care Survey and the National Hospital Ambulatory Medical Care Survey."[37(p390)] Confounding comorbidities such as inferior turbinate hypertrophy, rhinosinusitis, and pharyngeal occlusion, in addition to demographic variables, did not include BMI.[37] Their results corroborated those of Fass et al[38] in their investigation on the clinical predictors of heartburn in a cohort of 15 314 patients. In the subgroup of 3806 who reported heartburn using a questionnaire, increased BMI in addition to daytime sleepiness and snoring were reported as predictors. Contrary to those reports, several studies failed to substantiate the association between reflux disease and obesity in patients with sleep disorders. In a study by Wise et al,[39] the authors found no correlation between body mass index and dual-channel pH probe testing in a group of 37 patients with sleep-disordered breathing. Moreover, there was no correlation between presence of OSA in 28 subjects and reflux disease. However, the relatively high prevalence of LPRD in the snorers and OSA patients was notable.[39] Similarly, a study by Xiao et al[40] showed that LPRD was present in 51.4%, 43.8%, and 35% of obstructive sleep apnea hypopnea syndrome (HA), non-HA, and controls, respectively. The study was conducted on 53 patients using multichannel intraluminal 24-hour pH monitoring. BMI was the only predictor of OSAHS. Its correlation with LPR and GERD was not reported.

In summary, there is not enough evidence to support an association between LPRD and obesity. Future studies taking into account confounding variables such as OSA must be conducted in order to determine whether there is an association between these 2 entities.

How Does Obesity Affect Gastroesophageal Reflux Disease?

The correlation between obesity and GERD has been discussed extensively in the literature. Several mechanisms have been suggested to explain the higher prevalence of GERD in obese vs normal-weight subjects. Given the known interrelation between LPRD and GERD,[41-44] these same mechanisms may explain the symptoms and signs of LPRD in obese subjects.

1. *Increase in intra-abdominal pressure:* In a review by Barak et al[45] on the pathophysiologic and therapeutic implications of GERD in obesity, the authors highlighted the pathogenic role of abdominal pressure on the exacerbation of reflux. An increase in intra-abdominal pressure results in an increase in intravisceral pressure with subsequent displacement of the position of the lower esophageal sphincter. Pandolfino et al[46] investigated the impact of obesity-induced increased intragastric pressure on the esophagogastric junction and reported an association between BMI and gastroesophageal pressure gradient. The study was conducted on 285 patients using high-resolution manometry with 36 sensors. The pathogenic role of intra-abdominal pressure in relation to central obesity also has been described by Sugerman et al.[47] By measuring urinary bladder pressure as an estimation of the intra-abdominal pressure, the authors reported increase in intra-abdominal pressure secondary to central obesity with subsequent increase in pleural and cardiac filling pressure.[47] They concluded that central obesity causes an increase in intra-abdominal pressure with displacement of the diaphragm superiorly, resulting in hemodynamic and other changes.

2. *Alterations in lower esophageal sphincter pressure and transient relaxation time:* The lower esophageal sphincter consists of the distal esophageal

intrinsic smooth muscles and crural diaphragmatic skeletal muscles, and it is a major antireflux barrier. The presence of an incompetent LES "less than 4 mmHg above gastric pressure" or hypotensive LES "less than 10 mmHg above gastric pressure"[48(p1755)] allows an increase in the number of reflux episodes with potential subsequent erosion of the esophageal mucosal lining.[48] Similarly, the high frequency of transient lower esophageal sphincter relaxation observed in patients with GERD also can lead to injury to the esophageal mucosa. Transient relaxation is a physiologic phenomenon[49,50] that is nonswallow induced and occurs in the absence of esophageal peristalsis.[48] Although it occurs in normal individuals lasting up to 60 seconds, in patients with GERD, the frequency and duration of this physiologic phenomena are markedly increased.[50–52]

Both LES pressure and transient lower esophageal sphincter relaxation time are clinically important in understanding the interplay between obesity and GERD. The results of many studies on these variables in obese subjects are conflicting with no clear consensus.[8,10–12] In a study by Fisher et al[8] in 1999 on the correlation between obesity and reflux, the authors reported no significant correlation between body mass index, weight, and lower esophageal pressure. Similar findings have been reported by O'Brian,[12] with only 12% of patients with a mean weight of 170 lb having hypotensive lower esophageal sphincter pressure. However, Merrouche et al,[10] in their investigation on esophageal motility disorders in obese subjects, reported a decrease in LES pressure (less than 15 mm Hg) in 69% of the cases. The study was conducted on 100 patients using esophageal manometry in addition to endoscopy and 24-hour pH-metry. Similarly, Ayazi et al[11] investigated the association between BMI and esophageal acid exposure and found a higher prevalence of LES dysfunction in patients with higher BMI compared to normal-weight subjects with an odds ratio of 2.12. In summary, there is no consensus on whether there are obesity-induced alterations in LES pressure and transient lower esophageal sphincter relaxation time. Further studies are needed in order to elucidate the pathogenic role of obesity and these variables in GERD.

3. *Higher risk for hiatal hernia:* Many reports concur that obese patients are at a higher risk of having hiatal hernia.[10,15,53,54] Wilson et al[15] in 1999 reported excessive weight as an independent risk factor for the development of hiatal hernia in a group of patients undergoing upper endoscopic evaluation. This retrospective study conducted on 1389 cases of upper gastrointestinal endoscopy (EGD) revealed a significant increase in the probability of developing hiatal hernia with an increase in BMI and an odds ratio of 4.2 for esophagitis.[15] Similarly, Merrouche et al[10] reported hiatal hernia in 39.4% of 100 morbidly obese patients, 73% of whom had symptoms of GERD. These findings were supported by numerous studies on patients undergoing bariatric surgery. In a study on the role of preoperative gastroscopy in morbidly obese patients undergoing surgery, Estévez-Fernández et al[53] reported the presence of hiatal hernia in

18.1%, in addition to other gastric pathologies. Similarly, Saarinen et al,[54] in their investigation on the clinical findings of EGD in morbidly obese patients undergoing gastrectomy or gastric bypass, reported hiatal hernia and esophageal pathologies in 23% of cases.

The pathogenesis of hiatal hernia has been linked to disruption in the gastroesophageal junction, which in turn can lead to an increased risk for reflux and esophagitis as reported by Wilson et al.[15] This suggested mechanism has been substantiated by numerous authors. Stene-Larsen et al,[16] in their prospective study on 1224 patients, reported an association between hiatal hernia and reflux esophagitis and overweight. Moreover, 68% of patients with reflux esophagitis had evidence of hiatal hernia on upper endoscopy. Argyrou et al,[55] in their investigation on the polygenic basis of GERD, reported hiatal hernia and esophageal motor abnormalities, in addition to the genetic contribution, as important mechanisms in the development of GERD. Kishikawa et al[56] examined the relationship between gastric juice acidity and sliding hiatal hernia in 286 patients, 64 of whom had hiatal hernia. The authors found an association between the presence of hiatal hernia and increased gastric acid secretions, even after adjusting for confounding variable such as age. Similarly, Mochizuki et al[57] reported hiatal hernia as one of the associated factors with erosive esophagitis. The cohort study was conducted on 7552 patients who underwent endoscopy and 16.7% of whom had erosive esophagitis. The odds ratio for hiatal hernia in this subgroup of patients was 2.43, 95% CI: 1.43±4.05.

4. *Impaired gastric emptying:* Rapid gastric emptying was thought of initially as a deranged signal for satiety more commonly observed in obese patients.[58] However, recent studies have shown that obesity is associated with delayed gastric emptying[59-62] rather than altered satiety. In a study by Maddox et al[59] conducted on 62 subjects, the authors demonstrated delayed gastric and esophageal emptying of both solid and liquid meals in obese patients compared to controls. Moreover, there was a correlation between body mass index and gastric and esophageal emptying in the total group. The results of this investigation corroborated those of Mercer et al[63] on esophageal transit time in obese patients in comparison with lean volunteers. Using radionuclide scintigraphy and manometric measurements, the authors demonstrated prolongation of the esophageal transit time and increased gastroesophageal pressure gradient.

Numerous mechanisms have been suggested to explain delayed gastric emptying in obese patients.[63-65] These include a decrease in esophageal muscle maximum velocity, reduced gallbladder emptying following meals, alteration in mechanoreceptor sensitivity in gastric muscle with changes in smooth muscle behavior, and dysfunction in the autonomic nervous system as suggested by Peterson et al.[65] Irrespective of the mechanism, delay in gastric emptying is considered as one of the many causes of reflux disease. In a study by Quitadamo et al[66] on the relationship between obesity and GERD, the authors demonstrated a lower mean gastric half-emptying time (T1/2 GET) of 107.6 minutes in subjects with symptoms of GERD vs 116.5 minutes in asymptomatic subjects, vs 100.1 minutes in nonobese subjects. The study was performed on 113 patients between the ages of 4 and 17 years, and GET was measured using a radiation-free, noninvasive test during which breath samples were collected before and 30 minutes after meal ingestion. One suggested mechanism for the association between delayed gastric emptying and GERD is postprandial gastric distention with subsequent triggering of transient lower esophageal sphincter relaxation (TLESR),[67] during which more than 90% of reflux episodes occur.[52,68] Increase in the frequency and duration of TLESR by gastric distention is thought to be through stretch receptors.[69]

5. *Dietary changes:* High fat consumption, among other dietary changes such as the decrease in fruit and vegetable intake, is known to promote obesity.[70] The weight gain is based on fat-related properties such as satiety, as fat is less satiating than other food components such as carbohydrates and protein, and palatability because of its inherent aroma that brings flavor and thus makes it very palatable.[71] Fat also has high energy density, which promotes passive overconsumption,[72] along its own distinct metabolic pathway.[73] With the increase in dietary intake of fat in obese subjects, there is also an increase in GERD symptoms, namely heartburn and regurgitation, and an increase in the prevalence of esophagitis. El-Serag et al[74] investigated the association between various dietary food components

and symptoms of GERD using the gastroesophageal reflux disease questionnaire in a group of 164 patients. The average fat servings and total fat intake were significantly higher in patients with GERD symptoms. Moreover, the daily intake of total fat was also higher in patients with erosive esophagitis in comparison to those without erosive esophagitis.[74] Similar results were reported by Fox et al[75] in their study on the effect of dietary fat and caloric intake on symptoms of reflux. High dietary fat content was associated with higher frequency of reflux symptoms, but it had no statistically significant effect on esophageal acid exposure. The study was conducted on 15 subjects who followed 4 different dietary conditions over the course of 4 days during which esophageal acidity was measured using a wireless capsule.[75] The suggested mechanisms for dietary fat-induced GERD symptoms include increase in TLESRT, decrease in the esophageal gastric junction pressure, delayed gastric emptying, and increased visceral sensitivity.

6. *Alterations in sex hormonal level/ estrogen:* The prevalence of GERD and its associated morbidities differs between men and women. Nilsson et al[76] demonstrated higher prevalence of GERD-related symptoms in women compared to men, more so in women on estrogen replacement. A population-based cross-sectional study using public health surveys has shown a dose-response relationship between reflux symptoms and BMI. The association was higher in women compared to men, with odds ratios of 6.3 and 3.3, respectively. Moreover,

there was a significant difference in the association between reflux symptoms and BMI in premenopausal women vs postmenopausal women.[76] These results are consistent with several other reports that corroborate the strong link between sex hormones and reflux disease. A large cohort study by Close et al[77] that included 8831 menopausal women revealed a statistically significant association between hormonal therapy intake and GERD. Similar association also has been reported by Jacobson et al[78] in a group of 51 637 postmenopausal women. Almost 1 out of 4 reported GERD symptoms, and the odds ratio for the risk of GERD in women using estrogen was 1.46%. Moreover, there was a correlation between GERD symptoms and the duration and dosage of estrogen intake, which included over-the-counter products and selective estrogen receptor modulators.[78] A proposed mechanism by which estrogen may impact GERD is through relaxation of the lower esophageal sphincter smooth muscles secondary to an increase in nitric oxide synthesis, as reported in the discussion in the article by Nilsson et al[76] on obesity and estrogen as risk factors for GERD. Tsai et al[79] have documented that estradiol-induced lower esophageal sphincter relaxation is dose dependent and is associated with potassium channel. The investigation was carried out on porcine LES using isometric transducers in order to measure sphincter relaxation. Given that obesity is associated with an increase in estrogen production via estrone synthesis from fatty tissue, the estrogen-induced LES dysfunction leads to the conclusion that obese subjects are more likely to have reflux symptoms and signs.

7. *Alterations in the immune system:* In addition to the aforementioned mechanisms by which obesity can mediate reflux disease, there is growing evidence that a metabolic/immune mechanism involving inflammatory mediators is also responsible for the association between obesity and inflammatory conditions such as erosive esophagitis. Adipose tissue is well known to be a source of inflammatory mediators that are key components in modulating systemic inflammation and the immune system. The most commonly reported are leptin and adiponectin, tumor necrosis factor, and interleukin-6.[80] Increase in proinflammatory mediators has been implicated in the pathogenesis of esophageal inflammation and GERD-related symptoms. In the prospective study by Nam et al[81] conducted on 5329 patients undergoing esophagogastroduodenoscopy, the authors reported an association between erosive esophagitis and obesity. When the visceral adipose tissue exceeded 1500 cm^3, the odds ratio for erosive esophagitis reached 3. Moreover, as the stomach is a known target for leptin, the increase in leptin, in addition to the increase in cytokine TNF alpha and IL-1 in obese subjects, magnifies caustic injury and increases the prevalence of esophageal diseases.[82–86]

In summary, the causal relationship between obesity and reflux is based not only on a mechanical effect induced by the increase in intra-abdominal pressure and delayed gastric emptying but also on inflammatory-mediated pathways.

How Does Laryngopharyngeal Reflux Impact Voice?

Laryngopharyngeal reflux may impact voice directly and indirectly. A more comprehensive review on laryngeal manifestations of reflux and other gastroenterologic conditions can be found in Chapter 9 of this book.[1]

Indirect Effect

Laryngopharyngeal reflux may cause cough and repetitive throat clearing indirectly via vagal-mediated reflexes. In an animal study conducted by Ludemann et al[87] in which hydrochloric acid (HCI) and pepsin were infused in the pyriform sinuses of 16 New Zealand rabbits, the authors reported several mechanical effects induced by laryngeal chemoreflexes. These included biphasic stridor, paroxysm of cough, and apparent life-threatening events.[87] The repetitive clearing of throat and cough lead to abrupt and violent approximation of the vocal folds and arytenoid areas, resulting in various laryngeal pathologies and movement disorders.[19,88–92]

Direct Injury

The direct exposure of laryngeal mucosa to refluxed gastric juice and aerosol can cause reversible and irreversible injury to the epithelium by disrupting defense barriers.[93,94] The primary mechanisms of such injury are described here:

1. *Alteration in carbonic anhydrase secretion:* Carbonic anhydrase is a defensive enzyme that contributes to endogenous secretion of bicarbonate within epithelial cells.[26] As a result to exposure of the laryngeal mucosa to pepsin and acid, there is a decrease in intracellular carbonic anhydrase secretion with subsequent decrease in intraepithelial resistance.[25,95,96] Johnston et al[97] investigated the correlation between pepsin and CA-III depletion in laryngeal biopsies taken from 9 patients with reflux and 12 normal controls. Using antibodies specific for human pepsins, the authors demonstrated the presence of pepsin in 8 out of 9 biopsies and the presence of a negative correlation between pepsin and CAI-III. Similar results were reported by Gill et al[98] a year later in a larger cohort, further substantiating the protective role of CAI-III against laryngeal tissue injury.

2. *Decreased expression of E-cadherin:* E-cadherin is one of the many "calcium-dependent cell-cell adhesion" molecules[99(p1451)] that play a crucial role in sustaining the integrity of the epithelial lining by selectively binding to adherent molecules within its family.[99,100] In 2005, the group from Wake Forest University Health Sciences reported downregulation of E-cadherin in 54 laryngeal biopsies taken from 18 patients with LPR.[98] Similarly, a few years later, Reichel et al[101] demonstrated a reduction in the expression of E-cadherin in patients with LPR. Using an immunohistochemistry technique, the authors showed a significant difference in the expression of E-cadherin and not beta-catenin in patients with Ph-documented LPRD in comparison to those without LPRD. The decreased expression of E-cadherin, in parallel with that of CAI-III, reduces the resistance of the laryngeal mucosa.

3. *Altered expression of mucins:* Mucins serve as lubricators to the epithelial lining and protectors against external insults. Twenty mucin genes have been identified as responsible for the production of the various protein constituents of mucin, which provide the gel-like properties of mucus.[102] Dysfunction in intracellular pathways that regulate mucin gene expression may lead to epithelial barrier defects. In patients with LPRD, there is alteration in the expression of these genes. The most commonly reported are alterations in MUC5AC and MCU4.[102,103]

4. *Alteration in stress protein response:* Stress proteins are stress-induced proteins that contribute to cellular defense by repairing damaged proteins and controlling the transport of cellular polypeptides across cells.[104] Alteration in stress protein response has been shown to contribute to the development of mucosal injury. The study by Johnston et al[105] on the role of stress protein expression in laryngeal diseases related to reflux showed significantly less stress laryngeal protein 70 and stress protein 53 in patients with LPR compared to controls. Moreover, there was a significant association between the depletion of stress protein 70 and the presence of pepsin within the laryngeal epithelium. In conclusion, the authors asserted that alteration in the acid-mediated stress protein response contributes to laryngeal mucosal disease.

5. *A decrease in the concentration of salivary epidermal growth factors:* In addition to its volume and neutralizing capacity, saliva contains growth factors of paramount importance in cytoprotection of esophageal and laryngeal lining.[106] Salivary epidermal growth factor is a polypeptide linked to epithelial development and wound healing and has been shown to play a major protective role in patients with esophagitis and laryngitis.[25] Eckley and Costa[107] investigated the concentration of this factor in a group of 39 patients clinically diagnosed with LPR. The results showed a statistically significant difference in the concentration of epidermal growth factor in the LPR group in comparison to controls. Reduction in the concentration of salivary epidermal growth factor in patients with LPR is believed to contribute to the damage to the laryngopharyngeal mucosa.

As a result of the damage to laryngeal defense mechanisms in patients with GERD and LPRD reviewed above, there is impairment in the junctional complexes between epithelial cells with subsequent injury to the laryngeal mucosal lining, both at the microscopic and macroscopic levels.[108] Change in voice quality in affected patients has been attributed to dehydration and change in vocal folds' mucous consistency, microtrauma, secretion of inflammatory molecules, and hyperfunctional behavior.[108] As a result of phonotrauma, there are alterations in the viscoelastic and biomechanical properties of the vocal folds with subsequent development of benign and malignant masses.[109] A detailed review of the pathophysiology of dysphonia in patients with LPRD and on the association between reflux and laryngeal lesions can be found in the chapter "Reflux and Other Gastroenterologic Conditions That Can Affect Voice" of the fourth edition of the *Professional Voice*[1] and in other literature.

References

1. Sataloff RT, Castell DO, Katz PO, Sataloff DM, Hawkshaw MJ. Reflux and other gastroenterologic conditions that may affect the voice. In: Sataloff RT, ed. *Professional Voice: The Science and Art of Clinical Care.* 4th ed. San Diego, CA: Plural Publishing; 2017:907–998.
2. Nebel OT, Fornes MF, Castell DO. Symptomatic gastroesophageal reflux: incidence and precipitating factors. *Am J Dig Dis.* 1976;21(11):953–956.
3. Cohen S, Harris LD. The lower esophageal sphincter. *Gastroenterology.* 1972;63(6):1066–1073.
4. Spechler SJ. Epidemiology and natural history of gastro-oesophageal reflux disease. *Digestion.* 1992;51(suppl 1):24–29.
5. Locke GR III, Talley NJ, Fett SL, Zinsmeister AR, Melton LJ III. Risk factors associated with symptoms of gastroesophageal reflux. *Am J Med.* 1999;106(6):642–649.
6. Ruhl CE, Everhart JE. Overweight, but not high dietary fat intake, increases risk of gastroesophageal reflux disease hospitalization: the NHANES I Epidemiologic Follow-up Study. First National Health and Nutrition Examination Survey. *Ann Epidemiol.* 1999;9(7):424–435.
7. Langergren J, Bergstrom R, Nyren O. No relation between body mass and gastro-oesophageal reflux symptoms in a Swedish population based study. *Gut.* 2000;47(1):26–29.
8. Fisher BL, Pennathur A, Mutnick JL, Little AG. Obesity correlates with gastroesophageal reflux. *Dig Dis Sci.* 1999;44(11):2290–2294.
9. El-Serag HB, Ergun GA, Pandolfino J, Fitzgerald S, Tran T, Kramer JR. Obesity increases oesophageal acid exposure. *Gut.* 2007;56(6):749–755.
10. Merrouche M, Sabaté JM, Jouet P, et al. Gastroesophageal reflux and esophageal motility disorders in morbidly obese patients before and after bariatric surgery. *Obes Surg.* 2007;17(7):894–900.
11. Ayazi S, Hagen JA, Chan LS, et al. Obesity and gastroesophageal reflux: quantifying the association between body mass index, esophageal acid exposure, and lower esophageal sphincter status in a large series of patients with reflux symptoms. *J Gastrointest Surg.* 2009;13(8):1440–1447.
12. O'Brien TF Jr. Lower esophageal sphincter pressure (LESP) and esophageal function in obese humans. *J Clin Gastroenterol.* 1980;2(2):145–148.
13. Beauchamp G. Gastroesophageal reflux and obesity. *Surg Clin North Am.* 1983;63(4):869–876.
14. Lundell L, Ruth M, Sandberg N, Bove-Nielsen M. Does massive obesity promote abnormal gastroesophageal reflux. *Dig Dis Sci.* 1995;40(8):1632–1635.
15. Wilson LJ, Ma W, Hirschowitz BI. Association of obesity with hiatal hernia and esophagitis. *Am J Gastroenterol.* 1999;94(10):2840–2844.
16. Stene-Larsen G, Weberg R, Froyshov Larsen I, Bjortuft O, Hoel B, Berstad A. Relationship of overweight to hiatus hernia and reflux esophagitis. *Scand J Gastroenterol.* 1988;23(4):427–432.
17. Labenz J, Jaspersen D, Kulig M, et al. Risk factors for erosive esophagitis: a multivariate analysis based on the ProGERD study initiative. *Am J Gastroenterol.* 2004;99(9):1652–1656.
18. Hampel H, Abraham NS, El-Serag HB. Meta-analysis: obesity and the risk for gastroesophageal reflux disease and its complications. *Ann Intern Med.* 2005;143(3):199–211.
19. Koufman JA. The otolaryngologic manifestations of gastroesophageal reflux disease (GERD): a clinical investigation of 225 patients using ambulatory 24-hour pH monitoring and an experimental investigation of the role of acid and pepsin in the development of laryngeal injury. *Laryngoscope.* 1991;101(4, pt 2)(suppl 53):1–78.
20. Koufman JA, Wiener GJ, Wu WC, Castell DO. Reflux laryngitis and its sequelae: the diagnostic role of ambulatory 24-hour pH monitoring. *J Voice.* 1988;2(1):78–89.

21. Koufman JA, Amin MR, Panetti M. Prevalence of reflux in 113 consecutive patients with laryngeal and voice disorders. *Otolaryngol Head Neck Surg.* 2000;123(4):385–388.

22. Cohen JT, Bach KK, Postma GN, Koufman JA. Clinical manifestations of laryngopharyngeal reflux. *Ear Nose Throat J.* 2002; 81(9)(suppl 2):19–23.

23. Koufman JA. Laryngopharyngeal reflux 2002: a new paradigm of airway disease. *Ear Nose Throat J.* 2002;81(9)(suppl 2):2–6.

24. Koufman JA. Laryngopharyngeal reflux is different from classic gastroesophageal reflux disease. *Ear Nose Throat J.* 2002; 81(9)(suppl 2):7–9.

25. Eckley CA, Michelsohn N, Rizzo LV, Tadakoro CE, Costa HO. Salivary epidermal growth factor concentration in adults with reflux laryngitis. *Otolaryngol Head Neck Surg.* 2004;131(4):401–406.

26. Johnston N, Bulmer D, Gill GA, et al. Cell biology of laryngeal epithelial defenses in health and disease: further studies. *Ann Otol Rhinol Laryngol.* 2003;112(6):481–491.

27. Belafsky PC, Rees CJ. Laryngopharyngeal reflux: the value of otolaryngology examination. *Curr Gastroenterol Rep.* 2008;10(3): 278–282.

28. Halum SL, Postma GN, Johnston C, Belafsky PC, Koufman JA. Patients with isolated laryngopharyngeal reflux are not obese. *Laryngoscope.* 2005;115(6):1042–1045.

29. Jaspersen D, Kulig M, Labenz J, et al. Prevalence of extraesophageal manifestations in gastro-esophageal reflux disease: an analysis based on the ProGERDD study. *Aliment Pharmacol Ther.* 2003;17(12):1515–1520.

30. Demeter P, Pap A. The relationship between gastroesophageal reflux disease and obstructive sleep apnea. *J Gastroenterol.* 2004;39(9):815–820.

31. Eskiizmir G, Kezirian E. Is there a vicious cycle between obstructive sleep apnea and laryngopharyngeal reflux disease? *Med Hypotheses.* 2009;73(5):706–708.

32. Karkos PD, Leong SC, Benton J, Sastry A, Assimakopoulos DA, Issing WJ. Reflux and sleeping disorders: a systematic review. *J Laryngol Otol.* 2009;123(4):372–374.

33. Payne RJ, Kost KM, Frenkiel S, et al. Laryngeal inflammation assessed using the reflux finding score in obstructive sleep apnea. *Otolaryngol Head Neck Surg.* 2006;134(5): 836–842.

34. Nguyen AT, Jobin V, Payne R, Beauregard J, Naor N, Kimoff RJ. Laryngeal and velopharyngeal sensory impairment in obstructive sleep apnea. *Sleep.* 2005;28(5):585–593.

35. Xavier SD, Moraes JP, Eckley CA. Prevalence of signs and symptoms of laryngopharyngeal reflux in snorers with suspected obstructive sleep apnea. *Braz J Otorhinolaryngol.* 2013;79(5):589–593.

36. Rodrigues MM, Dibbern RS, Santos VJ, Passeri LA. Influence of obesity on the correlation between laryngopharyngeal reflux and obstructive sleep apnea. *Braz J Otorhinolaryngol.* 2014;80(1):5–10.

37. Gilani S, Quan SF, Pynnonen MA, Shin JJ. Obstructive sleep apnea and gastroesophageal reflux: a multivariate population-level analysis. *Otolaryngol Head Neck Surg.* 2016; 154(2):390–395.

38. Fass R, Quan SF, O'Connor GT, Ervin A, Iber C. Predictors of heartburn during sleep in a large prospective cohort study. *Chest.* 2005;127(5):1658–1666.

39. Wise SK, Wise JC, DelGaudio JM. Gastroesophageal reflux and laryngopharyngeal reflux in patients with sleep-disordered breathing. *Otolaryngol Head Neck Surg.* 2006;135(2):253–257.

40. Xiao YL, Liu FQ, Li J, et al. Gastroesophageal and laryngopharyngeal reflux profiles in patients with obstructive sleep apnea/hypopnea syndrome as determined by combined multichannel intraluminal impedance–pH monitoring. *Neurogastroenterol Motil.* 2012;24(6):e258–e265.

41. Groome M, Cotton JP, Borland M, McLeod S, Johnston DA, Dillon JF. Prevalence of laryngopharyngeal reflux in a population with gastroesophageal reflux. *Laryngoscope.* 2007;117(8):1424–1428.

42. Lai YC, Wang PC, Lin JC. Laryngopharyngeal reflux in patients with reflux esophagitis. *World J Gastroenterol.* 2008;14(28): 4523–4528.

43. Qua CS, Wong CH, Gopala K, Goh KL. Gastro-oesophageal reflux disease in chronic laryngitis: prevalence and response to acid-suppressive therapy. *Aliment Pharmacol Ther.* 2007;25(3):287–295.

44. Park S, Chun HJ, Keum B, et al. An electron microscopic study—correlation of gastroesophageal reflux disease and laryngopharyngeal reflux. *Laryngoscope.* 2010; 120(7):1303–1308.

45. Barak N, Ehrenpreis ED, Harrison JR, Sitrin MD. Gastro-oesophageal reflux disease in obesity: pathophysiological and therapeutic considerations. *Obes Rev.* 2002; 3(1):9–15.

46. Pandolfino JE, El–Serag HB, Zhang Q, Shah N, Ghosh SK, Kahrilas PJ. Obesity: a challenge to esophagogastric junction integrity. *Gastroenterology.* 2006;130(3):639–649.

47. Sugerman HJ, DeMaria EJ, Felton W, Nakatsuka M, Sismanis A. Increased intra-abdominal pressure and cardiac filling pressures in obesity-associated pseudotumor cerebri. *Neurology.* 1997;49(2):507–511.

48. Orlando RC. Overview of the mechanisms of gastroesophageal reflux. *Am J Med.* 2001;111(8A):174S–177S.

49. Holloway RH, Hongo M, Berger K, McCallum RW. Gastric distension: a mechanism for postprandial gastroesophageal reflux. *Gastroenterology.* 1985;89(4):779–784.

50. Mittal RK, Balaban DH. The esophagogastric junction. *N Engl J Med.* 1997;336(13): 924–932.

51. Kahrilas PJ, Shi G. Pathophysiology of gastroesophageal reflux disease: the antireflux barrier and luminal clearance mechanisms. In: Orlando RC, ed. *Gastroesophageal Reflux Disease.* New York, NY: Marcel Dekker; 2000:137–164.

52. Dodds WJ, Dent J, Hogan WJ, et al. Mechanisms of gastroesophageal reflux in patients with reflux esophagitis. *N Engl J Med.* 1982;307(25):1547–1552.

53. Estévez-Fernández S, Sánchez-Santos R, Mariño-Padín E, González-Fernández S, Turnes-Vázquez J. Esophagogastric pathology in morbid obese patient: preoperative diagnosis, influence in the selection of surgical technique. *Rev Esp Enferm Dig.* 2015; 107(7):408–412.

54. Saarinen T, Kettunen U, Pietiläinen KH, Juuti A. Is preoperative gastroscopy necessary before sleeve gastrectomy and Roux-en-Y gastric bypass? *Surg Obes Relat Dis.* 2018;14(6):757–762.

55. Argyrou A, Legaki E, Koutserimpas C, et al. Risk factors for gastroesophageal reflux disease and analysis of genetic contributors. *World J Clin Cases.* 2018;6(8):176–182.

56. Kishikawa H, Kimura K, Ito A, et al. Association between increased gastric juice acidity and sliding hiatal hernia development in humans. *PLoS One.* 2017;12(1):e0170416.

57. Mochizuki N, Fujita T, Kobayashi M, et al. Factors associated with the presentation of erosive esophagitis symptoms in health checkup subjects: a prospective, multicenter cohort study. *PLoS One.* 2018;13(5): e0196848.

58. Hunt JN, Cash R, Newland P. Energy density of food, gastric emptying and obesity. *Lancet.* 1975;2(7941):905–906.

59. Maddox A, Horowitz M, Wishart J, Collins P. Gastric and oesophageal emptying in obesity. *Scand J Gastroenterol.* 1989;24(5): 593–598.

60. Johansson C, Ekelund K. Relation between body weight and the gastric and intestinal handling of an oral caloric load. *Gut.* 1976; 17(6):456–462.

61. Lavigne ME, Wiley ZD, Meyer JH, Martin P, MacGregor IL. Gastric emptying rates of solid food in relation to body size. *Gastroenterology.* 1978;74(6):1258–1260.

62. Horowitz M, Collins PJ, Cook DJ, Harding PE, Shearman DJC. Abnormalities of gastric emptying in obese patients. *Int J Obes.* 1983;7(5):415–421.

63. Mercer CD, Rue C, Hanelin L, Hill LD. Effect of obesity on esophageal transit. *Am J Surg.* 1985;149(1):177–181.

64. Marzio L, Capone F, Neri M, Mezzetti A, DeAngelis C, Cuccurullo F. Gallbladder kinetics in obese patients. Effect of a regu-

lar meal and low-calorie meal. *Dig Dis Sci.* 1988;33(1):4–9.

65. Peterson HR, Rothschild M, Weinberg CR, Fell RD, McLeish KR, Pfeifer MA. Body fat and the activity of the autonomic nervous system. *N Engl J Med.* 1988;318(17): 1077–1083.

66. Quitadamo P, Zenzeri L, Mozzillo E, et al. Gastric emptying time, esophageal pH-impedance parameters, quality of life, and gastrointestinal comorbidity in obese children and adolescents. *J Pediatr.* 2018;194: 94–99.

67. Herregods TV, Bredenoord AJ, Smout AJ. Pathophysiology of gastroesophageal reflux disease: new understanding in a new era. *Neurogastroenterol Motil.* 2015;27(9): 1202–1213.

68. Dent J, Dodds WJ, Friedman RH, et al. Mechanism of gastroesophageal reflux in recumbent asymptomatic human subjects. *J Clin Invest.* 1980;65(2):256–267.

69. Penagini R, Carmagnola S, Cantu P, Allocca M, Bianchi PA. Mechanoreceptors of the proximal stomach: role in triggering transient lower esophageal sphincter relaxation. *Gastroenterology.* 2004;126(1):49–56.

70. Pearsons TJ, Power C, Logan S, Summerbell CD. Childhood predictors of adult obesity: a systematic review. *Int J Obes Relat Metab Disord.* 1999;23(suppl 8):S1–107.

71. Holt S, Miller JC, Petocz P, Farmakalidis E. A satiety index of common foods. *Eur J Clin Nutr.* 1995;49(9):675–690.

72. Prentice AM. Manipulation of dietary fat and energy density and subsequent effects on substrate flux and food intake. *Am J Clin Nutr.* 1998;67(3)(suppl):535S–541S.

73. Swinburn BA, Caterson I, Seidell JC, James WP. Diet, nutrition and the prevention of excess weight gain and obesity. *Public Health Nutr.* 2004;7(1A):123–146.

74. El-Serag HB, Satia JA, Rabeneck L. Dietary intake and the risk of gastro-oesophageal reflux disease: a cross sectional study in volunteers. *Gut.* 2005;54(1):11–17.

75. Fox M, Barr C, Nolan S, Lomer M, Anggiansah A, Wong T. The effects of dietary fat and calorie density on esophageal acid exposure and reflux symptoms. *Clin Gastroenterol Hepatol.* 2007;5(4):439–444.

76. Nilsson M, Johnsen R, Ye W, Hveem K, Lagergren J. Obesity and estrogen as risk factors for gastroesophageal reflux symptoms. *JAMA.* 2003;290(1):66–72.

77. Close H, Mason JM, Wilson D, Hungin AP. Hormone replacement therapy is associated with gastro-oesophageal reflux disease: a retrospective cohort study. *BMC Gastroenterol.* 2012;12:56.

78. Jacobson BC, Moy B, Colditz GA, Fuchs CS. Postmenopausal hormone use and symptoms of gastroesophageal reflux. *Arch Intern Med.* 2008;168(16):1798–1804.

79. Tsai CC, Tey SL, Chang LC, Su YT, Lin KJ, Huang SC. Estradiol mediates relaxation of porcine lower esophageal sphincter. *Steroids.* 2018;136:56–62.

80. Fonseca-Alaniz MH, Takada J, Alonso-Vale MI, Lima FB. Adipose tissue as an endocrine organ: from theory to practice. *J Pediatr (Rio J).* 2007;83(5)(suppl):S192–S203.

81. Nam SY, Choi IJ, Ryu KH, Park BJ, Kim HB, Nam BH. Abdominal visceral adipose tissue volume is associated with increased risk of erosive esophagitis in men and women. *Gastroenterology.* 2010;139(6):1902–1911.

82. Goiot H, Attoub S, Kermorgant S, et al. Antral mucosa expresses functional leptin receptors coupled to STAT-3 signaling, which is involved in the control of gastric secretions in the rat. *Gastroenterology.* 2001;121(6):1417–1427.

83. Ryan AM, Healy LA, Power DG, et al. Barrett esophagus: prevalence of central adiposity, metabolic syndrome, and a proinflammatory state. *Ann Surg.* 2008;247(6):909–915.

84. Mix H, Widjaja A, Jandl O, et al. Expression of leptin and leptin receptor isoforms in the human stomach. *Gut.* 2000;47(4):481–486.

85. Endo Y, Kumagai K. Induction by interleukin-1, tumor necrosis factor and lipopolysaccharides of histidine decarboxylase in the stomach and prolonged accumulation of gastric acid. *Br J Pharmacol.* 1998; 125(4):842–848.

86. Souza RF, Huo X, Mittal V, et al. Gastro-esophageal reflux might cause esophagitis through a cytokine-mediated mechanism rather than caustic acid injury. *Gastroenterology.* 2009;137(5):1776–1784.

87. Ludemann JP, Manoukian J, Shaw K, Bernard C, Davis M, al-Jubab A. Effects of simulated gastroesophageal reflux on the untraumatized rabbit larynx. *J Otolaryngol.* 1998;27(3):127–131.

88. Cherry J, Margulies SI. Contact ulcer of the larynx. *Laryngoscope.* 1968;78(11):1937–1940.

89. Delahunty JE, Cherry J. Experimentally produced vocal cord granulomas. *Laryngoscope.* 1968;78(11):1941–1947.

90. Morrison MD. Is chronic gastroesophageal reflux a causative factor in glottic carcinoma?. *Otolaryngol Head Neck Surg.* 1988;99(4):370–373.

91. Olson NR. Aerodigestive malignancy and gastroesophageal reflux disease. *Am J Med.* 1997;103(5A):97S–99S.

92. Yelken K, Yilmaz A, Guven M, Eyibilen A, Aladag I. Paradoxical vocal fold motion dysfunction in asthma patients. *Respirology.* 2009;14(5):729–733.

93. Habesoglu TE, Habesoglu M, Sürmeli M, et al. Histological changes of rat soft palate with exposure to experimental laryngopharyngeal reflux. *Auris Nasus Larynx.* 2010;37(6):730–736.

94. Erickson E, Sivasankar M. Simulated reflux decreases vocal fold epithelial barrier resistance. *Laryngoscope.* 2010;120(8):1569–1575.

95. Johnston N, Dettmar PW, Bishwokarma B, Lively MO, Koufman JA. Activity/stability of human pepsin: implications for reflux attributed laryngeal disease. *Laryngoscope.* 2007;117(6):1036–1039.

96. Axford SE, Sharp N, Ross PE, et al. Cell biology of laryngeal epithelial defenses in health and disease: preliminary studies. *Ann Otol Rhinol Laryngol.* 2001;110(12):1099–1108.

97. Johnston N, Knight J, Dettmar PW, Lively MO, Koufman J. Pepsin and carbonic anhy-drase isoenzyme III as diagnostic markers for laryngopharyngeal reflux disease. *Laryngoscope.* 2004;114(12):2129–2134.

98. Gill GA, Johnston N, Buda A, Pignatelli M, Pearson J, Dettmar PW, Koufman J. Laryngeal epithelial defenses against laryngopharyngeal reflux: investigations of E-cadherin, carbonic anhydrase isoenzyme III, and pepsin. *Ann Otol Rhinol Laryngol.* 2005;114(12):913–921.

99. Takeichi M. Cadherin cell adhesion receptors as a morphogenetic regulator. *Science.* 1991;251(5000):1451–1455.

100. Takeichi M. Morphogenetic roles of classic cadherins. *Curr Opin Cell Biol.* 1995;7(5):619–627.

101. Reichel O, Mayr D, Durst F, Berghaus. E-cadherin but not beta-catenin expression is decreased in laryngeal biopsies from patients with laryngopharyngeal reflux. *Eur Arch Otorhinolaryngol.* 2008;265(8):937–942.

102. Ali MS, Pearson JP. Upper airway mucin gene expression: a review. *Laryngoscope.* 2007;117(5):932–938.

103. Voynow JA, Gendler SJ, Rose MC. Regulation of mucin genes in chronic inflammatory airway diseases. *Am J Respir Cell Mol Biol.* 2006;34(6):661–665.

104. Welch WJ, Brown CR. Influence of molecular and chemical chaperones on protein folding. *Cell Stress Chaperones.* 1996;1(2):109–115.

105. Johnston N, Dettmar PW, Lively MO, et al. Effect of pepsin on laryngeal stress protein (Sep70, Sep53, and Hsp70) response: role in laryngopharyngeal reflux disease. *Ann Otol Rhinol Laryngol.* 2006;115(1):47–58.

106. Kongara KR, Soffer EE. Saliva and esophageal protection. *Am J Gastroenterol.* 1999;94(6):1446–1452.

107. Eckley CA, Costa HO. Salivary EGF concentration in adults with chronic laryngitis caused by laryngopharyngeal reflux. *Rev Bras Otorrinolaringol.* 2003;69(5):590–597.

108. Lechien JR, Saussez S, Harmegnies B, Finck C, Burns JA. Laryngopharyngeal reflux and voice disorders: a multifactorial model of

etiology and pathophysiology. *J Voice.* 2017;31(6):733–752.

109. Lechien JR, Schindler A, Robotti C, Lejeune L, Finck C. Laryngopharyngeal reflux disease in singers: pathophysiol-ogy, clinical findings and perspectives of a new patient-reported outcome instrument. *Eur Ann Otorhinolaryngol Head Neck Dis.* 2018; pii: S1879-7296(18)30126–1.

Nutrition and the Professional Voice

Jennifer A. Nasser, Nyree Dardarian,
Abigail D. Gilman, and Sobhana Rarijan

What Is Nutrition

As cited by the National Institutes of Health (NIH), nutrition is the "science of food, the nutrients and other substances therein, their action, interaction and balance in relation to health and disease, and the processes by which the organism ingests, absorbs, transports, utilizes and excretes food substances."[1] Using this definition, this chapter reviews the current guidelines for meeting nutrition needs for health and the latest literature on nutrition as it pertains to wellness, illness, and the professional voice user.

Basic Nutrition Needs for Health

The food that we consume provides nutrients that are essential for growth and survival of every human being. Our nutritional requirements include the *macronutrients* (carbohydrates, proteins, and fats), the *micronutrients* (vitamins and minerals),

and water.[2] The National Research Council established the first set of recommendations for dietary consumption by Americans in 1941.[3] These recommendations, called the Recommended Dietary Allowances (RDAs) for vitamins, minerals, protein, and energy, were developed from the perspective of preventing nutrient deficiency disorders and also intended to serve as a guide for good nutrition. By 1989, these recommendations had been revised 9 times and included 19 additional nutrients, for a total of 27 nutrient recommendations. Beginning in 1994, updated scientific knowledge and statistical understanding necessitated revision to include considerations for the prevention of chronic diseases as well as nutritional deficiencies. This led to the development of the Dietary Reference Intakes (DRIs) that features 4 reference values[4]: Estimated Average Requirements (EARs), Recommended Dietary Allowances (RDAs), Adequate Intakes (AIs) and Tolerable Upper Intake Levels (ULs) (Table 11–1). This is in contrast to the RDAs that were single values for each nutrient, adjusted for age, sex, and physiological condition. Thus, DRIs are

339

reference values for healthy people that identify the amount of nutrient needed to prevent deficiency diseases and also consider how much of this nutrient may reduce the risk of chronic diseases in healthy people. They also establish an upper level of safety for nutrients. A list of nutrients, their functions, recommended intakes, and food sources is presented in Table 11–1.

Table 11–1: The DRI Definitions

Estimated Average Requirement (EAR): The average daily nutrient intake level estimated to meet the requirements of half of the healthy individuals in a particular life stage and gender group. For energy, an Estimated Energy Requirement (EER) is used. The EER is the average dietary energy intake that is predicted to maintain energy balance in a healthy adult of a defined age, gender, weight, height, and level of physical activity consistent with good health. In children and pregnant and lactating women, the EER is taken to include the needs associated with the deposition of tissues or the secretion of milk at rates consistent with good health.

Recommended Dietary Allowance (RDA): The average daily dietary nutrient intake level sufficient to meet the nutrient requirements of nearly all (97%–98%) healthy individuals in a particular life stage and gender group.

Adequate Intake (AI): The recommended average daily intake level based on observed or experimentally determined approximations or estimates of nutrient intake by a group (or groups) of apparently healthy people that are assumed to be adequate; used when an RDA cannot be determined.

Tolerable Upper Intake Level (UL): The highest average daily nutrient intake level

that is likely to pose no risk of adverse health effects to almost all individuals in the general population. As intake increases above the UL, the potential risk of adverse effects may increase.

The US Department of Agriculture (USDA) considers these nutrient recommendations when establishing nutrition marketing tools and communications. A brief history of the USDA's key communications of nutrition recommendations below shows the evolution of the target messaging. In 1992, USDA released the widely known Food Guide Pyramid that translated nutritional recommendations into the types and amounts of food to eat each day. It took a whole diet approach indicating goals for 6 key food groups: bread/cereal/rice/pasta; fruit; vegetables; milk/yogurt/cheese; milk/poultry/fish/dry beans/eggs/nuts; and fats/oils/sweets. The recommendations included a range of daily amounts of each food group across 3 different calorie levels. In 2005, MyPyramid Food Guidance System replaced the Food Guide Pyramid. It was developed to parallel the recommendations provided in the 2005 Dietary Guidelines for Americans. Adding the "My" verbiage to the pyramid's image introduced a new idea of a personalized recommendations geared toward the individual. It included daily amounts of food intake at 12 different calorie levels, furthering the idea of individualization. It also included a more simplified illustration, depicting a stick figure climbing stairs to encourage exercise as a key component to overall health.[5] However, this illustration oversimplified the key messages and was soon replaced in June of 2011 with MyPlate.[6] The plate design was envisioned to grab the consumers' attention with the commonly recognized visual cue of a dinner plate[7] (Figure 11–1).

Table 11–1. Nutrients: Their Function, Recommended Intakes, and Sources

Nutrients	Function	Recommended Intake	Signs of Deficiency/Toxicity	Food Sources
Total water	• Maintains homeostasis in the body • Aids in transport of nutrients to cells • Removes and excretes waste products of metabolism	*AI:* Male: 3.7 L/day Female: 2.7 L/day	*Deficiency:* Dehydration Impaired cognitive function and motor control Decreased physical work capacity *Toxicity:* Hyponatremia resulting in heart failure and rhabdomyolosis (skeletal muscle tissue injury) which can lead to kidney failure	All beverages, drinking water, high moisture foods (watermelon, meats, soups/broth, etc)
Carbohydrates Total digestible (starch and sugar)	• Provide energy to cells in the body, particularly the brain • Source of kilocalories to maintain body weight • Spare protein • Helps breakdown fatty acids to prevent ketoacidosis	*RDA:* 130 g/day ᵃ*AMDR:* 45%–65% of total energy for adults	*Deficiency:* Increased production of keto acids Inadequate glycogen stores Bone mineral loss, hypercholesterolemia Increased risk of urolithiasis Adverse effect on general sense of well-being and central nervous system *Toxicity:* Increased risk of hyperinsulinemia, glucose intolerance, type 2 diabetes	Starch: Grains, vegetables (corn, pasta, rice, potatoes, breads) Natural sugars: fruits and juices Added sugars: soft drinks, candy, fruit drinks, and desserts

continues

341

Table 11–1. *continued*

Nutrients	Function	Recommended Intake	Signs of Deficiency/Toxicity	Food Sources
Total fiber (digestible fiber, functional fiber)	• Provide bulk and feeling of fullness • Improves laxation • Reduces risk of coronary heart disease • Maintains blood glucose levels and reduces blood cholesterol concentration	*AI:* Male (19–50 years): 38 g/day Male (>50 years): 30 g/day Female (19–50 years): 25 g/day Female (>50 years): 21 g/day	*Deficiency:* Inadequate fecal bulk *Toxicity:* Adverse GI symptoms	Grains (oats, wheat, unmilled rice) Functional fiber synthesized or isolated from plants or animals
Protein				
• Composed of 20 amino acids • 9 essential amino acids cannot be made within the body • 4 nonessential amino acids can be produced within the body • Conditional amino acids are usually not essential, except under times of stress or illness when the body cannot produce them	• Building block for all of life • Provides major structural component of all cells in the body • Functions as enzymes, hormones, nucleic acids, vitamins, and many other components of the body • Needed for growth, development, and repair • Essential for children, teens and pregnant women	*RDA:* 0.8 g/kg body weight (Needs may increase in times of stress, wound healing, growth, pregnancy) *AMDR:* 15%–20% of total energy for adults	*Deficiency:* Weight loss, weakness, lack of appetite, edema, diarrhea, and vomiting *Toxicity:* weight gain, kidney damage, dehydration	Animal sources: meat, poultry, eggs, dairy, seafood/shellfish Plant sources: beans, peas and legumes, seeds, soy products such as tofu and soy milk, whole grains, vegetables

Nutrients	Function	Recommended Intake	Signs of Deficiency/Toxicity	Food Sources
Fat				
(Saturated fat, unsaturated fat, trans-fatty acids)	• Supplies and stores energy • Needed for hormone production • Helps manage cholesterol levels • Regulates temperature • Needed for transport and absorption of fat-soluble vitamins	*AMDR:* 10%–20% of total energy for adults	*Deficiency:* Skin, hair, and nail disorders; impaired metabolism of fat and fat-soluble vitamins *Toxicity:* ketogenic state, weight gain/obesity, hypercholesterolemia, colon cancer cardiovascular disease	Unsaturated fats: vegetable oils that are liquid at room temperature (olive, peanut, canola, sunflower, safflower, flaxseed, etc), avocados, nuts, seeds, fish Saturated fats: fats solid at room temperature such as butter and lard, full fat dairy and cheese, visible fat on meats and poultry, sausage and other meat products Trans-fatty acids: hydrogenated or partially hydrogenated vegetable oils, processed and/or packaged foods and baked goods
Fat soluble vitamins				
Vitamin A (retinol, carotenoids)	• Essential for integrity of night vision • Promotes vision • Essential for normal growth, development, and maintenance of epithelial tissues • Supports reproduction • Promotes normal bone development and tooth formation • Functions as antioxidants	*RDA:* Male: 900 µg RAE/day Female: 700 µg RAE/day *UL*:* 3000 µg RAE/day (*The UL applies only to preformed retinol and not to vitamin A derived from carotenoids.)	*Deficiency:* Night blindness, xerophthalmia (blindness); dry, rough and scaly skin; increased susceptibility to infections *Toxicity:* fractures, osteoporosis, and bone abnormalities; spontaneous abortion and birth defects; liver damage; changes in skin and mucous membranes	Preformed retinol: liver, kidney, fish, eggs; fortified margarine, low-fat and nonfat milk and milk products Carotenoid precursors: spinach and other dark green leafy vegetables, yellow and orange fruits and vegetables

continues

Table 11–1. *continued*

Nutrients	Function	Recommended Intake	Signs of Deficiency/Toxicity	Food Sources
Vitamin D (Calciferol)	• Essential for normal growth and development • Supports bone and tooth growth • Influences absorption and metabolism of phosphorous and calcium	*AI**: Male/Female: 5 µg/day (19–50 years) 10 µg/day (51–70 years) 15 µg/day (>70 years) (*Based on assumption that person does not get enough sun exposure) *UL:* 50 µg/day	*Deficiency:* Rickets (bowed legs, beaded ribs) in children, osteomalacia or osteoporosis in adults *Toxicity:* Hypercalcemia forming kidney stones, hardening blood vessels	Fortified milk, margarine, butter, juices, cereals; veal, beef, egg yolks, liver and fatty fish Synthesized in the body with the help of sunlight
Vitamin E (Tocopherol, Tocotrienol)	• Powerful antioxidant • Protects cell membranes, unsaturated fatty acids, and vitamin A from oxidation • Protects red blood cells from hemolysis • Enhances immune function	*RDA:* Male/Female: 15 mg/day *UL:* 1000 mg/day	*Deficiency:* Impairment of nerve, muscle, and immune function; red blood cell breakage leading to hemolytic anemia *Toxicity:* Enhances the effects of anticlotting medication	Wheat germ, whole grains, vegetable oils, green leafy vegetables, nuts, seeds, liver, egg yolks, fatty meats
Vitamin K	• Coenzyme for prothrombin that assists in blood coagulation • Involved in bone metabolism • Regulates multiple enzyme systems	*AI:* Male: 120 µg/day Female: 90 µg/day	*Deficiency:* Hemorrhaging-impaired blood clotting Effect on bone health *Toxicity:* Jaundice in infants	Leafy green vegetables, cabbage-type vegetables Bacterial synthesis in the digestive tract

Nutrients	Function	Recommended Intake	Signs of Deficiency/Toxicity	Food Sources
Water soluble vitamins				
Vitamin B$_1$ (Thiamine)	• Essential role in carbohydrate and amino acid metabolism • Essential for growth, normal appetite, digestion and healthy nerves	*RDA:* Male: 1.2 mg/day Female: 1.1 mg/day	*Deficiency:* Beriberi Apathy, poor short-term memory, confusion, irritability Anorexia, weight loss Muscular weakness Enlarged heart, cardiac failure *Toxicity:* Headache, convulsions, muscular weakness, cardiac arrhythmia, allergic reactions	Whole grain, enriched cereals, breads, pasta Wheat germ, legumes, pork, tuna
Vitamin B$_2$ (Riboflavin)	• Essential role in carbohydrate, amino acid, and lipids metabolism • Required for growth • Plays enzymatic role in tissue respiration and acts as transporter of hydrogen ions • Coenzyme forms FMN and FAD	*RDA:* Male: 1.3 mg/day Female: 1.1 mg/day	*Deficiency:* Ariboflavinosis, fissuring of lips (cheilosis), cracks in the skin at the corner of mouth (angular stomatitis), seborrheic dermatitis, anemia *Toxicity:* None known	Milk and dairy products, organ meats, shrimp, eggs, green leafy vegetables, enriched grain products

continues

Table 11–1. *continued*

Nutrients	Function	Recommended Intake	Signs of Deficiency/Toxicity	Food Sources
Vitamin B₃ (Niacin)	• Part of coenzymes NAD and NADP used in energy metabolism • Involved in glycolysis and fat synthesis • Plays role in DNA replication, repair and cell differentiation	*RDA:* Male: 16 mg NE*/day Female: 14 mg NE*/day *UL:* 35 mg/day (*Allows for conversion of the amino acid tryptophan to niacin [1 mg niacin = 60 mg tryptophan])	*Deficiency:* Pellagra (diarrhea, dermatitis, dementia, death) Depression, apathy, fatigue, loss of memory; bilateral symmetrical rash on areas exposed to sun *Toxicity:* Painful flush, hives and rash; liver damage, impaired glucose tolerance Blurred vision, nausea, vomiting	Meat, liver, poultry, and fish; whole grains and enriched grains; nuts and protein-containing foods
Vitamin B₅ (Pantothenic acid)	• Part of coenzyme A–functions in the synthesis and breakdown of several vital compounds • Essential in intermediary metabolism of carbohydrate, fat, and protein	*AI:* Male/Female: 5 mg/day	*Deficiency:* Impairment in lipid synthesis and energy production; paresthesia and burning sensation in feet, depression, fatigue, weakness *Toxicity:* Mild intestinal distress, diarrhea	Widespread in all plant and animal foods; best sources: eggs, kidney, liver, salmon, and yeast
Vitamin B₆ (Pyridoxine, Pyridoxal, Pyridoxamine)	• As coenzymes PLP (pyridoxal phosphate) and PMP (pyridoxamine phosphate) aids in synthesis and breakdown of amino acids and fatty acids • Converts tryptophan to niacin and to serotonin • Assists in synthesis of blood cells	*RDA:* Male/Female (19–50 yrs): 1.3 mg/day Male (>50 years): 1.7 mg/day Female (>50 years): 1.5 mg/day *UL:* 100 mg/day	*Deficiency:* Anemia; seborrheic dermatitis; depression, confusion, convulsions *Toxicity:* Nerve damage causing numbness and weakness; skin lesions; depression, fatigue, irritability, headache	Most cuts of meat/fish/poultry, fortified cereals, oatmeal, chickpeas, legumes

Nutrients	Function	Recommended Intake	Signs of Deficiency/Toxicity	Food Sources
Vitamin B$_{12}$ (Cobalamin)	• Required for synthesis of nucleic acids and nucleoproteins • Involved in the metabolism of single-carbon fragments • Required for healthy nervous system • Reforms folate coenzyme • Assists with formation of blood	*RDA:* Male/Female: 2.4 µg/day	*Deficiency:* Pernicious anemia; memory loss, disorientation and dementia; tingling and numbness of extremities *Toxicity:* None known	Foods of animal origin (meat, fish, poultry, shellfish, milk, cheese, eggs), fortified cereals
Biotin	• Essential as enzyme cofactor in synthesis and breakdown of carbohydrates, fat, and proteins	*AI:* Male/Female: 30 µg/day	*Deficiency:* Hallucinations; numb or tingling sensation in extremities; depression, lethargy; anorexia, nausea; hepatic steatosis and hypercholesterolemia *Toxicity:* None known	Liver, egg yolk, fish, nuts and soybean, whole grains, most vegetables, mushrooms Synthesized by intestinal bacteria
Folic acid (Folate)	• Required for biosynthesis of nucleic acids, especially important in early fetal development • Essential for maturation of RBCs • Part of coenzymes THF (tetrahydrofolate) and DHF (dihydrofolate) used in DNA synthesis	*RDA:* Male/Female: 400 µg/day *UL:* 1000 µg/day	*Deficiency:* Macrocytic or megaloblastic anemia; neural tube defects in developing fetus; elevated homocysteine; glossitis; mental confusion, weakness, fatigue; shortness of breath *Toxicity:* Masks signs and symptoms of vitamin B$_{12}$ deficiency, especially signs of nerve damage	Green leafy vegetables, fortified grains, legumes, seeds, liver

continues

Table 11–1. *continued*

Nutrients	Function	Recommended Intake	Signs of Deficiency/Toxicity	Food Sources
Vitamin C (Ascorbic acid)	• Cofactor in collagen synthesis (strengthens blood vessel walls, forms scar tissues, provides matrix for bone growth) • Acts as antioxidant in extracellular fluids and lungs • Enhances immune function, strengthens resistance to infection • Assists in synthesis of hormones, neurotransmitters, and DNA • Enhances iron absorption	*RDA:* Male: 90 mg/day Female: 75 mg/day Smokers: +35 mg/day *UL:* 2000 mg/day	*Deficiency:* Scurvy (lesions in mesenchymal tissues, edema, hemorrhages, swollen bleeding gums, rheumatic pains, bone fragility, muscular atrophy) *Toxicity:* GI disturbances, diarrhea, kidney stones, nosebleeds, increased oxidative damage, aggravation of gout symptoms	Citrus fruits and juices, dark green vegetables, cabbage-type vegetables, strawberries, kiwi, tomatoes, potatoes, papaya, mangoes.
Calcium	• Required for vascular contraction and vasodilation, muscle function, nerve transmission, intracellular signaling and hormonal secretion • Serum levels highly regulated • Stored in bones and teeth to support structure and function	*RDA:* Male (19 to 51+ years): 1000 mg Female (19 to 51+ years): 1000 mg *UL:* 2500 mg	*Deficiency:* Osteopenia, Osteoporosis in adults Rickets in children *Toxicity:* Hypercalcemia causing renal insufficiency, vascular and soft tissue calcification, hypercalciuria, kidney stones, and constipation	Dairy sources: milk, yogurt, cheese Nondairy sources: Kale, broccoli, Chinese cabbage, sardines, tofu, fortified foods

Nutrients	Function	Recommended Intake	Signs of Deficiency/Toxicity	Food Sources
Magnesium	• Cofactor in 300+ enzymes to regulate wide variety of body functions • Required for energy production, oxidative phosphorylation, and glycolysis • Structural component of bones • Needed for synthesis of DNA, RNA, and glutathione	*RDA:* Male (19–30 years): 400 mg Male (30–51+ years): 420 mg Female (19–30 years): 310 mg Female (31–50+ years): 320 mg *UL:* 350 mg	*Deficiency:* Loss of appetite, nausea, vomiting, fatigue, weakness, hypocalcemia, or hypokalemia *Toxicity:* Diarrhea, hypotension, nausea, vomiting, facial flushing, retention of urine, ileus, depression, and lethargy	Green leafy vegetables, legumes, nuts, seeds, and whole grains; highest amounts are found in almonds, spinach, cashews, peanuts, shredded wheat cereal and soymilk
Phosphorus	• Involved in cell growth and repair • Role in breakdown of dietary carbohydrate and fats for energy • Integral component of adenosine triphosphate (ATP) • Forms backbone of DNA and RNA • Essential component of phospholipids	*RDA:* Male 19–51+ years: 700 mg/d Female 19–51+ years: 700mg/d *UL:* 4000 mg	*Deficiency:* Weight loss, muscle cramps, dizziness, stiff joints, bone pain *Toxicity:* impaired bone mineralization, increased cell death, impaired cell signaling, renal dysfunction, vascular calcification, and infertility	Milk, meat, poultry, fish, eggs, milk products, nuts, legumes, and cereal grains

continues

Table 11-1. *continued*

Nutrients	Function	Recommended Intake	Signs of Deficiency/Toxicity	Food Sources
Potassium	• Essential for heath and fluid homeostasis • Keeps body's cells functioning properly • Important electrolyte, works to regulate the balance of body fluids • Affects: nerve signaling, muscle contraction, tone of blood vessels, cardiovascular system • Lowers elevated blood pressure	*RDA:* Male/Female: 4700 mg	*Deficiency:* Hypokalemia include weak muscles, abnormal heart rhythms, slight rise in blood pressure *Toxicity:* prolonged diarrhea and/or vomiting, abnormal and dangerous heart rhythms (hyperkalemia)	Fruits, vegetables, low-fat dairy foods, reduced fat milk, coffee, chicken, beef, orange juice, grapefruit
Sodium	• Maintains and regulates normal fluid balance (body, tissues and cells) • Major role in normal cell and muscle functioning • Aids in the regulation of acid- base balance of the blood and tissues	*RDA:* Male/Female: 1500–2000 mg *UL:* 2300 mg	*Deficiency:* fainting, intolerance to heat, muscle cramps, swelling in the extremities, confusion *Toxicity:* Hypertension	Most foods, processed foods, soy sauce, cheese, chips, seafood

Nutrients	Function	Recommended Intake	Signs of Deficiency/Toxicity	Food Sources
Chromium	• Enhances action of insulin • Involved in macronutrient breakdown	*RDA:* Male (19–50 years): 35 mcg Male (50+ years): 30 mcg Female (19–50 years): 25 mcg Female (50+ years): 20 mcg	*Deficiency:* impaired ability to utilize glucose, increased insulin requirements, abnormal cholesterol metabolism, fatigue *Toxicity:* no toxicity exists	Meat and whole grain products, Brewer's yeast, broccoli, liver, beef, oysters, potatoes
Cobalt	• Involved in the formation and function of healthy red blood cells	No specific RDA	*Deficiency:* Pernicious anemia, weakness *Toxicity:* Rare	Organ meats, oysters, grains and cereals, milk, sea vegetables, spinach, broccoli cabbage
Copper	• Involved in enzymes that regulate pathways, such as energy production, iron metabolism, connective tissue growth and neurotransmission • Acts as an antioxidant	*RDA:* Male (19–50 years): 8 mg Male (51+ years): 8 mg Female (19–50 years): 18 mg Female (51+ years):8 mg *UL:* 10,000 mg	*Deficiency:* Anemia that is unresponsive to iron therapy *Toxicity:* Abdominal pain, nausea, vomiting, and diarrhea	Shellfish, liver, poultry, nuts, gelatin, whole grains, eggs, legumes, peas, avocados

continues

Table 11–1. *continued*

Nutrients	Function	Recommended Intake	Signs of Deficiency/Toxicity	Food Sources
Iron (Heme iron, Non-heme iron)	• Needed for the production of hemoglobin and oxygenation of red blood cells • Role in immune function and energy production	*RDA:* Male (19–50 years): 8 mg Male (51+ years): 8 mg Female (19–50 years): 18 mg Female (51+ years): 8 mg UL (14+ years): 45 mg	*Deficiency:* Fatigue, anemia, lack of stamina, headaches, decreased appetite; often associated with other nutrient deficiencies *Toxicity:* gastric upset, constipation, nausea, abdominal pain, vomiting, faintness	Heme sources (animal sources): oysters, beef liver, sardines, beef, eggs, fish Non-heme sources (plant and fortified sources): beans, lentils, tofu, chickpeas, asparagus, blackstrap molasses, prunes, raisins, enriched breads and cereals
Selenium	• Trace element • Plays role in reproduction, thyroid hormone metabolism, and DNA synthesis • Acts as an antioxidant • Needed for appropriate function of selenium-dependent enzymes, selenoproteins	*RDA:* Male/Female: (14–51+years): 55 mcg *UL:* (19+ years) : 400 mcg	*Deficiency:* Male infertility,, exacerbation of iodine deficiency, Keshan disease *Toxicity:* Hair and nail loss or brittleness, lesions of the skin and nervous system, nausea, diarrhea, skin rashes, mottled teeth, fatigue, irritability and nervous system abnormalities	Seafood, organ meat, muscle meats, cereals, other grains and dairy products Content in plant-based foods dependent on selenium content of the soil, as well as other soil characteristics
Silicon	• Functional role for silicon in human body not yet identified. • Involved in bone formation, seen in chicken and rats • Important for collagen formation	Not applicable	No evidence of deficiency or toxicity in humans	Plant-based foods, including whole grains and fresh vegetables

Nutrients	Function	Recommended Intake	Signs of Deficiency/Toxicity	Food Sources
Zinc	• Widely involved in cellular metabolism • Required for 100+ enzymes, immune function, protein synthesis, wound healing, DNA synthesis, growth and development • Required for sense of taste and smell	*RDA:* Male (14+ years): 11 mg Female (19+ years): 8 mg *UL:* (19+ years): 40 mg	*Deficiency:* Slowed growth, loss of appetite, impaired immune function, hair loss, diarrhea, delayed sexual maturation, delay wound healing, taste abnormalities *Toxicity:* Acute toxicity includes nausea, vomiting, loss of appetite, abdominal cramps, diarrhea, and headaches; chronic toxicity includes low copper status, altered iron function, reduced immune function, reduced levels of high-density lipoproteins	Oysters, red meat, poultry, beans, nuts, crab, lobster, whole grains, fortified breakfast cereal, dairy products Phytates, present in whole grains, bind zinc decreasing the bioavailability
Iodine	• Essential component of thyroid hormones (thyroxine T4 and triiodothyronine T3) which regulate protein synthesis, enzymatic activity and important for metabolism	*RDA:* Male (14+ years): 150 mcg Female (14+ years): 150 mcg *UL:* (19+ years): 1100 mcg	*Deficiency:* Adverse effects on growth and development, mental retardation, hypothyroidism, goiter *Toxicity:* goiter, elevated thyroid stimulating hormone, iodine-induced goiter hypothyroidism	Seaweed, seafood, dairy products, grain products, eggs Present in human breast milk and infant formulas

Notes: RDA, Recommended Dietary Allowance; AI, Adequate Intake; UL, Tolerable Upper Intake Levels; AMDR, Acceptable Macronutrient Distribution Range.

[a]AMDR is the range of intake for a particular energy source that is associated with reduced risk of chronic disease while providing intakes of essential nutrients. If an individual consumes in excess of the AMDR, there is a potential of increasing the risk of chronic diseases and/or insufficient intakes of essential nutrients.

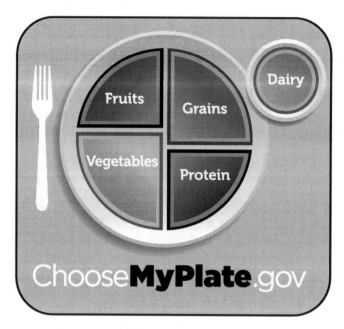

Figure 11–1. The USDA MyPlate.

MyPlate[6] is targeted to the general public and acts as a reminder for consumers to find a healthy eating style and habits, and to build these habits throughout the entire lifetime. The image helps consumers identify the appropriate portions and types of foods to include at every meal. The message stresses that all food and drinks matter, and combining the right variety of foods, as well as making small changes to current habits, can help lead to a healthy plate, and ultimately a healthy lifestyle.[7] MyPlate[6] suggests that every meal and snack should have a similar makeup: half of the plate comprising a Fruits and Vegetables group, one-quarter of the plate from the Protein group and the remaining quarter from the Grains group. It also recommends including food items from the Dairy group.

One-half of every plate should incorporate a variety of whole fruits and vegetables to help ensure adequate nutrient intake. Adults should consume 1.5 to 2 cups of fruit and 2.5 to 3 cups of vegetables every day.

Fruits and vegetables may be fresh, raw or cooked, frozen, canned, or dried/dehydrated and may be whole, cut-up, pureed, or in the form of 100% juice. Generally speaking, 1 cup of fruit 100% fruit juice, or ½ cup of dried fruit is considered as 1 serving from the Fruit group. One cup of raw or cooked vegetables or vegetable juice, or 2 cups of raw leafy greens count as 1 serving from the Vegetable group. One-quarter of the plate should be from the Protein foods group. Proteins should be from a variety of sources, focusing on leaner choices, with all visible fat removed. Lean protein choices include round steaks and roasts such as top round and round tip, loins such as pork loin or tenderloin, skinless chicken and poultry, seafood, nuts and beans and soy products such as tofu. Adults should have 5 to 6 ounce equivalents of protein per day. In general, 1 ounce of meat, poultry or fish, 1 egg, ¼ cup cooked beans, 1 tablespoon of peanut butter, or ½ ounce of nuts or seeds are considered as 1 ounce-equivalent from the Protein foods group.

The Grains group comprises the final quarter of the plate. Consumers should focus on making at least half of their grains whole-grain products. Whole-grains contain the entire grain kernel (bran, germ, and endosperm), parts of which are often removed in the refining process. Eating whole-grain products provides additional vitamins and fiber that are not present in refined, white grains. Whole-grain options include whole-wheat flour, bulgur, oatmeal, brown rice, whole cornmeal, and corn (popcorn). Adults should consume 3 to 3.5 ounce equivalents per day. One ounce equivalent is approximately 1 slice of bread, 1 cup of cereal, or ½ cup of cooked rice, pasta, or cereal. Food items from the Dairy group should also be included at meals, with a shift toward low-fat or fat-free rather than whole-fat choices. Adults should consume 3 cups of dairy per day. One serving from the Dairy Group is equivalent to 1 cup of milk, yogurt, or soymilk (soy beverage), 1.5 ounces of natural cheese, or 2 ounces of processed cheese. This recommendation includes choices from fluid milk and milk products, such as milk, yogurt, and cheese. If dairy or lactose is avoided, individuals should consume calcium-rich foods such as kale and other dark leafy greens, fortified foods, canned fish, and soy products. Although these recommendations are for the general public, the exact amount of food from each food group depends on age, sex, and level of physical activity.

The USDA additionally publishes The Dietary Guidelines for Americans every 5 years to direct health professionals and policy makers to the scientific evidence regarding food, nutrition, and health. The first set of recommendations, the Dietary Goals for the American People, was published in 1977 by the US Senate Select Committee on Nutrition and Human Needs.[8] These recommendations focused on energy balance to avoid overweight, and they recommended that Americans consume less energy and expend more energy. Nutrition recommendations have evolved to include more specific guidelines to live a healthy and nutritious lifestyle. The eighth and most recent edition, recommendations for 2015 to 2020,[9] contains 5 key guidelines that parallel the messages touted by the MyPlate.[6] The first guideline emphasizes that individuals should follow a healthy eating pattern across the life span. Choosing a healthy eating pattern at an appropriate calorie level will help maintain a healthy body weight and overall healthy lifestyle. The second guideline recommends that individuals focus on variety, nutrient density, and amount of food consumed. Choosing a variety of foods ensures adequate nutrient intake. The third guideline suggests limiting calories from added sugars and saturated fats, and reducing overall sodium intake. It highlights that excess consumption of these foods may lead to excess weight and chronic disease while limiting these can help establish a healthy eating pattern. The fourth recommendation advises a shift to healthier food and beverage choices leading to a healthier eating pattern. The final guideline suggests supporting healthy eating patterns for everyone. It encourages all levels of society to participate in contributing to changes toward a healthy eating pattern. This includes individuals, families, schools, communities, and corporations.[9]

Medical Nutrition Issues of the Professional Voice User

Poor nutrition status undergirds the development and prognosis of a number of illnesses, including the common causes of death, namely ischemic heart disease, stroke, cancer, and diabetes. Unlike heart disease, stroke, and cancer, which are illnesses that can interrupt an individual's career, diabetes is an illness that must be managed while someone is carrying on his or her career. This is also true of illnesses involving the gastrointestinal tract such as gastroesophageal reflux disorder (GERD). These illnesses can directly affect the professional use of the voice. The remainder of this section will focus its attention on diabetes and GERD as they can affect the day-to-day life of the professional voice user and, for which, there is peer-reviewed evidence upon which to base nutrition interventions for their treatment.

Diabetes

Diabetes is a disease related to the absence of insulin (type 1) or to decreased carbohydrate-related sensitivity to insulin (type 2). Type I diabetes requires the use of exogenous insulin and careful coordination of food intake, insulin dosing, and physical activity. As such it can present a challenge to professional voice users, especially those involved in lengthy, high energy performances such as musical theater, opera, and rock singers. Management of type 1 diabetes begins with knowing the blood glucose level and the glucose response to insulin dosing, followed by glucose response to insulin in conjunction with food intake and in conjunction with physical activity. The care of those with type 1 diabetes is handled best by specialists in the field (both physicians and nonphysician diabetes educators and clinicians) and will not be addressed in this chapter. However, type 2 diabetes and its precursor, pre-diabetes, are conditions intimately related to lifestyle habits and responsive to lifestyle treatment (diet and physical activity). Recent NIH funded studies, the Diabetes Prevention Program,[10,11] and

the LOOK AHEAD Study,[12] have demonstrated that lifestyle intervention is superior to medication alone in the management of pre-diabetes and type 2 diabetes. According to statistics from the Centers for Disease Control and Prevention, incidence of type 2 diabetes in the United States is roughly more than 8% of the population (~19 million people diagnosed, 7 million people undiagnosed). An additional 35% of the population has pre-diabetes, and they have an increased risk of developing type 2 diabetes, heart disease, and stroke.[13] Most of those with pre-diabetes, defined as fasting blood glucose between 100 mg/dL and 125 mg/dL (5.6 mm/L6.9 mm/L), or a random non-fasting blood glucose between 140 mg/dL and 200 mg/dL, or hemoglobin A1C levels between 5.7% and 6.4%, have high waist circumferences (greater than 35 inches in women [88 cm], greater than 40 inches [102 cm] in men) and body mass indices (BMI) of 30 or greater. The symptoms of diabetes include excessive thirst, frequent urination, increased hunger, fatigue, and poor wound healing, to mention a few. Excessive thirst, frequent urination, and fatigue can have direct effects on professional use of the voice, and patients complaining of these symptoms, or of difficulty staying hydrated when they use their voice, should be screened for diabetes as well as other disorders. This is especially important given that Hamdan et al[14] report increased hoarseness grade scores (on the GRBAS[grade, roughness, breathiness, asthenia, strain]) for those with type 2 diabetes exhibiting poor glycemic control and neuropathy, and those with diabetes are at greater risk for vocal cord paralysis.[15] According to the American Diabetes Association,[16] effective lifestyle interventions for type 2 diabetes include 30 minutes of aerobic exercise at least 5 days per week combined with resistance training 2 times per week, and a diet high in whole grains, fruits and vegetables, fiber, lean meat, and low-fat dairy.[17] Carbohydrate restriction is not required, but it is recommended that refined carbohydrates and sweets be used sparingly. As type 2 diabetes progresses, or in those who cannot follow an intensive lifestyle intervention, medication may be needed to maintain blood glucose control. However, practicing healthy eating and physical activity helps to increase the effectiveness of medications used to treat type 2 diabetes, and in some cases can allow for lower doses to be used. Since these drugs have side effects that can themselves create lifestyle challenges (such as increased gastrointestinal motility, urination, and weight gain) for professional performers, it makes good health sense to optimize healthy eating practices and physical activity to limit the amount of medication needed to have good blood glucose control.

Over the last 30 years, much interest has been directed at gastric bypass surgery as a method for alleviating type 2 diabetes, inducing weight loss and preventing the progression of pre-diabetes to type 2 diabetes.[18–20] The reduction in blood glucose after gastric bypass surgery is superior to that seen with equivalent weight loss by caloric restriction[21]; however, the decision to undergo gastric bypass surgery is a serious one and only one small study to date has addressed potential detrimental effects on the voice following gastric bypass surgery.[22] More research is needed in this area to determine the best treatment for type 2 diabetes in professional voice users.

Gastroesophageal Reflux Disorder

The gastrointestinal (GI) tract has a particularly important role to play in ensuring proper nutrition health as it is the conduit for entry of nutrients into the body. Malfunctions of the GI tract can present day to day and present longer-term challenges in managing one's health and career. An illness of major concern for professional voice users is GERD. GERD is characterized by reflux of stomach acid into the esophagus and has the potential to develop into laryngopharyngeal reflux (LPR)[23] as discussed in Chapter 9. Since the larynx is not equipped to handle contact with hydrochloric acid (stomach acid), GERD and LPR can physically damage the larynx. Symptoms of stomach acid–induced laryngeal damage include hoarseness, laryngitis, sensation of "lump in the throat," excessive mucus, and coughing among others. With respect to voice usage, Ross et al[24] report that there is increased abnormal perceptual voice characteristics (musculoskeletal tension, hard glottal attack, glottal fry, restricted tone placement, and hoarseness) as well as increased shimmer in those with LPR compared to the controls. Treatment of GERD and comorbid LPR usually involves use of various medications to reduce stomach acid and raise lower esophageal sphincter (LES) pressure[25] as well as numerous other treatment approaches discussed in Chapter 9.

Nutritional interventions for GERD and LPR have the same goals as drug interventions as they also target reduction in stomach acid and maintenance of LES pressure. Foods known to increase gastric acid secretion include alcohol, caffeine, chocolate, garlic, onions, high-fat/high-carbohydrate foods, and peppermint as well as carbonated beverages.[26] Some recent studies[27,28] suggest that meal patterns, in addition to meal composition, can exacerbate or alleviate GERD symptoms. Significant differences were reported between number of meals per day and reflux[28] with 2 meals per day and plenty of inter-meal liquids providing reflux relief compared to the traditional 3 meals per day. Meal patterns regular and irregular (which were not defined well in the paper) also were shown to produce differing effects on reflux symptoms. The effect of meal pattern disappeared, however, when the analysis was controlled for BMI[27] lending support to obesity itself being a predisposing condition that supports development of GERD and LPR. Nelms et al[25] as well as the Johns Hopkins Voice Center website[29] recommend weight loss as an additional approach to alleviating GERD, as well as avoiding eating within 3 hours of bedtime or lying down and avoiding creation of intra-abdominal pressure after eating by the wearing of tight fitting clothes, bending over, or straining. Other dietary modifications are discussed in Chapter 9. In summary, GERD and LPR present challenges to the professional voice user that can be addressed by healthy eating and medication.

Nutrition for the Professional Singer

Professional singers can be compared to professional athletes, and as such have special nutritional needs, different from those seen in the general population. Dietary behaviors are a crucial component to enhance the performance of singers and other vocalists. Consuming an optimal balance of energy, macronutrients, micronutrients, fluid, and electrolytes helps maximize performance. However, among performing artists, dietary requirements depend on factors such as the frequency, intensity, and type of performance. This section outlines the energy, nutrient, and fluid recommendations for healthy adult professional singers. A registered dietitian/nutritionist can customize these general recommendations to accommodate individual differences in body composition, health and performance goals, and dietary likes and dislikes. Accurate determination of energy, nutrient, and fluid needs will provide a good foundation for the overall health of the professional singer. Nutrition guidelines for pre- and post-performance are also an integral component to enhancing the wellness of the student or professional singer.

Energy and Hydration

For performers, adequate energy intake is the balance of energy expended and energy consumed to optimize overall health. Nutrient demands of a performer are similar to those of a professional athlete. Long rehearsals and demanding performance schedules often lead to behaviors that include skipping meals and/or long periods of time between meals. As a result, elevated energy demands coupled with inadequate nutrient intake lead to impaired performance.[30] Total daily energy expenditure (TDEE) is represented by 4 subcomponents: basal metabolic rate, thermic effect of food, non-energy activity thermogenesis, and exercise energy thermogenesis (Figure 11–2[31]). The terms

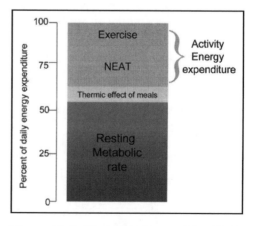

Figure 11–2. The components of Total Daily Energy Expenditure.

Kilocalorie (kcal) and Calorie are often used interchangeably when describing energy derived from food sources. The Kilocalorie represents the amount of heat needed to raise 1 kilogram of water 1°C. Calories consumed from foods and fluids provide the energy to maintain weight, replenish glycogen stores, and repair damaged tissue. Daily caloric requirements fluctuate depending on the frequency, intensity, time, and type of performance. Determining individualized energy requirements is a crucial component of the diet prescription. Energy and fluid imbalances can be detrimental to performance. Early fatigue, cognitive decline, and poor thermoregulation are a few of the potential consequences.

Energy Expenditure

Resting metabolic rate (RMR) is the largest component of total daily expenditure, representing nearly 60% to 75% of an individual's energy needs over a 24-hour period. Resting metabolic rate is synonymous with resting energy expenditure (REE), and these terms will be used interchangeably throughout the chapter. Resting metabolic rate accounts for the energy required to maintain the body's cellular processes for life such as heartbeat and respiration, while in an awake and post-absorptive state. The RMR for adult females is approximately 10% to 15% lower than males due to a higher proportion of fat to muscle mass. Another difference between healthy weight females and males is the average decline in RMR per decade between the ages of 10 and 96 years, 2% and 2.9%, respectively.[32] The decrease in metabolic rate accelerates around the age of 50 years in females and 40 years in males.[33,34] The loss of fat free mass associated with menopause may explain the later and more accelerated decline in metabolic rate for females.[33,34] Using 2400 Calories as

the recommended energy requirement for the average healthy female or male, a 2% to 2.9% decline in energy requirements per decade would translate to a 48 to 72 daily Calorie restriction. Though 48 to 72 Calories seems trivial, the clinical significance is the compounding effects of the metabolic decline. Maintenance of muscle throughout the lifecycle can help sustain metabolism, or lessen the decline. The thermic effect of food represents approximately 10% to 25% of TDEE and is used to express the energy expended for digestion.

Physical activity, categorized as non-exercise thermogenesis and exercise energy expenditure, poses the greatest variable when determining TDEE. Energy requirements for non-exercise-related activities of daily living vary depending on an individual's lifestyle. An active person would expend more energy a day simply by sitting less and walking more than someone who is sedentary, thereby increasing his or her non-exercise activity thermogenesis. Exercise energy expenditure varies based on the frequency, intensity, duration, and type of physical activity.

Several methods are used to determine energy needs. These methods include using stable isotopes (ie, doubly labeled), or indirect calorimetry (ie, whole room calorimeter or metabolic cart). The measurement of energy expenditure is costly, requiring expensive equipment and skilled staff. Therefore, several prediction equations have been developed to estimate resting metabolic rate. Most of the predictive equations used to estimate energy needs incorporate height, sex, weight, and age as variables. The Harris-Benedict[35] and Mifflin-St. Jeor[36] equations (MSJE) are commonly used in clinical practice to estimate REE (Table 11–2). The Harris-Benedict[35] is more accurate in predicting REE in healthy and active individuals. The Mifflin St. Jeor[36] equation is

Table 11–2. Determining Resting Energy Expenditure (REE) Using Predictive Equations

Equation	Sex	Formula
Mifflin-St. Jeor (Mifflin et al, 1990)[36]	Male	(10 × wt) + (6.25 × ht) − (5 × age) + 5
	Female	(10 × wt) + (6.25 × ht) − (5 × age) − 161
Harris-Benedict (Harris, 1919)[35]	Male	(13.75 × wt) + (5 × ht) − 6.67 × age) + 66.47
	Female	(9.56 × wt) + (1.85 × ht) − (4.68 × age) + 655.1

most accurate for overweight and obese individuals using their actual weight.

Once resting energy expenditure has been calculated, the results are used to determine TDEE multiplying by selected activity factors. Activity factors are similar for both equations. Energy requirement is then used to determine the macronutrient distribution of the diet.

Macronutrients

Carbohydrates, fats, and protein are the nutrients that contribute to the energy or Calories in the diet. A recommendation for each of the nutrients for a healthy individual is typically expressed as a percentage of his or her TDEE. The Acceptable Macronutrient Distribution Ranges (AMDRs)[37] outlines the recommended proportions of carbohydrate, fat, and protein in a healthy diet. The AMDR should remain in the range of 45 to 65 of total Calories from carbohydrates. The recommendations for fat and protein are 20% to 35% and 10% to 35%, respectively.

Carbohydrates are the primary source of energy for the body and brain. In humans, carbohydrates are stored in the muscle, liver, and circulating blood as glycogen. Dietary consumption of carbohydrates helps to maintain these stores, providing quick and

accessible energy for everyday tasks. Carbohydrates are ultimately catabolized to glucose, the preferred source of energy for the brain, muscles, and central nervous system. Adequate carbohydrate consumption ensures optimal energy metabolism and prevents fatigue, before and during practices and performances.

The primary function of carbohydrates is to produce energy in the form of adenosine triphosphate (ATP).[38] Adenosine triphosphate fuels the endergonic cellular reactions that affect mechanical energy for muscle movement. It is also an important coenzyme required for body temperature regulation under stress. All carbohydrates follow the glycolytic pathway, whereby energy is attained through aerobic and/or anaerobic respiration. The reactions from the oxidation of glucose in the glycolysis pathway and subsequent pyruvate result in total production of 36 ATP molecules.[38] Oxidation of alternative substrates can result in muscle breakdown and the accumulation of adverse by-products such as lactic acid and ketones; therefore, maintaining optimal carbohydrate consumption is recommended for those in the performing arts. The minimum requirement for carbohydrates in the diet is 130 grams per day.[37]

Fat is the most highly concentrated energy source that fuels the body. Unlike carbohydrates and protein, which provide only 4 Calories per gram, fat provides 9 Calories per gram. Fats are essential for the digestion, insulation, joint lubrication, fat-soluble vitamin transport, molecular signaling, cellular membrane structure, and thermal regulation. Fatty acids are metabolized to acetyl-Coenzyme A (acetyl-CoA) for energy in the beta-oxidation cycle, with the assistance of carbohydrates, which play a vital role in this metabolic pathway. At the termination of the beta-oxidation cycles, each fatty acid yields 14 molecules of ATP. Similar to dietary carbohydrate recommendations, fat recommendations are based on total energy intake, body weight, and activity levels. In addition to function, fat adds flavor to foods and provides sustained satiety after eating. According to the Dietary Guidelines for Americans, less than 35% of total Calories should come from fats, and less than 10% of those Calories per day should come from saturated fats.[9] Omega-3 fatty acids have been researched for their potential antiinflammatory and healing properties, and have been recommended to replace saturated fat in the diet, along with monounsaturated and polyunsaturated fats. The Recommended Daily Allowance for omega-3 (linolenic) fatty acid has not been established. However, the Food and Nutrition Board of the US Institute of Medicine recommends an Adequate Intake (AI) for adult males and females of 1.6 and 1.1 g/day, respectively. For health benefits, unsaturated fats from nuts, oils, and coldwater fish are preferred to saturated and trans-fats from animal products, processed and fried foods, and supplements.

Carbohydrates and fats are the primary sources of energy in a healthy diet. The consumption of lean, high-quality proteins in the diet ensures the delivery of all the essential amino acids used for growth and optimal body function. Proteins in the body function as enzymes, hormones, antibodies, collagen, and structural materials. Proteins help to maintain fluid and acid-base balance of bodily fluids. Insufficient protein intake will impair the body's ability to function optimally; however, excess protein offers no advantage. The AMDR for protein is 10% to 35% of total daily energy requirements, or 0.8 grams of protein per kilogram per day of healthy body weight.[37]

Hydration

The balance between fluid intake and losses is regulated to maintain homeostasis by the hypothalamus, hormones, and nutrients. Fluid imbalances can cause detrimental consequences such as dehydration or intoxication. Often indicated by thirst, the first sign of dehydration is caused by inadequate water intake. Dehydration rapidly progresses to more severe symptoms (weakness, exhaustion, delirium, and death). As little as 1% to 2% loss of total body weight in fluid results in fatigue. Recommendations for fluid vary depending on diet, exercise, and environmental conditions. Based on a 2000-Calorie energy requirement, the AI for fluid is approximately 8 to 12 cups per day. Although water is a healthy choice, dietary sources of fluid are not limited to water. Most fruits and vegetables contain up to 90% water. Meats and cheeses also contain water, though they also are a source of energy and should be consumed in accordance with the Recommendations of the Dietary Guidelines for Americans.

For professional singers, adequate hydration may improve vocal function or voice quality.[39] van Wyk et al[39] examined the effect of systemic hydration on the voice quality of university students studying music ($n = 12$). Hypohydrated (no fluid intake

2 hours prior to and during rehearsal) participants demonstrated a significant grade of hoarseness ($P = 0.046$), a possible indicator of vocal fatigue and an increase in jitter percentage ($P = 0.041$). When hydrated, jitter decreased and singers were able to sustain sound, and both duration and phonation yielded significant improvements.

Nutrient Timing for Performances

Nutrition strategies implemented pre-, during, and post-performance should address various factors that can cause fatigue, deterioration, and poorer recovery outcomes (Table 11–3). It is important that the professional vocalist is comfortable throughout the event by diminishing feelings of hunger or consuming foods that reduce gastrointestinal discomfort that might reduce enjoyment of the event. It is important to optimize nutritional support for health and further adaptation to the rigorous rehearsal, traveling, and performance schedules. These strategies include adequate hydration and nutrient consumption before, during, or between performances in order to reduce the impact of these factors. No single food improves health, voice, or skill on stage, although some foods do support performance better than others. Many performers engage in pre-performance rituals that include food preferences and behaviors. Individual food practices or routines are acceptable as long as they are not harmful.

24 Hours Pre-Performance Meal

Nutrition and hydration preparation should begin at least 24 hours before the performance. Consuming a healthy diet rich in fruits and vegetables, whole grains, lean proteins, and low-fat dairy is ideal. Fluid consumption to achieve euhydration should begin 24 hours pre-event in order to allow adequate time for excess fluid to be voided. A simple method to evaluate hydration is by assessing urine color. Urine pale yellow in color is a good indicator of adequate hydration status, and should be the goal 24 hours prior to performance time.

Day-of-Performance Meals

It is important to spread meals throughout the day to avoid overeating after the performance, often a challenge for professional singers. Recommendations for pre-performance meals are designed to provide sufficient portion sizes and proportions of macronutrients and fluids in order to (1) sustain energy and prevent early fatigue that can result in a decrease in voice quality, (2) diminish feelings of hunger, and (3) optimize hydration. The main meal should be consumed 3 to 4 hours before the performance to allow time for the stomach to empty. Carbohydrate-rich meals that are low in fat and low in fiber are recommended to sustain energy and avoid gastric discomfort throughout the performance. Meal size should decrease in size closer to the start of the performance. The recommendation for fluid intake in the 2 to 4 hours before the performance is 5 to 10 mL/kg of body weight (BW) or approximately 1 to 2 cups of fluid to maintain hydration, and then sips of fluid throughout the performance when applicable. If the performance lasts more than 90 minutes, a high-carbohydrate snack is recommended between acts or during intermissions to diminish hunger late at night. Examples of high-carbohydrate snacks include fruit juices and whole fruits that are easily available and digestible. Yogurt, nuts, soda, and baked goods, although usually desirable, are best avoided during the performance because of the

Table 11–3. Performance Day Meal Planning Using the US Department of Agriculture MyPlate Daily Checklist for 2200 Calories a Day

Food Group	Guidelines	24 Hours Pre-Performance	3–4 Hours Pre-Performance	During Performance	30 Minutes–1 Hour Post-Performance
Fruits	Whole fruits that are fresh, frozen, canned, or dried	½ cup	½ cup	½ cup	½ cup
Vegetables	Variety of colors include dark green, red, and orange	1 cup	As desired		As desired
Grains	Make half of your selections whole grain	2–3 ounces	2–3 ounces	1–2 ounces	1–2 ounces
Protein	Include seafood, beans, and peas, unsalted nuts, soy products, eggs, lean meats, and poultry	3–4 ounces	1–2 ounces		2–3 ounces
Dairy	Select low-fat or fat-free milk, yogurt, and soy drinks	1 cup			1 cup (*substitute for protein group)
Fluid	Choose water or Calorie-free options	~to hydration	~2–3 cups	~1–2 cups	~2–3 cups

Source: Adapted from the US Department of Agriculture MyPlate Daily Checklist.

higher fat and/or protein-to-carbohydrate ratio. Simple carbohydrates are metabolized and used as energy faster in the absence of fat and protein. Proper hydration and energy balance have the potential to delay fatigue and improve performance.

Similar to athletes, recommendations for post-event nutrition impact recovery time. This is especially important during back-to-back rehearsals and performances. After the performance, rehydration and nutrition strategies can be implemented to support fuel availability for following performances. Recent research suggests the rate of glycogen synthesis is only ~5% per hour during the 4- to 6-hour recovery period.[30] To restore muscle glycogen stores and improve muscle protein synthesis (MPS), the post-performance meal should include at least ~1 to 1.2 grams per kilogram per hour of a carbohydrate source, and 15 to 25 grams of protein.[40] The preferred window for recovery nutrition is 30 to 60 minutes after a performance. The earlier carbohydrates, protein, and fluid are ingested, the faster the energy stores in the muscle are restored, and muscle repair and growth are stimulated.

Nutrition and Travel

Traveling for performances is a part of life for many performers, and it introduces challenges for meeting nutritional goals for optimal health and wellness. Disruptions in eating schedules can occur when travel time is long or includes crossing time zones. Performers, like athletes, are at a greater risk of failing to meet nutritional needs, acquiring infections, and being affected by gastrointestinal disturbances while on the road.[41]

Meal and fluid options during travel may be limited, requiring the performer to depend on hotels, restaurants, airlines, and fast food outlets for food. Particular food preferences, allergies, and intolerances will limit food options further during travel and can be challenging without adequate planning before departure. Performers are advised to request their dietary requirements with facilities and establishments before arrival. Performers can pack nonperishable foods to be used if adequate or nutritious food is not available. Researching local food customs of unfamiliar destinations allows performers to plan ahead and make informed choices to ensure that their nutritional needs are supported. Special attention should be paid to food safety, personal hygiene, and sanitation practices to reduce the risk of infection and gastrointestinal disturbances common when traveling. Hand washing helps prevent the spread of many diseases and conditions including diarrhea and respiratory infections, and possibly skin and eye infections.[42]

Maintenance of adequate hydration status is recommended during travel. Increasing the amount of fluid consumed, 15 to 20 mL an hour during a flight will restore exacerbated moisture losses during respiration in response to dry air conditions on board.[41] Dehydration may heighten fatigue and other symptoms associated with jet lag.[43] Alcohol causes increased urine output and should be avoided.

Dietitian/Nutritionist and Treatment of the Professional Voice User

The registered dietitian/nutritionist (RDN) is the health professional trained in the science of nutrition, food science, and nutrition counseling behavior and is uniquely qualified to integrate these sciences with the relationship of diet to health and disease. Becoming registered as a RDN requires completion of an accredited preclinical program and 1200 hours of accredited and supervised internship followed by satisfactory performance on a nationally administered examination.

The RDN's scope of practice in medical nutrition involves assessment of nutrition status, recommendation of necessary dietary treatment, treatment monitoring and evaluation, and nutrition education. In addition to providing medical nutrition care, the RDN is especially qualified to assist the professional voice user with incorporating "health living and eating" conditions into his or her daily work situation. A number of supermarkets employ RDNs to provide health eating assistance to shoppers. Additionally, many RDNs belong to national and/or international Dietetic Practice Groups that can provide referrals for continuity of care as the voice professional meets his or her work-related travel requirements. With respect to nutrition education, the RDN can provide continuing updates on the scientific evidence that supports or refutes the latest "dietary fads" and consumer-directed diet-health information. In short, the RDN can provide skilled clinical care and education to the professional voice user and serve as a knowledgeable colleague to other clinicians in their care of the professional voice user.

References

1. Council on Foods and Nutrition. Nutrition teaching in medical schools. *JAMA.* 1963; 183(11):955–957.

2. Mahan LK, Escott-Stump S, Raymond JL. *Krause's Food and the Nutrition Care Process.* St Louis, MO: Elsevier Health Sciences; 2012.

3. Subcommittee on the Tenth Edition of the RDAs, Food and Nutrition Board, Commission on Life Sciences, National Research Council. *Dietary Recommended Allowances.* 10th ed. Washington, DC: National Academy Press; 1989.

4. Otten JJ, Hellwig JP, Meyers LD. *Dietary Reference Intakes: the Essential Guide to Nutrient Requirements.* National Academies Press; 2006. https://fnic.nal.usda.gov/dietary-guidance/dietary-reference-intakes/dri-nutrient-reports

5. Tagtow A, Haven J, Maniscalco S, Bailey DJ, Bard S. MyPlate celebrates 4 years. *J Acad Nutr Diet.* 2015;115(7):1039–1040.

6. US Department of Agriculture, Choose MyPlate. *MyPlate.* 2016. http://www.choosemyplate.gov/MyPlate

7. Center for Nutrition Policy and Promotion. A Brief History of USDA Food Guides; 2011. http://www.choosemyplate.gov

8. US Senate Select Committee on Nutrition and Human Needs. *Dietary Goals for the United States.* 2nd ed. Washington, DC: US Government Printing Office; 1977.

9. *Dietary Guidelines for Americans 2015–2020.* Washington, DC: US Department of Agriculture (USDA), Human Nutrition Information Service; 2015.

10. Ratner RE and Diabetes Prevention Program Research. An update on the Diabetes Prevention Program. *Endocr Pract.* 2006; 12(suppl 1):20–24.

11. Knowler WC, Barrett-Connor E, Fowler SE, et al. Reduction in the incidence of type 2 diabetes with lifestyle intervention or metformin. *N Engl J Med.* 2002;346(6):393–403.

12. Dutton GR, Lewis CE. The Look AHEAD Trial: implications for lifestyle intervention in type 2 diabetes mellitus. *Prog Cardiovasc Dis.* 2015;58(1):69–75.

13. Centers for Disease Control and Prevention. *National diabetes fact sheet: national estimates and general information on diabetes and prediabetes in the United States, 2011.* Atlanta, GA: US Department of Health and Human Services, Centers for Disease Control and Prevention. 2011 Jan;201(1).

14. Hamdan AL, Jabbour J, Nassar J, Dahouk I, Azar ST. Vocal characteristics in patients with type 2 diabetes mellitus. *Eur Arch Otorhinolaryngol.* 2012;269(5):1489–1495.

15. Schechter GL, Kostianovsky M. Vocal cord paralysis in diabetes mellitus. *Trans Am Acad Ophthalmol Otolaryngol.* 1972;76(3):729–740.

16. American Diabetes Association. www.diabetes.org

17. Position Statement of the American Diabetes Association: Nutrition recommendations and interventions for diabetes. *Diabetes Care.* 2008;31(suppl 1):S61–S78.

18. Pories WJ, Caro JF, Flickinger EG, Meelheim HD, Swanson MS. The control of diabetes mellitus (NIDDM) in the morbidly obese with the Greenville Gastric Bypass. *Ann Surg.* 1987;206(3):316–323.

19. Pories WJ, Swanson MS, MacDonald KG, et al. Who would have thought it? An operation proves to be the most effective therapy for adult-onset diabetes mellitus. *Ann Surg.* 1995;222(3):339–350; discussion 350–352.

20. Long SD, O'Brien K, MacDonald KG Jr, et al. Weight loss in severely obese subjects prevents the progression of impaired glucose tolerance to type II diabetes. A longitudinal interventional study. *Diabetes Care.* 1994; 17(5):372–375.

21. Laferrère B, Teixeira J, McGinty J, et al. Effect of weight loss by gastric bypass surgery versus hypocaloric diet on glucose and incretin levels in patients with type 2 diabetes. *J Clin Endocrinol Metab.* 2008;93(7):2479–2485.

22. Hamdan AL, Safadi B, Chamseddine G, et al. Effect of weight loss on voice after bariatric surgery. *J Voice.* 2014;28(5):618–623.

23. Hawkshaw MJ, Pebdani P, Sataloff RT. Reflux laryngitis: an update, 2009-2012. *J Voice.* 2013;27(4):486–494.

24. Ross JA, Noordzji JP, Woo P. Voice disorders in patients with suspected laryngopharyngeal reflux disease. *J Voice.* 1998;12(1):84–88.

25. Nelms M. Diseases of the upper gastrointestinal tract. In: Nelms M, Sucher KP, Long S, eds. *Nutrition Therapy and Pathophysiology.* Belmont, CA: Thomson Brooks/Cole; 2007: 433–436.

26. Gaynor EB. Otolaryngologic manifestations of gastroesophageal reflux. *Am J Gastroenterol.* 1991;86(7):801–808.

27. Esmaillzadeh A, Keshteli AH, Feizi A, et al. Patterns of diet-related practices and prevalence of gastro-esophageal reflux disease. *Neurogastroenterol Motil.* 2013;25(10): 831–838.

28. Randhawa MA, Mahfouz SA, Selim NA, Yar T, Gillessen A. An old dietary regimen as a new lifestyle change for gastroesophageal reflux disease: a pilot study. *Pak J Pharm Sci.* 2015;28(5):1583–1586.

29. Johns Hopkins Voice Center. www.gbmc. org/refluxchangestothelarynx.

30. Thomas DT, Erdman KA, Burke LM. Position of the Academy of Nutrition and Dietetics, Dietitians of Canada, and the American College of Sports Medicine: Nutrition and Athletic Performance. *J Acad Nutr Diet.* 2016;116(3):501–528.

31. Trexler ET, Smith-Ryan AE, Norton LE. Metabolic adaptation to weight loss: implications for the athlete. *J Int Soc Sports Nutr.* 2014;11(1):1.

32. Roberts SB, Dallal GE. Energy requirements and aging. *Public Health Nutr.* 2005; 8(7A):1028–1036.

33. Poehlman ET, Goran M, Gardner A, et al. Determinants of decline in resting metabolic rate in aging females. *Am J Physiol Endocrinol Metab.* 1993; 264:E450–E455.

34. Poehlman ET. Energy expenditure and requirements in aging humans. *J Nutr.* 1992; 122:2057–2065.

35. Harris J, Benedict F. *A Biometric Study of Basal Metabolism in Man.* Philadelphia, PA: Lippencott; 1919.

36. Mifflin MD, St Jeor ST, Hill LA, et al. A new predictive equation for resting energy expenditure in healthy individuals. *Am J Clin Nutr.* 1990;51(2):241–247.

37. Institute of Medicine. *Food and Nutrition Board. Dietary Reference Intakes for Energy, Carbohydrate, Fiber, Fat, Fatty Acids, Cholesterol, Protein, and Amino Acids (Macronutrients).* Washington, DC: The National Academies Press; 2005.

38. Berning JR, Steen SN. *Nutrition for Sport and Exercise.* 2nd ed. Gaithersburg, MD: Aspen Publishers; 1998.

39. van Wyk L, Cloete M, Hattingh D, et al. The effect of hydration on the voice quality of future professional vocal performers

[published online February 9, 2016]. *J Voice*. doi:10.1016/j.jvoice.2016.01.002

40. Dick RW, Berning JR, Dawson W, et al. Athletes and the arts—the role of sports medicine in the performing arts. *Curr Sports Med Rep*. 2013;12(6):397–403.

41. Reilly T, Waterhouse J, Burke LM, et al. Nutrition for travel. *J Sports Sci*. 2007;25(suppl 1): S125–S134.

42. Centers for Disease Control and Prevention. *Handwashing: clean hands save lives*. Atlanta, GA: US Department of Health and Human Services; 2016. http://www.cdc.gov/handwashing/why-handwashing.html

43. Ranchordas MK, Rogersion D, Ruddock A, Killer SC, Winter EM. Nutrition for tennis: practical recommendations. *J Sports Sci Med*. 2013;12(2):211–224.

12

Effect of Weight Loss on Voice

Abdul-Latif Hamdan, Robert Thayer Sataloff, and Mary J. Hawkshaw

The effect of weight loss on voice is scarcely discussed in the literature. Only a few studies have been published and they contain only limited discussion of the mechanisms by which weight reduction may impact phonation.[1-3] This chapter summarizes the reports on the impact of weight loss on voice and discusses how weight loss can affect phonation and describes weight cycling and its metabolic impact.

Impact of Weight Loss on Voice

Most of the information on the impact of weight loss on voice is derived from studies on patients who had undergone bariatric surgery.[1-3] Solomon et al[1] in 2011 reported a comprehensive voice evaluation of 8 obese patients with a "body mass Index BMI greater than 35 kg/m^{2}"[1(p31)] who underwent bariatric surgery and compared them with 8 nonobese patients who underwent other types of abdominal procedures. In their visual perceptual analysis, the authors described normal laryngeal stroboscopic examination except for the presence of reduced mucosal waves in half the partici-

pants of each group. Interestingly, marked supraglottic constriction, mediolaterally and anteroposteriorly, was observed in 1 obese patient and which improved following weight loss. The auditory-perceptual evaluation revealed a significant difference in loudness between the 2 groups with nonobese subjects judged as being louder than obese subjects. However, it is important to note that all the averaged data from the 3 listeners who made the assessments were within normal limits. There were also mild variations in the ratings of strain and pitch across the different sessions, but none of which exceeded the normative values. There was no significant difference in the acoustic measures across sessions either preoperatively or postoperatively. Similarly, there were no significant changes in aerodynamic measures preoperatively and across sessions, except for the phonatory threshold pressure (PTP) at 30% and 80% of the fundamental frequency range. Despite no significant difference between the obese group and nonobese group, a correlation between PTP and body mass index (BMI) was reported. The authors alluded to the pathogenic role of BMI in phonation, suggesting that it becomes easier to phonate with a decrease in weight. Aside from this finding on longitudinal analysis, the results of Solomon et al[1] support the lack of difference in any phonatory parameter between obese and nonobese subjects over the course of 6 months during which 4 assessment sessions occurred.

Three years later, Hamdan et al[2] reported the effect of weight loss on voice in a group of 9 female obese patients who underwent bariatric surgery. Assessment using subjective and objective measures was performed preoperatively and at 3 and 8 months postoperatively. There was no statistically significant difference in any of the auditory perceptual measures using the GRBAS scale. Moreover, there was no significant difference in the acoustic parameters or laryngeal stroboscopic findings preoperatively vs postoperatively. The only significant difference before and after surgery involved self-reported phonatory symptoms. There was a change in voice quality in 3 of the 9 patients, described as an increase in pitch, a decrease in loudness, and an increase in phonatory effort. In the discussion, the authors attributed the increase in pitch to the inverse correlation between body weight and fundamental frequency as reported by Evans et al[4] ($r = -.34$, $p = .02$), whereas the increase in phonatory effort was attributed to the overall body fatigability secondary to the substantial weight loss. Weight loss often is accompanied by protein malnutrition and other micronutrient deficiencies, among which are vitamin D, vitamin B12, and minerals such as zinc and copper.[5,6]

In 2017, de Souza et al[3] investigated the effect of weight loss on voice in a group of 25 obese women (mean BMI 44.88 kg/m^2) who underwent bariatric surgery, Rouxen-Y bypass, in comparison to 23 normal subjects. The authors reported an increase in the mean fundamental frequency and in maximum phonation time of all vowels /ɑ/, /i/, and /u/. These changes were attributed to the decrease in vocal tract fat deposition in parallel with the reduction in neck circumference by 6 cm and to the improvement in breathing following a decrease in the mean BMI by 11.60 kg/m^2.[3]

In all the aforementioned studies, it is important to note that there is no information on weight-induced changes in vocal tract measures, pulmonary function testing, or sex hormone levels despite the strong link between these variables and phonation. In order to plan future research, it is useful to review the mechanisms by which weight loss might alter voice quality.

Why Would Weight Loss Affect Voice?

Weight loss may affect voice through the same mechanisms by which obesity and excess weight can affect adversely phonation. These can be stratified under 4 categories: (1) the effect of weight loss on vocal tract morphology, (2) the effect of weight loss on breathing in subjects with and without respiratory diseases, (3) the effect of weight loss on sex hormones levels, and (4) the effect of weight loss on the prevalence and possibly severity of laryngopharyngeal reflux disease.

Effect of Weight Loss on Vocal Tract Morphology

Despite the numerous reports on the correlation between pharyngeal size, contour, and body mass index,[7-9] little has been written on weight loss–induced vocal tract changes. Solomon et al,[1] in their study on the effect of weight loss on voice, reported 2 findings of clinical significance: one is the association between PTP and BMI, and second is the constriction of vocal tract structures in 1 obese subject that resolved following weight loss. The authors proposed that with weight loss, there is a decrease in tissue bulk and hence laryngeal resistance. With the decrease in laryngeal resistance, there is also a reduction in the pressure needed to the set the vocal folds into vibration. The explanation provided by Solomon et al[1] regarding PTP and laryngeal resistance is based on the premise that weight loss causes an alteration in the size or volume of upper airway structures. This observation is supported by the study of Da Cunha et al,[10] who reported vocal straining toward the end of sound emission in their perceptual evaluation of 45 obese patients. The authors attributed this "stress phonation" and vocal strangulation to excess fat deposition along the vocal tract, in addition to impairment in breathing. Similarly, de Souza et al[3] reported significant improvement in maximum phonation time and an increase in F0 that they speculated were due to the decrease in neck circumference (42 cm vs 36 cm) and reduction in vocal tract structures.

Despite the fact that no vocal tract or intraluminal airway measurements were made in any of the discussed above, the reasoning suggested by Solomon et al[1] and de Souza et al[3] regarding vocal tract changes is in agreement with many reports on obesity-induced anatomical variation of the vocal tract and the reversibility of these variations.[7,11–15] It is known that fat concentration in the upper airway is higher in obese subjects in comparison to nonobese subjects. Fat deposition and distribution vary at different sites of the upper airway. Horner et al,[7] using radiologic imaging, reported excessive fat deposition in obese subjects with and without obstructive sleep apnea (OSA). The sites most commonly affected were the palatopharyngeal area, the space anterior to the laryngopharyngeal complex,

tongue, and palate.[7] The study by Turnbull et al[11] also showed a significant correlation between obesity and fat volume in the lateral pharyngeal wall, tongue, and palate and apnea hypopnea syndrome (AHS). The study was conducted using magnetic resonance imaging on 53 morbidly obese patients scheduled for bariatric surgery. Schwab et al,[12] in their investigation on the anatomical variations that carry significant risk for OSA, asserted the enlargement of pharyngeal lymphoid tissue in obese patients and that it is potentially dangerous. An increase in "the ratio of airway soft tissue to craniofacial space"[12(p1295)] also poses a risk for apnea in these patients. The study was conducted on 137 adolescents (87 obese and 50 of lean weight) using magnetic resonance imaging (MRI) where the smallest cross-sectional area at different sites of the upper airway were measured.[12] Thickening of nasopharyngeal tissues and enlargement of base of tongue also have been described in obese subjects by Shakakibara et al[13] using cephalometric measurements.

In summary, all of these studies suggest a strong link between vocal tract morphology and obesity. Importantly, the obesity-induced vocal tract changes are reversible through weight loss. Several studies indicate that weight loss in morbidly obese patients results in widening or enlargement of the upper airway and/or in reduction of pharyngeal tissues.[8,14–15] Shelton et al[8] reported regression in the size of pharyngeal adipose tissue in 2 obese subjects after weight loss. Pahkala et al[14] also reported improvement in preoperative differences in upper airway morphology in 32 overweight subjects after surgery. These subjects were divided into an intervention group who followed an intensive weight reduction program with an increase in physical activity vs a control group who had only exercise and dietary counseling. Following a 1-year lifestyle intervention to decrease weight, there was a marked decrease in the pharyngeal fat pad from 194 mm^2 to 158 mm^2 in the intervention group and from 169 mm^2 to 141 mm^2 in the control group.[14] Similarly, Busetto et al[15] reported an increase in upper airway passage size in 17 morbidly obese patients who underwent intragastric balloon insertion. With a drop of 7.2 kg/m^2 in 6 months following the date of intervention, the mean pharyngeal cross-sectional area increased in both upright and supine position, but it remained lower than in the nonobese group (2.19 ± 0.37 cm^2 vs 2.65 ± 0.55 cm^2, respectively in the sitting position and 1.78 ± 0.32 cm^2 vs 2.38 ± 0.39 cm^2, respectively in the supine position.[15]

In summary, given the importance of vocal tract morphology in voice production, it is reasonable to infer that changes in upper airway measures secondary to weight loss may lead to changes in voice quality. Future investigation is needed to elucidate the interplay between weight loss or gain, vocal tract changes, and voice.

Effect of Weight Loss on Pulmonary Function

Another possible mechanism by which weight loss might impact voice is through its effect on breathing. There are numerous reports in the literature that confirm the strong link between obesity and respiration.[16–21] Obese subjects may experience dyspnea and shortness of breath even in the absence of lung diseases.[16–18] Moreover, the effect of central obesity, often referred to as the android type, is worse than that of the genoid type characterized by deposition of fat in the gluteal and hip regions.[22,23] These respiratory symptoms reported in obese subjects often are accompanied by abnormal pulmonary function testing.[20,21] In a large study by Leone et al,[20] central obesity was found to be a good predictor of poor lung function. The most commonly reported findings were reduction in total lung capacity and forced vital capacity, in addition to elevated respiratory rate.

Several mechanisms have been proposed to explain the correlation between obesity and breathing disturbances. These include mechanical impairment with reduction in the movement of the diaphragm,[24,25] reduced chest and lung compliance,[26,27] abnormal neural respiratory drive,[28] altered lung perfusion and ventilation,[29–31] and a proinflammatory state secondary to the release of inflammatory mediators by fat cells.[32,33]

Several authors have suggested that weight loss may reverse the adverse effects of obesity on breathing. In 2010, Xavier et al[34] reported improvement in pulmonary function following reduction in weight in 20 patients who underwent the Fobi-Capella operation (also known as the banded gastric bypass). Using spirometry, the authors reported a significant difference in respiratory rate, expiratory reserve volume, and functional residual capacity after surgery.[34] A year later, Wei et al[35] further corroborated the favorable effect of bariatric surgery on respiration. In their analysis of 94 patients with BMI greater than 32 kg/m^2, the authors reported a correlation between anthropometric measures such as waist-to hip-ratio and pulmonary function, particularly functional vital capacity and functional expiratory volume in the first second (FEV1). In 2012, the evolution of respiratory muscle strength following gastroplasty was also investigated by Parreira et al[36] in a longitudinal study on obese patients with a BMI of 43 ± 4 kg/m^2. By measuring maximum inspiratory pressure and maximum expiratory pressure, the authors reported an improvement in inspiratory muscle strength over the course of 36 months following surgery. In a more recent retrospective data analysis conducted on asthmatic patients who underwent bariatric surgery, Guerron et al[37] reported an exponential decrease in asthma medication.

With all this evidence on the positive effect of bariatric surgery on breathing, and given the critical role of breathing both as a power source and modulator of voice, it is reasonable to infer that weight reduction may improve voice quality.

Effect of Weight Loss on Sex Hormones

Adipose tissue is an endocrine organ involved actively in body metabolism. It is partially responsible for sex hormone production in both genders and at various stages of life.[38,39] As discussed in Chapter 6 on obesity, sex hormones, and voice, there is an association between sex hormones and BMI. Glass et al in 1977[40] reported a reduction in sex hormone binding globulin (SHBG) and testosterone and an increase in estradiol level in obese subjects. These sex hormone changes also were described by Stanik et al[41] in a group of obese men whose weight was 18% or more above the ideal body weight for age and sex. There was a significant increase in estrone E1 in 22 of the 24 subjects and a decrease in serum testosterone in 50% of the subjects. The increase in the level of estradiol and estrone associated with obesity was partially attributed to the increased conversion to estrogen of androstenedione and testosterone in the adipose tissue. This conversion is catalyzed by 2 important enzymes, active aromatase and 17, beta-hydroxysteroid dehydrogenase, the concentration of which depends on the number and size of adipose cells.[42] As such, aromatization of

androstenedione and testosterone in adipose tissue is considered as a main source of peripheral estrogen in obese men.[43] As in obese men, there are also alterations in sex hormones in obese women. There is elevation in free testosterone level with concomitant reduction in SHBG.[44-46] Several authors reported a hyperandrogenic state in obese women secondary to the increase in testosterone, androstenedione, and androstenediol.[47,48] The correlation between the aforementioned sex hormones and visceral fat concentration in obese women also has been investigated by Leenen et al.[49] Using magnetic resonance imaging, the authors reported an association between the abundance of visceral fat and elevated levels of free testosterone.[49] This association has been described by numerous authors who further corroborated the link between androgenic hormones and abdominal fat in women.[50-55]

Following weight loss, there is marked change in sex hormone levels. With a decrease in visceral fat concentration, there is an increase in SHBG and free 17, beta-estradiol/free T ratio.[49] Bastounis et al[56] investigated the effect of weight loss on sex hormones in a group of 57 morbidly obese patients who underwent vertical banded gastroplasty. The authors demonstrated that following a mean weight loss of 70 ± 10 kg, there was a significant increase in both total testosterone and SHBG levels and a decrease in estradiol levels in men. In women, there was an increase in SHBG and a decrease in testosterone, free testosterone, and androstenedione. The decrease in estrogen level in men was attributed to the increase in SHBG and to the decrease in the peripheral conversion of androgen to estrogen.[56] In 2012, Woodard et al[57] reported normalization of serum testosterone levels following surgically induced weight loss. The study was conducted on 64 patients with BMI of 48.2 kg/m^2 who underwent Roux-en-Y-gastric bypass. Lee et al[58] in 2018, in their meta-analysis on the effect of bariatric surgery on sex hormones and which included 1022 patients, measured the increase in total and free testosterone levels following surgery. The results showed a significant increase in testosterone and SHBG and a decrease in total estradiol. Di Vincenzo et al[59] also reported elevation of testosterone and reduction in estradiol following a decrease in weight by 17.2 ± 6.7 kg in a group of 29 men with BMI of 43.4 ± 8.5 kg.

In summary, weight reduction normalizes sex hormones in obese subjects. As the larynx is a hormonal target, alterations in sex hormone levels due to weight loss may affect the voice.

Effect of Weight Loss on Gastroesophageal Reflux Disease

Numerous studies substantiate the adverse effect of obesity on the gastroenterologic system.[60-64] Subjects with high BMI are reported to have prolonged esophageal acid exposure in comparison to subjects with low BMI.[62-64] Obesity has been associated with symptoms of reflux and increased reflux disease-related hospitalization.[60,61] It has been identified as a significant risk factor for esophagitis[65] with an odds ratio of 1.8.[66] In a large meta-analysis by Hampel et al,[67] the authors reported a significant association between BMI, esophagitis, and esophageal adenocarcinoma. Several mechanisms have been proposed to explain the high prevalence of reflux symptoms and comorbidities in obese subjects. These include increased intra-abdominal and intragastric pressure secondary to the excessive central adiposity, dysfunction in lower esophageal pressure, displacement of the gastroesopha-

geal junction with the increased risk for hiatal hernia,[64,68,69] delayed gastric emptying with autonomic nervous system dysfunction,[70,71] alteration in transient lower esophageal sphincter relaxation time,[72,73] and the dietary habits associated with obesity.[74,75] With all the aforementioned significant associations between obesity and GERD, it is reasonable to conclude that weight reduction might lead to improvement in the symptoms of reflux and hence might have a favorable effect on voice. Though there are no studies on the impact of weight loss on voice in the context of GERD, there are numerous studies on the effect of surgery-induced and/or diet-induced weight loss on GERD, but with no clear consensus.[76-81] The effect of a very low-caloric diet (420 kcal/d) or low-calorie diet (less than 1000–1500 kcal/d) on GERD is controversial. De Bortoli et al[76] reported a significant improvement in GERD symptoms in patients with proven GERD who were enrolled on a hypocaloric diet in addition to proton pump inhibitors (PPIs) in comparison to patients on standard-of-care diet and on PPIs. Nevertheless, in a systematic review on the effects of conservative treatment for obesity on GERD, De Groot et al[77] reported improvement in reflux symptoms and decrease in esophageal acid exposure following a low-carbohydrate diet in only 1 study[78] and no response following dietary intervention in many others.[79-81]

Similarly, based on a review of multicenter, randomized controlled trials by Schlottmann et al,[82] the effects of surgery-induced weight loss on GERD are controversial and depend on the type of surgery performed.[83] The most commonly reported are the Roux-en-Y gastric bypass and sleeve gastrectomy with a 3-fold increase in use of the latter technique over the last few years. Despite the safety and effectiveness of these surgeries in reducing weight and associated comorbidities, there has been mounting evidence on associated esophageal dysfunction postoperatively secondary to disruption of the anatomic reflux barriers. Based on a study by El Labban et al[84] on 60 patients who underwent bariatric surgery, symptoms of reflux such as heartburn, regurgitation, and vomiting increased significantly after surgery, more so in those who had sleeve gastrectomy. The patients were followed up 6 months and more postoperatively using gastrointestinal symptoms questionnaires. In a review by Savarino et al[85] on associated esophageal dysfunction in patients undergoing bariatric surgery, the authors reported objective measures of esophageal dysfunction in association with laparoscopic adjustable gastric banding and laparoscopic sleeve gastrectomy. In other studies on bariatric surgery and gastroesophageal reflux disease, sleeve resection also has been associated with de novo Barrett's esophagus in 17.2% and de novo GERD in almost 50% of the cases.[86,87] The decrease in the lower esophageal pressure and the change in angulation of the angle of His are believed to be the main causes for worsening of GERD symptoms in operated patients.[88]

The "Yo-Yo" Diet and Its Metabolic Effect

A low-caloric diet (LCD) and very low-caloric diet (VLCD) (less than 800 kcal/d) are commonly used strategies to reduce weight. Several readily available commercial and weight-loss programs have yielded greater weight reduction in comparison to simple weight control diets.[89] The degree of weight loss can reach up to 25% of the initial weight when lifestyle modification is adopted in combination with a very low-caloric diet. However, long-term failure is

very common as 1 out of 2 subjects regain up to 50% of their initial weight loss a year or 2 following their diet.[90] Despite the limited adverse events described in dieting patients, namely the increase in uric acid, alopecia, constipation, and transient cold intolerance, there are many healthy metabolic alterations.[91-97] List et al[97] described a beneficial effect of weight loss on cellular senescence, and numerous authors reported the decrease in risk factors for cardiovascular diseases following diet.[91-93] Of relevance to phonation are the hormonal, breathing, and GERD-associated changes. In a meta-analysis by Corona et al[98] that included 2 studies on low-caloric diet, the authors highlighted the diet-induced weight loss effects on sex hormones, particularly the increase in total testosterone and sex hormone binding globulin, and the decrease in estradiol. Svendsen et al[99] examined the effect of a low-caloric diet on androgen level, lipid metabolism, and fat distribution in 10 women with BMI greater than 28 kg/m^2 and reported a significant decrease in free testosterone with a decrease in abdominal and subcutaneous fat distribution. Weight loss also has been reported to have a positive effect on the respiratory and gastrointestinal systems. In a study by Bhammar et al[100] on the effect of moderate weight loss on breathing in a group of 29 women with a BMI of 36 ± 4 kg/m^2, the authors reported improvement in pulmonary function, with an increase in end-expiratory lung volume and O_2 cost of breathing.

Notwithstanding the well-documented positive effects of a low- or hypocaloric diet on various systems in the body, the long-term effects do not seem to be as encouraging as many patients regain weight.[101-104] In a review by Amigo and Fernández[101] on the long-term effect of a low-caloric diet on weight control, the authors describe how the majority return to their original weight and a subgroup eventually become even more overweight. This weight cycling effect, often referred to as the "yo-yo"[101(p323)] effect, is the process of losing and gaining weight repeatedly. Various determining factors in this transformation have been described, and these include both biologic factors such as change in basal metabolism and psychological factors. In a study by Jebb et al[102] on 11 women with BMI of 311.44 kg/m² enrolled in 3 cycles of dieting, the authors reported an initial decrease in basal metabolic rate that was not progressive toward the end. However, Steen et al[104] reported a decrease in the resting energy expenditure in 14% in a group of wrestlers. The underlying mechanisms behind the decrease in weight loss after the second cycle of dieting are unknown. In addition to metabolic alterations, poor diet compliance with increased preference for fat has been suggested.[105] Numerous reports indicate a change in fat distribution despite the many studies that showed no alteration in body composition among cyclers vs noncyclers.[106,107] Fat redistribution with abdominal deposition measured using a waist-to-hip ratio has been described by Rodin et al[108] in women on weight cycling.

The "yo-yo" diet has gained a lot of attention over the years in view of the associated comorbidities and rise in mortality. With the increase in weight and body fat redistribution, there is an increased risk for adverse health issues. In addition to its association with eating disorders and binge eating, weight cycling has been linked to numerous morbidities and health outcomes.[109–113] These include cardiovascular diseases, hypertension, diabetes, and psychopathologic conditions. Based on a review by Brownell and Rodin,[109] the "relative risk of increased weight variability is similar to the risk attributed to obesity and to several of the cardiovascular risk factors."[109(p1329)] With

mounting evidence on the pathogenic role of weight cycling in systemic diseases, several authors consider this weight variability as a risk for increased mortality. In more than 1 study, it has been shown that weight variability correlates with increased mortality from all causes and in particular from coronary artery diseases.[110–112] Schofield et al[113] reported the damaging effect of weight fluctuation in a murine model. By switching to 3 types of diet, the authors described an increase in the deposition of internal fat in comparison to those that maintained a high-fat diet. In conclusion, they alluded to the increased risk of metabolic syndrome and its subsequent systemic effects in association with excess adipose tissue.[113] These findings are in partial alignment with the study by Olszanecka-Glinianowicz et al[114] on the systemic effect of weight loss and regain in a group of 16 women who had initial weight loss (more than 5%) that was followed by an increase after 5 years.

Despite all the above reports on the impact of weight cycling on metabolic and systemic diseases, its effect on voice has not been investigated. Based on the similarity in the relative risk of weight variability and obesity on several systems in the body, we can extrapolate that weight cycling might carry the same adverse effects on voice as those reported in obesity. Future investigation is needed.

References

1. Solomon NP, Helou LB, Dietrich-Burns K, Stojadinovic A. Do obesity and weight loss affect vocal function? *Semin Speech Lang.* 2011;32(1):31–42.
2. Hamdan AL, Safadi B, Chamseddine G, Kasty M, Turfe ZA, Ziade G. Effect of weight loss on voice after bariatric surgery. *J Voice.* 2014;28(5):618–623.

3. de Souza LBR, Dos Santos MM, Pernambuco LA, de Almeida Godoy CM, da Silva Lima DM. Effects of weight loss on acoustic parameters after bariatric surgery. *Obes Surg.* 2018;28(5):1372–1376.

4. Evans S, Neave N, Wakelin D. Relationships between vocal characteristics and body size and shape in human males: an evolutionary explanation for a deep male voice. *Biol Psychol.* 2006;72(2):160–163.

5. Schuetz P, Peterli R, Ludwig C, Peters T. Fatigue, weakness and sexual dysfunction after bariatric surgery—not an unusual case but an unusual cause. *Obes Surg.* 2004; 14(7):1025–1028.

6. Bal BS, Finelli FC, Shope TR, Koch TR. Nutritional deficiencies after bariatric surgery. *Nat Rev Endocrinol.* 2012;8(9): 544–556.

7. Horner RL, Mohiaddin RH, Lowell DG, et al. Sites and sizes of fat deposits around the pharynx in obese patients with obstructive sleep apnoea and weight matched controls. *Eur Respir J.* 1989;2(7):613–622.

8. Shelton KE, Woodson H, Gay S, Suratt PM. Pharyngeal fat in obstructive sleep apnea. *Am Rev Respir Dis.* 1993;148(2):462–466.

9. Mortimore IL, Marshall I, Wraith PK, Sellar RJ, Douglas NJ. Neck and total body fat deposition in nonobese and obese patients with sleep apnea compared with that in control subjects. *Am J Respir Crit Care Med.* 1998;157(1):280–283.

10. Da Cunha MG, Passerotti GH, Weber R, Zilberstein B, Cecconello I. Voice feature characteristic in morbid obese population. *Obes Surg.* 2011;21(3):340–344.

11. Turnbull CD, Wang SH, Manuel AR, et al. Relationships between MRI fat distributions and sleep apnea and obesity hypoventilation syndrome in very obese patients. *Sleep Breath.* 2018;22(3):673–681.

12. Schwab RJ, Kim C, Bagchi S, et al. Understanding the anatomic basis for obstructive sleep apnea syndrome in adolescents. *Am J Respir Crit Care Med.* 2015;191(11): 1295–1309.

13. Shakakibara H, Tong M, Matsushita K, Hirata M, Konishi Y, Suetsugu S. Cepha-lometric abnormalities in non-obese and obese patients with obstructive sleep apnoea. *Eur Respir J.* 1999;13(2):403–410.

14. Pahkala R, Seppä J, Ikonen A, Smirnov G, Tuomilehto H. The impact of pharyngeal fat tissue on the pathogenesis of obstructive sleep apnea. *Sleep Breath.* 2014;18(2): 275–282.

15. Busetto L, Enzi G, Inelmen EM, et al. Obstructive sleep apnea syndrome in morbid obesity: effects of intragastric balloon. *Chest.* 2005;128(2):618–623.

16. Parameswaran K, Todd DC, Soth M. Altered respiratory physiology in obesity. *Can Resp J.* 2006;13(4):203–210.

17. Bernhardt V, Babb TG. Exertional dyspnoea in obesity. *Eur Respir Rev.* 2016;25(142): 487–495.

18. Carpio C, Villasante C, Galera R, et al. Systemic inflammation and higher perception of dyspnea mimicking asthma in obese subjects. *J Allergy Clin Immunol.* 2016; 137(3):718–726.

19. Sahebjami H. Dyspnea in obese healthy men. *Chest.* 1998;114(5):1373–1377.

20. Leone N, Courbon D, Thomas F, et al. Lung function impairment and metabolic syndrome: the critical role of abdominal obesity. *Am J Respir Crit Care Med.* 2009; 179(6):509–516.

21. Littleton SW. Impact of obesity on respiratory function. *Respirology.* 2012;17(1): 43–49.

22. Davis KE, Neinast MD, Sun K, et al. The sexually dimorphic role of adipose and adipocyte estrogen receptors in modulating adipose tissue expansion, inflammation, and fibrosis. *Mol Metab.* 2013;2(3): 227–242.

23. Collins LC, Hoberty PD, Walker JF, Fletcher EC, Peiris AN. The effect of body fat distribution on pulmonary function tests. *Chest.* 1995;107(5):1298–1302.

24. Unterborn J. Pulmonary function testing in obesity, pregnancy, and extremes of body habitus. *Clin Chest Med.* 2001;22(4): 759–767.

25. Sampson MG, Grassino AE. Load compensation in obese patients during quiet tidal

breathing. *J Appl Physiol Respir Environ Exerc Physiol.* 1983;55(4):1269–1276.

26. Pelosi P, Croci M, Ravagnan I, et al. The effects of body mass on lung volumes, respiratory mechanics, and gas exchange during general anesthesia. *Anesth Analg.* 1998;87(3):654–660.

27. Naimark A, Cherniack RM. Compliance of the respiratory system and its components in health and obesity. *J Appl Physiol.* 1960;15:377–382.

28. Chlif M, Keochkerian D, Choquet D, Vaidie A, Ahmaidi S. Effects of obesity on breathing pattern, ventilatory neural drive and mechanics. *Respir Physiol Neurobiol.* 2009;168(3):198–202.

29. Hedenstierna G, Santesson J, Norlander O. Airway closure and distribution of inspired gas in the extremely obese, breathing spontaneously and during anaesthesia with intermittent positive pressure ventilation. *Acta Anaesthesiol Scand.* 1976;20(4): 334–342.

30. Rivas E, Arismendi E, Agustí A, et al. Ventilation/perfusion distribution abnormalities in morbidly obese subjects before and after bariatric surgery. *Chest.* 2015;147(4): 1127–1134.

31. Dempsey JA, Reddan W, Rankin J, Balke B. Alveolar-arterial gas exchange during muscular work in obesity. *J Appl Physiol.* 1966;21(6):1807–1814.

32. Fernández-Sánchez A, Madrigal-Santillán E, Bautista M, et al. Inflammation, oxidative stress, and obesity. *Int J Mol Sci.* 2011; 12(5):3117–3132.

33. Ozata M, Mergen M, Oktenli C, et al. Increased oxidative stress and hypozincemia in male obesity. *Clin Biochem.* 2002; 35(8):627–631.

34. Xavier MAF, Ceneviva R, Terra Filho J, Sankarankutty AK. Pulmonary function and quality of life in patients with morbid obesity six months after bariatric surgery. *Acta Cir Bras.* 2010;25(5):407–415.

35. Wei YF, Tseng WK, Huang CK, Tai CM, Hsuan CF, Wu HD. Surgically induced weight loss, including reduction in waist circumference, is associated with improved pulmonary function in obese patients. *Surg Obes Relat Dis.* 2011;7(5):599–604.

36. Parreira VF, Matos CM, Athayde FT, Moraes KS, Barbosa MH, Britto RR. Evolution of respiratory muscle strength in postoperative gastroplasty. *Rev Bras Fisioter.* 2012;16(3):225–230.

37. Guerron AD, Ortega CB, Lee HJ, Davalos G, Ingram J, Portenier D. Asthma medication usage is significantly reduced following bariatric surgery [published online October 17, 2018]. *Surg Endosc.*

38. Kley HK, Solbach HG, McKinnan JC, Kruskemper HL. Testosterone decrease and oestrogen increase in male patients with obesity. *Acta Endocrinol (Copenh).* 1979;91(3):553–563.

39. Luglio HF. Estrogen and body weight regulation in women: the role of estrogen receptor alpha (ER-α) on adipocyte lipolysis. *Acta Med Indones.* 2014;46(4):333–338.

40. Glass AR, Swerdloff RS, Bray GA, Dahms WT, Atkinson RL. Low serum testosterone and sex-hormone-binding-globulin in massively obese men. *J Clin Endocrinol Metab.* 1977;45(6):1211–1219.

41. Stanik S, Dornfeld LP, Maxwell MH, Viosca SP, Korenman SG. The effect of weight loss on reproductive hormones in obese men. *J Clin Endocrinol Metab.* 1981;53(4):828–832.

42. Deslypere JP, Verdonck L, Vermeulen A. Fat tissue: a steroid reservoir and site of steroid metabolism. *J Clin Endocrinol Metab.* 1985;61(3):564–570.

43. Kim JH, Cho HT, Kim YJ. The role of estrogen in adipose tissue metabolism: insights into glucose homeostasis regulation. *Endocr J.* 2014;61(11):1055–1067.

44. Palmer BF, Clegg DJ. The sexual dimorphism of obesity. *Mol Cell Endocrinol.* 2015;402:113–119.

45. Bernasconi D, Del Monte P, Meozzi M, et al. The impact of obesity on hormonal parameters in hirsute and nonhirsute women. *Metabolism.* 1996;45(1):72–75.

46. Grenman S, Rönnemaa T, Irjala K, Kaihola HL, Grönroos M. Sex steroid, gonadotropin, cortisol and prolactin levels in healthy, massively obese women: correlation with

abdominal fat cell size and effect of weight reduction. *J Clin Endocrinol Metab.* 1986; 63(6):1257–1261.

47. Samojlik E, Kirschner MA, Silber D, Schneider G, Ertel NH. Elevated production and metabolic clearance rates of androgens in morbidly obese women. *J Clin Endocrinol Metab.* 1984;59(5):949–954.

48. Lopez M, Tena-Sempere M. Estradiol and brown fat. *Best Pract Res Clin Endocrinol Metab.* 2016;30(4):527–536.

49. Leenen R, Van Der Kooy K, Seidell JC, Deurenberg P, Koppeschaar HP. Visceral fat accumulation in relation to sex hormones in obese men and women undergoing weight loss therapy. *J Clin Endocrinol Metab.* 1994;78(6):1515–1520.

50. Evans DJ, Hoffmann RG, Kalkhoff RK, Kissebah AH. Relationship of androgenic activity to body fat topography, fat cell morphology, and metabolic aberrations in premenopausal women. *J Clin Endocrinol Metab.* 1983;57(2):304–310.

51. Haffner SM, Katz MS, Stern MP, Dunn JF. Relationship of sex hormone binding globulin to overall adiposity and body fat distribution in a biethnic population. *Int J Obes.* 1989;13(1):1–9.

52. Kirschner MA, Samojlik E, Drejka M, Szmal E, Schneider G, Ertel N. Androgen-estrogen metabolism in women with upper body versus lower body obesity. *J Clin Endocrinol Metab.* 1990;70(2):473–479.

53. Kirschner MA, Samojlik E. Sex hormone metabolism in upper and lower body obesity. *Int J Obes.* 1991;15(2):101–108.

54. Evans DJ, Barth JH, Burke CW. Body fat topography in women with androgen excess. *Int J Obes.* 1988;12(2):157–162.

55. Seidell JC, Cigolini M, Charzewska J, et al. Androgenicity in relation to body fat distribution and metabolism in 38-year-old women-the European fat distribution study. *J Clin Epidemiol.* 1990;43(1):21–34.

56. Bastounis EA, Karayiannakis AJ, Syrigos K, Zbar A, Makri GG, Alexiou D. Sex hormone changes in morbidly obese patients after vertical banded gastroplasty. *Eur Surg Res.* 1998;30(1):43–47.

57. Woodard G, Ahmed S, Podelski V, Hernandez-Boussard T, Presti J Jr, Morton JM. Effect of Roux-en-Y gastric bypass on testosterone and prostate-specific antigen. *Br J Surg.* 2012;99(5):693–698.

58. Lee Y, Dang JT, Switzer N, et al. Impact of bariatric surgery on male sex hormones and sperm quality: a systematic review and meta-analysis [published online October 31, 2018]. *Obes Surg.*

59. Di Vincenzo A, Silvestrin V, Bertoli E, et al. Short-term effects of surgical weight loss after sleeve gastrectomy on sex steroids plasma levels and PSA concentration in men with severe obesity [published online November 17, 2018]. *Aging Male.*

60. Locke GR III, Talley NJ, Fett SL, Zinsmeister AR, Melton LJ III. Risk factors associated with symptoms of gastroesophageal reflux. *Am J Med.* 1999;106(6):642–649.

61. Ruhl CE, Everhart JE. Overweight, but not high dietary fat intake, increases risk of gastroesophageal reflux disease hospitalization: the NHANES I Epidemiologic Follow-up Study. First National Health and Nutrition Examination Survey. *Ann Epidemiol.* 1999;9(7):424–435.

62. Fisher BL, Pennathur A, Mutnick JL, Little AG. Obesity correlates with gastroesophageal reflux. *Dig Dis Sci.* 1999;44(11):2290–2294.

63. El-Serag HB, Ergun GA, Pandolfino J, Fitzgerald S, Tran T, Kramer JR. Obesity increases oesophageal acid exposure. *Gut.* 2007;56(6):749–755.

64. Merrouche M, Sabaté JM, Jouet P, et al. Gastro-esophageal reflux and esophageal motility disorders in morbidly obese patients before and after bariatric surgery. *Obes Surg.* 2007;17(7):894–900.

65. Labenz J, Jaspersen D, Kulig M, et al. Risk factors for erosive esophagitis: a multivariate analysis based on the ProGERD study initiative. *Am J Gastroenterol.* 2004;99(9):1652–1656.

66. Wilson LJ, Ma W, Hirschowitz BI. Association of obesity with hiatal hernia and esophagitis. *Am J Gastroenterol.* 1999;94(10):2840–2844.

67. Hampel H, Abraham NS, El-Serag HB. Meta-analysis: obesity and the risk for gastroesophageal reflux disease and its complications. *Ann Intern Med.* 2005;143(3): 199–211.

68. Barak N, Ehrenpreis ED, Harrison JR, Sitrin MD. Gastro-oesophageal reflux disease in obesity: pathophysiological and therapeutic considerations. *Obes Rev.* 2002; 3(1):9–15.

69. Pandolfino JE, El-Serag HB, Zhang Q, Shah N, Ghosh SK, Kahrilas PJ. Obesity: a challenge to esophagogastric junction integrity. *Gastroenterology.* 2006;130(3):639–649.

70. Maddox A, Horowitz M, Wishart J, Collins P. Gastric and oesophageal emptying in obesity. *Scand J Gastroenterol.* 1989;24(5): 593–598.

71. Peterson HR, Rothschild M, Weinberg CR, Fell RD, McLeish KR, Pfeifer MA. Body fat and the activity of the autonomic nervous system. *N Engl J Med.* 1988;318(17): 1077–1083.

72. Kahrilas PJ, Shi G. Pathophysiology of gastroesophageal reflux disease: the antireflux barrier and luminal clearance mechanisms. In: Orlando RC, ed. *Gastroesophageal Reflux Disease.* New York, NY: Marcel Dekker; 2000:137–164.

73. Dodds WJ, Dent J, Hogan WJ, et al. Mechanisms of gastroesophageal reflux in patients with reflux esophagitis. *N Engl J Med.* 1982;307(25):1547–1552.

74. El-Serag HB, Satia JA, Rabeneck L. Dietary intake and the risk of gastro-oesophageal reflux disease: a cross sectional study in volunteers. *Gut.* 2005;54(1):11–17.

75. Fox M, Barr C, Nolan S, Lomer M, Anggiansah A, Wong T. The effects of dietary fat and calorie density on esophageal acid exposure and reflux symptoms. *Clin Gastroenterol Hepatol.* 2007;5(4):439–444.

76. De Bortoli N, Guidi G, Martinucci I, et al. Voluntary and controlled weight loss can reduce symptoms and proton pump inhibitor use and dosage in patients with gastroesophageal reflux disease: a comparative study. *Dis Esophagus.* 2016;29(2):197–204.

77. De Groot NL, Burgerhart JS, Van De Meeberg PC, De Vries DR, Smout AJ, Siersema PD. Systematic review: the effects of conservative and surgical treatment for obesity on gastro-oesophageal reflux disease. *Aliment Pharmacol Ther.* 2009;30(11–12): 1091–1102.

78. Austin GL, Thiny MT, Westman EC, Yancy WS Jr, Shaheen NJ. A very low-carbohydrate diet improves gastroesophageal reflux and its symptoms. *Dig Dis Sci.* 2006; 51(8):1307–1312.

79. Frederiksen SG, Johansson J, Johnsson F, Hedenbro J. Neither low-calorie diet nor vertical banded gastroplasty influence gastro-oesophageal reflux in morbidly obese patients. *Eur J Surg.* 2000;166(4):296–300.

80. Kjellin A, Ramel S, Rossner S, Thor K. Gastroesophageal reflux in obese patients is not reduced by weight reduction. *Scand J Gastroenterol.* 1996;31(11):1047–1051.

81. Mathus-Vliegen LM, Tytgat GN. Twenty-four-hour pH measurements in morbid obesity: effects of massive overweight, weight loss and gastric distension. *Eur J Gastroenterol Hepatol.* 1996; 8(7):635–640.

82. Schlottmann F, Herbella FA, Patti MG. Bariatric surgery and gastroesophageal reflux. *J Laparoendosc Adv Surg Tech A.* 2018; 28(8):953–955.

83. Ponce J, DeMaria EJ, Nguyen NT, et al. American Society for Metabolic and Bariatric Surgery estimation of bariatric surgery procedures in 2015 and surgeon workforce in the United States. *Surg Obes Relat Dis.* 2016;12(9):1637–1639.

84. El Labban S, Safadi B, Olabi A. The effect of Roux-en-Y gastric bypass and sleeve gastrectomy surgery on dietary intake, food preferences, and gastrointestinal symptoms in post-surgical morbidly obese Lebanese subjects: a cross-sectional pilot study. *Obes Surg.* 2015;25(12):2393–2399.

85. Savarino E, Marabotto E, Savarino V. Effects of bariatric surgery on the esophagus. *Curr Opin Gastroenterol.* 2018;34(4):243–248.

86. Genco A, Soricelli E, Casella G, et al. Gastroesophageal reflux disease and Bar-

rett's esophagus after laparoscopic sleeve gastrectomy: a possible, underestimated long-term complication. *Surg Obes Relat Dis.* 2017;13(4):568–574.

87. Mandeville Y, Van Looveren R, Vancoillie PJ, et al. Moderating the enthusiasm of sleeve gastrectomy: up to fifty percent of reflux symptoms after ten years in a consecutive series of one hundred laparoscopic sleeve gastrectomies. *Obes Surg.* 2017;27(7): 1797–1803.

88. Nadaleto BF, Herbella FA, Patti MG. Gastroesophageal reflux disease in the obese: pathophysiology and treatment. *Surgery.* 2016;159(2):475–486.

89. Gudzune KA, Doshi RS, Mehta AK, et al. Efficacy of commercial weight-loss programs: an updated systematic review. *Ann Intern Med.* 2015;162(7):501–512.

90. Tsai AG, Wadden TA. The evolution of very-low-calorie diets: an update and meta-analysis. *Obesity (Silver Spring).* 2006; 14(8):1283–1293.

91. Wadden TA, Foster GD, Letizia KA, Stunkard AJ. A multicenter evaluation of a proprietary weight reduction program for the treatment of marked obesity. *Arch Intern Med.* 1992;152(5):961–966.

92. Anderson JW, Brinkman-Kaplan V, Hamilton CC, Logan JE, Collins RW, Gustafson NJ. Food-containing hypocaloric diets are as effective as liquid-supplement diets for obese individuals with NIDDM. *Diabetes Care.* 1994;17(6):602–604.

93. Anderson JW, Brinkman-Kaplan VL, Lee H, Wood CL. Relationship of weight loss to cardiovascular risk factors in morbidly obese individuals. *J Am Coll Nutr.* 1994; 13(3):256–261.

94. Last AR, Wilson SA. Low-carbohydrate diets. *Am Fam Physician.* 2006;73(11): 1942–1948.

95. Wing RR, Blair E, Marcus M, Epstein LH, Harvey J. Year-long weight loss treatment for obese patients with type II diabetes: does including an intermittent very-low-calorie diet improve outcome? *Am J Med.* 1994;97(4):354–362.

96. Wing RR, Marcus MD, Salata R, Epstein LH, Miaskiewicz S, Blair EH. Effects of a very-low-calorie diet on long-term glycemic control in obese type 2 diabetic subjects. *Arch Intern Med.* 1991;151(7):1334–1340.

97. List EO, Jensen E, Kowalski J, Buchman M, Berryman DE, Kopchick JJ. Diet-induced weight loss is sufficient to reduce senescent cell number in white adipose tissue of weight-cycled mice. *Nutr Healthy Aging.* 2016;4(1):95–99.

98. Corona G, Rastrelli G, Monami M, et al. Body weight loss reverts obesity-associated hypogonadotropic hypogonadism: a systematic review and meta-analysis. *Eur J Endocrinol.* 2013;168(6):829–843.

99. Svendsen PF, Jensen FK, Holst JJ, Haugaard SB, Nilas L, Madsbad S. The effect of a very low calorie diet on insulin sensitivity, beta cell function, insulin clearance, incretin hormone secretion, androgen levels and body composition in obese young women. *Scand J Clin Lab Invest.* 2012;72(5):410–419.

100. Bhammar DM, Stickford JL, Bernhardt V, Babb TG. Effect of weight loss on operational lung volumes and oxygen cost of breathing in obese women. *Int J Obes (Lond).* 2016;40(6):998–1004.

101. Amigo I, Fernández C. Effects of diets and their role in weight control. *Psychol Health Med.* 2007;12(3):321–327.

102. Jebb SA, Goldberg GR, Coward WA, Murgatroyd PR, Prentice AM. Effects of weight cycling caused by intermittent dieting on metabolic rate and body composition in obese women. *Int J Obes.* 1991;15(5): 367–374.

103. Kroke A, Liese AD, Schulz M, et al. Recent weight changes and weight cycling as predictors of subsequent two-year weight change in a middle-aged cohort. *Int J Obes Relat Metab Disord.* 2002;26(3):403–409.

104. Steen SN, Oppliger RA, Brownell KD. Metabolic effects of repeated weight loss and regain in adolescent wrestlers. *JAMA.* 1988;260(1):47–50.

105. Drewnowski A, Holden-Wiltse J. Taste responses and food preferences in obese

women: effects of weight cycling. *Int J Obes Relat Metab Disord.* 1992;16(9):639–648.

106. vanDale D, Saris WHM. Repetitive weight loss and weight regain: effects on weight reduction, resting metabolic rate, and lipolytic activity before and after exercise and/or diet treatment. *Am J Clin Nutr.* 1989;49(3):409–416.

107. Wadden TA, Bartlett S, Letizia KA, Foster GD, Stunkard AJ, Conill A. Relationship of dieting history to resting metabolic rate, body composition, eating behavior, and subsequent weight loss. *Am J Clin Nutr.* 1991;56(1)(suppl):203S–208S.

108. Rodin J, Radke-Sharpe N, Rebuffe-Scrive M, Greenwood MR. Weight cycling and fat distribution. *Int J Obes.* 1990;14(4):303–310.

109. Brownell KD, Rodin J. Medical, metabolic, and psychological effects of weight cycling. *Arch Intern Med.* 1994;154(12):1325–1330.

110. Lee IM, Paffenbarger RS Jr. Change in body weight and longevity. *JAMA.* 1992;268(15):2045–2049.

111. Lissner L, Bengtsson C, Lapidus L, Larrson B, Bengtsson B, Brownell KD. Body weight variability and mortality in the Gothenburg Prospective Studies on men and women. In: Bjorntorp P, Rossner S, eds. *Obesity in Europe 88: Proceedings of the First European Congress on Obesity.* London, UK: Libbey; 1989:55–60.

112. Lissner L, Odell PM, D'Agostino RB, et al. Variability of body weight and health outcomes in the Framingham population. *N Engl J Med.*1991;324(26):1839–1844.

113. Schofield SE, Parkinson JR, Henley AB, Sahuri-Arisoylu M, Sanchez-Canon GJ, Bell JD. Metabolic dysfunction following weight cycling in male mice. *Int J Obes.* 2017;41(3):402–411.

114. Olszanecka-Glinianowicz M, Chudek J, Szromek A, Zahorska-Markiewicz B. Changes of systemic microinflammation after weight loss and regain—a five-year follow up study. *Endokrynol Pol.* 2012;63(6):432–438.

13

Conclusion

Abdul-Latif Hamdan, Robert Thayer Sataloff, and Mary J. Hawkshaw

A thorough review of the literature leads us to conclude that there is no consensus on the association between obesity and voice. The hypothesis that obese individuals have distinctive vocal characteristics has not been proven despite the known impact of obesity on various systems in the body. The predictive role of voice in estimating body size is controversial and the acoustic cues used in the appraising associations between weight and voice remain ill defined.

However, it is important to note that all components of the phonatory apparatus are affected by obesity. It is well established that the vocal tract, the bottleneck in vocal emission, is a target for fat deposition in obese subjects. With an increase in body mass index, there is an increase in the concentration of adipose tissue in various sites, including the pharyngeal fat pad with subsequent narrowing of the airway. Similarly, obese subjects experience breathlessness and dyspnea together with alteration in pulmonary function even in the absence of lung diseases, and these changes are likely to undermine the power source of the voice. Obesity does not seem to accentuate asthma, and the pathogenic role of obesity in chronic obstructive lung disease is still

uncertain. Obesity is linked strongly to sex hormones, which are key to laryngeal development, as well as voice maturation and stability over time. Adipose tissue is a source of estrogen synthesis and estrogen plays an important role in modulating fat deposition and distribution, as well as in affecting voice. Although there is a negative correlation between androgens and body mass index (BMI), an adverse impact of reduced testosterone level on voice in adult obese men has not been proven. There is also little evidence to support any association between obesity-related laryngopharyngeal reflux disease and voice, although there is ample evidence that LPR affects voice and that obesity worsens reflux. Despite the ubiquity of studies on the causal relationship between gastroesophageal reflux disease and obesity, there is scarcity of reports on the extraesophageal manifestations of reflux in obese subjects.

In summary, the association between voice characteristics and body weight needs further investigation. The information on obesity and voice currently available to the readers is largely inconclusive. Similarly, the effects of weight loss on voice remains uncertain. Future research is needed to identify relationship between body mass index, weight fluctuation, and voice. Additional evidence-based data are essential in order to provide optimal clinical care to voice patients, an increasing percentage of whom, like the rest of the population, are overweight or obese.

Index

mechanical impairment of, 164–165
obesity and, 4
respiratory neural drive and, 165
Broca area, 39
Bronchitis
reflux and, 202
secondhand smoke and, 79
tobacco tar and, 77
Bronchoconstriction, small airway, 144
Broyles ligament, 16, 18, 25
Bruxism, 98
Buccopharyngeal tract, 121

C

C albicans, 175
Calcium
absorption of, 261
channel blocking agents, esophageal
pressures and, 246
replacement, PPI side effects, 260
Calorie, 359
Campylobacter jejuni, 263
Cancer, 219–221
obesity and, 3
smoking induced, 79
Carcinoma, 219–221
Barrett's esophagus and, 219
cheek, smoking tobacco and, 79
Cardiac
angina, 201
events, PPIs and, 264
muscles, obesity and, 2
Cardiovascular disorders, obesity and, 169
Carotid arteries, 40
Cartilages, voice, 13–20
Cartilages of Santorini, 18
Cartilages of Wrisberg, 18
C difficile, 261, 262, 263, 264, 268
Celiac disease (CD), 242
Center for Celiac Research, 242
Centers for Disease Control and Prevention
(CDC), 76, 356
Central apnea, 221
Central nervous system (CNS), myenteric
plexus and, 195
Cerebellar
disease, ataxic dysarthria and, 112
flocculus, 37

Cerebellum, 40
Cerebral palsy
hyperkinetic dysarthria and, 112
spastic dysarthria, 112
Cheek carcinoma, smoking tobacco and, 79
Cheerleading, voice abuse and, 72
Chest compliance, lungs and, 165
Children, LPR and, 221
Chorea, hyperkinetic dysarthria and, 112
Chronic
bronchitis, smoking tobacco and, 77
cough
LPR and, 205
reflux and, 202
sore throat
postnasal drip and, 202
reflux laryngitis and, 202
Chronic Obstructive Pulmonary Disease
(COPD)
dysphonia in, 175
LPR and, 206
obesity and, 169, 172–175
vocal dysfunction in, 175–176
Cimetadine, 220
Cimetidine, H2-receptor antagonists and,
249–250
Cirrhosis, PPIs and, 263
Cisapride, 251, 252
Clopidogrel, 266
PPIs and, 261
Clostridium difficile, 261, 265
Coated tongue, reflux laryngitis and, 202
Collagen, in lamina propria, 21
Collis gastroplasty, 283
Combined multichannel intraluminal
impedance (MII), 231–232
Community-acquired pneumonia, PPI side
effects, 261
Conducting, voice abuse and, 72–73
Conductive hearing loss, 98
Contact urticaria, 242
Contractions, tertiary, 190
Corniculate cartilages, 18
Corticobulbar fibers, 37
Corticosteroids, granulomas and, 215
Costal cartilage, 44
Coughing, 74
Craniofacial bony structures, obese patients
and, 125

P

Palate-pharyngeal fat, distribution of, obstructive sleep apnea (OSA), 123
Pantoprazole, 252–260, 266, 268
Paraglottic space, thyroid cartilage and, 20
Parkinson disease, hypokinetic dysarthria, 112
Passive smoke, 79
Patient history questionnaire, 66
  age, 66–67
  allergy/cold symptoms, 74
  amount of voice training, 69–70
  bodily injury, 82–83
  body, weakness/tremor/fatigue/loss of control, 74
  bowels/belly and, 80–81
  breathing problems, 75
  career and goals, 69
  commitments, 68–69
  environmental irritants, 75
  foods and voice, 80
  form, 88–95
  hearing, 74
  hearing loss, 82
  jaw/dental problems, 82
  medications, 84–85
  menstrual cycle/menopause/hormones, 82
  misusing/abusing awareness, 72
    during speaking, 72–73
  physical condition of, 73–74
  reflux laryngitis and, 80
  smoke and, 76–80
  stress, 81
  surgery, 83
  therapy, 81
  voice
    conditions of use of, 70–71
    practice/exercise, 71
    weakness/tremor/fatigue/loss of control, 74
  voice problem identification, 67–68
  weight/tiredness/cold, 81–82
  whiplash, 82–83
Pectoralis muscles, 46, 48
Pepsin
  oral/tracheal secretions and, 204
  tracheoesophageal puncture sites and, 205
Peptic strictures, 199

Performance, 144
Perfusion, 165–166
Periaqueductal gray (PAG) matter, 38–39
Perichondrium, epiglottic cartilage and, 18
Peristalsis, 189–190
  control of esophageal, 194–197
Pharyngeal
  fat, 5
  lumen, 5
  monitoring, 232–234
  obstruction, 154
  stage of swallowing, 187–188
  wall, lymphoid tissue in, 98
Pharyngolaryngeal reflux, sugarless gum and, 269–270
Pharynx, cancer of, 79
pH monitoring, 230–231
  ambulatory, 226–231, 236
  telemetry, 226–231
Phonation
  ability examination, 105–106
  obesity and, 4
  physical condition and, 73–74
  quotient, 1, 107
Phonation threshold pressure (PTP), following exercise, 168
Phonatory physiology, 49–52
Phonatory threshold pressure (PTP), 369
Phonetogram, 106
Phosphopeptide-amorphous calcium phosphate, teeth and, 205
Photoelectroglottography, 105
Physical examination, 105
  acoustic analysis, 107–108
  aerodynamic measures, 106–107
  described, 97
  electroglottography (EGG), 105
  eye/ear/nose/throat, 98–99
  laryngeal, 99–103
  electromyography, 108–109
  phonatory ability measures, 105–106
  psychoacoustic evaluation, 108
  respiratory assessment, 146
  singing voice evaluation, 109–112
  strobovideolaryngoscopy, 103–105
  vocal fold vibration, 105
Piriform sinuses, 18
Pitch
  menopausal women and, 135